to
Newborn Infants

Volume 1

AIIMS Protocols in Neonatology

Core Protocols

Third Edition

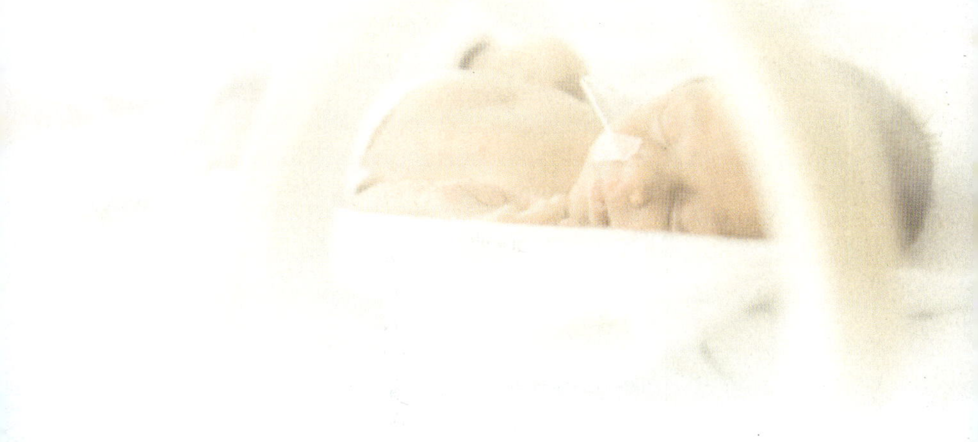

Volume 1

AIIMS Protocols in Neonatology

Core Protocols

Third Edition

Ramesh Agarwal
MD DM (Neonatology)
Professor*

Ashok Deorari
MD FAMS
Principal and Dean, Himalayan Institute of Medical Sciences
Swami Rama Himalayan University, Dehradun
Former Professor and Head*

Vinod K Paul
MD PhD DNB FAMS FIAP FNNF
Member, NITI Aayog, Government of India
Former Professor and Head*

M Jeeva Sankar
MD DM
Additional Professor*

Anu Sachdeva
MD DM
Additional Professor*

***Department of Pediatrics**
WHO Collaborating Centre for Education and Research in Newborn Care
All India Institute of Medical Sciences, New Delhi, India
www.newbornwhocc.org

[PDFs of the protocols are available online: www.newbornwhocc.org]

CBSPD

CBS Publishers & Distributors Pvt Ltd

New Delhi • Bengaluru • Chennai • Kochi • Kolkata • Lucknow • Mumbai
Gujarat • Hyderabad • Jharkhand • Nagpur • Patna • Pune • Uttarakhand

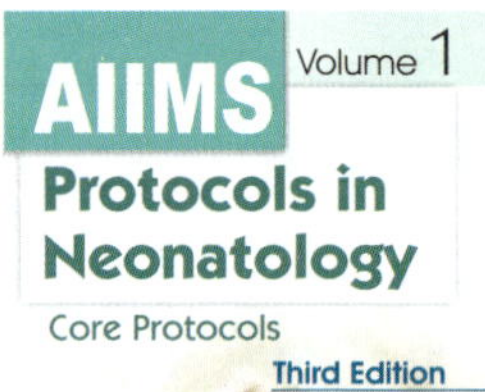

Disclaimer

Science and technology are constantly changing fields. New research and experience broaden the scope of information and knowledge. The authors have tried their best in giving information available to them while preparing the material for this book. Although all efforts have been made to ensure optimum accuracy of the material, yet it is quite possible some errors might have been left uncorrected. The publisher, the printer and the authors will not be held responsible for any inadvertent errors, omissions or inaccuracies.

The protocols are context-specific, and readers are advised to modify and adapt the protocols for their settings.

ISBN: 978-93-5466-921-7

Third Edition: 2024

Reprint: 2025, 2026, **2027**

First Edition 2015

Second Edition 2019

Published by Satish Kumar Jain and produced by Varun Jain for

CBS Publishers & Distributors Pvt Ltd

4819/XI Prahlad Street, 24 Ansari Road, Daryaganj, New Delhi 110 002, India
Ph: 011-23289259, 23266838 Website: www.cbspd.com
e-mail: delhi@cbspd.com

Corporate Office: 204 FIE, Industrial Area, Patparganj, Delhi 110 092, India
Ph: 011-4934 4934 Fax: 011-4934 4935 e-mail: publishing@cbspd.com; publicity@cbspd.com

Branches

- **Bengaluru:** Seema House 2975, 17th Cross, KR Road, Banasankari 2nd Stage, Bengaluru 560 070, Karnataka, India
  Ph: +91-80-26771678/79 Fax: +91-80-26771680 e-mail: bangalore@cbspd.com
- **Chennai:** 18/8B, Subbaraya Street, Shenoy Nagar, Chennai 600 030, Tamil Nadu, India
  Ph: +91-44-42032115, 45022115 e-mail: chennai@cbspd.com
- **Kochi:** 42/1325, 1326, Power House Road, Opposite KSEB, Ernakulum Kochi 682 018, Kerala, India
  Ph: +91-484-4059061-65 Fax: +91-484-4059065 e-mail: kochi@cbspd.com
- **Kolkata:** 147, Hind Ceramics Compound, 1st Floor, Nilgunj Road, Belghoria, Kolkata 700 056, West Bengal, India
  Ph: +91-33-25633055/56 e-mail: kolkata@cbspd.com
- **Lucknow:** Basement, Khushnuma Complex, 7 Meerabai Marg (behind Jawahar Bhawan), Lucknow 226 001, UP, India
  Ph: +91-522-4000032 e-mail: tiwari.lucknow@cbspd.com
- **Mumbai:** PWD Shed, Gala no 25/26, Ramchandra Bhatt Marg, Next to JJ Hospital Gate no. 2, Opp. Union Bank of India, Noorbaug, Mumbai 400 009, Maharashtra, India
  Ph: +91-22-66661880/89 e-mail: mumbai@cbspd.com

Representatives

- **Gujarat** • **Hyderabad** • **Jharkhand** • **Nagpur** • **Patna** • **Pune** • **Uttarakhand**

For trade terms please contact customercare@cbspd.com
For general enquiries please contact info@cbspd.com

Printed at: HT Media Ltd, Greater Noida, UP, India

The volumes in the set

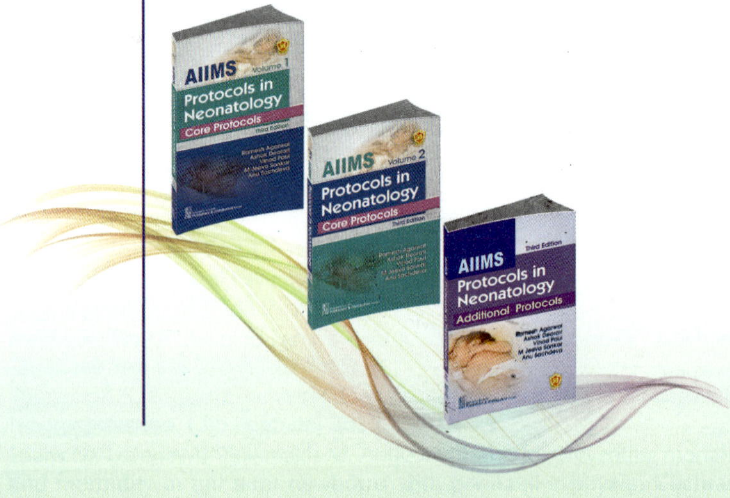

Contributors

Aathira Ravindranath DM
Consultant Pediatric
Gastroenterologist
Apollo BGS Hospital, Mysuru
aathira.r@gmail.com

Abin Sheref Mohammed MBBS
Junior Resident
Department of Pediatrics
All India Institute of Medical Sciences
New Delhi
Abinsheref.1997@gmail.com

Aditi Sinha PhD
Additional Professor
Department of Pediatrics
All India Institute of Medical Sciences
New Delhi
aditisinhaaiims@gmail.com

Akash Sharma
Consultant Neonatologist and
Pediatrician
In-charge NICU, Surya Hospitals
Jaipur, drakash.jpr@gmail.com

Akash Singhal MD
Senior Resident
Department of Neonatology
All India Institute of Medical Sciences
New Delhi

Alec Reginald Errol Correa DM
Medical Geneticist
Lifecell International
Pune
aleccorrea88@hotmail.com

Alisha Gupta MCh
Ex-Senior Resident
Department of Pediatric Surgery
All India Institute of Medical Sciences
New Delhi
doc.alishagupta@gmail.com

Amanpreet Sethi DM
Assistant Professor
Department of Pediatrics
Guru Gobind Singh Medical College
Faridkot, Punjab
sethi.amanpreet702@gmail.com

Amit Upadhyay DM
Consultant Neonatologist
Nutema Hospital, Meerut
au.llrm@gmail.com

Anapti Anil MD
Senior Resident
Department of Obstetrics and
Gynaecology
All India Institute of Medical Sciences
New Delhi, anapti.garg9@gmail.com

Anjan Kumar Dhua MCh
Additional Professor
Department of Pediatric Surgery
All India Institute of Medical Sciences
anjandhua@hotmail.com

Ankit Meena DM
Senior Resident
Department of Pediatrics
All India Institute of Medical Sciences
New Delhi
ankit.aiims.meena@gmail.com

Ankita MBBS
Junior Resident
Department of Pediatrics
All India Institute of Medical Sciences
New Delhi
ankiagar23@gmail.com

Ankit Verma MD
Assistant Professor
Department of Pediatrics
All India Institute of Medical Sciences
New Delhi
ankitverma0486@gmail.com

Ankitha Ravishankar MBBS
Junior Resident
Department of Pediatrics
All India Institute of Medical Sciences
New Delhi
ankitha.ravishankar@gmail.com

Anubhuti Rana MD
Assistant Professor
Department of Obstetrics and Gynaecology
All India Institute of Medical Sciences
New Delhi, anubhuti_rana@yahoo.com

Aparna Chandrasekaran DM
Chief Neonatologist
Krishna Institute of Medical Sciences (KIMS), Cuddles
Kondapur, Hyderabad
appubanu@gmail.com

Aparna K Sharma MD
Professor
Department of Obstetrics and Gynaecology
All India Institute of Medical Sciences
New Delhi
kaparnasharma@gmail.com

Arunambika Chinnappan MD
Senior Resident
Department of Neonatology
All India Institute of Medical Sciences
Bhubaneswar
arunambika.chinnappan@gmail.com

Arun Sasi DM
Consultant Neonatologist
Royal Children's Hospital, Melbourne
Mercy Hospital for Women, Melbourne
Adjunct Clinical Lecturer
Department of Obstetrics and Gynecology
University of Melbourne
Melbourne, Australia

Arvind Bagga MD
Director and Sr Consultant
Department of Pediatric Nephrology
Indraprastha Apollo Hospitals
New Delhi, arvindbagga@hotmail.com

Ashish Jain DM
Associate Professor and Head
Department of Neonatology
Maulana Azad Medical College
New Delhi
neoashish2008@gmail.com

Ashutosh Kapoor DM
Consultant Neonatologist and Pediatrician
In-charge NICU
Chandan Hospital, Lucknow
ashukap22@gmail.com

Biswaroop Chakrabarty DM
Additional Professor
Department of Pediatrics
All India Institute of Medical Sciences
New Delhi
biswaroopchakrabarty@gmail.com

Chandrakumar Natarajan DM
Senior Consultant and Head
Department of Neonatology
KKCTH Hospital
Nungambakkam, Chennai
drchandrakumar@gmail.com

Deena Thomas DM
Consultant Neonatologist
Muthoot Hospital
Kozhencherry, Kerala
deenathomas87@gmail.com

Deepak Chawla DM
Professor
Government Medical College and Hospital, Chandigarh
drdeepakchawla@gmail.com

Deepika Kainth DM
Assistant Professor
All India Institute of Medical Sciences
New Delhi
aiims.deepika@gmail.com

Delona Treesa Joseph MBBS
Senior Resident
Department of Pediatric Surgery
All India Institute of Medical Sciences
New Delhi
delonatreeza@gmail.com

Deula Candida D'Cruz MD
Senior Resident
Department of Pediatrics
All India Institute of Medical Sciences
New Delhi
deulacandidadcruz@gmail.com

Devi S Saranya MD
Senior Resident
Division of Genetics
Department of Pediatrics
All India Institute of Medical Sciences
New Delhi
devisaranyas92@gmail.com

Dhinakaran Raman DM
Consultant Neonatologist
Prashanth Hospital
Velachery, Chennai
dhina.mmc@gmail.com

Dilip Kumar MBBS
Junior Resident
Department of Pediatrics
All India Institute of Medical Sciences
New Delhi

Girish Gururaj DM
Apollo Hospital, Mysuru

Gitanjali Jain MD
Senior Resident
Department of Neonatology
All India Institute of Medical Sciences
New Delhi
gitanjali_jain@yahoo.co.in

Haleemath Afrah MBBS
Junior Resident
Department of Pediatrics
All India Institute of Medical Sciences
New Delhi
helloafrah@gmail.com

Harshita Nori MD
Senior Resident
Department of Neonatology
All India Institute of Medical Sciences
New Delhi
harshita.nori@gmail.com

Jagjit Singh Dalal DM
Senior Professor and Head
Department of Neonatology
Pandit BD Sharma PGIMS
Rohtak
jagjit.dr@gmail.com

Kamal Arora DM
Professor
Division of Neonatology
Department of Pediatrics
Dayanand Medical College and
Hospital, Ludhiana
dockamalpaeds@yahoo.com

Kapil Sikka MS
Professor
Department of Otorhinolaryngology
and Head–Neck Surgery
All India Institute of Medical Sciences
New Delhi
kapil_sikka@yahoo.com

Krishna Mohan Gulla MD, FNB (PICU) DM
Resident
Division of Pediatric Pulmonology
and Intensive Care
All India Institute of Medical Sciences
New Delhi
mohangulla35@gmail.com

Lalit Takia DM
Assistant Professor
Department of Pediatrics
All India Institute of Medical Sciences
New Delhi, lalitpgims@gmail.com

Likhita P MBBS
Junior Resident
Department of Pediatrics
All India Institute of Medical Sciences, New Delhi
likhu13@gmail.com

Lumchio Levis Murry MSc (Nursing)
Associate Professor
All India Institute of Medical Sciences
New Delhi, levis.murry@gmail.com

Madhulika Kabra MD
Professor
All India Institute of Medical Sciences
New Delhi
madhulikakabra@hotmail.com

Madhumati Bose
Certified Neonatal Oro-Motor Assessment Scale
Consultant on Autism for State Initiative on Disabilities (SID), Kerala; Honorary Consultant
All India Institute of Medical Sciences
Holy Family Hospital, New Delhi
madhumatibose@gmail.com

Mahesh V DM (Pediatric Nephrology)
Assistant Professor
Department of Pediatrics
All India Institute of Medical Sciences
Mangalagiri, Andhra Pradesh
vmaahi46@gmail.com

Manas Upadhyay DM
Consultant Neonatologist
Cuttack, Odisha
manl013456@gmail.com

Manisha Jana MD, FRCR
Professor
All India Institute of Medical Sciences
New Delhi
manishajana@gmail.com

Manju Saksena PhD
Physician Scientist
All India Institute of Medical Sciences
New Delhi
manjusaksena@gmail.com

Mayank Priyadarshi DM
Assistant Professor
Department of Neonatology
All India Institute of Medical Sciences
Rishikesh, Uttarakhand
priyadarshi.aiims@gmail.com

Mehak Sehgal MCh (Pediatric Surgery)
Ex-Senior Resident
All India Institute of Medical Sciences
New Delhi
mehak.sehgal91@gmail.com

Mohammad Tousifullah DM
Consultant Neonatologist
Jaswant Rai Speciality Hospital
Meerut, drmdtousif@gmail.com

Mudit Agarwal MBBS
Junior Resident
Department of Pediatrics
All India Institute of Medical Sciences
New Delhi
mudit.agarwal07@gmail.com

Mukul Kumar Mangla DM
Senior Medical Officer
Safadarjung Hospital and VMMC
New Delhi
drmanglamukul@yahoo.com

Narendra Kumar Bagri MD
Additional Professor
Division of Pediatric Rheumatology and Clinical Immunology
Department of Pediatrics
All India Institute of Medical Sciences
New Delhi
drnarendrabagri@gmail.com

Neerja Gupta DM
Additional Professor
Division of Genetics
Department of Pediatrics
All India Institute of Medical Sciences
New Delhi, neerja17aiims@gmail.com

Nidhi Garg MD
Senior Resident
Department of Neonatology
All India Institute of Medical Sciences
New Delhi
ng5620@gmail.com

Parminder Singh Rooprai MD
Senior Resident
Department of Neonatology
All India Institute of Medical Sciences
New Delhi
param_rules@yahoo.co.in

Pavneet Kaur MD
Junior Resident
Department of Pediatrics
All India Institute of Medical Sciences
New Delhi
dr.pavneetkaurthind@gmail.com

Poonam Coshic MBBS, MBA (Healthcare Administration)
Chief Medical Officer
Blood Bank (H)
All India Institute of Medical Sciences
New Delhi
poonamcoshic@gmail.com

Pradeep Kumar Sharma DM
Senior Consultant
Deep Hospital, Ludhiana
psaiims@yahoo.co.in

Prashant Jauhari DM
Additional Professor
Department of Pediatrics
All India Institute of Medical Sciences
New Delhi
pjauhari0@gmail.com

Pratima Anand DM
Neonatologist
Department of Neonatology
Lady Hardinge Medical College and Associated Hospitals
New Delhi
anandpratima@gmail.com

Pragya Tyagi MASLP
Audiologist
Department of Otorhinolaryngology and Head–Neck Surgery
All India Institute of Medical Sciences
New Delhi
pragyatyagi@hotmail.com

Praveen George Paul MD, DM
Senior Resident
Department of Pediatric Endocrinology
All India Institute of Medical Sciences
New Delhi
praveenpaul388@gmail.com

Priyanka Gupta MD, DM
Senior Resident
Department of Pediatric Endocrinology
All India Institute of Medical Sciences
New Delhi
prigupta552@gmail.com

Priyanka Khandelwal DM (Pediatric Nephrology), International Pediatric Nephrology Fellow
Department of Pediatrics
Great Ormond Street Hospital for Children
London,
drpriyanka8588@gmail.com

Priyanka Singh MD
Senior Resident
Department of Neonatology
All India Institute of Medical Sciences
New Delhi
priyanka09singh@gmail.com

Puneet Kumar Choudhary DM
Senior Resident
Department of Pediatrics
All India Institute of Medical Sciences
New Delhi
shinepuneet@gmail.com

Purna Chandra Guggilum DM
Senior Resident
Department of Pediatrics
All India Institute of Medical Sciences
New Delhi
chandra.puri12@gmail.com

Rahul Kumar MBBS
Junior Resident
Department of Pediatrics
All India Institute of Medical Sciences
New Delhi
mailtorahulkumarsuman@gmail.com

Raja Ashok Koganti DM (Neonatology)
Consultant Neonatologist
Ankura Hospital for Women and Children, Vijayawada
drrajaashok@gmail.com

Rajiv Aggarwal Fellowship in Neonatology
Director and Senior Consultant
Department of Pediatrics and Neonatology
Narayana Health City, Bengaluru
drrajivaggarwal@hotmail.com

Rajni Sharma MD
Additional Professor
All India Institute of Medical Sciences
New Delhi
email:drrajnisharma@yahoo.com

Rakesh Lodha MD
Professor
Department of Pediatrics
All India Institute of Medical Sciences
New Delhi
rlodha1661@gmail.com

Ranjith Kumar Manokaran DM
Associate Professor
Sri Ramachandra Institute of Higher Education and Research
Porur, Chennai
doct.ranjith@gmail.com

Ravneet Kaur DM
Associate Consultant
Division of Medical Genetics
Fortis Hospital
Mohali, Punjab
docravneet@gmail.com

Richie Dalai DM
Assistant Professor
Department of Neonatology
All India Institute of Medical Sciences
Patna
richie.aiims@gmail.com

Rinchen Zangmo MD
Ex-Assistant Professor
Department of Obstetrics and Gynaecology
All India Institute of Medical Sciences
New Delhi
rinchhen.zn@gmail.com

Rishika Potharaju MBBS
Junior Resident
Department of Pediatrics
All India Institute of Medical Sciences
New Delhi

Rohan Malik DM
Additional Professor
All India Institute of Medical Sciences
New Delhi
dr.rohanmalik@gmail.com

Sachit Anand MCh
Assistant Professor
Department of Pediatric Surgery
All India Institute of Medical Sciences
New Delhi
kanu.sachit@gmail.com

Sai Srinivas Gurram MD
Senior Resident
Department of Neonatology
All India Institute of Medical Sciences
New Delhi
srinivassai982@gmail.com

Satish Mishra DM
Consultant Neonatologist and Pediatrician
NEO Center for Advanced Neonatology and Child Health
Sagar, Madhya Pradesh
drmishrasatish@gmail.com

Satya Prakash MD, DM
Senior Resident
Department of Neonatology
All India Institute of Medical Sciences
New Delhi
satyaprakash1994@gmail.com

Saurabh Kumar Gupta
MD (Pediatrics), DM (Cardiology)
Professor
Department of Cardiology
All India Institute of Medical Sciences
New Delhi
drsaurabhmd@gmail.com

Seema Singhal MD
Additional Professor
Department of Obstetrics and Gynaecology
All India Institute of Medical Sciences
New Delhi
drseemasinghal@gmail.com

Shamnad Madathil MD, DM
Consultant Neonatologist
Baby Memorial Hospital
Kozhikode
shamnadmadathil@gmail.com

Shashank S Koundinya MBBS
Junior Resident
Department of Pediatrics
All India Institute of Medical Sciences
New Delhi
shashankskoundinya007@gmail.com

Shridhar Gopalakrishnan
DM (Neonatology)
Professor
Department of Pediatrics
Armed Forces Medical College, Pune
shri27cat@gmail.com

Sindhu Sivanandan DM
Consultant Neonatologist and Clincal Lead
Kauvery Hospital, Chennai
drsindhusivanandan@gmail.com

Srikanth Kulkarni DM (Neonatology)
Consultant Neonatologist
Rainbow Children's Hospital
Marathahalli
Bengaluru
sskulkarni151@gmail.com

Srinivasavaradan S Govindarajan MD, DM
Senior Resident
Department of Pediatric Nephrology
All India Institute of Medical Sciences
New Delhi
kavisrini.1993@gmail.com

Subhash Chandra Shaw DM
Professor
Department of Pediatrics
Army Hospital Research and Referral
Delhi
drscshaw@rediffmail.com

Subramanian Sreeram DM
Consultant
Paramitha Children Hospital and NEO BBC Children Hospital
Hyderabad
drsreeraman@yahoo.co.in

Suman Chaurasia MD, PhD
Assistant Professor
All India Institute of Medical Sciences
Rishikesh, Uttarakhand
sumanyss@gmail.com

Suma S DM
Consultant Neonatologist
Bai Jerbai Wadia Hospital for Children
Mumbai, suma.sund@gmail.com

Sunil Kushwah MD, DM
Senior Resident
Department of Pediatric Nephrology
Post Graduate Institute of
Medical Education and Research
(PGIMER), Chandigarh
drsunilkushwah04@gmail.com

Sunil Saharan MD
Assistant Professor
Division of Congenital Interventional Cardiology, New York University
Langone Medical Center, New York
sunilsaharan@gmail.com

Surjeet Kumar Bhardwaj MD, DM (Neonatology)
Assistant Professor
Department of Pediatrics
DrYSPGMC, Nahan, HP
drsurjeet99@gmail.com

Suvasini Sharma DM
Associate Professor
Lady Hardinge Medical College,
New Delhi
sharma.suvasini@gmail.com

Tanushree Sahoo MD, DM
Assistant Professor
Department of Neonatology
All India Institute of Medical Sciences
Bhubaneswar
tanushree_sony206@yahoo.co.in

Tejo Pratap Oleti DM
Senior Consultant and Head
Department of Neonatology
Fernandez Hospital, Hyderabad
tejopratap@gmail.com

Umang Bhardwaj MD
Senior Resident
Department of Neonatology
All India Institute of Medical Sciences
New Delhi
umangbhardwaj51@gmail.com

Vandana Jain MD
Professor
All India Institute of Medical Sciences
New Delhi
drvandanajain@aiims.edu

Vasudha Kohli MD
Senior Resident
Department of Pediatrics
All India Institute of Medical Sciences
New Delhi
kohli.vasudha@gmail.com

Venkatesan Sampath Kumar MS
Associate Professor
Department of Orthopaedics
All India Institute of Medical Sciences
New Delhi
venkatortho4@gmail.com

Venkatnarayan Kannan DM
Officer on Special Duty
NITI Aayog, Government of India
New Delhi
venkatnarayan_kannan@yahoo.co.in

Vishesh Jain MCh
Assistant Professor
Department of Pediatric Surgery
All India Institute of Medical Sciences
New Delhi
dr.vishesh79@gmail.com

Vivek Kumar MD
Consultant (Research)
Department of Pediatrics
All India Institute of Medical Sciences
New Delhi
vivekneoaiims@gmail.com

Vivek Tiwari MS
Senior Orthopaedic Consultant
Apollo Sage Hospital, Bhopal
vivek_tiwari50@yahoo.com

V Prakash MD
All India Institute of Medical Sciences
New Delhi

Preface to the Third Edition

We take immense pleasure in presenting the third edition of *AIIMS Protocols in Neonatology*. In this updated edition, we have introduced 39 new protocols and deleted nine protocols from the second edition, expanding the compendium to encompass 106 protocols. Our primary aim is to provide valuable resources that enhance our readers' education and patient care.

These protocols are thoughtfully categorized into two distinct packages: Core Protocols, spanning two volumes, cater to the management of common neonatal conditions, while Additional Protocols are dedicated to practitioners handling critically ill neonates and to DM and DNB fellows. This categorization empowers readers to delve into all protocols or focus exclusively on the Core ones.

Our unwavering commitment throughout the development of this edition has been to ensure that these protocols are firmly rooted in evidence-based practices. Our team has diligently reviewed the extensive body of literature, including guidelines from reputed bodies such as the World Health Organization (WHO), American Academy of Pediatrics (AAP), American College of Obstetrics and Gynecology (ACOG), National Institute of Clinical Excellence (NICE), Government of India, and National Neonatology Forum (NNF), meticulously contextualized the information, and presented it in a user-friendly format.

We emphasize that the protocols primarily apply to our own or similar institutions and *may have to be adapted to the users' context*. We highly recommend appropriate diligence in this regard.

Creating this edition has demanded a monumental collaborative effort. Faculty members, fellows, residents from our division, colleagues from other divisions within our department and various departments across our institution, and colleagues from other institutions have invested their time and expertise into its development. We extend our heartfelt gratitude to all those who have contributed to this endeavor.

We are grateful to the readers of the second edition who provided us with their valuable feedback. Your insights have been instrumental in refining this edition. We have diligently incorporated relevant changes and rectified any errors to make this version more comprehensive and reliable.

We extend our heartfelt gratitude to Mr YN Arjuna and the dedicated team at CBS, our new publisher, for their exceptional commitment and hands-on involvement in supervising the entire publication process of this third edition.

We acknowledge the possibility of mistakes in this edition. We value your feedback, as it has been invaluable in the past. Please send any observations or suggestions to us via email at ra.aiims@gmail.com, jeevasankar@gmail.com, or dranuthukral@gmail.com.

Ramesh Agarwal
Ashok Deorari
Vinod K Paul
M Jeeva Sankar
Anu Sachdeva

Preface to the First Edition

Protocols are instrumental for adoption of evidence-based practices and elimination of unnecessary or potentially harmful practices. Protocol based approach makes sure that there is a uniform clinical practice irrespective of disparate players and their views. Unit protocols also facilitate learning of the trainee doctors and nurses.

Protocols have been an integral part of NICU life at AIIMS right since its inception. As part of its philosophy of unrestricted sharing of the knowledge and resources, the neonatology faculty at AIIMS decided way back to publish the protocols in Indian Journal of Pediatrics. There was an overwhelming response from the neonatal fraternity to the extent that AIIMS protocols practically became part of majority of the neonatal units in India as well as other countries in South East Asia. For postgraduate students, it served as first hand resource for learning neonatology. The AIIMS protocols have been cited for over 400 times across the globe including in many major publications of recent times.

Initially, we published the protocols in Indian Journal of Pediatrics, which were periodically updated. Subsequently, the journal published them in form of a manual that enhanced their usability and outreach. The full texts of the protocols were made available on our website (wwwnewbornwhocc.org), which was one of the reasons of its popularity receiving nearly 200,000 hits over the last few years.

This publication is a manifestation of our desire to bring out a physician manual that contains relevant protocols based on context specific and updated evidence as well as other necessary resources and tools for day-to-day neonatology practice in level 2 and 3 neonatal units in South East Asia. The current manual has 33 protocols. These are focused on the operational aspects of a condition rather than discussing the theory. There are summaries of relevant evidence and management algorithms at appropriate places. There is a substantial amount of additional resource material such as resuscitation algorithm, hand hygiene poster, BP charts, drugs to be avoided in G6PD deficiency, online resources for self-learning and drugs use in pregnancy and lactation. There is a section that deals with main findings on chest X-ray of common conditions. A section on drug dosages has also been included.

India produces over 1200 postgraduate theses in pediatrics every year; however, the quality of research is too low to teach research methods to the students and generate a good piece of evidence. We have included a section that provides a number of research questions and optimum design to be used and relevant outcomes to be studied.

AIIMS protocols have been an outcome of intense efforts of the faculty, scientists and many past and present residents and fellows over a long time. All of them have shown an extraordinary commitment for this cause. We wish to acknowledge the immense contribution of Drs M Jeeva Sankar, Anu Thukral, Deepak Chawla, Kamal Arora and Aparna Chandrasekaran who not only contributed substantially in terms of contents but also in process of editing. We wish to thank Mr YN Arjuna of CBS Publishers who patiently accommodated our changing philosophy and style.

No book is flawless and we are unlikely to be exception. We would really appreciate your constructive criticism (ra.aiims@gmail.com).

Ramesh Agarwal
Ashok Deorari
Vinod K Paul

Contents

Section 6: Gastrointestinal and Hepatobiliary Tract and Nutrition

Section 7: Infections

Section

1

Fetal and Perinatal Care

1. Care during Pregnancy and Common Obstetric Illnesses and their Effect on the Fetus and Neonate
2. Antenatal Corticosteroid Therapy for Preterm Birth

CHAPTER

1 Care during Pregnancy and Common Obstetric Illnesses and their Effect on the Fetus and Neonate

The World Health Organization (WHO) recommends that all pregnant women should have their first antenatal visit in the first 12 weeks and then at 20, 26, 30, 34, 36, 38 and 40 weeks gestation.[1] The National Institute of Health and Care Excellence (NICE) Guidance recommends that nulliparous antenatal women have ten antenatal visits and parous women have seven visits.[2]

The current protocol summarizes the essential steps in routine antenatal care, including history and examination. It lists the common symptoms during pregnancy, obstetric conditions, and their effect on the fetus and newborn.

ROUTINE ANTENATAL CARE

A. History

First/booking visit should include evaluating the following:

- Menstrual history including last menstrual period, obstetric history, medical history, medications including supplements, overall mental health, any history of allergy, smoking, alcohol intake or drug abuse, support at home, occupation.
- Review past obstetric, medical, and surgical records
- Ask about the history of domestic abuse.

Subsequent visits should include evaluating the following:

Risk assessment of:

- General health, well-being, and any concerns about birth
- Reviewing the care plan for the pregnancy
- Identifying women requiring additional care, and
- Updating the antenatal card with fresh complaints, examination findings, and investigations at each visit.

B. Examinations, Investigations, and Advice

At the First Contact

- Determine gestational age and detect multifetal gestation.

- Measure weight and height, calculate body mass index.
- Advise blood tests for blood grouping and Rh typing, complete blood count, HIV, hepatitis B and syphilis, and blood sugar.
- Offer first-trimester aneuploidy screening. This includes ultrasound for nuchal translucency and nasal bone and a double marker test for serum-free beta hCG and PAPP-A.[3]
- Advise continuing folic acid supplement in the first trimester to prevent neural tube defects.[4] The recommended dose is 400 μg per day; however, 5 mg preparation is advised due to availability issues.
- Advise on avoiding alcohol and active and passive smoking.

At Subsequent Visits:

Advise pregnant women to

- Take iron and calcium supplements from the second trimester of pregnancy until the onset of labor[5] and at least three months after delivery. Iron and calcium supplements are widely available in various formulations. The recommended dose for prophylaxis is 60 mg of elemental iron and 1200 mg of calcium per day.[5]
- Advise antenatal women to avoid sleeping on their backs after 20 weeks of pregnancy.[2]
- Advice hemoglobin assessment at 32 weeks for anemia.

Offer the following:

Anomaly scans at 18–20 weeks for detection of congenital anomalies and localization of the placenta.[2]

- Abdominal examination for fundal height from 24 weeks of gestation.
- Vaccination against tetanus and influenza.
- COVID vaccination as per the local protocol.
- Anti-D injection to prevent rhesus alloimmunization to rhesus-negative women at 28 weeks of pregnancy.

Common Symptoms during Pregnancy and their Management

The common symptoms during pregnancy include:

Nausea and vomiting: This common symptom can persist until 16–22 weeks of pregnancy.[2] Women with symptoms should avoid large meals and fatty food. Medications can be prescribed with dietary management. Care must be taken to avoid missing hyperemesis gravidarum, a dreaded but rare complication in the first trimester.

Vaginal discharge: This is normal in pregnancy unless it is profuse, associated with a foul smell, or vaginal soreness.

Obstetric Conditions during Pregnancy and their Effect on Fetus and Newborn

Most obstetric conditions have fetal implications; thus, the neonatologist must be updated during the antenatal period and whenever a delivery is planned.

1. Preeclampsia and Hypertensive Disorders in Pregnancy

Preeclampsia is a multisystem progressive disorder characterized by the new onset of hypertension and proteinuria or the recent onset of hypertension plus significant end-organ dysfunction with or without proteinuria, typically presenting after 20 weeks of gestation or postpartum. Several subtypes of preeclampsia may exist, with various pathophysiological pathways leading to maternal and fetal mortality and morbidity.[6] The most commonly described subtypes are early onset (<34 weeks of gestation) and late-onset (34 weeks of pregnancy). The clinical features overlap, but the spectrum of disease and outcomes differ: Early-onset disease has been associated with more severe placental and maternal/fetal clinical findings and, in turn, poorer maternal/fetal outcomes.

Management: Tablet aspirin 150 mg once a day from 12 weeks of pregnancy till delivery for those at risk of preeclampsia.[6] A comprehensive workup must be done to find the cause and look for end-organ involvement. The blood pressure should be recorded, and a urine dipstick test be done at every routine physical appointment. A target blood pressure of 135/85 mm Hg should be the aim in all hypertensive disorders of pregnancy. Tablet labetalol given to a maximum of 2400 mg daily in divided doses is the drug of choice. Nifedipine can be given where labetalol is contraindicated, and alpha methyldopa can be prescribed as per availability.[9] Auscultate the fetal heart at every antenatal appointment. Conduct an ultrasound for fetal assessment at diagnosis if facilities are available and, if normal, repeat every two weeks. Conduct a CTG at diagnosis and then only if clinically indicated. In women with chronic hypertension, ultrasound for fetal growth, amniotic fluid volume assessment, and umbilical artery Doppler should be done at 28 weeks, 32 weeks, and 36 weeks.

Planning delivery: Delivery can be planned between 37–38 weeks of gestation if BP is within 160/110 mm Hg with or without medication.[6]

Table 1.1: Indication for early delivery (before 37 weeks) in hypertensive disorders of pregnancy[6]
Uncontrolled blood pressure despite three or more antihypertensives in appropriate doses
Oxygen saturation <90%
Progressive worsening of liver or kidney function, hemolysis, or decreased platelet count
Presence of neurological features (intractable headache, repeated scotomata, or eclampsia)
Placental abruption
Reversed end-diastolic flow in the umbilical artery Doppler velocimetry in the fetus
A nonreassuring CTG

Indications for delivery before 37 weeks are mentioned in Table 1.1. Intravenous magnesium sulfate ($MgSO_4$) for neuroprotection and prevention of eclampsia, and a course of antenatal corticosteroids if early delivery is planned in preterm preeclampsia.[9] Women with chronic hypertension must be advised about exercise, healthy eating, and low salt intake.[9]

Specific management of severe hypertension, severe preeclampsia, or eclampsia

1. Anticonvulsant: If delivery is planned within 24 hours, or when one or more of the features of severe preeclampsia are present (severe headaches, visual scotomata, nausea or vomiting, epigastric pain, decreased urine output, severe hypertension, progressive deterioration in laboratory parameters (rising creatinine or liver transaminases, or falling platelet count) intravenous $MgSO_4$ must be administered with a loading dose of 4 g intravenously over 5–15 minutes, followed by infusion of 1 g/hour for 24 hours. In recurrent convulsions: a further dose of 2–4 g is given intravenously over 5–15 minutes.[8]
2. Antihypertensive include labetalol (oral or IV), nifedipine, and intravenous hydralazine.

Effect on fetus and newborn: Preeclampsia is associated with systemic and pulmonary vascular dysfunction in the offspring. The systemic vascular defect predisposes to chronic hypertension and stroke later in life, beginning from childhood.[11] There is an increased risk of fetal growth restriction and preterm birth.[10]

2. Gestational Diabetes Mellitus (GDM)

Gestational diabetes mellitus (GDM) develops in pregnant people whose pancreatic function is insufficient to overcome the insulin resistance associated with the pregnant state. Patients with GDM are at high risk of developing type 2 diabetes later in life, which is unsurprising since the pathophysiologic path of inadequate insulin secretion in the setting of insulin resistance during pregnancy also underlies type 2 diabetes outside of pregnancy. Screening for GDM must be done in all antenatal women. All antenatal women should be offered blood sugar fasting and post-meal at the first visit. Women with additional risk factors (Table 1.2) offer a glucose tolerance test (GTT) with 75 g glucose at the first antenatal visit. offer GTT with 75 g glucose to all antenatal women not previously diagnosed with diabetes at 24–28 weeks of gestation.[7]

This depends on the degree of control required. Medical nutrition therapy with regular exercise for 30 minutes every day is advisable. Oral hypoglycemic agent metformin is preferred. Rapidly acting insulin analogs are safe in pregnancy. Long-acting insulin analog: Isophane is the first choice. Type 2 diabetic women already on other long-acting insulin like detemir and glargine can continue with the same if sugars are well controlled. Blood sugar monitoring can be done at home with a finger prick test using a glucometer. Women are advised to keep a check on fetal movements. Delivery in adequately controlled diabetes is ideally done at 40 completed weeks. Women with macrosomia should be explained the risk of shoulder dystocia with vaginal delivery.

Effect on fetus and newborn: GDM is associated with an increased risk of congenital malformations, preterm delivery, cesarean delivery, macrosomia and large for gestational age newborns, respiratory distress syndrome, admission to a neonatal intensive care unit, neonatal hypoglycemia, and hyperbilirubinemia.[7,8]

Table 1.2: Risk factors for GDM needing GTT at first visit[7]
BMI >30 kg/m^2
Previous macrosomic neonate weighing 4.5 kg or more
Previous gestational diabetes
History of diabetes in the family
History of polycystic ovarian syndrome
Planning delivery and other management

3. Cholestasis of Pregnancy

The diagnosis of intrahepatic cholestasis of pregnancy should be considered in pregnant women with normal itching, appearing skin, and raised peak random total bile acid concentration of 19 µmol/L or more. Pruritus is characteristic as it involves palms and soles, particularly at night. It is diagnosed with unexplained pruritus in pregnancy associated with abnormal liver function tests (LFTs) and or increased bile acids, both resolving after delivery.[9] LFTs should be repeated in women with persistent pruritus and normal biochemistry.

Planning delivery and other management: The incidence of iatrogenic prematurity is increased; the usual delivery timing is 37–38 weeks.

Topical emollients like calamine lotion are safe during pregnancy. Ursodeoxycholic acid (UDCA) improves symptoms and deranged liver function. Water-soluble vitamin K (5–10 mg daily) should be administered when prothrombin time is prolonged. Continuous fetal monitoring in labor is required.

Effect on fetus and newborn: There are no reliable methods for preventing fetal death in obstetric cholestasis. There is an increased risk of iatrogenic and spontaneous preterm birth, increased incidence of meconium-stained liquor, a marginally increased risk of NICU admissions, and a slight risk of stillbirth at term.[9]

4. Antepartum Hemorrhage

Antepartum hemorrhage (APH) is bleeding from or into the genital tract from 24 weeks of pregnancy and before the neonate delivery.[10] The two most important causes of antepartum hemorrhage are placenta previa and placental abruption.

Placenta praevia: Placenta praevia is diagnosed when the placenta lies directly over the internal os. The incidence of placenta previa and accreta is increasing due to increased cesarean sections, advanced maternal age, and assisted reproductive techniques (ART) for conception.[10] The routine anomaly scan should localize the placenta so that women at risk of placenta previa can be identified. If the placenta is less than 20 mm from the internal os or praevia at the routine fetal anomaly scan, a repeat USG with a transvaginal sonogram (TVS) is advised at 32 weeks to look for the persistence of the previous finding. In case of the persistent low-lying placenta or placenta praevia at 32 weeks with no symptoms, another TVS is recommended at around 36 weeks of gestation. If findings remain the same at 36 weeks, it is labeled as placenta previa.

Planning delivery and other management: A single course of antenatal corticosteroids is recommended at less than 34 weeks. Delivery is to be conducted in a facility with blood transfusion services and a critical care facility. In the absence of symptoms, the ideal time of termination is 37 weeks. Tocolysis may be considered for 48 hours to facilitate the administration of antenatal corticosteroids if there is no maternal or fetal compromise. Immediate cord clamping is advisable to prevent fetal blood loss if the placenta is transected during cesarean section. Bleeding is controlled with medical measures followed by tamponade and surgical or interventional radiological techniques where possible.

Placenta accreta spectrum disorders: Major risk factors for these disorders include a history of accreta in a previous pregnancy, previous cesarean delivery, and other uterine surgery, including repeated endometrial curettage. The risk rises with the number of prior cesarean sections. Delivery is planned at 35–36 weeks in the absence of symptoms.

Placental abruption: The risk factors for abruption include prior abruption, hypertensive disorders of pregnancy, assisted reproductive techniques, PPROM, polyhydramnios, abdominal trauma, smoking, and drug abuse. Vaginal examination is mandated only after confirmation that the placenta is not low-lying. The abdominal examination suggests a tense woody feel of the uterus.

Planning delivery and other management: A single course of antenatal corticosteroids is recommended at less than 34 weeks. Delivery is to be conducted in a facility with blood transfusion services and a critical care facility. All women with APH with bleeding heavier than spotting must be admitted. In case of fetal demise, vaginal delivery is the recommended mode of delivery, but cesarean may need to be considered for some. If the fetus has any signs of compromise, an emergency cesarean section with simultaneous maternal resuscitation is necessary.

5. Fetal Growth Restriction (FGR)

FGR is defined as the failure of the fetus to reach its genetically predetermined growth potential.[11] A risk assessment for FGR must

Table 1.3: Recommendations on diagnosing FGR[12]	
Recommendation	*Grade*
Fetal size alone is insufficient to identify FGR unless AC or EFW is below the 3rd percentile.	C
A drop in fetal growth velocity, i.e. a drop in AC or EFW of >2 quartiles or >50 percentiles, should alert the physician to possible FGR	C
Doppler velocimetry of the uteroplacental and fetoplacental circulations may be used to distinguish between SGA and FGR.	Good practice point
Multimodal assessment is recommended for the evaluation of pregnancies with suspected FGR	Good practice point
cCTG or BPP scoring should be used in combination with Doppler velocimetry	A

be done at the booking visit and again in the second trimester. The grade recommendation of different parameters for diagnosing FGR is depicted in Table 1.3. Perform symphysis fundal height (SFH) measurement at each antenatal visit after 24 weeks at least two weeks intervals in singleton pregnancy unless the woman has regular growth scans.[11]

Planning delivery and other management: A growth scan should be ordered in case of discrepancies between the gestation period. Progressively increasing pulsatility index in the umbilical artery (UA) corresponds to a progressive reduction in the placental surface area available for nutrient exchange and increased fetal afterload resistance. This is associated with placental vascular insufficiency reflected by absent and, in the end-stage phase, reversed end-diastolic flow (REDF) in the UA. Reduced fetal MCA-PI results from vasodilatation, the so-called 'brain-sparing' effect. Doppler velocimetry plays a central role in the identification, surveillance, and management of FGR because it allows for the identification of uteroplacental insufficiency and/or fetal cardiovascular adaptation to hypoxemia. In the absence of contraindications, induction of labor is indicated. During labor, continuous fetal heart rate monitoring is recommended.

Indications of Delivery[11]

1. Any gestational age in the presence of maternal indications like severe preeclampsia
2. Spontaneous repeated unprovoked FHR decelarations

3. Abnormal biophysical profile score of 4 or less.
4. Abnormal ductus venosus waveform.
5. STV <2.6 at 26–28 weeks, STV <3 at 29–32 weeks, STV <3.5 between 32 and 34 weeks, and STV <4.5 after 34 weeks.
6. REDF in the umbilical artery beyond 30 weeks
7. AEDF in umbilical artery: 32–34 weeks
8. Between 36 and 37 weeks: Deliver if UA PI is >95th centile or AC/EFW <3rd centile
9. Between 38 and 39 weeks: Deliver if cerebral blood flow redistribution.

Indications for Elective Caesarean Delivery

- Abnormal cCTG STV
- Ductus venosus Doppler alteration
- Absent or reversed UA-EDF
- Altered BPP
- Maternal indication

Effect on fetus and newborn: The risk of being born prematurely leads to complications, including respiratory distress syndrome, necrotizing enterocolitis, intracranial hemorrhage, retinopathy of prematurity, and patent ductus arteriosus. Short-term complications occur soon after birth and include respiratory distress, perinatal asphyxia, meconium aspiration syndrome, hypoglycemia, polycythemia, hyperbilirubinemia, sepsis, hypocalcemia, hypothermia, and immunological incompetence. Long-term complications include increased perinatal mortality, increased risk of adverse neurodevelopmental outcomes, increased risk of obesity, cardiovascular diseases, metabolic syndrome, dyslipidemia, diabetes mellitus, and renal diseases later in life.

REFERENCES

1. WHO recommendations on antenatal care for a positive pregnancy experience. Geneva: World Health Organization; 2016. (https://www. who. int/publications/i/item/9789241549912, accessed 14 January 2021).
2. NICE guideline on Antenatal Care, Published: 19 August 2021. www.nice. org.uk/guidance/ng201.
3. Alldred SK, Takwoingi Y, Guo B, Pennant M, Deeks JJ, Neilson JP, et al. First trimester ultrasound tests alone or in combination with first-trimester serum tests for Down's syndrome screening. Cochrane Database Syst Rev [Internet]. 2017;3(3):CD012600. Available from: http://dx.doi.org/10.1002/14651858. CD012600.

4. Centers for Disease Control and Prevention. CDC grand rounds: additional opportunities to prevent neural tube defects with folic acid fortification. MMWR – Morbidity & Mortality Weekly Report. 2010;59(31):980–4.
5. Hofmeyr GJ, Lawrie TA, Atallah ÁN, Torloni MR. Calcium supplementation during pregnancy for preventing hypertensive disorders and related problems. Cochrane Database Syst Rev. 2018 Oct 1;10(10): CD001059.
6. National Institute for Health and Care Excellence. Hypertension in pregnancy: diagnosis and management: NICE guideline [NG133]. Accessed Jan 15, 2023. https://www.nice.org.uk/guidance/ng133/chapter/Recommendations#management-of-chronic-hypertension-in-pregnancy.
7. NICE guideline on diabetes in pregnancy: management from preconception to the postnatal period). Last updated 16 December 2020. www.nice.org.uk/guidance/ng3. Published 25 February 2015.
8. Ye W, Luo C, Huang J, Li C, Liu Z, Liu F. Gestational diabetes mellitus and adverse pregnancy outcomes: systematic review and meta-analysis. BMJ. 2022 May 25;377:e067946. doi 10.1136/bmj-2021-067946.
9. Girling J, Knight CL, Chappell L; Royal College of Obstetricians and Gynaecologists. Intrahepatic cholestasis of pregnancy: Green-top Guideline No. 43 June 2022. BJOG. 2022 Dec;129(13):e95–e114.
10. Jauniaux E, Alflrevic Z, Bhide AG, Belfort MA. Placenta Praevia and Placenta Accreta: Diagnosis and Management. Green top guideline 27a. BJOG Sept. 2018;
11. Lees CC, Stampalija T, Baschat A, da Silva Costa F, Ferrazzi E, Figueras F, Hecher K, Kingdom J, Poon LC, Salomon LJ, Unterscheider J. ISUOG Practice Guidelines: diagnosis and management of the small-for-gestational-age fetus and fetal growth restriction. Ultrasound Obstet Gynecol. 2020 Aug;56(2):298–312.
12. Gordijn SJ, Beune IM, Thilaganathan A, Papageorghiou A, Baschat AA, Baker PN, Silver RM, Wynia K, Ganzevoort W. Consensus definition of fetal growth restriction: A Delphi procedure. Ultrasound Obstet Gynecol 2016;48:333–9.

CHAPTER

2

Antenatal Corticosteroid Therapy for Preterm Birth

Globally, complications of preterm birth are the leading cause of under-5 mortality, accounting for 20% under-5 deaths in 2015.[1] Preterm infants who survive are at a risk of wide range of morbidities. Administration of antenatal corticosteroids (ACS) to mother for enhancing fetal lung maturity before any anticipated preterm birth is one of the most important strategies to improve the preterm neonatal outcomes.

BENEFITS

The updated Cochrane (2020) reaffirms the reduction of perinatal death, neonatal death, respiratory distress syndrome and intraventricular-periventricular hemmorhage by 15% (RR 0.85, 95% CI 0.77–0.93), 22% (RR 0.78, 0.70–0.87), 29% (RR 0.71, 0.65–0.78) and 42% (RR 0.58, 0.45–0.75), respectively.[2]

FIRST COURSE

We give the first course of ACS therapy in women at risk of preterm birth from 24^{+0} weeks to 34 weeks of gestation (irrespective of singleton or multiple pregnancy and the growth restriction of the fetus) when all the following conditions are met:[3]

i. Gestational age assessment can be accurately undertaken
ii. Preterm birth is considered imminent as evidenced by onset of true labor pains
iii. There is no clinical evidence of maternal infection

It is important that health facilities providing ACS therapy to women with preterm labor has adequate childbirth care including the capacity to recognize and manage preterm labor and birth and the preterm newborn can receive adequate care (including resuscitation, thermal care, feeding support, infection treatment and safe oxygen use).

There is variation in the recommended gestation range for administration of the first course of ACS: ACOG 2017[4] and NICE 2016[5] recommend this gestation range as 24^{+0} to 33^{+6} weeks while WHO[3] and Government of India as 24–34 weeks of gestation.

Drugs and Dosage[3]

Two drugs can be used for ACS therapy:

1. **Dexamethasone:** 6 mg every 12 hours for a total of 4 doses (24 mg).
2. **Betamethasone:** a mixture (1:1) of betamethasone acetate (long acting) and betamethasone phosphate (fast acting): 12 mg every 24 hours, a total of 2 doses (24 mg).

As the combination preparation of betamethasone is not available in India (the available preparation is betamethasone phosphate) and is costly as an imported product, dexamethasone is the drug of choice given its comparable efficacy and safety, wide availability, and low cost.[6]

i. Give the first dose of ACS in imminent delivery. Even a single dose given within 24 hours of delivery is associated with significant reduction in neonatal morbidity and mortality.[3]
ii. Multiple fetal pregnancies (twins, triplets) should receive the same dose as singleton.[3]
iii. Mothers diagnosed with pregestational and gestational diabetes should be administered complete course of ACS. Interventions to optimize the maternal blood glucose levels should be ensured.[3]
iv. Mothers already on oral steroids like prednisolone should also receive the standard course of ACS.

Contraindications

Chorioamnionitis is the only absolute contraindication. Maternal diabetes, preeclampsia and hypertension are **NOT** contraindications for using ACS.

Repeat Course

Consider a repeat course in women with:

a. Pregnancy of less than 34^{+6} weeks
b. Still at risk of preterm labor within next 7 days, and
c. Prior dose of ACS given more than 14 days ago.[4]

Only single repeat course is recommended, avoid multiple courses.

Interval between the first course and repeat course is still debatable. WHO recommends it to be 7 days instead of 14 days.[3] RCOG and Government of India guidelines, 2014 do not recommend the repeat course.

Late Preterm ($34^{0/7}$ to $36^{6/7}$ Weeks)

We do not use ACS in late preterm of $34^{0/6}$ to $36^{6/7}$ weeks' gestation.

Current evidence does not support use of ACS in late preterm pregnancies. A systematic review[7] showed short-term benefits in neonatal morbidities: lower risk of transient tachypnea of the newborn (RR 0.56, 95% CI 0.37–0.86), severe RDS (0.55, 0.33–0.91), use of surfactant, and mechanical ventilation, and lower time of receiving oxygen, and a shorter duration of stay in NICU. However, there was no difference in neonatal mortality. WHO and Government of India guidelines recommend against the administration of corticosteroids for lung maturity beyond 34 weeks of gestation.

Periviable Gestation (22–24 Weeks)

The decision to administer corticosteroids in gestation below 24 weeks should be individualized considering the neonatal unit's capability to provide care to such babies and parental wishes.

Evidence supports the benefits of ACS in preterm neonates born at 22–24 weeks' gestation. A meta-analysis showed reduced mortality (OR 0.48; 95% CI 0.42–0.55) and peri-intraventricular hemorhage and periventricular leucomalacia (OR 0.70, 95% CI 0.63–0.79) in these neonates.[8]

Elective Cesarean Sections in more than 34 Weeks' Gestation

ACS is not recommended in women undergoing planned cesarean section at late preterm gestations ($34–36^{+6}$ weeks)

Table 2.1: Guideline recommendations for antenatal corticosteroids
RCOG Updated August 2021 1. Clinicians should offer a single course of antenatal corticosteroids to women between 24^{+0} and 34^{+6} weeks of gestation who are at risk of preterm birth. 2. Antenatal corticosteroids can be considered for women between 23^{+0} and 23^{+6} weeks of gestation who are at risk of preterm birth. 3. The decision to administer corticosteroids at gestations less than 24^{+0} weeks should be made at a senior level taking all clinical aspects into consideration. 4. Antenatal corticosteroids should be given to all women at risk of iatrogenic or spontaneous preterm birth up to 34^{+6} weeks of gestation.

(Contd.)

Table 2.1: Guideline recommendations for antenatal corticosteroids (*Contd.*)

5. Senior opinion should be sought if a rescue course is to be considered. A rescue course of two doses of 12 mg betamethasone or four doses of 6 mg dexamethasone should only be considered with caution in those pregnancies where the first course was given at less than 26^{+0} weeks of gestation and another obstetric indication arises later in pregnancy.

ACOG 2017

1. A single course of corticosteroids is recommended for pregnant women between $24^{0/7}$ weeks and $33^{6/7}$ weeks of gestation who are at risk of preterm delivery within 7 days, including for those with ruptured membranes and multiple gestations. It also may be considered for pregnant women starting at $23^{0/7}$ weeks of gestation who are at risk of preterm delivery within 7 days, based on a family's decision regarding resuscitation, irrespective of membrane rupture status and regardless of fetal number.
2. A single course of betamethasone is recommended for pregnant women between $34^{0/7}$ weeks and $36^{6/7}$ weeks of gestation at risk of preterm birth within 7 days, and who have not received a previous course of antenatal corticosteroids.
3. Regularly scheduled repeat courses or serial courses (more than two) are not currently recommended.
4. A single repeat course of antenatal corticosteroids should be considered in women who are less than $34^{0/7}$ weeks of gestation who are at risk of preterm delivery within 7 days, and whose prior course of antenatal corticosteroids was administered more than 14 days previously. Rescue course corticosteroids could be provided as early as 7 days from the prior dose, if indicated by the clinical scenario.

WHO September 2022

Antenatal corticosteroid therapy is recommended for women with a high likelihood of preterm birth from 24 weeks to 34 weeks of gestation when the following conditions are met.

1. Gestational age assessment can be accurately undertaken.
2. There is a high likelihood of preterm birth within 7 days of starting therapy.
3. There is no clinical evidence of maternal infection.
4. Adequate childbirth care is available (including capacity to recognize and safely manage preterm labour and birth).
5. The preterm newborn can receive adequate care (including resuscitation, kangaroo mother care, thermal care, feeding support, infection treatment and respiratory support including continuous positive airway pressure [CPAP] as needed).

Antenatal corticosteroid therapy is not recommended for women undergoing planned caesarean section at 34 weeks 0 days to 36 weeks 6 days.

A single repeat course of antenatal corticosteroids is recommended for women who have received a single course of antenatal corticosteroids at least 7 days prior and, on clinical assessment, have a high likelihood of giving birth preterm in the next 7 days.

REFERENCES

1. Liu L, Oza S, Hogan D, et al. Global, regional, and national causes of under-5 mortality in 2000-15: an updated systematic analysis with implications for the Sustainable Development Goals. Lancet 2016; 388:3027–35.
2. McGoldrick E, Stewart F, Parker R, Dalziel SR. Antenatal corticosteroids for accelerating fetal lung maturation for women at risk of preterm birth. Cochrane Database Syst Rev. 2020 Dec 25;12(12).
3. World Health Organization. WHO recommendations on interventions to improve preterm birth outcomes [Internet]. Geneva: World Health Organization, 2015. last accessed 7th July 2022 available at https://apps.who.int/iris/bitstream/handle/10665/183037/9789241508988_eng.pdf;jsessionid=083E9259BFC77088EBF77E4B3EB994C9?sequence=1
4. Committee on Obstetric Practice. Committee Opinion No. 713: Antenatal Corticosteroid Therapy for Fetal Maturation. Obstet Gynecol. 2017 Aug;130 (2): e102-e109.doi: 10.1097/AOG.0000000000002237. PMID: 28742678.
5. Preterm labour and birth National Institute for Health and Care Excellence published 20th November 2015 last accessed 9th July 2022 available at https://www.nice.org.uk/guidance/ng25
6. Ciapponi A, Klein K, Colaci D, Althabe F, Belizán JM, Deegan A, Veroniki AA, Florez ID. Dexamethasone versus betamethasone for preterm birth: a systematic review and network meta-analysis. Am J Obstet Gynecol MFM. 2021 May;3 (3): 100312.
7. Htun ZT, Hairston JC, Gyamfi-Bannerman C, Marasch J, Duarte Ribeiro AP. Antenatal Corticosteroids: Extending the Practice for Late-Preterm and Scheduled Early-Term Deliveries? Children (Basel). 2021 Apr 1;8 (4):272.
8. Deshmukh M, Patole S. Antenatal corticosteroids for neonates born before 25 weeks—A systematic review and meta-analysis. PLOS ONE. 2017 May 9;12(5):e0176090.

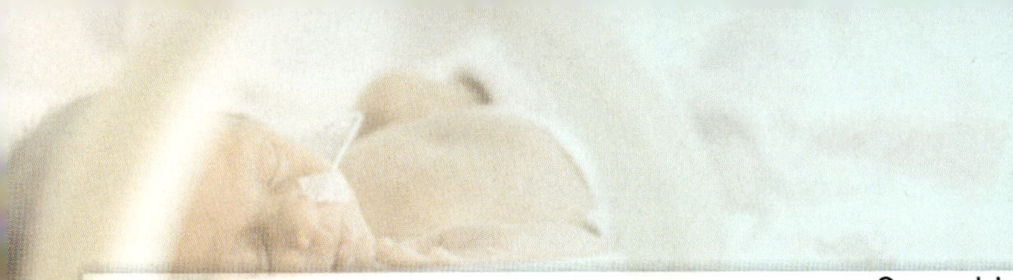

Section

2

Issues in Care of Normal and High-risk Newborns

3. Care of Normal Newborn
4. Common External Markers
5. Thermal Management
6. Golden-hour Management of High-risk Newborn
7. Birth Injury

CHAPTER

3

Care of Normal Neonate

Normal neonate in this protocol has been defined as:

- Birth weight greater than 2500 g and gestation 37 weeks or more.
- No major malformation or birth trauma.
- Birth weight between 10th and 90th percentiles as per AIIMS intrauterine growth charts.[1]
- The absence of maternal illness or intrapartum event that may put a neonate at risk of illness (e.g. gestational diabetes, antepartum hemorrhage, etc.).
- Normal Apgar scores; no need for resuscitation at birth.
- No postnatal illness such as respiratory distress, sepsis, dyselectrolytemia, hypoglycemia, or polycythemia.

CARE AT BIRTH

Personnel and equipment to be present at delivery:[2] One health provider (physician or nurse) trained in neonatal resuscitation must be physically available at birth of all infants irrespective of their risk status (high or low). *It is not good enough to have someone on call.*

More advanced neonatal resuscitation may be required if the delivery is anticipated to be high risk because of risk factors identified before birth. In these cases, at least two persons should be present solely to manage the neonate. The goal should be to provide a 'resuscitation team' with a specified leader and each member's identified role. There should be separate teams for multiple births.

The resuscitation corner must be in the delivery room itself. The health professional designated to care for the neonate at birth should check for "*Resuscitation Preparedness*" at the birthing place well in time before the neonate is delivered (Table 3.1). One may refer to the 'Neonatal Resuscitation Programme' (NRP) guidelines for details of resuscitation (www.aap.org/nrp).[2]

Table 3.1: Checklist for *"Resuscitation Preparedness"*	
For providing warmth	Preheat the warmer by turning on manual mode for at least 20 minutes. At least three prewarmed towels and a blanket should be available.
Thermoregulation	Plastic bag or plastic wrap, heated mattress, and cap for small neonates.
For positioning	Prepare shoulder rolls and keep it ready.
For clearing airway	10–12 F suction catheter, suction set at 80–100 mm Hg, meconium aspirator.
For ventilation	Check the availability and the functioning of the self-inflating bags. Check for availability of all sizes of the masks 00, 0, and 1, 8F feeding tube, and 20 ml syringe.
For oxygen delivery	Oxygen tubing or T-piece resuscitator that can deliver the free flow oxygen. Pulse oximeter, oxygen blender.
For intubation	Laryngoscope with blades of sizes 0 and 1, endotracheal tubes, sizes: 2.5, 3.0, 3.5, stethoscope.
For medication	Access to 1:10,000 epinephrine and normal saline, supplies for administrating medications and placing an emergency umbilical venous catheter, neonatal case record sheet for documentation.
For transportation	The transport incubator should be stationed in the birthing place for transportation in all high-risk deliveries.

Time of birth: The attending physician/nurse should note the time of birth. It is essential to call out the time of delivery loudly. This helps record accurate time and alerts other personnel in case any help is needed.

Standard precautions and asepsis at birth: In all cases, the personnel attending the delivery must exercise all the universal/ standard precautions. All fluid products from the neonate/ mother should be treated as potentially infectious. Gloves, masks, and gowns should be worn when resuscitating the newborn. Protective eyewear or face shields should be worn during procedures likely to generate blood or other bodily fluids droplets.

It is essential to prevent infection at birth by observing five cleans:

1. **Clean hands:** Appropriate hand hygiene and wearing sterile gloves.

2. **Clean surface:** Use a clean and sterile towel to dry and cover the neonate.
3. **Clean cut:** The umbilical cord should be cut with a clean and sterile blade/scissor.
4. **Clean tie:** The cord should be clamped with a clean and sterile clamp or tie.
5. **Clean cord:** One should not apply anything to the cord.

Prevention and management of hypothermia: Immediately after birth, the newborn is at maximum risk of hypothermia. This may have a detrimental effect on the infant's health as the admission temperature of non-asphyxiated newborns has been shown to be a strong predictor of mortality at all gestational ages.[2] Take special care to prevent and manage hypothermia. It should be ensured that the delivery room temperature is 25–28°C and free from air draft.[3] The pediatrician should receive the neonate directly (*no middle person should be allowed*) in a prewarmed sterile linen sheet. The infant should be dried thoroughly, including the head and face areas. Any wet linen should not remain in contact with the infant.

Skin-to-skin contact (STS): Any infant born vaginally and requiring only routine steps should be placed on the mother's abdomen or chest immediately after the birth for the initial one hour of life to ensure early skin-to-skin (STS) contact with the mother.[4] This will maintain the newborn's temperature, promote early breastfeeding, and decrease the mother's pain and bleeding. The mother-neonate dyad should not be left alone and should be observed for breathing, color, and temperature every 15 minutes.

Delayed clamping of the umbilical cord: Umbilical cord clamping must be delayed for at least 30–60 seconds to allow additional blood transfer from the placenta to the infant. This delayed cord clamping is associated with improved hematologic status, iron status, and clinical anemia in term infants at 2–6 months.[5]

Drying of the neonate: The neonate should be dried at birth with a clean and sterile cloth. The drying should be gentle and only wipe out the blood and the meconium and not be vigorous enough to remove the vernix caseosa (white greasy material on the skin). The vernix protects the skin of the infant and helps maintain temperature. This gets absorbed on its own after some time. Paraffin or any other emollient is not recommended for cleaning at birth.

Clamping of the cord: The umbilical cord should be clamped 2–3 cm away from the abdomen using a commercially available clamp, a clean and autoclaved thread, or a sterile rubber band. The stump should be away from the genitals to avoid contamination. When the commercial clamps are unavailable, the rubber band could be a better option than a thread, as once the cord starts shriveling; the rubber band would still maintain its grip while the thread might loosen up. Inspect the cord every 15–30 minutes for the initial few hours after birth to detect any oozing from the cord early.

Routine stomach wash: Routine stomach wash in neonates to prevent gastritis (amniotic fluid or meconium) is not done.

Care of the eye: At birth, the neonates' eyes should be cleaned with separate swabs. Sterile water or normal saline may be used for this purpose. The swipe to clean the eyes should be gentle and done from the inner canthus area to the outer canthus. Cleaning the eyes daily is not recommended as a routine. There is insufficient evidence to recommend the routine antibiotic prophylaxis to prevent ophthalmia neonatorum in the Indian setting.

Placement of identity band: The birthing places with high birth rates should take utmost care to ensure the identity of the mother-neonate dyad by an appropriate method as per the hospital policy. Each infant must have an identity band containing the mother's name, hospital registration number, gender, and birth weight of the infant. The reliability of the footprints for identification has not been investigated.

Recording of apgar scores: The Apgar scores should be recorded at 1 minute and 5 minutes of birth. This score has a limited value in guiding resuscitation and initial stabilization. The prediction of the subsequent outcomes by Apgar scores is also poor. However, Apgar scores may help in deciding the need for nursery admission.

A recent review by Ramaswamy et al. (2022)[3] exploring delivery room interventions to prevent hypothermia in term and late preterm neonates found one cluster RCT that compared an operation theatre room temperature of 23°C with 20°C for births from caesarian section. The higher room temperature was associated with higher incidence of normothermia (RR 1.26, 95% CI 1.11–1.42), higher body temperature (MD 0.30°C, 95% CI 0.23–0.37) and lower risk of moderate hypothermia (RR 0.26, 95% CI 0.16–0.42).

A review by Moore et al. (2016)[4] found that skin-to-skin contact between the mother and her neonate immediately after birth improves breastfeeding rate at 1–4 months and its duration by over 60 days, and helps the mother to breastfeed successfully on first attempt. Further, newborns who receive STS have higher blood glucose and similar temperature as compared to those receiving standard care. No important negative effects were identified.

A Cochrane review[5] including 15 trials (3911 mother and infant pairs) showed that delayed cord clamping, compared to early cord clamping, was associated with the following effects in term infants:

- Higher mean birthweight (WMD 101 g, 95% CI 45–157).
- Higher hemoglobin concentration at 24–48 hours (WMD 1.5 g/dl, 95% CI 1.21–1.78).
- Increased requirement of phototherapy for jaundice (RR 1.61, 95% CI 1.04–2.44).
- Lower incidence of iron deficiency at 3–6 months (RR 0.38, 95% CI 0.15–0.96).

CARE OF NEONATE DURING THE INITIAL FEW HOURS AFTER BIRTH

Weight: The neonate should be weighed after STS/stabilization, and the temperature should be documented to be normal. A sterile preheated sheet (or a single-use paper towel) should be placed on a 5–10-g sensitivity weighing machine. After zeroing, the neonate is gently placed on the weighing machine, and the weight is recorded. Weighing the neonate is a complex skill and requires adequate training of health providers.

Initiation of breastfeeds: Breastfeeding should be initiated at the earliest time possible, preferably during STS contact. The time of initiation of breastfeeding should be documented. The health provider should actively assist the mother in putting the neonate on the breast irrespective of the mode of delivery. Breastfeeding counseling alone without proactive support is unlikely to result in high rates of successful breastfeeding.

Vitamin K: Vitamin K should be administered to all neonates (0.5 mg for neonates less than 1000 grams and 1 mg for neonates more than 1000 grams).[6] It is preferable to administer vitamin K1; however, vitamin K3 may be administered if unavailable.[7] This should be administered as an IM injection using the 26 G (1/2 inch) needle and a 1 ml syringe on the anterolateral aspect of the thigh.

First examination: The neonate should be thoroughly examined by the attending person from head to toe, and the findings should be recorded in the neonatal record sheet. Looking at midline structures for malformations (e.g. cleft lip, neck masses, chest abnormality, omphalocele, meningocele, cloacal abnormality, etc.) is vital. Give special attention to identifying and documenting the anal opening. There is no need for routine catheter passage in the stomach, nostrils, and rectum to detect esophageal atresia, choanal atresia, and anorectal malformation, respectively. The axillary temperature of the neonate should be recorded before the neonate is shifted out from the birthing place. The neonate should be examined for birth injuries in cases with difficult extraction.

Communication with the family: Before leaving the birthing place, the health professional should communicate with the mother and the family members. One should ensure that the family members and the mother get to witness the gender and identity number of the neonate. The following facts should be told to the family:

1. The gender of the neonate
2. Birth weight
3. The well-being of the neonate.

Rooming in: A normal newborn should never be separated from the mother. In the initial few hours of life, the neonate is very active, and the closeness of the neonate to the mother will facilitate early breastfeeding and bonding. Studies have shown that any separation during these initial hours may adversely impact various outcomes, including exclusive breastfeeding rates at discharge.[8]

Care of the cord: The umbilical stump should be kept dry and devoid of application. Fold the nappy below the stump to avoid any contamination. Recent evidence supports the application of 4% chlorhexidine in community settings with high neonatal mortality and unhygienic cord practices.[9]

Oil massage: The benefits of the oil application have been described for low birth weight neonates in both developed and developing countries. However, a lack of data exists for the oil application and/or massage in term neonates.[10] Oil massage is a low-cost traditional practice well ingrained in different cultures, with no reported adverse outcome. The same may be allowed in a gentle way and with clean hands. Do not use oils with additives or irritant oils (such as mustard oil) for this purpose.

Exclusive breastfeeding: A proactive and systematic approach should be followed to initiate, support, and maintain breastfeeding. The various advantages of breastfeeds should be discussed with the mother to motivate her to breastfeed. The availability of a dedicated lactation nurse or counselor would significantly increase the chances of successful breastfeeding.

Bath: Recent evidence suggests that delaying the first newborn bath until at least 24 hours of life may prevent hypothermia and reduce mortality risk. [11] Avoid dip baths during the hospital stay, as this increases the risk of hypothermia. The sponging of the neonate should be done once a day with clean water, as per the requirement. The dip bath may be undertaken once the cord has fallen and the neonate is discharged from the hospital.

Powder application: Currently, there is no evidence to suggest regular powder use and the same should be avoided.

Position of sleep: No Indian study has addressed the issue of the relation of sleep position to the occurrence of sudden infant death syndrome (SIDS). There is substantial evidence in the literature from developed countries of an association between prone position and SIDS independent of the other variables.[12] Healthy-term newborns should preferably be made to sleep on their backs.

Traditional practices that should be discouraged: Applying kajal/surma in the eyes, putting oil in the ear, or applying the cow-dung on the cord must be discouraged.

Timing of discharge in a normal newborn: The mother and neonate must stay in the hospital for at least 48–72 hours (for the establishment of breastfeeding and observation for any morbidity, including jaundice). However, an early discharge within 24–48 hours may be considered for non-primigravida mothers with a history of successful breastfeeding.

The following criteria should be met in all the neonates before discharge planning:

- The routine formal examination of the newborn has been performed and documented.
- The newborn has received the immunization as per schedule.
- The newborn has undergone screening as per unit protocols, e.g. critical heart diseases, hearing defects, eye abnormalities, and congenital hypothyroidism.

- The mother is confident and trained to take care of the neonate.
- The newborn is not having any significant jaundice or other illness requiring close observation by a health provider.
- The newborn is breastfeeding adequately. The adequacy of feeds can be determined by
  - Passage of urine 6–8 times every 24 hours
  - Neonate sleeping well for 2–3 hours after feeds
  - There is no excessive weight loss (usually, neonates do not lose more than 8–10% in the initial 3–4 days)
- The mother has been counseled regarding routine newborn care, and her queries are answered.
- Neonates should have a follow up visit at 48 hours of discharge if discharged before 48 hours or if there was feeding or other issues at discharge. Evaluate breastfeeding and jaundice in these neonates
- Follow-up advice should be communicated to the mother of the neonate.

ADVICE ON DISCHARGE: NORMAL NEWBORN

1. **Exclusive breastfeeds:** All mothers should be advised to exclusively breastfeed their neonates until 6 months of age. The short-term and long-term advantages of breast milk should be discussed with the mother to facilitate success.
2. **Vitamin D supplementation:**[13] A daily dose of 400 IU/day has been shown to achieve 25(OH)D levels >50 nmol/L in most breastfed term infants. The supplementation should continue for one year.
3. **Immunization:** The mother should be explained the immunization schedule, and the date of the following vaccination should be mentioned on the discharge card.
4. The follow-up date for the neonates discharged early (within 48 hours) for assessment of jaundice should be communicated to the parents.
5. The danger signs should be documented, and the mother should be educated to recognize the same and report early when they are recognized:[14, 15]
   a. Not feeding well.
   b. History of convulsions.
   c. No spontaneous movement.
   d. Fast breathing (RR >60/min).

e. Severe chest in-drawing.
f. A temperature of more than 37.5°C or below 35.5°C.
g. Any jaundice in the first 24 hr of life OR yellow palms and soles at any age.

Skin-to-skin (STS) Contact at Birth in Term Neonates

- Assess the neonate as per neonatal resuscitation guidelines:
  - The neonates that are delivered vaginally and eligible for Routine Care must receive STS contact with their mother for initial one hr of life.
- Rarely, a neonate in STS contact may show a sign of illness (respiratory distress) or develop some complication (smothering). DO NOT leave the mother and neonate dyad alone. MONITOR them during this period.

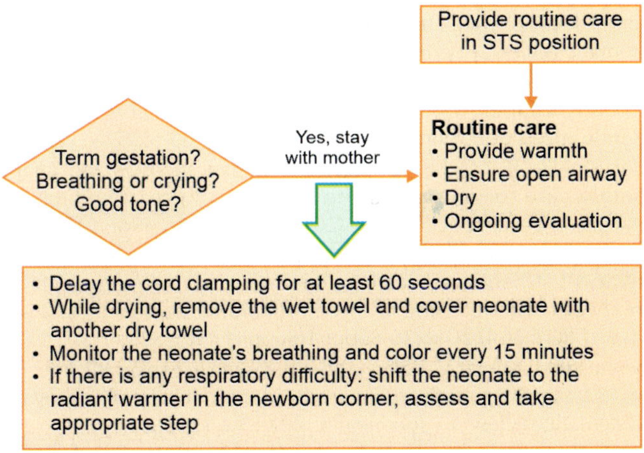

- Continue STS for one hr in the birthing room by putting neonate over chest between the breasts.
- Perform quick examination for obvious malformation.
- Show the neonate to the mother and counsel her.
- Put identity band.
- Initiate breastfeeding.
- Do not leave the mother-neonate dyad alone and monitor breathing and color q 15 minutes.
- If mother has to be shifted to postnatal ward: shift with neonate in STS and continue STS for 1 hour.
- After 1 hour: weigh the neonate and give injection vitamin K and initiate rooming-in.

REFERENCES

1. Thomas D, Anand P, Thukral A, Agarwal R, Deorari A, Sankar MJ. Secular Trends in Birthweights in Two Epochs Over 40 Years in a Tertiary Care Center. Indian Pediatr. 2022;59(8):603–7.
2. Gary M. Weiner, Jeanette Zaichkin. Textbook of Neonatal Resuscitation. 8th edition. United States, American Academy of Pediatrics, 2021.
3. Ramaswamy VV, de Almeida MF, Dawson JA, et al. Maintaining normal temperature immediately after birth in late preterm and term infants: A systematic review and meta-analysis. Resuscitation. 2022;180:81–98.
4. Moore ER, Bergman N, Anderson GC, Medley N. Early skin-to-skin contact for mothers and their healthy newborn infants. Cochrane Database Syst Rev. 2016;11(11): CD003519. Published 2016 Nov 25.
5. McDonald SJ, Middleton P, Dowswell T, Morris PS. Effect of timing of umbilical cord clamping of term infants on maternal and neonatal outcomes. Cochrane Database Syst Rev. 2013;2013(7):CD004074. Published 2013 Jul 11.
6. Sankar MJ, Chandrasekaran A, Kumar P, Thukral A, Agarwal R, Paul VK. Vitamin K prophylaxis for prevention of vitamin K deficiency bleeding: a systematic review. J Perinatol. 2016;36 Suppl 1(Suppl 1):S29-S35.
7. Chawla D, Deorari AK, Saxena R, Paul VK, Agarwal R, Biswas A et al.Vitamin K1 versus Vitamin K3 for prevention of subclinical vitamin deficiency: A Randomized Controlled Trial. Indian Pediatr 2007:22:817–22.
8. Jaafar SH, Ho JJ, Lee KS. Rooming-in for new mothers and infants versus separate care for increasing the duration of breastfeeding. Cochrane Database of Systematic Reviews 2016, Issue 8. Art. No.: CD006641. DOI: 10.1002/14651858.CD006641.pub3.
9. Sankar MJ, Chandrasekaran A, Ravindranath A, Agarwal R, Paul VK. Umbilical cord cleansing with chlorhexidine in neonates: a systematic review. J Perinatol. 2016;36 Suppl 1(Suppl 1):S12-S20.
10. Priyadarshi M, Kumar V, Balachander B, Gupta S, Sankar MJ. Effect of whole-body massage on growth and neurodevelopment in term healthy newborns: A systematic review. J Glob Health. 2022;12:12005.
11. Priyadarshi M, Balachander B, Gupta S, Sankar MJ. Timing of the first bath in term healthy newborns: A systematic review. J Glob Health. 2022;12:12004.
12. Priyadarshi M, Balachander B, Sankar MJ. Effect of sleep position in term healthy newborns on sudden infant death syndrome and other infant outcomes: A systematic review. J Glob Health. 2022;12:12001.
13. Zittermann A, Pilz S, Berthold HK. Serum 25-hydroxyvitamin D response to vitamin D supplementation in infants: a systematic review and meta-analysis of clinical intervention trials. Eur J Nutr. 2020;59(1):359–69.
14. Young Infants Clinical Signs Study Group. Clinical signs that predict severe illness in children under age two months: a multicentre study. Lancet. 2008;371:135–42.
15. World Health Organization, Special Programme of Research, Research Training in Human Reproduction (World Health Organization). WHO recommendations on maternal and newborn care for a positive postnatal experience. World Health Organization; 2022 Mar 29.

CHAPTER

4

Common External Markers

Name of marker	*Background*	*Clinical features*	*Management*
Port wine stain	• Low flow vascular (capillary) malformation. • Constitute 0.3% of cutaneous vascular anomalies • Types Isolated (most common), non-isolated/ syndromic[1]	• Painless, pink or reddish flat well demarcated blanchable patch • Mostly unilateral • Complication: Skin thickening, glaucoma risk, occult neural tube defect (lumbosacral stains) and localized overgrowth	• Diagnosis: clinical, no routine MRI brain in asymptomatic isolated facial stain. • Eye examination for glaucoma • Pulsed dye laser (PDL) therapy to prevent complication and for cosmetic reasons
Hemangioma			
Congenital hemangioma (CH)	• CHs are vascular tumors that fully developed at birth. • Constitute 0.3% of cutaneous vascular anomalies. • Three types: RICH[2] (Rapidly involuting congenital hemangioma)	• Pink or violaceous patch or plaque or exophytic mass with overlying telangiectasias and peripheral halo, present since birth. • RICHs are most common, occur commonly as solitary lesion and majority of them involute by 14 months of age	• Diagnosis: clinical, may consider Doppler USG in suspicious lesions. • Hepatic USG: If large lesion (>5 cm or multiple lesions (>5) • CH: GLUT-1 negative on IHC staining • Treatment: RICH: Daily application of emollients during involution

(Contd.)

(*Contd.*)

Name of marker	*Background*	*Clinical features*	*Management*
	NICH (Non-involuting congenital hemangioma) and partial involuting congenital hemangirma (PICH)	• Complication: Pain, ulceration, bleeding thrombocytopenia, DIC coagulopathy, CCF	• For residual lesion/ complication/ cosmetic reasons: surgically excision or with pulsed dye laser (PDL) • Majority of RICH are self involuting (75%) and have good prognosis
Infantile hemangioma (IH)[3]	• Most common vascular tumor of infancy. • Majority appear after few weeks of birth. • Constitute 4.5% of cutaneous vascular anomalies • Depending upon dermal involvement: Superficial, deep and mixed type • Depending upon risk of complication: Low risk (focal, small and thin superficial) and high risk • IH: GLUT-1 positive on IHC staining	• Premonitory telangiectatic lesion → rapidly proliferate to red colored plaque or papulo-nodular structure and grow over 9–12 months → involutes (majority involute by 4 years of age) • Large facial or lumbosacral segmental associated with PHACE syndrome and LUMBAR syndrome respectively • Complications: Ulceration, bleeding, air ways obstruction, functional impairment, disfigurement, scarring, hepatic	• Diagnosis: clinical, may consider Doppler USG in uncertain lesions. • Hepatic USG: if multiple lesions (>5) present • MRI/MRA: if structural anomalies suspected. • Treatment:, Majority of small/ focal IH do not need treatment. • Inpatient treatment in infants 8 weeks of corrected age. • High risk IH: Early treatment (within 4–6 weeks of age) with propranalol (start 1 mg/kg/day in 1 st wk→weekly Increase→to maximum 2–3 mg/ kg/day for 6–12 months. • Give propranolol with/after feed. Rule out contraindication to

(*Contd.*)

(Contd.)

Name of marker	*Background*	*Clinical features*	*Management*
		involvement, congestive cardiac failure and consumptive hypothyroidism	β blockers. Do pre-drug and post-drug monitoring of HR (±ECG) and BP • Low risk focal IH/ thin superficial IH: 0.5% Timolol 1 drop BD 6–9 months • Other modalities: Steroids (oral prednisolone, intralesional triamcinolone • Residual lesions: Surgery or pulsed dye laser (PDL) • Parental counselling • Lid/facial IH: regular eye follow up
Tuft of hair			
	• Present in >50% of closed spinal dysraphism (CSD)	• Triangular or V-shaped area of hypertrichosis in midline, may be associated with skin appendages, hyperpigmentation or lipoma.	• Early diagnosis of CSD by USG lumbosacral spine, MRI[4] (investigation of choice) • Management involves treatment of underlying CSD
Single umbilical artery (two vessel cord)[5]			
	• Prevalence: 0.3–1% in live births • Types: Isolated (most common) and non-isolated	• Single large UA • Isolated SUA: increased risk of perinatal morbidities and mortality, poly- or oligohydramnios,	• Society for Maternal-Fetal Medicine recommends weekly antenatal fetal surveillance beginning at 36 0/7 weeks of gestation

(Contd.)

(*Contd.*)

Name of marker	*Background*	*Clinical features*	*Management*
	(associated with malformations and aneuploidies (20–36%).)	• low 5 min APGAR, placental (small) and cord abnormalities.	• No routine postnatal renal scan for isolated SUA • Detailed neonatal examination after birth is must.
Preauricular tags (PAT)			
	• Most common benign congenital ear anomaly • Present in about 0.6% of neonates • Types Isolated (most common), nonisolated/ syndromic.	• Mound of skin, subcutaneous fat with or without cartilaginous component • Commonly located anterior to tragus or on helix or cheek.	• Isolated preauricular tags: do not need any treatment. • For cosmetic purpose, these may be excised. • Hearing screening is a must • Postnatal renal scans: Isolated PAT do not need routine renal scan.[6] However, consider it if preauricular sinus or abnormal antenatal scan or dysmorphic features present.

REFERENCES

1. Sabeti S, Ball KL, Bhattacharya SK, Bitrian E, Blieden LS, Brandt JD, Burkhart C, Chugani HT, Falchek SJ, Jain BG, Juhasz C, Loeb JA, Luat A, Pinto A, Segal E, Salvin J, Kelly KM. Consensus Statement for the Management and Treatment of Sturge-Weber Syndrome: Neurology, Neuroimaging, and Ophthalmology Recommendations. Pediatr Neurol. 2021;121:59–66.
2. Boon LM, Enjolras O, Mulliken JB. Congenital hemangioma: evidence of accelerated involution. J Pediatr. 1996 Mar;128(3):329–35.
3. Krowchuk DP, Frieden IJ, Mancini AJ, Darrow DH, Blei F, Greene AK, Annam A, Baker CN, Frommelt PC, Hodak A, Pate BM, Pelletier JL, Sandrock D, Weinberg ST, Whelan MA; Subcommittee on the Management of Infantile

Hemangiomas. Clinical Practice Guideline for the Management of Infantile Hemangiomas. Pediatrics. 2019 ;143:e20183475.
4. Sewell MJ, Chiu YE, Drolet BA. Neural tube dysraphism: review of cutaneous markers and imaging. Pediatr Dermatol. 2015 Mar-Apr;32(2):161–70.
5. Ebbing C, Kessler J, Moster D, Rasmussen S. Isolated single umbilical artery and the risk of adverse perinatal outcome and third stage of labor complications: A population-based study. Acta Obstet Gynecol Scand. 2020;99:374–80.
6. Kugelman A, Tubi A, Bader D, Chemo M, Dabbah H. Pre-auricular tags and pits in the newborn: the role of renal ultrasonography. J Pediatr. 2002;141:388–91.

CHAPTER

5

Thermal Management

Despite being homeothermic, environmental temperatures can easily overwhelm a newborn's ability to maintain body temperature. Thermal protection of the newborn is a set of continuing measures, which starts at birth, to ensure that the neonate maintains a normal body temperature (Table 5.1).[1]

THERMONEUTRAL ENVIRONMENT

Thermoneutral environment (TNE) refers to a narrow environmental temperature range at which the neonate has a minimum basal metabolic rate (BMR) and maintains normal body temperature. NE varies by gestation and postnatal age (Table 5.2). The infants, therefore, should be kept in TNE so that their energy is utilized

Table 5.1: Temperature ranges

Normal axillary temperature	36.5–37.5°C
Mild hypothermia or cold stress	36–36.4°C
Moderate hypothermia	32–35.9°C
Severe hypothermia	<32°C
Hyperthermia	>37.5°C

Table 5.2: Thermoneutral zone[2]

Weight of the neonate	*Recommended ambient temperature*			
	35°C	*34°C*	*33°C*	*32°C*
<1500 g	1–10 days old	11 days to 3 weeks	3–5 weeks	>5 weeks
1500–1999 g		1–10 days	11 days to 4 weeks	>4 weeks
2000–2499 g		1–2 days old	3 days to 3 weeks	>3 weeks
≥2500 g			1–2 days old	≥3 days old

for growth and other vital functions. As opposed to TNE, thermoregulatory environment (TRE) refers to environmental temperature beyond TNE range, at which the neonate increases its BMR to maintain normal body temperature.

RECORDING TEMPERATURE

The following minimum schedule for taking the temperature of the newborn is recommended:

1. Immediately after completion of initial care of the newborn
2. Arrival in the nursery or postnatal ward.
3. For healthy neonates with their mothers, no further routine measurement is required.

Having identified that an infant is at risk, appropriate nursing measures should be taken immediately. However, it should be explained to the mother that the temperature should be checked if the neonate's feet feel cold. Temperature should be monitored every 1–2 hours for a sick neonate, twice daily for neonates weighing 1500–2499 g, and four times daily for neonates below 1500 g.

Methods of Recording Temperature

Touch Method

Abdominal skin, hands, and feet are touched with the back of the health provider's hand to note the warmth. Abdominal temperature is representative of the core temperature. The interpretation is as follows:

- Neonate's feet and hands are warm: Thermal comfort
- Hands and feet are cold, but the abdomen is warm: Cold stress
- Hands and feet, as well as the abdomen, are cold: Hypothermia

Thermometers

WHO recommends using a low-reading thermometer that can record up to 30°C. The American Academy of Pediatrics (AAP) recommends against using mercury thermometers, given the poisonous nature of mercury.[3] It is best to use a digital thermometer.

Thermister Probe

Skin temperature can be recorded by a thermister probe (available in radiant warmer and incubator). The probe is attached to the skin over the upper abdomen.

Concept of Warm Chain

The warm chain is a set of ten interlinked steps carried out at birth and later, which reduce the chances of hypothermia in newborns:

1. **Thermal care in the delivery room:** After birth, the newborn's temperature can drop at 0.1°C and 0.3°C per minute for core and skin, respectively. The delivery room should be clean, warm (at least 25–28°C), and free from air drafts from open windows, doors, and fans.

   If the room temperature is less than the desired, a room heater should be used to warm the room. The radiant warmer should be switched on in advance (at least 20–30 mins) and put on manual mode with 100% heater output. All the linen (towels, blankets, caps, and neonates' clothes) should be pre-warmed.
2. **Warm resuscitation:** The neonate should be resuscitated using warm supplies, equipment, and drugs. Cold items should be avoided from coming in contact with the neonate.
3. **Immediate drying:** After birth, the neonate should be immediately dried with a dry and warm towel, starting with the head. After drying thoroughly, the neonate should be covered with another dry and warm towel, and the head should be covered with a warm cap.
4. **Skin-to-skin contact:** An otherwise healthy neonate should be kept in skin-to-skin (STS) contact with the mother immediately after delivery.[4] In contrast, the mother is being attended to for placental delivery, episiotomy suturing, and during postnatal ward transfer for a few hours. If the neonate develops cold stress, he should be immediately placed in STS contact with his mother.

Early Skin-to-skin contact: What is the evidence?
A Cochrane review has shown that early skin to skin contact started soon after birth until the end of first breastfeeding improved breastfeeding rates and duration. In addition, neonates have better cardiorespiratory stability and higher blood glucose levels.[4]

5. **Breastfeeding:** Breastfeeding should begin as soon as possible after birth, preferably within an hour. This ensures an adequate supply of energy sources.
6. **Postpone bathing /weighing:** Bathing should be postponed in all neonates until stable enough (ideally, it should be given

at home after discharge. For neonates <2 kg, it should be given once the neonate attains a weight of 2 kg). Weighing should be done after covering the neonate adequately and making zero corrections for clothing.

7. **Appropriate clothing:** Newborns should be covered with 1–2 layers of clothes, and caps, socks, and mittens are provided.
8. **Mother and neonate together (bedding in):** The mother and the neonate should be nursed on the same bed for thermal protection and breastfeeding.
9. **Warm transportation:** Thermal protection should be ensured in transport-home or another hospital/ward. Stable neonates can be transported in the STS position, including preterm and low birth weight. Sick and small (VLBW) neonates should be transported using an incubator. The temperature should be checked before and after transport. All peripheral hospitals caring for high-risk mothers should undergo in-utero transfer as early as possible.
10. **Training and awareness:** All the healthcare personnel involved in newborn care should be adequately trained and informed about the principles of the warm chain.

THERMAL MANAGEMENT IN PRETERM NEONATES

Apart from the routine measures, extra care is required for preterm neonates:

Polythene occlusive wraps: NRP 2015 recommends using polythene wraps and thermal mattresses for all neonates <32 weeks. This technique involves covering the neonate in a food grade polyethylene bag or wrap just after birth (without drying). The neonate is then placed on a radiant warmer for resuscitation as required. Wrapping reduces evaporative heat loss while allowing radiant heat delivery to the neonate.[5]

Polythene occlusive wraps: What is the evidence?

A Cochrane review has confirmed the efficacy of plastic bags in addition to radiant warming in improving the NICU admission temperature of premature neonates <28 weeks gestation.[6]

All preterm neonates <34 weeks should be nursed in a radiant warmer/incubator. When transferred to an open cot/mother, the preterm neonates provide kangaroo mother care.

Incubators: Incubators are preferred over radiant warmer for the care of preterm neonates <32 weeks.[7] Incubators ensure better thermal protection than radiant warmer in these neonates by decreasing the insensible water loss (IWL) and convective heat losses. Radiant warmers, in contrast, increase the IWL in such infants.

a. **Mechanisms:** The modern incubator incorporates a transparent plastic hood with various access ports. A warming device is positioned below the bed surface, and the air is blown over the heater. The warm air is circulated using a quiet fan to attain a uniform temperature within the hood. A low rate of air circulation, ideally not more than 20–30 L/min, minimizes convective heat losses. The noise level should be kept below 60 dB. Double-wall incubators, which have an additional wall, had the advantage of decreasing the irradiative heat loss from the neonate compared to single-wall incubators.[8]

b. **Practical tips**
   - In air mode, the desired environment temperature around the neonate is set, and the heater output adjusts itself to maintain this. The appropriate set temperature is decided by using the thermoneutral temperature charts
   - In servo mode, the desired skin temperature is 36.5–36.8°C. The feedback system modifies heater output to keep the neonate's temperature constant
   - The temperature probe should be positioned appropriately. Dislodgement of the probe can overheat the neonate. For sick neonates, servo mode is preferred as it minimizes the temperature fluctuations in the neonate.
   - Air mode is preferred for procedures and when the incubator's door is opened. When switching to air mode, set the air temperature equal to the average incubator air temperature in servo mode.

c. **Humidification:** Humidity (80%) can be started in neonates <28 weeks gestation for the initial seven days, followed by weaning by 5% each day for the next seven days.[9] It minimizes insensible water losses and helps in better thermal protection and fluid management. The humidification chamber should be filled with sterile water, cleaned, and dried daily. There is an increased risk of sepsis (particularly *Pseudomonas*) with humidity.[9]

Radiant warmers: Radiant warmer (RW) is a convenient 'open care' system for managing preterm neonates >32 weeks. It allows easy access to neonates for procedures and monitoring but has the disadvantage of increasing the insensible water losses. Maintenance and cost of RW are low.

a. **Principle:** The radiant warmers produce heat using a quartz crystal heating element. The heat is uniformly reflected onto the surface of the neonate by parabolic reflectors.
b. **Modes:** The Servo mode of control is preferred over the manual mode. Servo control modulates heater output based on skin temperature in real-time. Set the skin temperature at 36.5–36.8°C. The room temperature should be around 25°C for the optimum functioning of RW. A sick neonate can be provided with a cap, socks, and mitten, keeping the chest and abdomen area bare for easy observation. Stable neonates can be covered except the face with appropriate clothing while the neonate is under RW.

   Manual mode allows the operator to determine the heater output. It is used during resuscitation, for rapid re-warming of a hypothermic neonate, and if the neonate has a fever (to prevent frequent alarms). It is not routinely used because of the risk of overheating or hypothermia.
c. **Practical tips**
   - If on manual mode, the neonate's temperature should be checked frequently (every 15 minutes).
   - There should not be more than one neonate under an RW, as this may allow cross-infection and unequal heat distribution.
   - For small neonates cared in RW, cling wraps mode of polythene sheets can be used for covering the bassinet, which will help in reducing the insensible water loss

Hybrid incubators:[10] Advanced neonatal incubators combine two warming modes: the incubator and the radiant warmer. In the incubator mode, movable plastic walls enclose the infant. In contrast, in the warmer mode, these walls drop down, and the radiant warmer rise overhead on a motorized pylon which maintains the temperature of the neonate during procedures. They provide the benefits of a humidifier system and easy accessibility to the neonate during care procedures.

Kangaroo mother care: KMC is an effective way of keeping neonates warm. KMC is no-cost, accessible, and applicable at home, with multiple advantages (*see* Chapter 52: Kangaroo Mother Care).

Heated water-filled mattress: It is an economical but unsafe device for keeping LBW/sick neonates. Generally, they are of five liters of water capacity. An electric heating plate and control unit fit into a compartment in the bottom of the mattress, keeping the water temperature at 35–38°C. This is not routinely used because of practical difficulties.

PCM devices: It consists of a sealed pouch containing phase-changing material. These can maintain the neonate's temperature for 4–6 hours. These devices require large-scale validation for their efficacy and practical difficulties.

HYPOTHERMIA

The World Health Organization (WHO) defines neonatal hypothermia as an axillary temperature below 36.5°C (97.7°F) among newborns below 28 days. The prevalence rates of hypothermia range from 32 to 85% in hospital settings of developing countries.[12]

Clinical Presentation of Hypothermia

Signs of hypothermia are usually absent or nonspecific in neonates. It can be discussed under the four different situations

a. Early signs of hypothermia are because of peripheral vasoconstriction, including pallor, acrocyanosis, cool extremities, and decreased peripheral perfusion. There can be irritability.
b. Late signs include features of CNS depression like lethargy, bradycardia, apnea, poor feeding, hypotonia, weak suck or cry, and emesis. There may be respiratory distress because of increased pulmonary artery pressure. Abdominal signs like increased gastric residuals, abdominal distention, or emesis can occur.
c. Prolonged hypothermia leads to increased metabolism leading to hypoglycemia, hypoxia, metabolic acidosis, coagulation failure, and sometimes persistent pulmonary hypertension in newborns. ARF, in extreme cases, carries a high mortality.
d. Chronic periods of cold stress lead to weight loss and poor weight gain.

Important: Hypothermia may be a sign of infection in neonates.

Management

Management of a hypothermic neonate depends on the degree of hypothermia. The management algorithm is elaborated in Flowchart 5.1.

Outcome

Neonatal hypothermia is an independent predictor of neonatal mortality across all gestational ages. In addition, hypothermia in

Flowchart 5.1: Management of hypothermic neonate

Newborn with symptoms/signs of hypothermia

↓

Measure axillary temperature*

↓

Temperature 36–36.4°C **Cold stress**	Temperature 32–35.9°C **Moderate hypothermia**	Temperature <32°C **Severe Hypothermia**
• Cover the neonate adequately with warm clothes; remove cold/wet clothes • Warm the environment including room/ bed • Ensure STS contact with mother. • Breastfeeding	• Provide extra-heat by room heater, applying warm towel or using phase changing mattresses • Rewarm in an incubator or radiant warmer, if available. • Maintain STS contact with mother • Warm room/bed • Take measures to reduce heat loss	• Immediately admit • Rapid rewarming using a radiant warmer or incubator until 34°C followed by slow rewarming to 36.5°C • Take all measures to reduce heat loss • Start IVF at 60–80 mL/kg of 10% dextrose. • Monitor blood glucose. • Possible oxygen if needed • Give Inj vitamin K 1 mg to term and 0.5 mg in preterm neonates. • If not improving, consider sepsis

*In all cases, monitor the axillary temperature every 0.5–1 hours till it reaches 36.5°C, then hourly for the next 4 hours, two hourly for 12 hours after that.

very low birth weight neonates has been associated with an increased risk of intraventricular hemorrhage, bronchopulmonary dysplasia, neonatal sepsis, and retinopathy of prematurity.[11]

HYPERTHERMIA

Hyperthermia is also a common problem with neonates. It is common in dry and warm areas. A temperature of more than 37.5°C is defined as hyperthermia in newborns.

Causes

- Too hot environment
- The neonate has too much of clothes
- Dehydration
- Sepsis—especially in term neonates

Symptoms

Early: Irritable, tachycardia, tachypnea, flushed face, hot and dry kin
Late: Apathy, lethargy, and coma
Severe hyperthermia can lead to shock, convulsions, and even death.

Management

Place the neonate in a normal environment (25–28°C) away from the heat source. Undress the neonate partially/fully. Give frequent breastfeeding or expressed breast milk by *katori* spoon. The neonate can be sponged with tap water if the temperature is >39. Measure the temperature hourly till it becomes normal. Evaluate for underlying cause if there is no response.

REFERENCES

1. World Health Organization. Maternal and Newborn Health/Safe Motherhood. (1997). Thermal protection of the newborn: a practical guide.
2. Hey E. Thermal neutrality. Br Med Bull. 1975 Jan;31(1):69–74.
3. American Academy of Pediatrics, Altmann TR, Hill DL. Caring for Your Baby and Young Child: Birth to Age 5. American Academy of Pediatrics; 2019.
4. Moore ER, Bergman N, Anderson GC, Medley N. Early skin-to-skin contact for mothers and their healthy newborn infants. Cochrane Database Syst Rev. 2016 Nov 25;11(11):CD003519.
5. Weiner GM, Zaichkin J, Kattwinkel J, American Academy of Pediatrics, American Heart Association, editors. Textbook of neonatal resuscitation. 7th edition. Elk Grove Village, IL: American Academy of Pediatrics; 2016.
6. McCall EM, Alderdice F, Halliday HL, Jenkins JG, Vohra S. Interventions to prevent hypothermia at birth in preterm and/or low birth weight infants. Cochrane Database Syst Rev. 2010 Mar 17;(3):CD004210.
7. Flenady V, Woodgate PG. Radiant warmers versus incubators for regulating body temperature in newborn infants. Cochrane Database of Systematic Reviews 2003, Issue 4. Art. No.:CD000435.
8. Laroia N, Phelps D, Roy J. Double wall versus single wall incubator for reducing heat loss in low birth weight infants in incubators. Cochrane Database of Systematic Reviews 2007, Issue 2. Art. No.:CD004215.
9. Harpin VA, Rutter N. Humidification of incubators. Arch Dis Child. 1985 Mar;60(3):219–24.
10. Gleason CA, Juul SE, editors. Avery's diseases of the newborn. Tenth edition. Philadelphia, PA: Elsevier; 2018. 1627 p.
11. Lunze K, Bloom DE, Jamison DT, Hamer DH. The global burden of neonatal hypothermia: a systematic review of a major challenge for newborn survival. BMC Med. 2013 Jan 31;11:24.

CHAPTER

6

Golden-hour Management of High-risk Newborn

'Golden-hour' (first 60 minutes of life) management refers to implementing evidence-based practices focused resuscitation, and stabilization at birth and within the first hour of life. Specific interventions include thermal protection, gentle ventilation, avoidance of hyperoxia, timely administration of surfactant, and early initiation of nutrition. Team performance and communication form the backbone of golden-hour care.

BEFORE DELIVERY

Organizing a team: Preterm neonates, particularly those born before 32 weeks' gestation, may need resuscitation at birth. A team of 3–4 members, including a neonatologist or senior neonatal fellow, one or two pediatric residents, and a nurse, should always be ready for resuscitation and management during golden hour. The roles and responsibilities of team members should be assigned, and equipment should be pre-arranged using a checklist.

Parental counseling: Parents confronted with delivering a preterm neonate experience anxiety and fear. Antenatal counseling is best done by a team comprising both neonatologists and obstetricians. The physician should provide information on survival and anticipated morbidity relevant to the gestational age in simple terms. The use of a written template and decision aids for counseling is recommended. The morbidity statistics of extremely low birth weight (ELBW) infants from a birth cohort of 2013–2018 delivered at AIIMS are given in Table 6.1.[1]

Decision-making at limits of viability: Gestational age of the fetus is an essential determinant of viability and influences major interventions at birth. Hence, every effort should be made to confirm the exact gestational age based on LMP (last menstrual period) and

Table 6.1: Morbidity statistics for extremely low-birth-weight neonates delivered in AIIMS, New Delhi, between 2013 and 2018

Morbidity	*Risk*
Respiratory distress syndrome	80%
Bronchopulmonary dysplasia (any severity)	40%
Severe intraventricular hemorrhage	20%
Patent ductus arteriosus requiring treatment	30%
Major neurodevelopmental impairment (cerebral palsy, motor or mental developmental quotient <70 on DASII, visual or hearing impairment, or epilepsy) at 18 months corrected age	<28 weeks; 40% <1000 g; 30%

first-trimester ultrasound. Other factors that positively influence the neonatal outcome at peri-viable gestation include; female sex, singleton gestation, not being SGA, exposure to antenatal steroids, absence of perinatal complications like chorioamnionitis, and being born in a tertiary care center.[2]

India has no national guidelines regarding resuscitation at limits of viability. The survival of neonates 25 weeks' gestation is uniformly good across various developed countries[3,4] and therefore full resuscitation is recommended. If the gestation is between 24^{+0} and 24^{+6} weeks (gray zone), resuscitation depends on shared decision-making with parents.[5] Our center offers comfort care for neonates with gestation 23 weeks. Although survival of neonates less than 500 grams is less, decision-making should not solely rely on birth weight alone as viable neonates with intrauterine growth restriction can have birth weights less than 500 grams.

One should never forget the inaccuracies associated with gestational age and birth weight estimations, with first-trimester dating ultrasound variation of ±7 days and estimates of fetal weight variation of ±15%. Thus, in many situations, the clinician should continually reassess the neonate's response to resuscitative efforts. For example, if a neonate born at 24 weeks' gestation is severely compromised at birth, redirection to comfort care after provisional NICU admission can be made. If the neonate is vigorous at birth or responds well to initial resuscitation, active management with ongoing evaluation after admission to NICU is advised.

Antenatal steroids: A single course of corticosteroids (betamethasone 12 mg, two doses given 24 hours apart, or dexamethasone 6 mg, four doses given 12 hours apart IM) is recommended for pregnant women between 24 and 34 weeks of gestation.[6] Even in periviable gestations (23–26 weeks), antenatal corticosteroids[7] do have a role in decreasing neonatal mortality and IVH and should be used where applicable. A single repeat course of steroids can be given to pregnant women <34 weeks' gestation with an impending preterm delivery within the next seven days and who received an earlier course more than 14 days ago.[8] As even a single dose of antenatal steroid significantly reduces neonatal morbidity and mortality, the first dose should be administered even if the chances of completing an entire course appear unlikely.

Antenatal magnesium sulfate ($MgSO_4$) for neuro-protection: The prevalence of cerebral palsy (CP) in very-low-birth-weight infants is 60 per 1000 infants, and about a third of new CP cases are associated with prematurity before 32 weeks' gestation.[13] Six randomized trials involving 6000 women have shown the neuroprotective benefits of $MgSO_4$ in reducing the risk of CP in preterm infants when provided for pregnant women <32 weeks gestation with imminent preterm birth (preterm birth likely within the next 24 hours) irrespective of the cause of preterm birth or the number of fetuses in-utero.[9] The drug is administered as a 4 g IV loading dose over 30 minutes, followed by a 1 g/hour maintenance infusion until birth. Therapy should be discontinued if delivery does not occur or a maximum infusion period of 24 hours is reached. The treatment is safe for neonates without increased risk of resuscitation at birth. Mothers receiving $MgSO_4$ require monitoring for adverse effects like respiratory depression.

Evidence for antenatal magnesium sulfate[9]

Magnesium sulfate administered to pregnant women at risk of imminent preterm birth reduces the risk of cerebral palsy (RR 0.68; 95% CI 0.54–0.87). It also decreases substantial gross motor dysfunction (inability to walk without assistance) (RR 0.61; 95% CI 0.44–0.85) at two years of age.[10] The benefits were noted regardless of gestational age, cause of birth, or total dose administered.

DURING DELIVERY

Resuscitation and initial stabilization of a preterm neonate during the "golden hour" should follow the Neonatal Resuscitation Program guidelines and requires adequate preparation and teamwork. Preterm neonates are at high risk of hypothermia, and each degree drop in admission temperature is associated with increased odds of mortality by 28% and late-onset sepsis by 11%. Preterm neonates have surfactant deficiency, poor respiratory drive, weak and compliant chest wall, fragile brain capillary network, and higher sensitivity to oxygen-induced free radical damage. Hence specific interventions at birth should focus on (Table 6.2).

Table 6.2: Delivery room management of very preterm neonates

Situation		*Recommendations*
Anticipatory preparation		• Use pre-resuscitation checklist. • Check equipment and organize a team. • Prepare a resuscitation kit. • Call for additional help if necessary.
Delivery room management	Delayed cord clamping	• In uncomplicated preterm birth, delayed cord clamping should be attempted for a minimum time of 30 seconds after delivery.
	Thermore-gulation	• Maintain DR temperature of at least 26°C for all deliveries <32 weeks. Switch off the air conditioner in the DR. • Pre-warm the radiant warmer to 100% heater output for at least 10 minutes before delivery. • Use polythene bags/wraps for all neonates <32 weeks' gestation. Do not dry the neonate. Do not remove the bag until the neonate is transferred to the NICU axnd normal temperature is recorded. • Cover the head with a plastic bag. Use of hat is recommended. • Use a transport incubator to transfer neonates from DR to NICU. Pre-warm the baby boundaries and the transport incubator before use. • Measure axillary temperature within 10 minutes of NICU admission.
	Respiratory management and oxygen targeting	• Neonates are resuscitated as per NRP guidelines. • Spontaneously breathing preterm infants <32 weeks' gestation at high risk of RDS should be supported with CPAP of 5 cm H_2O using T-Piece as soon as respiratory distress is noted. • Infants needing positive pressure ventilation are provided with PIP and PEEP using a T-Piece device. Initial settings on the device are 15/5. If rapid heart rate or chest movement improvement is not obtained, higher pressures to achieve effective ventilation may be used.

(Contd.)

Table 6.2: Delivery room management of very preterm neonates *(Contd.)*

Situation		*Recommendations*
		• Avoid the use of self-inflating bags for delivering PPV in preterm infants <32 weeks to prevent uncontrolled delivery of tidal volume. • Use a pulse oximeter and blended oxygen to target oxygen saturation. • Begin resuscitation with FiO_2 between 21–30% and titrate every minute to target the NRP saturation targets.
	Supportive care	• Maintain a normal body temperature of 36.5–37.5°C. • Start early parenteral nutrition after inserting the central line in ELBW neonates. • Early initiation of enteral feeding with mother's milk. • Titrate oxygen administration by monitoring oxygen saturation using pulse oximetry. Target oxygen saturation should be between 90 and 95%. • Monitor blood pressure and perfusion. • Protocols for pain management and developmentally supportive care.

Evidence

1. Delayed cord clamping in preterm neonates is associated with a 30% reduction in in-hospital mortality, decreased need for transfusions for anemia (RR 0.61, 95% CI 0.46–0.81) and less intraventricular hemorrhage of all grades (RR 0.59, 95% CI 0.41–0.85). Other physiological benefits include better circulatory stability, better lung fluid clearance, increased cardiac output, and better tissue oxygen delivery.[11]
2. Thermoregulation: Plastic wraps applied within 10 minutes of birth to preterm or low-birth-weight neonates improve core body temperature on NICU admission and up to two hours after birth (body temperatures were 0.58°C higher compared to usual thermal care). The incidence of hypothermia was 23% lower (95% CI 0.62–0.72) with the use of plastic bags. The risk of pulmonary hemorrhage was less, but there is insufficient evidence to suggest a reduction in in-hospital mortality or other significant morbidities.[12]
3. Delivery room CPAP: Early CPAP among very preterm neonates (especially those <28 weeks' gestation) as compared to intubation and surfactant administration is associated with a reduction in the incidence of BPD at 36 weeks, (RR 0.89, 95% CI 0.79–0.99), need for mechanical ventilation (RR 0.50, 95% CI 0.42–0.59) and surfactant in the CPAP group (typical RR 0.54, 95% CI 0.40–0.73).[13]

1. Delayed cord clamping
2. Thermoregulation
3. Gentle respiratory support, and
4. Hyperoxia avoidance

Delayed cord clamping: NRP recommends delayed umbilical cord clamping for at least 30 seconds for preterm infants not requiring immediate resuscitation after birth.[16] There are no recommendations regarding delayed cord clamping in a non-vigorous infant, where resuscitative efforts take priority. Performing delayed cord clamping in preterm neonates who require immediate resuscitation at birth is a challenge and future studies are required to investigate the feasibility and safety of resuscitating neonates with an intact cord. Umbilical cord milking in preterm infants is not recommended, as a higher rate of severe intraventricular hemorrhage was noted in the umbilical cord milking group in a large RCT.

Thermoregulation: Prevention of heat loss requires multiple strategies, including increasing the temperature of the delivery room, preheating the radiant warmer, and using food-grade plastic bags or wraps. The neonate should be covered or placed inside the plastic bag without drying, and the head should be covered with a hat to prevent evaporative heat loss. The plastic wrap should be removed only after ensuring a normal axillary temperature in the NICU.

Using an exothermic heat mattress also improves temperature stabilization, but caution is needed when both plastic bags and exothermic mattresses are used simultaneously due to the risk of hyperthermia. Although studies show that plastic bags improve admission temperatures of preterm neonates, there is insufficient evidence that it improves important clinical outcomes like mortality or neurodevelopment.

Monitoring the neonate's temperature in the delivery room and using a pre-warmed transport incubator further reduce heat loss at birth. NRP recommends that the temperature of a neonate be maintained between 36.5°C and 37.5°C from birth till initial stabilization and admission temperature be recorded as a predictor of outcomes and a quality indicator of good resuscitation.

Respiratory support in the delivery room: Respiratory support aims to help establish functional residual capacity (FRC) in the lung to ensure adequate gas exchange. This is facilitated by assisting ventilation in the least invasive manner and providing just the right amount of oxygen.

Devices for respiratory support in the delivery room: The T-piece device delivers peak inspiratory and positive end-expiratory pressure (PEEP) more consistently than a resuscitation bag[21]. Many countries report usage rates of 45–50% in the delivery room. Advantages of the T-piece device include its ease of use and ability to deliver continuous positive airway pressure or PEEP. Its limitations are the need for a pressurized gas source to drive the device, the need to turn the pressure knob to increase the PIP repeatedly, and the possibility of inadvertently delivering higher levels of PEEP.

Setting up the T-piece device: While setting the machine for preterm deliveries <32 weeks, we prefer flow rates of (5–8) lpm and PIP and PEEP of 15 and 5 cm H_2O, respectively. The FiO_2 is set between 21 and 30%. The preferred level of delivery room CPAP is 5 cm H_2O. CPAP level of 8 cm H_2O or above is associated with a high risk of pneumothorax and should be avoided.

After completing the initial steps, a spontaneously breathing neonate with respiratory distress should be offered CPAP than intubation and positive pressure breaths. Early CPAP rather than intubation in the delivery room among neonates <28 weeks' gestation has been shown in meta-analyses to produce a small but clinically significant reduction in the incidence of BPD at 36 weeks' postmenstrual age, the need for mechanical ventilation as well as surfactant.[13] However, positive pressure breaths (PPV) should be delivered *if the neonate is apneic or gasping or if the heart rate is less than 100 bpm*. A trial of PPV should also be considered if oxygen saturation is below the target range despite free flow oxygen and or CPAP in a spontaneously breathing neonate with a heart rate 100 bpm.

Role of sustained inflation (SI): Sustained Inflation refers to the delivery of PIP for a longer duration, typically from 5 to 15 seconds, with pressures varying from 20 to 30 cm H_2O for 1–3 breaths for preterm neonates exhibiting signs of respiratory distress (rescue) at birth. While studies showed short-term benefits with SI, like the reduced need for mechanical ventilation in the first 72 hours of life, there was no effect on the incidence of significant outcomes like BPD or overall mortality. Of note, pressure, time duration, and frequency of SI breaths used differed significantly in various studies, and the interface as well (endotracheal tube, face mask, or nasopharyngeal tube). NRP does not recommend using SI for resuscitation except in individual clinical circumstances or research settings.

Avoidance of hyperoxia: Oxygen blenders capable of delivering titrated oxygen and a pulse oximeter must be available for all high-risk deliveries. The pulse oximeter sensor should first be placed on the right hand or wrist and then connected to the monitor to rapidly acquire the pleth signal. The blender should be set between 21 and 30% and subsequent oxygen administration should be based on the inter-quartile range of saturations targets as described for healthy term neonates.

Initial stabilization in the NICU: Continuing care in the NICU should focus on thermoregulation, respiratory support, and early initiation of nutrition. Spontaneously breathing preterm neonates with respiratory distress are most effectively treated with CPAP until the criteria for surfactant therapy are met. Early (<2 hours) selective surfactant therapy that is given by the "INSURE" approach (INtubation, SURfactant, Extubation) or less invasive surfactant administration (LISA) is preferred. Neonates <32 weeks' gestation are administered caffeine therapy for the treatment of apnea of prematurity or before extubation from mechanical ventilation. Caffeine therapy has been shown in RCT to reduce the risks of both short-term morbidities such as bronchopulmonary dysplasia (BPD) and severe retinopathy of prematurity and long-term neurodevelopmental impairment at 18 months and improve gross motor function at five years.[14] We initiate early caffeine therapy for neonates <28 weeks' gestation, irrespective of their respiratory support. Observational studies have shown that early caffeine initiation (0–3 days of life) is associated with less incidence of BPD, patent ductus arteriosus, and a shorter duration of mechanical ventilation.[15]

Central line insertion and early nutrition: Umbilical venous cannulation is established at birth to initiate intravenous fluids or early parenteral nutrition in neonates <1000 grams (as per unit policy) to get the lines in by 30 minutes of age. The first blood sugar is checked with line insertion and other blood work.

Interventions to minimize stress: At every opportunity, efforts should focus on reducing pain and stress by providing developmentally supportive care. These include noise reduction, gentle handling, coupling procedures, attention to skin care, and early parental participation.

Implementation of quality initiatives to improve outcomes: Several institutions that have implemented a protocolized approach to management in the "golden hour" have demonstrated improved outcomes among preterm neonates like better admission temperature and blood glucose level, a marked decrease in intraventricular hemorrhage, and faster time for umbilical catheter insertion and surfactant administration. QI studies have also demonstrated improved clinical outcomes, such as a reduction in late-onset sepsis and bronchopulmonary dysplasia and a trend toward reduction in early blood transfusion and ventilation duration.[16]

REFERENCES

1. Sahoo T, Anand P, Verma A, et al. The outcome of extremely low birth weight (ELBW) infants from a birth cohort (2013–2018) in a tertiary care unit in North India. J Perinatol. 2020: 40, 743–9.
2. Salihu HM, Salinas-Miranda AA, Hill L, Chandler K. Survival of pre-viable preterm infants in the United States: a systematic review and meta-analysis. Semin Perinatol. 2013;37(6):389–400.
3. Stoll BJ, Hansen NI, Bell EF, et al. Neonatal outcomes of extremely preterm infants from the NICHD Neonatal Research Network. Pediatrics. 2010;126(3):443–56.
4. Fischer N, Steurer MA, Adams M, Berger TM, Swiss Neonatal N. Survival rates of extremely preterm infants (gestational age <26 weeks) in Switzerland: impact of the Swiss guidelines for the care of infants born at the limit of viability. Arch Dis Child Fetal Neonatal Ed. 2009;94(6):F407–13.
5. Berger TM, Bernet V, El Alama S, et al. Perinatal care at the limit of viability between 22 and 26 completed weeks of gestation in Switzerland. 2011 revision of the Swiss recommendations. Swiss Med Wkly. 2011;141:w13280.
6. McGoldrick E, Stewart F, Parker R, Dalziel SR. Antenatal corticosteroids for accelerating fetal lung maturation for women at risk of preterm birth. Cochrane Database Syst Rev. 2020 Dec 25;12(12):CD004454.
7. Wapner RJ. Antenatal corticosteroids for periviable birth. Semin Perinatol. 2013;37(6):410–3.
8. American College of O, Gynecologists' Committee on Obstetric P, Society for Maternal- Fetal M. Committee Opinion No.677: Antenatal Corticosteroid Therapy for Fetal Maturation. Obstet Gynecol. 2016;128(4):e187–94.
9. Wolf HT, Huusom LD, Henriksen TB, Hegaard HK, Brok J, Pinborg A. Magnesium sulphate for fetal neuroprotection at imminent risk for preterm delivery: a systematic review with meta-analysis and trial sequential analysis. BJOG. 2020 Sep;127(10):1180–8.
10. Doyle LW, Crowther CA, Middleton P, Marret S, Rouse D. Magnesium sulphate for women at risk of preterm birth for neuroprotection of the fetus. Cochrane Database Syst Rev. 2009(1):CD004661.

11. Rabe H, Gyte GM, Díaz-Rossello JL, Duley L. Effect of timing of umbilical cord clamping and other strategies to influence placental transfusion at preterm birth on maternal and infant outcomes. Cochrane Database Syst Rev. 2019 Sep 17;9(9):CD003248.10.
12. Jani P, Mishra U, Buchmayer J, Walker K, Gözen D, Maheshwari R, D'Çruz D, Lowe K, Wright A, Marceau J, Culcer M, Priyadarshi A, Kirby A, Moore JE, Oei JL, Shah V, Vaidya U, Khashana A, Godambe S, Cheah FC, Zhou W, Xiaojing H, Satardien M. Thermoregulation and golden hour practices in extremely preterm infants: an international survey. Pediatr Res. 2022 Sep 8:1–9.
13. Subramaniam P, Ho JJ, Davis PG. Prophylactic nasal continuous positive airway pressure for preventing morbidity and mortality in very preterm infants. Cochrane Database Syst Rev. 2016(6):CD001243.
14. Schmidt B, Roberts RS, Davis P, et al. Caffeine therapy for apnea of prematurity. N Engl J Med. 2006;354(20):2112–21.
15. Patel RM, Leong T, Carlton DP, Vyas-Read S. Early caffeine therapy and clinical outcomes in extremely preterm infants. J Perinatol. 2013;33(2):134–40.
16. Croop SEW, Thoyre SM, Aliaga S, McCaffrey MJ, Peter-Wohl S. The Golden Hour: a quality improvement initiative for extremely premature infants in the neonatal intensive care unit. J Perinatol. 2020 Mar;40(3):530–9.

CHAPTER

7

Birth Injury

Birth injury or trauma is a loss of the neonate's body structure or function due to adverse events during the birth process.[1] This consists of a broad range of major to minor injuries due to mechanical forces during labor or cesarean sections. Injuries caused by intrauterine diagnostic and therapeutic interventions like Intra-uterine transfusion and amniocentesis are not considered birth injuries.

A neonate with risk factors for birth injury or trauma should be thoroughly examined, including a complete neurological examination. Most birth injuries recover spontaneously without permanent sequelae. The various common birth injuries and their risk factors and subsequent complications are shown in Table 7.1.

Table 7.1: Common birth injuries, risk factors, and associated complications

S.no.	*Birth Injury*	*Risk factors*	*Complications*	*Prognosis*
		Head and Neck Injury		
1.	Cephalhematoma/ Sub-galeal hemorrhage	Forceps; Vacuum extraction; Macrosomia; Precipitous delivery	Prolonged jaundice; Hypotension due to blood loss (subgaleal bleed); Anemia; Secondary infection.	• Cephalhematoma usually resolves within 4–6 weeks. • Subgaleal bleed: Monitor for hypovolemia.
2.	Skull fracture (Linear and depressed)	Vacuum extraction; Forceps application (Parietal or Frontal bone);	Associated Intracranial bleeds (Subdural or Sub-arachnoid);	• A depressed fracture usually requires neurosurgical intervention.

(Contd.)

Table 7.1: Common birth injuries, risk factors, and associated complications (*Contd.*)

		Breech delivery (Occipital bone)	Leptomeningeal cyst following dural tear	
3.	Sternocleido-mastoid (SCM) injury (Sternocleido-mastoid tumor)	Abnormal intrauterine positioning leads to rupture of muscle fibers with subsequent development of hematoma, then fibrosis followed by shortening	Torticollis with a head tilt towards the injury site; Developmental dysplasia of the hip (DDH) is also associated in 10% of cases	• Stretching exercises of the affected muscle may lead to recovery within 3–4 months in around 80% of cases. • Persistent deformity may require surgery or Botulinum toxin.
		Nerve injury		
4	Facial nerve injury	Forceps application; Uterine fibroids	Most common cranial nerve injury. Peripheral facial nerve palsy (Lower motor neuron type) involving the entire ipsilateral facial side is more common.	Excellent recovery occurs by three weeks of age in almost all cases.
		Brachial plexus injury		
	1. Duchenne–Erb palsy (C5, C6 nerve root injury with occasional C7 involvement): 90% cases	Macrosomia; Malpresentation; Shoulder dystocia; Forceps or vacuum application	1. Weakness in shoulder abduction, elbow flexion, and external rotation leading to	• Duchenne–Erb palsy with intact grasp reflex has a good spontaneous recovery in 80% of cases.

(*Contd.*)

Table 7.1: Common birth injuries, risk factors, and associated complications (*Contd.*)

	2. Total brachial plexus injury (C5, C6, C7, C8, T1 nerve root injury): 10% cases 3. Klumpke's Palsy (C7, C8 T1 nerve root injury): very rare		a "Waiter's Tip" posture. The grasp is usually intact. 2. Extensive flaccid paralysis of the entire arm with absent grasp reflex 3. Weakness of hand and wrist muscles with Horner syndrome	• Total brachial palsy has a poor outcome, with recovery in 30–50% of cases.
		Bone injury		
5.	Clavicle fracture: Most commonly injured bone during delivery	Macrosomia; Shoulder dystocia; Breech presentation	Pseudoparalysis of the affected arm with asymmetric Moro's reflex	Complete healing occurs in most cases with proper splinting
6.	Long bone fractures: a. Humerus b. Femur	1. Humerus fracture: Breech presentation; Obstructed labor 2. Femur fracture: Breech presentation	1. Swelling and pseudoparalysis of the affected arm 2. Swelling and pseudoparalysis of the affected leg	• Recovery is usually good after closed reduction and casting for two weeks. • Recovery is good without limb shortening after splinting with hip-spica cast.

REFERENCE

1. Dumpa V, Kamity R. Birth Trauma. 2022 Aug 29. In: StatPearls [Internet]. Treasure Island (FL): StatPearls Publishing; 2023 Jan. PMID: 30969653.

Section

3

Central Nervous System

CHAPTER

8

Post-resuscitation Management of Asphyxiated Neonates

Perinatal asphyxia (PA) is a major cause of neonatal and under-5 mortality, particularly in developing countries. As per the latest estimates, PA accounts for 9.4% (i.e. 0.72 millions) of total under-5 child mortality worldwide. Along with prematurity and systemic infections, PA is one of the three most common causes of neonatal deaths.[1] It is also an important cause of stillbirths—of the total 2.7 million stillbirths that occur globally, about 1.2 million occur during the intrapartum period, largely due to asphyxia.[2] The National Neonatal Perinatal Database (NNPD; 2002–2003) reported PA to be the most common cause of stillbirths, accounting for 45.1% of all such cases.[4] Almost all (98.2%) asphyxia related deaths occur in first week of life, with 73% of asphyxia related deaths occurring within 24 hours of birth.[3] Therefore, providing adequate post-resuscitation care is essential to reduce neonatal and child mortality.

INCIDENCE

As per the NNPD (2002–2003), the incidence of PA—defined as Apgar score of <7 at 1 minute of life—was 8.4% of all live births.[5] Oxygen was the most commonly used resuscitative measure in 9.5%, bag and mask ventilation in 6.3%, chest compressions in 0.8%, and use of medications in 0.5%. PA was responsible for 28.8% of all neonatal deaths. Manifestations of hypoxic–ischemic encephalopathy (HIE) were seen in approximately 1.4% of live births. Asphyxia is also responsible for lifelong neuromotor disability in a large number of children.

DEFINITIONS

The terms used to evaluate a newborn with brain damage are as follows:

1. **Perinatal hypoxia, ischemia, and asphyxia:** Hypoxia refers to lower oxygen levels, ischemia to decreased blood flow, and asphyxia to decreased gas exchange in the fetus or newborn.

Table 8.1: Definitions of perinatal asphyxia	
	Definition
World Health Oragnization[6]	Failure to initiate and sustain breathing.
NNPD Network[5]	• **Moderate PA:** Slow/gasping breathing or an Apgar score of 4–6 at 1 minute of age. • **Severe PA:** No breathing or an Apgar score of 0–3 at 1 minute of age.
American Academy of Pediatrics and American College of Obstetrics and Gynecology[7]	Presence of all of following criteria: • Profound metabolic or mixed acidemia (pH <7.0) in umbilical cord blood. • Persistence of low Apgar scores less than 3 for more than 5 minutes. • Signs of neonatal neurologic dysfunction (e.g. seizures, encephalopathy, tone abnormalities). • Evidence of multiple organ involvement (such as that of kidneys, lungs, liver, heart and intestine).

2. **Perinatal/neonatal depression:** This term refers to the physical state of a newborn within the first hour of life following birth and is unrelated to the newborn's prenatal and postnatal conditions. It describes the clinical state of newborns, such as hypotonia, poor mental status, and/or cardiovascular and respiratory disturbances.
3. **Neonatal encephalopathy:** It is the clinical term for abnormal mental state, level of consciousness, brain stem damage, and motor dysfunction. It need not always be irreversible; it could also result from reversible causes such as maternal medicines, hypoglycemia, or medications given during cesarean section under general anesthesia.
4. **Hypoxic–ischemic encephalopathy (HIE):** This term refers to the objective proof that hypoxia and ischemia are causing the clinical characteristics of encephalopathy that were previously defined.

There is no single, well-accepted definition of PA (Table 8.1). The definition is context specific and can be sensitive (e.g. those given by WHO and NNPD for the purpose of deciding immediate care of newborn) or specific (such as the one given by AAP for the purpose of giving a label or predicting the long-term outcome).

Consequences of Asphyxia

PA is a multi-organ-system disorder affecting virtually every organ-system in the body including brain, heart, lungs, kidneys and intestine. Care of asphyxiated infant therefore should be oriented towards determining the severity of dysfunction of critical organ systems and provide appropriate support to allow recovery to happen. Many of these complications are potentially fatal. In term infants with asphyxia, renal, CNS, cardiac and lung dysfunction occur in 50%, 28%, 25% and 25% cases, respectively.[8] The extent of organ system dysfunction determines the early outcome of an asphyxiated neonate (Table 8.2).

Hypoxic ischemic encephalopathy (HIE) is often the prime concern while managing asphyxiated neonates because it is not only associated with high risk of mortality but also carries a significant risk of serious long-term neuromotor sequelae among survivors.

A detailed classification of HIE in term neonates was proposed by Sarnat and Sarnat.[9] A simpler and practical classification of HIE by severity of manifestations provided by Levene is recommended for routine use (Table 8.3).[10] Recent addition to this list is the Thompson score, which is based on features of HIE and has a maximum (worst) score of 22. A score of 15 or more has shown a positive predictive

Table 8.2: Organ system dysfunction in perinatal asphyxia

CNS	Hypoxic–ischemic encephalopathy, intracranial hemorrhage, seizures, long-term neurological sequelae
Cardiac	Myocardial dysfunction, valvular dysfunction, rhythm abnormalities, congestive cardiac failure
Renal	Hematuria, acute tubular necrosis, renal vein thrombosis
Pulmonary	Delayed adaptation, respiratory failure, meconium aspiration, surfactant depletion, primary pulmonary hypertension
GI tract	Necrotizing enterocolitis, hepatic dysfunction
Hematological	Thrombocytopenia, coagulation abnormalities
Metabolic	Acidosis, hypoglycemia, hypocalcemia, hyponatremia

Table 8.3: Classification of HIE (Levene)

Features	*Mild*	*Moderate*	*Severe*
Consciousness	Irritable	Lethargy	Comatose
Tone	Hypotonia	Marked hypotonia	Severe hypotonia
Seizures	No	Yes	Prolonged
Sucking/ respiration	Poor suck	Unable to suck	Unable to sustain spontaneous respiration

value of 92%, negative predictive value of 82%, sensitivity of 71% and specificity of 96% for abnormal outcome at 12 months of age.[11]

Evolution of HIE Changes

HIE evolves gradually beginning from the time of insult to hours and days later (Table 8.4). The initial hypoxic–ischemic event results in infarction of the brain tissue (primary energy failure). The subsequent injury–secondary injury–is mediated by reperfusion and free radicals in an area surrounding the necrotic area (penumbra). The penumbra undergoes a programmed neuronal death (apoptosis) even after the hypoxic insult is over. The time gap between these two phases could be 6–24 hours and provides a window to institute specific therapeutic intervention.

MANAGEMENT OF A NEONATE WITH PERINATAL ASPHYXIA

Management of asphyxiated neonates is mainly supportive and involves maintaining optimum oxygenation, ventilation, perfusion, metabolic milieu and control of seizures.

Table 8.4: Clinical features of severe HIE and the timeframe

Time frame	*Clinical features*
Birth to 12 hours	• Decreased alertness and tone • Convulsions • Periodic breathing or respiratory failure • Intact pupillary and oculomotor responses
12–24 hours	• Change in alertness level • Apneic spells • Increase in convulsions • Jitteriness • Weakness in proximal limbs • In term neonates, upper limbs more involved than lower limbs; in preterm, lower limbs more involved
24–72 hours	• Further decrease in alertness • Pupillary and oculomotor disturbances • Respiratory arrest • In preterm neonates, intraventricular hemorrhage and periventricular hemorrhagic infarction
After 72 hours	• Persistent and diminishing stupor • Abnormal sucking, swallowing, gag and tongue movements • Hypotonia more common than hypertonia • Weakness in proximal limbs

Delivery Room Care

- For neonates born at term and near term (35 weeks) gestation, resuscitation should start with 21% oxygen.
- For preterm neonates born at less than 35 weeks of gestation, resuscitation should start with 21–30% oxygen; further oxygen concentration should be titrated to achieve target saturations.[12]
- For non-vigorous neonates born through meconium-stained amniotic fluid, the 2015 Neonatal Resuscitation Program (NRP) does not recommend routine intubation for suctioning of meconium, citing more harm due to intubation along with delay in providing adequate ventilation.[12]
- Obtain arterial cord blood for analysis: After cutting the cord, apply additional clamp on umbilical cord on placental side keeping a cord segment of 10–15 cm between two clamps.
- Take a heparinized syringe and puncture the cord (clamped segment, once placenta is out and resuscitation is over) to take blood sample from umbilical artery.

Presence of metabolic acidosis (pH <7.00 and base deficit greater than 16 mmol/L) indicates relatively long-standing asphyxia (many minutes to hours), while presence of respiratory acidosis in absence of metabolic acidosis indicates presence of acute asphyxia (minutes) as in cord prolapse, acute abruption of placenta, etc.

Cord blood gas in asphyxia: what is the evidence?

A recent meta-analysis has shown a good association of cord ABG abnormalities (pH<7.0 and base deficit ≥16 mmol/l) with short-term (mortality, HIE, IVH or PVL) and long-term adverse outcomes (cerebral palsy).[13]

NICU Care

Transfer the Neonate to NICU, If

- Apgar score at 1 minute is <3.
- Required prolonged bag and mask ventilation (60 seconds or more).
- Required chest compressions.

Even neonates transferred to mother should be monitored frequently in the first 48–72 hours for development of features suggestive of HIE.

Care in NICU

1. **Maintain normal temperature**
   - After drying, place the baby under the radiant warmer.

- Maintain normal body temperature.
- Avoid hyperthermia.[14]

2. **Maintain normal oxygenation and ventilation**
   - Assess the infant for adequacy of oxygenation and ventilation and provide support as needed.
   - Keep under oxygen hood if needed; maintain saturations between 90 and 95%; avoid any hypoxia or hyperoxia
   - Assisted ventilation is required if there is apnea, or spontaneous respiration is inadequate or there is continuing hypoxia or hypercarbia.
   - Measure arterial blood gas, if any respiratory or perfusion abnormalities are present (maintain pO_2 between 60 and 90 mm Hg and pCO_2 at 35–45 mm Hg). Avoid both hypocarbia (reduces cerebral perfusion) and hypercarbia (increases cerebral perfusion and intracranial pressure and predisposes to intracranial bleed).

3. **Maintain normal tissue perfusion**
   - Ensure normal perfusion i.e. capillary refill time of less than 3 seconds, absence of tachycardia and metabolic acidosis, normal blood pressure, and adequate urine output.
   - Start intravenous fluids in all neonates with Apgar scores <4 at 1 minute or <7 at 5 minutes of age or if the neonate is sick (respiratory distress, encephalopathy or abnormal tone).
   - In sick neonates, place arterial line for guiding management of blood pressure. BP should be tightly maintained in upper normal range according to gestation and postnatal age specific BP charts avoiding wider fluctuation.[15]
   - If tissue perfusion is inadequate, infuse normal saline or Ringer's lactate at 10 mL/kg over 5–10 min.
   - Administer dobutamine (preferred) or dopamine to maintain adequate cardiac output, as required.
   - Do not restrict fluid routinely because it may predispose to hypoperfusion; restrict fluids only if there is hyponatremia (sodium <120 mEq/L) secondary to syndrome of inappropriate secretion of ADH (SIADH) or if there is renal failure.
   - Do echocardiography in infants needing ionotropic support to assess decreased contractibility due to asphyxia related cardiogenic shock. This helps to guide appropriate management strategy.[16]

4. **Maintain normal hematocrit and metabolic milieu**
   - Check blood glucose levels and maintain blood glucose levels between 75 mg/dl and 100 mg/dl.
   - Check hematocrit; correct anemia and maintain hematocrit between 45 and 55%. If the venous hematocrit is above 65%, bring it down to 55% by partial exchange transfusion using normal saline.
   - Check blood gases to detect metabolic acidosis; maintain pH above 7.30.
   - In case of severe asphyxia (see AAP criteria in Table 8.1), provide calcium in a maintenance dose of 4 mL/kg/day of 10% calcium gluconate for 1–2 days as a continuous infusion or as 1:1 diluted boluses, slowly under cardiac monitoring; maintain serum calcium concentration in the normal range.
5. **Treat seizures**
   - Refer to protocol on 'Neonatal seizures'.
6. **Nutrition**
   - Start oral feeding once the neonate is hemodynamically stable, is off vasopressor support, and has normal abdominal examination findings (no distension and normal bowel sounds).

Role of Special Investigations

The role of special investigations is to provide information on long-term prognosis.

Electroencephalography (EEG)

EEG is not indicated routinely in all asphyxiated neonates, but it helps in diagnosis and management of seizures and prognosticating for long-term outcomes. The prognosis is likely to be poor, if the EEG shows any one of the following:

1. Long periods of inactivity (>10 seconds).
2. Brief period of bursts (<6 seconds) with small amplitude bursts.
3. Interhemispheric asymmetry and asynchrony.
4. Isoelectric and low voltage (<5 microvolts).[17]

Amplitude-integrated electroencephalography (aEEG) is a simple, reliable, non-invasive technique which can be applied at the bedside in NICU for monitoring EEG continuously. Following abnormalities in aEEG would indicate poor prognosis:

- Wide fluctuations in the amplitude with the baseline voltages dropping to near zero.
- Peak amplitudes under 5 mV.
- Seizure spikes.

While a normal aEEG may not necessarily mean that the brain is normal, a severe or moderately severe aEEG abnormality may indicate brain injury and poor outcome. The time of onset of sleep wake cycling (SWC) also has a prognostic value. If SWC returns before 36 hours of age, the prognosis is likely to be good.[18]

Cranial Ultrasound (US)

Cranial US is not good for detecting changes of HIE in term neonates. However, hypoechoic areas can be seen in very severe cases (having large areas of infarction).

In preterm neonates, US can detect periventricular leukomalacia and intraventricular–periventricular hemorrhage during the first week of life. US is more useful than CT in providing adjunct prognostic information in preterm neonates.

Computed Tomography (CT)

CT has a role in initial evaluation, if MRI is not readily accessible. In acute stage of HIE, CT in term babies show generalized low attenuation of brain parenchyma. However, several weeks after asphyxial insult CT readily picks up diffuse cortical neuronal injury, injury to basal ganglia and thalamus, focal and multifocal ischemic brain injury as well as periventricular leukomalacia. CT has a limited role in identification of parasagittal cerebral injury.

Magnetic Resonance Imaging (MRI)

MRI is the best imaging modality for determining prognosis in term neonates. Diffusion weighted MRI can detect abnormalities within 24–48 hours after birth (optimal time is 2–3 days), whereas conventional MRI can show abnormalities in the first 3–4 days (though optimal time is later during the first week of life). An altered signal at the level of posterior limb of the internal capsule and abnormalities of thalami and basal ganglia in term neonates and that of white and grey matter at term equivalent age in preterm neonates are strong predictors of subsequent risk of poor neurodevelopmental outcome.[19] Another common pattern of injury is injury to the watershed regions.

Prognostic test in neonates with asphyxia: what is the evidence?

In a recent meta-analysis of 29 studies describing 13 prognostic tests in 1306 term neonates with hypoxic-ischemic encephalopathy, aEEG in the first 6 hours showed maximum sensitivity and specificity (93% and 90% respectively).[20]

SPECIFIC MANAGEMENT

1. Therapeutic Hypothermia (TH)

Institution of moderate therapeutic hypothermia (TH; 33–34°C) in infants of at least 35 weeks' gestation with moderate to severe encephalopathy initiated within 4–6 hours and continued for 72 hours of age in ICU settings has been shown to reduce mortality and neuro-morbidity by 18 months of age.[21] TH can be instituted by selectively cooling the head or the whole body. It is a safe modality in settings where intensive care facilities to manage sickest neonates are available.

TH has now become the standard of care in developed countries. However, this is not the case in low to middle income countries (LMIC), where the patient profile is different (concomitant IUGR, infection and nutritional deficiencies), there is a paucity of intensive care, and many births occur out of hospital. Indeed, a few studies have shown increased mortality following TH in these settings.[22,23]

Therapeutic hypothermia: What is the evidence?

The Cochrane review (8 RCTs; 638 term neonates with moderate/ severe encephalopathy and evidence of intrapartum asphyxia) showed that TH reduced combined outcome of mortality or major neurodevelopmental disability by 24% at 18 months of age.[24]

Evidence for Therapeutic Hypothermia from LMIC (Helix Trial)[31]

Evidence from Hypothermia for moderate or severe neonatal encephalopathy in low-income and middle-income countries (HELIX)Trial.

Countries Involved: India, Sri Lanka, Bangladesh.

Study Participants: Late preterm neonates (≥36 weeks) and term neonates with moderate to severe encephalopathy.

Enrolled participants (n): 408.

Intervention: Therapeutic hypothermia for 72 hours.

Primary outcome: Death or moderate to severe disability at 18–22 months.

Major results:

a. No effect on death or moderate to severe disability [50% vs 47% (RR:1.06; 95% CI 0·87–1·30; p=0·55)].
b. Increased risk of death before discharge in the intervention group [36% vs 24%; RR: 1·50; 95% CI: 1·10–2·04)].

Mechanism of Action of TH

TH has been shown to be protective at critical cellular and vascular sites of cerebral injury following asphyxia. It acts by the following mechanisms to reduce the extent of brain injury:[25]

1. Decreased cerebral metabolism and blood flow: Decrease in energy requirement and cerebral edema.
2. Decreased brain lactic acid, glutamate, and nitric oxide concentrations: Less excitotoxic and oxidative injury.
3. Inhibits protease activation, mitochondrial failure, free radical damage, lipid peroxidation: Less apoptosis and necrosis.

Selection of Neonates for TH (Table 8.5)

Table 8.5: Selection criteria of neonates for therapeutic hypothermia (NNF India 2021[32])

Whom to treat?	Neonates with the following characteristics: • Gestational age: ≥36 weeks • Age: <6 hours • Admission temperature: 36–37.4°C And following features: • Evidence of perinatal asphyxia as shown by any one of the following: A. pH <7 or Base excess >–16 in cord blood gas or arterial blood gas within 1 hour of birth. B. Apgar score <5 at 10 minutes of age. C. Positive pressure ventilation for at least 10 minutes. D. History of acute peripartum event like cord prolapse, uterine rupture. • Evidence of moderate to severe encephalopathy.
Whom not to treat?	Neonates with the following conditions: • Major congenital malformation. • Severe IUGR. • Severe coagulopathy. • Severe Intracranial bleed.
Where TH should be administered?	Level 3 NICU having a multidisciplinary team and following facilities can offer TH: • Bedside EEG, Cranial ultrasonography. • Access to MRI imaging, CT scan. • 24 hour monitoring of vital parameters like heart rate, respiration, blood pressure, temperature and saturation. • Desirable Nurse to patient ratio 1:2 or 1:1. • Long term follow up for at least 18 months.

(Contd.)

Table 8.5: Selection criteria of neonates for therapeutic hypothermia (NNF India 2021[32]) (*Contd.*)

Which device should be used for TH?	Only servo-controlled devices should be used for providing hypothermia.
What should be the appropriate duration?	72 hours

Cooling Devices Used for TH

1. Whole body cooling devices
   a. High technology devices: Examples–Tecotherm™, Blanketrol™, Meditherm™
   b. Low technology devices: Example–Miracradle™
2. Selective head cooling device: Examples–Olympic cool cap system™

High Technology Devices

These devices usually have a circulating water/coolant system. The water/coolant flows over and around the heating/cooling element located in the circulating reservoir. The heated or cooled water/coolant then flows out of the reservoir to the circulating pump, through connecting hoses over a water temperature sensor to the blanket. The water circulates through the blanket(s) and returns to the unit.

Low Technology Devices

These devices use the phase change material (PCM) technology to induce therapeutic hypothermia. PCMs are special thermal energy storage materials that store and release heat at a particular temperature. The thermal energy transfer occurs when the material changes phase from solid to liquid or liquid to solid.

In our unit, we use 'Blanketrol III Hyper-hypothermia' temperature management system which is a servo-controlled whole-body hypothermia device.

How to Initiate Whole Body Hypothermia

1. Counsel the parents about indications, benefits and risks of therapy.
2. Prepare the cooling system for operation.
3. Set the cooling blanket temperature of 33.5°C.
4. Monitor and document the infant's pre-cooling vital signs.

5. Place the infant on the warmer in the supine position with the entire head and body resting on the cooling blanket.
6. Place and secure central and arterial lines before starting hypothermia.
7. Gently insert the patient rectal probe 2 cm into the infant's rectum, and secure to the infant's leg with tape.
8. The infant must lie directly on the cooling blanket, wearing a diaper only.

Monitoring after Initiating TH

The frequency of monitoring and investigations after initiating TH is shown in Table 8.6:

Rewarming

1. Increase the infant's core temperature by 0.5°C every hour until 36.5°C has been reached.

Table 8.6: Monitoring (frequency)

Parameter	*Day 1*	*Day 2*	*Day 3*
Vitals monitoring including invasive blood pressure monitoring	Q 1 hour	Q 1 hour	Q 1 hour
Neurological monitoring	Q 12 hours	Q 12 hours	Q 12 hours
Urine output	Q 6 hours	Q 6 hours	Q 6 hours
ECG	Continuously	Continuously	Continuously
aEEG	Continuously	Continuously	Continuously
Skin integrity	Q 6 hours	Q 6 hours	Q 6 hours
Investigations			
Glucose	Q 6 hours	Q 6 hours	Q 6 hours
Blood gas	Q 6 hours or as indicated by condition of baby	Q 12 hours or as indicated	Q 12 hours or as indicated
Renal function test	Once	Once	Once
Electrolytes	Once	Once	Once
Complete hemogram	Only if required	Only if required	Only if required
Neurosonogram	If abnormal	If abnormal	If abnormal

2. When the infant's core temperature is 36.5°C, remove the patient from the cooling blanket/device.
3. Re-activate the radiant warmer, monitor and document the infant's temperature with the skin probe.
4. Problems while rewarming: seizures and hypotension.

Supportive Therapy during TH

Sedative/analgesics	Morphine (preferred) or fentanyl should be given by infusion during therapeutic hypothermia.
Enteral feeds	Start MEN, if hemodynamically stable.
Antibiotics	Prophylactic antibiotics should not be given.
Anticonvulsants	Anticonvulsants should be given in the presence of seizures; electric seizures in absence of clinical correlates should be treated.
Platelet concentrate	If platelet count is less than 100,000/cmm.
Fresh frozen plasma	Only if there is active bleeding.

Adverse Effects of TH[24]

The common adverse effects include sinus bradycardia (heart rate <80/min) and thrombocytopenia (platelet count $<150 \times 10^9$/L).

2. Prophylactic Phenobarbitone

Some interest has been generated in the protective role of prophylactic phenobarbitone in newborns with perinatal asphyxia. A dose of 40 mg/kg administered prophylactically was associated with a better neurodevelopmental outcome at 3 years of age.[26] However, the Cochrane review that included 5 RCTs reported no difference in the risk of death, neurodisability.[26] Another study using 40 mg/kg within 1st hour showed a significant reduction in HIE with no difference in complications.[26] Recommendation for use of prophylactic phenobarbitone still awaits further studies.

Prophylactic phenobarbitone in HIE: What is the evidence?

The systematic review by Evans DJ showed no significant difference in the risk of the combined outcome of death or severe neurodevelopmental disability (typical RR 0.78, 95% CI 0.49, 1.23).[26]

3. Drugs under Investigation

A large number of drugs are under investigation for neuroprotection in HIE. They need to be used in the early period of hypoxic–ischemic injury along with therapeutic hypothermia. They act by causing blockade of free radical generation (allopurinol, oxypurinol, melatonin), scavenging of oxidants (superoxide dismutase, glutathione, N-acetyl cysteine), calcium channel blockade (flunarizine, nimodipine), blockage of NMDA receptors (magnesium, Xenon, dextromethorphan) and blockage of inflammatory mediators (phospholipase A2, indomethacin, erythropoietin).[27] A recent multicenter 'Total body hypothermia plus Xenon' (TOBY-XE) trial reported no effect of this intervention on reduced thalamic lactate to N-acetyl aspartate ratio, a surrogate marker of good neurodevelopmental outcome.[28]

Follow-up

It is essential to follow all the neonates with the moderate and severe asphyxia, especially those with stage II and III HIE staging. They should have a complete neurological assessment and early intervention, if needed during the follow-up. A formal psychometric assessment at 18 months should be performed in them.

Long-term Outcome

Among the neonates who survive severe HIE, the sequelae include mental retardation, epilepsy, and cerebral palsy of varying degrees. The latter can be in the form of hemiplegia, paraplegia, or quadriplegia. Such infants need careful evaluation and support. They may need to be referred to specialized clinics capable of providing coordinated comprehensive follow-up care.

Predictors of mortality and neurological morbidity after perinatal hypoxic ischemic insult:

1. Extended very low APGAR scores (at 20 minutes or more).
2. Time to establish spontaneous respiration (for 30 or more minutes).
3. Neonatal neurological examination (severe HIE).
4. Brain imaging (USG, MRI).
5. Other investigations (EEG, aEEG, evoked potentials like BERA).

The incidence of long-term complications depends on the severity of HIE. Up to 80% of neonates with stage III HIE die whereas rest 20% have neurological sequelae. Up to 80% of infants who survive severe HIE develop serious complications, 10–20% develop moderately serious disabilities, and up to 10% are normal. The incidence of death is up to 5% and that of neurological sequelae is up to 24% after moderate birth asphyxia. Among the infants who survive moderately severe HIE, 30–50% may suffer from serious long-term complications, and 10–20% with minor neurological morbidities. Infants with mild HIE tend to be free from death or any neurological sequelae.[29, 30]

A recent study on long-term outcomes of whole body hypothermia for HIE revealed the rate of combined end point of death or an IQ score of less than 70 at 6–7 years of age to be lower among neonates undergoing whole body hypothermia (47%) than those undergoing usual care (62%).[25]

REFERENCES

1. Liu L, Johnson HL, Cousens S, Perin J, Scott S, Lawn JE, Rudan I, Campbell H, Cibulskis R, Li M, Mathers C, Black RE. Global, regional, and national causes of child mortality: an updated systematic analysis for 2010 with time trends since 2000. Lancet 2012;379:2151–61.
2. Lawn JE, Blencowe H, Oza S, You D, Lee AC, Waiswa P, Lalli M, Bhutta Z, Barros AJ, Christian P, Mathers C, Cousens SN; Lancet Every Newborn Study Group. Every Newborn: progress, priorities, and potential beyond survival. Lancet 2014;384:189–205.
3. Lawn JE, Blencowe H, Pattinson R, Cousens S, Kumar R, Ibiebele I, Gardosi J, Day LT, Stanton C; Lancet's Stillbirths Series steering committee. Stillbirths: Where? When? Why? How to make the data count? Lancet 2011;377:1448–63.
4. Sankar MJ, Natarajan CK, Das RR, Agarwal R, Chandrasekaran A, Paul VK. When do newborns die? A systematic review of timing of overall and cause-specific neonatal deaths in developing countries. J Perinatol 2016;36 Suppl 1:S1-S11.
5. Report of the National Neonatal Perinatal Database (National Neonatology Forum, India) 2003.
6. World Health Organization. Perinatal mortality: a listing of available information. FRH/MSM.96.7.Geneva:WHO,1996.
7. Committee on fetus and newborn, American Academy of Pediatrics and Committee on obstetric practice, American College of Obstetrics and Gynecology. Use and abuse of the APGAR score. Pediatr 1996;98:141–2.
8. Perlman JM, Tack ED, Martin T, Shackelford G, Amon E. Acute systemic organ injury in term infants after asphyxia. Am J Dis Child 1989;143:617–20.
9. Sarnat HB, Sarnat MS: Neonatal encephalopathy following fetal distress: A clinical and electroencephalographic study. Arch Neurol 1976;33:695–706.
10. Levene MI. The asphyxiated newborn infant. In: Levene MI, Lilford RJ. Fetal and neonatal neurology and neurosurgery. Edinburgh: Churchill Livingstone 1995:405–26.
11. Thompson CM, et al: The value of a scoring system for hypoxic encephalopathy in predicting neurodevelopmental outcome. Acta Paediatr 1997;86:757.

12. Wyckoff MH, Aziz K, Escobedo MB, et al. Part 13: Neonatal Resuscitation: 2015 American Heart Association guidelines update for cardiopulmonary resuscitation and emergency cardiovascular care. Circulation 2015;132: S543–60.
13. Malin GL, Morris RK, Khan KS. Strength of association between umbilical cord pH and perinatal and long term outcomes: systematic review and meta-analysis. BMJ 2010; 340: c1471.
14. Laptook A, Tyson J, Shankaran S, McDonald S, Ehrenkranz R, Fanaroff A, Donovan E, Goldberg R, O'Shea TM, Higgins RD, Poole WK; National Institute of Child Health and Human Development Neonatal Research Network. Elevated temperature after hypoxic-ischemic encephalopathy: risk factor for adverse outcomes. Pediatrics 2008;122:491–9.
15. Zubrow A B, Hulman S, Kushner H, Falkner B. Determinants of blood pressure in infants admitted to neonatal intensive care units: a prospective multicentre study. J Perinatol 1995;15:472–9.
16. Ranjit M S. Cardiac abnormalities in birth asphyxia. Indian J Paediatr 2000;67:529–32.
17. Menache CC, Bourgeois BF, Volpe JJ. Prognostic value of neonatal discontinuous EEG. Pediatr Neurol 2002;27:93–101.
18. Osredkar D, Toet MC, van Rooij LG, van Huffelen AC, Groenendaal F, de Vries LS. Sleep wave cycling on amplitude integrated electroencephalography in term newborns with hypoxic ischaemic encephalopathy. Pediatrics 2005;115:327–32.
19. Lianne J, Woodward, Anderson PJ, Austin NC, Howard K, Inder TE. Neonatal MRI to predict neurodevelopmental outcomes in preterm infants. N Engl J Med 2006;355:685–94.
20. van Laerhoven H, de Haan TR, Offringa M, Post B, van der Lee JH. Prognostic tests in term neonates with hypoxic-ischemic encephalopathy: a systematic review. Pediatrics 2013;131:88–98.
21. Edwards AD, Brocklehurst P, Gunn AJ, Halliday H, Juszczak E, Levene M, Strohm B, Thoresen M, Whitelaw A, Azzopardi D. Neurological outcomes at 18 months of age after moderate hypothermia for perinatal hypoxic ischaemic encephalopathy: synthesis and meta-analysis of trial data. BMJ 2010 9;340:c363.
22. Thayyil S, Chandrasekaran M, Taylor A, Bainbridge A, Cady EB, Chong WK, Murad S, Omar RZ, Robertson NJ. Cerebral magnetic resonance biomarkers in neonatal encephalopathy: a meta-analysis. Pediatrics 2010;125:e382–95.
23. Bhardwaj SK, Bhat BV. Therapeutic hypothermia using gel packs for term neonates with hypoxic ischemic encephalopathy in resource-limited settings: a randomized controlled trial. J Trop Pediatr 2012;58:382–8.
24. Jacobs SE, Berg M, Hunt R, Tarnow-Mordi WO, Inder TE, Davis PG. Cochrane Database Syst Rev 2013;1:CD003311.
25. Shankaran S. Hypoxic-ischemic Encephalopathy and Novel Strategies for Neuroprotection. Clin Perinatol 2012;39:919–29.
26. Evans DJ, Levene MI, Tsakmakis M. Anticonvulsants for preventing mortality and morbidity in full term newborns with perinatal asphyxia. Cochrane Database Syst Rev 2007 Jul 18;(3):CD001240.

27. McAdams RM, Juul SE. Neonatal Encephalopathy: Update on Therapeutic Hypothermia and Other Novel Therapeutics. Clin Perinatol 2016;43:485–500.
28. Azzopardi D, Robertson NJ, Bainbridge A, et al. Moderate hypothermia within 6 h of birth plus inhaled xenon versus moderate hypothermia alone after birth asphyxia (TOBY-Xe): a proof-of-concept, open-label, randomised controlled trial. Lancet Neurol 2015; 15:145–53.
29. Rutherford MA, et al. Abnormal magnetic resonance signal in the internal capsule predicts poor neurodevelopmental outcome in infants with hypoxic ischaemic encephalopathy. Pediatrics 1998; 102:323.
30. Robertson C, Finer N. Term infants with hypoxic ischaemic encephalopathy: outcome at 3.5 years. Dev Med Child Neurol 1985; 27:473–84.
31. Thayyil S, Pant S, Montaldo P et al. Hypothermia for moderate or severe neonatal encephalopathy in low-income and middle-income countries (HELIX): a randomised controlled trial in India, Sri Lanka, and Bangladesh. Lancet Glob Health. 2021 Sep;9(9): e1273-e1285.
32. Position Statement and Guidelines For Use of Therapeutic Hypothermia to treat Neonatal Hypoxic Ischemic Encephalopathy In India. National Neonatology Forum, 2021.

CHAPTER

9 Neonatal Seizures

Neonatal seizures (NS) are the most distinctive clinical manifestations of neurological dysfunction in neonates. Infants with NS are at a high risk of death during the neonatal period and neurological impairment/epilepsy disorders in later life. Though mortality due to NS has decreased from 40% to about 7–20% over the years, the prevalence of long-term neurodevelopmental sequelae has largely remained unchanged[1,2] Close to 30% neonates with NS develop cerebral palsy, 15–35% develop epilepsy and 50% have developmental delay.[2,3] They pose a significant clinical challenge for physicians in low- and middle-income countries (LMIC). Delayed recognition of NS is possibly a major contributor to its poor outcomes, considering that NS can be very difficult to recognize clinically.

EPIDEMIOLOGY

The National Neonatal Perinatal Database (NNPD; 2002–03), which collected data from 18 tertiary care units across the country, reported an incidence of 10.3 per 1000 live-births;[4] recent reports from low- and middle-income countries report an incidence of 36–90 per 1000 live births, whereas the incidence in high-income countries is 1–3 per 1000 live births.[2] The incidence was found to increase with decreasing gestation and birth weight. Preterm infants had almost twice the incidence when compared to term neonates (20.8 vs. 8.4 per 1000 live-births) while very low birth weight infants had more than 4-fold higher incidence (36.1 per 1000 live-births).[4]

DEFINITION

Seizure is defined clinically as paroxysmal alterations in neurologic function, i.e. motor, behavior and/or autonomic function.[5] NS can be of the following types:[6]

1. **Electrographic seizure:** Paroxysmal abnormality in cortical electrical activity that evolves over time.

2. **Electroclinical seizure:** Electrographic seizure with associated clinical signs. These kind of seizures can only be identified by EEG monitoring, and some studies indicate that EEG-only seizures may constitute as much as 70–80% of NS.[7,8]

CLASSIFICATION

Four clinically evident types of NS have traditionally been recognized:[5]

Subtle seizures: The clinical manifestations are mild motor, behavioral or autonomic paroxysms and may often be missed. They are the most common type, constituting about 50% of all seizures. Some kinds of subtle seizures in full-term newborns do not have an EEG correlate, i.e. they are *clinical only.* Common examples of subtle seizures include:

1. **Ocular:** Tonic horizontal deviation of eyes (more common in term) or sustained eye opening with ocular fixation (more common in preterm) or cycled fluttering
2. **Oral–facial–lingual movements:** Chewing, tongue-thrusting, lip-smacking, etc.
3. **Limb movements:** Cycling, paddling, boxing-jabs, hooking etc.
4. **Autonomic phenomena:** Tachycardia or bradycardia.
5. **Apnea** may be a rare manifestation of seizures, particularly in term infants. Apnea due to seizure activity has an accelerated or a normal heart rate when evaluated 20 seconds after onset. Bradycardia is thus not an early manifestation in convulsive apnea but may occur later due to prolonged hypoxemia.

Clonic seizures: They involve rhythmic movements of muscle groups with a rapid phase followed by a slow return. They occur at a frequency of 1–3 jerks/second and are commonly associated with EEG changes. Clonic seizures may be focal clonic (localized, not associated with loss of consciousness), multifocal clonic (simultaneous/sequential jerking in multiple locations; non-Jacksonian migration) or generalized clonic seizures (rare in neonates).

Tonic seizures: This refers to a sustained flexion or extension of axial or appendicular muscle groups. These seizures may be focal or generalized and often resemble decerebrate (tonic extension of all limbs) or decorticate posturing (flexion of upper limbs and extension of lower limbs). Generalized tonic seizures are not associated with EEG changes in around 85% cases and may represent a 'brainstem release' phenomena secondary to severe brain injury.

Myoclonic seizures: They manifest as single or multiple lightning-fast jerks of the upper or lower limbs and are usually distinguished from clonic movements because of rapid frequency of myoclonic jerks, absence of slow return, and predilection for flexor muscle groups. Common changes seen on EEG include burst suppression pattern, focal sharp waves, and hypsarrhythmia.

Myoclonic seizures carry the worst prognosis in terms of neurodevelopmental outcome and seizure recurrence. Focal clonic seizures have the best prognosis.

*A note on the ILAE 2021 classification of neonatal seizures.

The ILAE has recently given a new classification for neonatal seizures, wherein seizures are defined only as electroclinical or electrical, but clinical events without an EEG correlate were defined as non-seizure episodes. Further, new descriptive terms were used to classify seizures such as 'sequential seizures' and 'automatisms.' However, in view of paucity of EEG availability in most neonatal units in our setting and ambiguity surrounding the new classification, we continue to use the clinical classification of seizures currently.

ETIOLOGY OF NEONATAL SEIZURES

Majority of neonatal seizures are acute symptomatic seizures with only 10–15% occurring as the first manifestation of an epilepsy syndrome.[1,9] Etiology of NS differs in LMIC with hypoxic–ischemic encephalopathy, intracranial infections and transient metabolic disturbances (hypoglycemia and hypocalcemia) being much more common as compared to those in HIC.[2,10] However, etiology can vary between different centers depending upon the patient population (term vs. preterm), level of monitoring (only clinical vs. electrical and clinical seizures), etc.

Hypoxic–ischemic encephalopathy (HIE): HIE secondary to perinatal asphyxia is the most common cause of NS. Most seizures due to HIE (about 50–65%) have onset within the first 12–24 hours of life, while the rest manifest by 24–48 hours of life. Additional problems like hypoglycemia, hypocalcemia, and intracranial hemorrhage may coexist in neonates with perinatal asphyxia and should always be excluded. Perinatal variables such as Apgar scores do not predict occurrence of seizures. Subtle seizures are the most common type of seizures in neonates with HIE.

Metabolic causes: Common metabolic causes of seizures include hypoglycemia, hypocalcemia (both early and late onset), hypomagnesemia and hypo- and hypernatremia. Rare causes include several inborn errors of metabolism (non-ketotic hyperglycinemia, urea cycle defects, mitochondrial disorders, Zellweger syndrome, etc.), pyridoxine-dependent seizures, folinic acid-responsive seizures, etc.

Infections: Bacterial meningitis usually causes seizures in the latter part of the first week of life and should be excluded in all neonates with seizures. Meningoencephalitis secondary to intrauterine infections (TORCH group, syphilis) may also present as seizures in the neonatal period.

Intracranial hemorrhage and vascular causes: Seizures due to subarachnoid, intraparenchymal or subdural hemorrhage occur more often in term neonates, while seizures secondary to intraventricular hemorrhage (IVH) occur in preterm neonates. Most seizures due to intracranial hemorrhage occur between 2 and 7 days of age. Seizures occurring in a term 'well baby' on day 2–3 of life is often due to subarachnoid hemorrhage. Ischemic stroke and CSVT are also well-known causes of neonatal seizures but are often missed due to lack of clinical suspicion and neuroimaging.

Developmental defects: Cerebral dysgenesis and neuronal migration disorders are rare causes of seizures in the neonatal period.

Miscellaneous: These include polycythemia, maternal narcotic withdrawal, drug toxicity (e.g. theophylline, doxapram), local anesthetic injection into scalp, and phacomatosis (e.g. tuberous sclerosis, incontinentia pigmentii). Accidental injection of local anesthetic into scalp may be suspected in the presence of fixed and dilated pupil and absence of doll's eye reflex. Multifocal clonic seizures on the 5th day of life may be related to low zinc levels in the CSF fluid (benign idiopathic neonatal convulsions).

Seizures due to SAH and late onset hypocalcemia carry a good prognosis for long-term neurodevelopmental outcome while seizures related to hypoglycemia, cerebral malformations, and meningitis have a high risk for adverse outcome.

APPROACH TO AN INFANT WITH NEONATAL SEIZURES

History

Seizure history: A complete description of the seizure should be obtained from the parents/attendant. History of associated eye movements, restraint of episode by passive flexion of the affected limb, change in skin color (mottling or cyanosis), autonomic phenomena, and whether the infant was conscious or sleeping at the time of seizure should be elicited. If possible, the attendant should be asked to video record the event to understand the nature of the seizures. The day of life on which the seizures first occur may provide an important clue to its diagnosis. While seizures occurring on day 1–3 might be related to perinatal asphyxia, intracranial hemorrhage, and metabolic causes, those occurring on day 4–7 are more often due to sepsis, meningitis, metabolic causes, and developmental defects.

Antenatal history: History suggestive of intrauterine infection, maternal diabetes, and narcotic addiction should be elicited in the antenatal history. A history of sudden increase in fetal movements may be suggestive of intrauterine convulsions.

Perinatal history: Perinatal asphyxia is the most common cause of neonatal seizures and a detailed history including history of fetal distress, decreased fetal movements, instrumental delivery, need for resuscitation in the labor room, Apgar scores, and abnormal cord pH (<7) and base deficit (>12 mEq/L) should be obtained.

Feeding history: Clinical features like lethargy, poor activity, drowsiness, and vomiting after initiation of breastfeeding may be suggestive of inborn errors of metabolism. Late onset hypocalcemia should be considered in the presence of top feeding with cow's milk.

Family history: History of consanguinity in parents, family history of seizures or intellectual disability and early fetal/neonatal deaths would be suggestive of inborn errors of metabolism. History of seizures in either parent or sibling(s) in the neonatal period may suggest benign familial neonatal convulsions (BFNC).

Examination

Vital signs: Heart rate, respiration, blood pressure, capillary refill time and temperature should be recorded in all neonates.

General examination: Gestation, birth weight, and weight for age should be recorded as they may provide important clues to the etiology—for example, seizures in a term 'well baby' may be due to subarachnoid hemorrhage while seizures in a large-for-date neonate may be secondary to hypoglycemia. The neonate should also be examined for the presence of any obvious malformations or dysmorphic features. Jitteriness may be an associated finding in seizures due to hypoglycemia or hypocalcemia.

CNS examination: Presence of a bulging anterior fontanelle may be suggestive of meningitis or intracranial hemorrhage. A detailed neurological examination should include assessment of consciousness (alert/drowsy/comatose), tone (hypotonia or hypertonia), and fundus examination for chorioretinitis.

Systemic examination: Presence of hepatosplenomegaly or an abnormal urine odor may be suggestive of IEM. The skin should be examined for the presence of any neurocutaneous markers. Presence of hypopigmented macules or ash-leaf spot is suggestive of tuberous sclerosis.

Investigations

Essential Investigations

Table 9.1 depicts the investigations that should be considered in all neonates with seizures. CSF examination should be done in all cases, as seizures may be the first sign of meningitis. It should not be omitted even if another etiology such as hypoglycemia is present. CSF study may be withheld if severe cardio-respiratory compromise is present or omitted in neonates with severe birth asphyxia (documented abnormal cord pH/base excess and onset of seizures within 12–24 hours of life).

Table 9.1: Investigations required in a neonate with seizures

Essential investigations (required in all with few exceptions)*	*Additional investigations*
• Blood sugar • Serum sodium and calcium • Cerebrospinal fluid (CSF) examination • Cranial ultrasound (US) and • Electroencephalography (EEG) and/or amplitude-integrated EEG	• Hematocrit (if plethoric and/or at risk for polycythemia) • Serum bilirubin (if icteric) • Serum magnesium • Arterial blood gas and anion gap (lethargy, vomiting, family history, etc.) • Imaging: CT and/or MRI (if no etiology found after essential investigations) • TORCH screen for congenital infections • Work-up for inborn errors of metabolism

*Given in the text

One should carry out all these investigations even if one or more investigations are positive, as multiple etiologies may coexist, e.g. sepsis, meningitis and hypoglycemia.

Additional Investigations

These may be considered in neonates who do not respond to a combination of phenobarbitone and phenytoin or earlier in neonates with specific features. These include neuroimaging (CT, MRI), screen for congenital infections (TORCH), and for inborn errors of metabolism (IEM). If an IEM is suspected (intrapartum seizures, refractory seizures, findings of HIE without any hypoxic insult, progressive worsening), an arterial blood gas should be obtained. Additional investigations may also be required to identify the cause of metabolic abnormality such as hypoglycemia or hypocalcemia.

Imaging: Cranial USG is an excellent tool for detection of intraventricular and parenchymal hemorrhage but lacks sensitivity for SAH and subdural hemorrhage. It should be done in all infants with seizures. CT scan should be done in term infants where subarachnoid hemorrhage is suspected and in infants with suspected intrauterine infections to identify intracranial calcification. Magnetic resonance imaging (MRI) is indicated in HIE, cerebral dysgenesis, lissencephaly, and other neuronal migration disorders.

Electroencephalogram (EEG): Conventional continuous EEG (cEEG) has both diagnostic and prognostic role in seizures. It is recommended in all neonates in whom seizures are suspected. It helps in confirmation of clinical seizures and helps us to avoid unwanted use of anticonvulsants. Clinically silent seizures can be identified only by means of an EEG. Further, EEG helps to detect electromechanical dissociation, i.e. persistence of electrical seizures after starting anti-seizure medications. It also helps in discontinuation of AEDs after resolution of symptomatic seizures.[11] cEEG should be performed for at least one hour. Interictal EEG is useful for prognostication of neonates with seizures, with certain background abnormalities denoting a high risk for neurological sequelae. These include burst-suppression pattern, low voltage invariant pattern, and electrocerebral inactivity.

Amplitude integrated EEG (aEEG): aEEG is a bedside investigation is often preferred over cEEG in NICUs, since it easier to apply and interpret. As with conventional EEG, background abnormalities like burst-suppression or continuous low voltage pattern in aEEG also help in prognosticating the infant with seizures, particularly in the setting of HIE. Seizure activity on aEEG is characterized by a rapid rise in both the lower and upper margins of the trace. Some seizures that are focal or relatively brief are, however, missed by this technique.[5]

Screen for congenital infections: TORCH screen and VDRL should be considered in the presence of hepatosplenomegaly, thrombocytopenia, intrauterine growth restriction, small-for-gestational age, or chorioretinitis.

Metabolic screen: This includes blood and urine ketones, urine reducing substances, blood ammonia, anion gap, urine and plasma aminoacidogram, serum and CSF lactate/pyruvate ratio.

Management

1. Initial Medical Management

The first step in the management of seizures is to ensure airway, breathing, and circulation and to nurse the baby in a thermoneutral environment. Oxygen should be started, IV access should be secured, and blood should be collected for glucose and other investigations. A brief relevant history should be obtained and quick clinical examination should be performed. These steps should not require more than 2–5 minutes.

2. Correction of Hypoglycemia and Hypocalcemia

If point-of-care glucose test shows hypoglycemia or if there is no facility to test blood sugar immediately, 2 ml/kg of 10% dextrose should be given as a bolus injection followed by a continuous infusion of 6–8 mg/kg/min.

If hypoglycemia has been treated or excluded as a cause, the neonate should receive 2 ml/kg of 10% calcium gluconate IV over 10 minutes under strict cardiac monitoring. If serum calcium levels are suggestive of hypocalcemia, the newborn should receive calcium gluconate at 8 ml/kg/d for 3 days. If seizures continue despite correction of hypocalcemia, 0.25 ml/kg of 50% magnesium sulfate should be given intramuscularly.

3. Anti-seizure Medications (ASMs)

Anti-seizure medications (ASMs) should be considered in the presence of even a single clinical seizure because clinical observations tend to grossly underestimate electrical seizures and facilities for continuous EEG monitoring are not universally available. If aEEG is being used, eliminating all electrical seizure activity should be the goal of ASM therapy.[3] ASM should be given if seizures persist even after correction of hypoglycemia/hypocalcemia (Fig. 9.1).

3.1 Phenobarbitone (PB)

It is the drug of choice in neonatal seizures. The dose is 20 mg/kg/IV slowly over 20 minutes (not faster than 1 mg/kg/min), this achieves a blood level of ~ 20 μg/ml. Close respiratory monitoring is required during administration of PB. If seizures persist after completion of the loading dose, additional doses of phenobarbitone 10 mg/kg may be used every 20–30 minutes until a total dose of 40 mg/kg has been given. The maintenance dose of PB is 3–5 mg/kg/day in 1–2 divided doses, starting 12 hours after the loading dose. Recent evidence shows that the risk of seizure recurrence may not be high even in the absence of maintenance doses of PB in late preterm and term infants with seizures.[12]

First-line ASM: Evidence and recommendations

A Cochrane review found only one RCT that showed comparable seizure control rate with phenobarbital and phenytoin (RR 1.03, 95% CI 0.96–1.62), controlling seizures in only half of cases.[13]

Another randomized trial conducted in India concluded that phenobarbitone was much more effective for seizure control (72%) as compared to phenytoin (14%) [$p < 0.001$].[14]

Based on the available evidence, the 2011 WHO guidelines on neonatal seizures recommend phenobarbitone as the first-line agent for management of neonatal seizures.[15]

3.2 Phenytoin (PHT)

Phenytoin is indicated if the maximal dose of phenobarbitone (40 mg/kg) fails to resolve seizures or earlier if adverse effects like respiratory depression, hypotension or bradycardia ensue with phenobarbitone. The dose is 20 mg/kg IV at a rate of not more than 1 mg/kg/min under cardiac monitoring. PHT should be diluted in normal saline because it is incompatible with dextrose. A repeat dose of 10 mg/kg may be tried in refractory seizures. The maintenance dose is 3–5 mg/kg/day (maximum of 8 mg/kg/day) in 2–4 divided doses. Oral suspension has very erratic absorption and should be avoided in neonates.

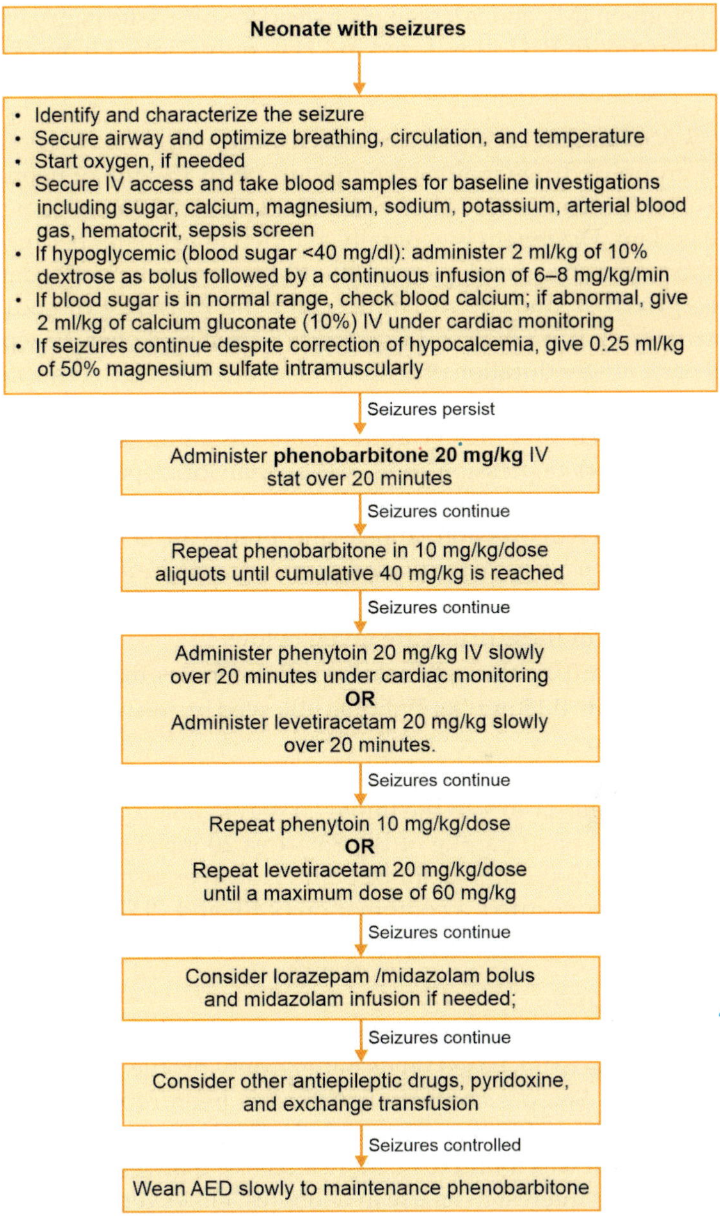

Fig. 9.1: Acute management of neonatal seizures

Fosphenytoin, the prodrug of PHT, does not cause the same degree of hypotension or cardiac abnormalities, has high water solubility (can be given IM), and is less likely to lead to soft-tissue injury when compared with PHT. It is dosed in PHT equivalents; 1.5 mg/kg of fosphenytoin is equivalent to 1 mg/kg of PHT.

3.3 Benzodiazepines

This group of drugs may be required in up to 15–20% of neonatal seizures. The commonly used benzodiazepines are lorazepam and midazolam. Diazepam is generally avoided in neonates because of its short duration of antiepileptic effect but very prolonged sedative effect, narrow therapeutic index, and the presence of sodium benzoate as a preservative. Lorazepam is preferred over diazepam as it has a longer duration of action and results in less adverse effects (sedation and cardiovascular effects). Midazolam is faster acting than lorazepam and may be administered as an infusion. It causes less respiratory depression and sedation than lorazepam. However, when used as continuous infusion, the infant has to be monitored for respiratory depression, apnea, and bradycardia *(equipment for resuscitation and assisted ventilation should be available at the bedside of all neonates given multiple doses of AED).*

The doses of these drugs are given below:

Lorazepam: 0.05 mg/kg IV bolus over 2–5 minutes; may be repeated

Midazolam: 0.15 mg/kg IV bolus followed by infusion of 0.1–0.4 mg/kg/hour.

The expected control rate of neonatal clinical seizures to anticonvulsants is 40% to the initial 20 mg/kg loading dose of PB, 70% to a total of 40 mg/kg of PB, 85% to a 20 mg/kg of PHT, and 95–100% to 0.05–0.1 mg/kg lorazepam[5]. However, as far as electrical seizures are concerned, a combination of PB and PHT will achieve seizure control in only around 60% cases.[5]

3.4 Levetiracetam

Levetiracetam is increasingly being used in neonates as a first-line or second-line drug, based on its better safety profile and less drug interactions. Seizure control of >80% has been reported with a dose of 20–50 mg/kg/day[16], however in the recent NeoLEV-2 RCT, phenobarbital was found to be more effective than levetiracetam.[17] There is great interest in its use in neonates. However, randomized studies have not been performed. On the contrary, a recent meta-analysis reported there was no significant difference in efficacy between levetiracetam and phenobarbitone, but levetiracetam use was associated with fewer side effects.[18] Even though evidence regarding efficacy is conflicting, given the better safety profile in terms of respiratory and cardiovascular compromise, levetiracetam may be an appropriate second-line agent for neonatal seizures.

Second-line ASM: Evidence and recommendations

A Cochrane review[13] found one study that randomized infants who failed to respond to phenobarbital to receive either lidocaine or midazolam as second-line agents. There was a trend for lidocaine to be more effective in reducing seizure burden (RR 0.40, 95% CI 0.14–1.17) but both groups had similarly poor long-term outcomes assessed at one year.

Based on the available evidence, the WHO guidelines on neonatal seizures recommend either midazolam or lidocaine as the second-line AED in neonatal seizures.[15]

However, given the lack of robust evidence and constraints involved in providing respiratory support and/or monitoring in most neonatal units in India, it seems appropriate to use phenytoin as the second-line agent in neonates with seizures.

Recent evidence has shown that levetiracetam has a good safety profile,[18] with a systematic review showing no difference in efficacy when compared to phenobarbitone and a recent randomized trial reporting higher efficacy of levetiracetam for term asphyxiated newborns.[18,19] PB has some side effects, such as hypotension and respiratory depression, and it can accelerate neuronal apoptosis in the immature brain. Thus, it may be appropriate to use levetiracetam as a second line agent, until more evidence is available regarding its efficacy with the first line drug phenobarbitone.

3.5 Antiseizure medications for seizures refractory to above treatment

In exceptional circumstances when the seizures are refractory to PB, PHT, and midazolam, the following drugs may be tried:

Lidocaine: It is usually administered as a bolus dose of 4 mg/kg IV followed by an infusion rate of 2 mg/kg/hr. It is tapered over several days. Adverse effects include arrhythmias, hypotension, and seizures. It should not be administered with phenytoin.

Paraldehyde: A dose of 0.1–0.2 ml/kg/dose may be given IM or 0.3 mL/kg/dose mixed with coconut oil in 3:1 may be used by rectal route. Additional doses may be used after 30 minutes and q 4–6 hourly. Adverse effects include pulmonary hemorrhage, pulmonary edema, hypotension, and liver injury.

Sodium valproate: Per rectal or IV route may be used in acute condition. The dose is 20–25 mg/kg followed by 5–10 mg/kg every 12 hours. It should, however, be used with caution in newborns given the uncertain risk of hepatotoxicity.

Vigabatrin: It has been used in neonates with infantile spasms, at a dose of 50 mg/kg/day.

Topiramate: It shows promise in neonatal seizures because of its potential neuroprotective effect against injury caused by seizures. It has been used for refractory infantile spasms in infants. The higher volume of distribution compared with other drugs requires higher initial and maintenance doses of approximately 3 mg/kg.

3.6 Other therapies

Pyridoxine: A therapeutic trial of pyridoxine is reserved as a last resort in refractory seizures. Intravenous route is the preferred method; however, suitable IV preparations are not universally available. Hence intramuscular (IM) route may have to be used (1 ml of injection Neurobion has 50 mg pyridoxine and 1 ml each may be administered both the sides in either the gluteal region or anterolateral aspect of thigh). It should be given with continuous monitoring, as hypotension and apnea can occur.

Exchange transfusion: This is indicated in life-threatening metabolic disorders, accidental injection of local anesthetics, transplacental transfer of maternal drugs (e.g. chlorpropamide), and bilirubin encephalopathy.

3.7 Maintenance anti-epileptic therapy

Principles of ASM used in older children and adults are applicable to neonates also. Monotherapy is the most appropriate strategy to control seizures. Attempts should be made to stop all anti-epileptic drugs and wean the baby to only phenobarbitone at 3–5 mg/kg/day. If seizures are uncontrolled or if clinical toxicity appears, a second ASM may be added. The choice may vary from phenytoin, carbamazepine, and valproic acid.

3.8 When to discontinue ASMs?

This is highly individualized and no specific guidelines are available. The goal is to discontinue ASMs as early as possible. We usually try to discontinue all medications at discharge if clinical examination is normal, irrespective of etiology and EEG. A recent retrospective comparative effectiveness study demonstrated that discontinuation of ASMs at discharge for acute symptomatic neonatal seizures had no difference in functional neurodevelopmental outcomes and risk of epilepsy at 24 months of age when compared with continuation of ASMs at discharge.[20] If neurological examination is persistently

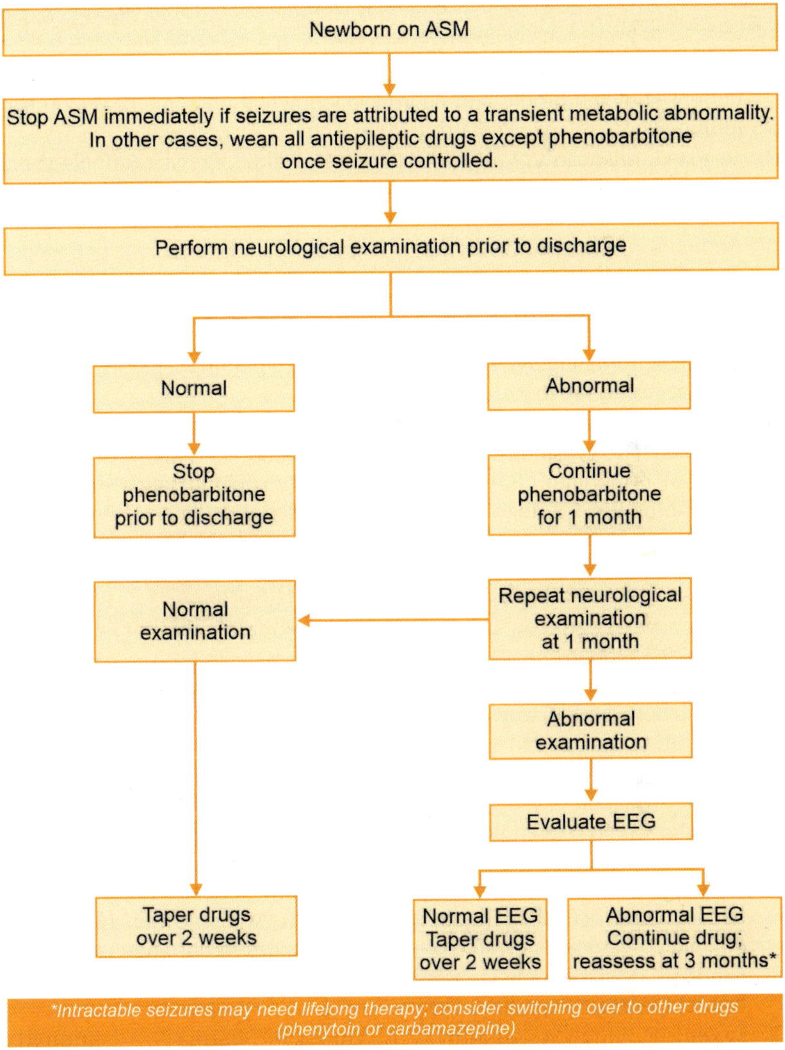

Fig. 9.2: Weaning of antiseizure medications

abnormal at discharge, ASM is continued, and the baby is reassessed after one month. If the baby is normal on examination and seizure free at 1 month, phenobarbitone is discontinued over 2 weeks. If neurological assessment is not normal, an EEG is obtained. If EEG is not overtly paroxysmal, phenobarbitone is tapered and stopped. If EEG is overtly abnormal, the infant is reassessed in the same manner at 3 months and then 3-monthly till 1 year of age (Fig. 9.2).

REFERENCES

1. Tekgul H, Gauvreau K, Soul J, Murphy L, Robertson R, Stewart J, et al. The current etiologic profile and neurodevelopmental outcome of seizures in term newborn infants. Pediatrics. 2006 Apr;117(4):1270–80.
2. Vegda H, Krishnan V, Variane G, Bagayi V, Ivain P, Pressler RM. Neonatal Seizures-Perspective in Low-and Middle-Income Countries. Indian J Pediatr. 2022 Mar;89(3):245–53.
3. Andreolli A, Turco EC, Pedrazzi G, Beghi E, Pisani F. Incidence of Epilepsy after Neonatal Seizures: A Population-Based Study. Neuroepidemiology. 2019;52(3–4):144–51.
4. National Neonatal Perinatal Database. Report for the year 2002–03 [Internet]. Available from: http://www.newbornwhocc.org/pdf/nnpd_report_2002-03.PDF (accessed Jan 8, 2012).
5. Volpe J. Volpe's Neurology of the Newborn. 6th edition. 2018.
6. Tsuchida TN, Wusthoff CJ, Shellhaas RA, Abend NS, Hahn CD, Sullivan JE, et al. American clinical neurophysiology society standardized EEG terminology and categorization for the description of continuous EEG monitoring in neonates: report of the American Clinical Neurophysiology Society critical care monitoring committee. J Clin Neurophysiol Off Publ Am Electroencephalogr Soc. 2013 Apr;30(2):161–73.
7. Clancy RR, Legido A, Lewis D. Occult neonatal seizures. Epilepsia. 1988;29(3):256–61.
8. Murray DM, Boylan GB, Ali I, Ryan CA, Murphy BP, Connolly S. Defining the gap between electrographic seizure burden, clinical expression and staff recognition of neonatal seizures. Arch Dis Child Fetal Neonatal Ed. 2008 May;93(3):F187–191.
9. Pisani F, Spagnoli C, Falsaperla R, Nagarajan L, Ramantani G. Seizures in the neonate: A review of etiologies and outcomes. Seizure. 2021 Feb;85:48–56.
10. Venkataraman Reddy K, Soren C, Jagtap S, Pardhasaradhi Y, Satish S. Clinico-Etiological Profile Of Neonatal Seizures In Term Neonates [Internet]. New Indian Journal of Pediatrics. [cited 2023 Feb 19]. Available from: https://nijp.org/clinico-etiological-profile-of-neonatal-seizures-in-term-neonates/
11. Sands TT, McDonough TL. Recent Advances in Neonatal Seizures. Curr Neurol Neurosci Rep. 2016 Oct;16(10):92.
12. Saxena P, Singh A, Upadhyay A, Gupta P, Sharma S, Vishnubatla S. Effect of Withholding Phenobarbitone Maintenance in Neonatal Seizures: A Randomized Controlled Trial. Indian Pediatr. 2016 Dec 15;53(12):1069–73.
13. Abiramalatha T, Thanigainathan S, Ramaswamy VV, Pressler R, Brigo F, Hartmann H. Antiseizure medications for neonates with seizures. Cochrane Database Syst Rev [Internet]. 2022 [cited 2023 Feb 20];2022(3). Available from: https://www.readcube.com/articles/10.1002%2F14651858.cd014967.
14. Pathak G, Upadhyay A, Pathak U, Chawla D, Goel SP. Phenobarbitone versus phenytoin for treatment of neonatal seizures: an open-label randomized controlled trial. Indian Pediatr. 2013 Aug;50(8):753–7.

15. World Health Organization. Guidelines on neonatal seizures [Internet]. Geneva: World Health Organization; 2011 [cited 2023 Feb 22]. 95 p. Available from: https://apps.who.int/iris/handle/10665/77756.
16. Khan O, Chang E, Cipriani C, Wright C, Crisp E, Kirmani B. Use of intravenous levetiracetam for management of acute seizures in neonates. Pediatr Neurol. 2011 Apr;44(4):265–9.
17. Sharpe C, Reiner GE, Davis SL, Nespeca M, Gold JJ, Rasmussen M, et al. Levetiracetam Versus Phenobarbital for Neonatal Seizures: A Randomized Controlled Trial. Pediatrics. 2020 Jun;145(6):e20193182.
18. Qiao MY, Cui HT, Zhao LZ, Miao JK, Chen QX. Efficacy and Safety of Levetiracetam vs. Phenobarbital for Neonatal Seizures: A Systematic Review and Meta-Analysis. Front Neurol. 2021 Nov 18;12:747745.
19. Susnerwala S, Joshi A, Deshmukh L, Londhe A. Levetiracetam or Phenobarbitone as a First-Line Anticonvulsant in Asphyxiated Term Newborns? An Open-Label, Single-Center, Randomized, Controlled, Pragmatic Trial. Hosp Pediatr. 2022 Jun 8;12(7):647–53.
20. Glass HC, Soul JS, Chang T, Wusthoff CJ, Chu CJ, Massey SL, et al. Safety of Early Discontinuation of Antiseizure Medication After Acute Symptomatic Neonatal Seizures. JAMA Neurol. 2021 Jul 1;78(7):817–25.

CHAPTER

10

Preterm Brain Injury

The two most common forms of brain injury noted in preterm infants are intraventricular hemorrhage (IVH) and periventricular leukomalacia (PVL).[1] These lesions are more common in the smallest and the most premature infants and contribute significantly to mortality, morbidity during hospital stay, and long-term neurodevelopmental impairment. The overall incidence of IVH among VLBW neonates is 20–25% but two thirds of them are of mild to moderate severity (grade 1–2). Severe forms of hemorrhage (grade 3 and periventricular hemorrhagic infarction [PVHI]), although rare, have higher incidence among extremely preterm neonates. About 25% of infants between 501 and 750 g and 14% between 751 and 1000 g develop severe forms of hemorrhage.[2]

INTRAVENTRICULAR HEMORRHAGE (IVH)

The site of IVH in preterm infants is the fragile capillary network of the germinal matrix, which is located between the caudate and thalamic nuclei at the level of or slightly posterior to the foramen of Munro. The germinal matrix is a highly vascularized structure that also serves as the area for origination of neuronal and glial precursors. It begins to involute after 34 weeks of gestation which explains why IVH occurs predominantly in very preterm neonates.

Grades and Diagnosis

Grade I refers to hemorrhage confined to the subependymal germinal matrix with no blood clot in the ventricular lumen while grade II is hemorrhage occupying 10–50% of the lateral ventricles without any ventricular enlargement. Grade III is hemorrhage occupying >50% of the lateral ventricle and associated with ventriculomegaly. Grade IV hemorrhage is a separate notation in Volpe's classification called periventricular hemorrhagic infarction; which is IVH associated with ipsilateral parenchymal hemorrhage.[3]

Ultrasonography is the primary imaging modality for the screening and diagnosis of IVH and parenchymal hemorrhage in neonates because of the ideal acoustic window offered by the anterior fontanelle, easy and quick image acquisition at the bedside, and lack of radiation hazard. It has high sensitivity and specificity for diagnosis of IVH.

Clinical Presentation

There are three presentations of IVH—clinically silent, saltatory and catastrophic, of which the most common is clinically silent presentation. The preterm neonate is often asymptomatic and the only clinical sign may be an unexplained fall in hematocrit. In the saltatory presentation, the symptoms evolve over days to weeks and may present with lethargy, apnea, tone abnormalities and tight popliteal angle on examination. The most striking but the least common is the catastrophic presentation, with rapid evolution over hours and manifests with severe apnea, seizures, altered sensorium, decorticate or decerebrate posturing, hypotension and even death. Because most neonates with IVH are asymptomatic, screening is mandatory in high-risk neonates (see 'Protocol on cranial ultrasound'). Generally, all neonates at high risk for IVH (gestational age <32 weeks or birth weight <1500 g) should undergo screening. More mature preterm infants (32 wks) should also be screened if they experience a turbulent postnatal course (shock requiring inotropes, unexplained anemia, or severe RDS requiring mechanical ventilation).

Consequences

The hemorrhage into the lateral ventricle spreads throughout the ventricular system and into the subarachnoid space where it can trigger obliterative arachnoiditis. The CSF flow can be impaired both inside the ventricles (at the aqueduct of Sylvius) and outside it (at the arachnoid granulations). The consequences of IVH are three-fold (in the temporal order of occurrence):

1. **Damage to germinal matrix** and thereby injury to the glial and neuronal precursors
2. **Periventricular hemorrhagic infarction (PVHI):** noted in 15% of all IVH among VLBW neonates, denotes a parenchymal lesion occurring on the same side as severe IVH. PVHI is actually a venous infarct due to obstruction of the terminal vein by the large IVH (often grade III).

3. **Post-hemorrhagic hydrocephalus (PHH):** Obstruction to the flow of CSF due to particulate matter in the hemorrhage leads to acute ventriculomegaly while progressive dilatation is secondary to obstructive arachidonitis. The rapidity and severity of ventriculomegaly is related to the size of IVH.

Progression

Approximately half of all IVH occur on day 1 of life, an additional 25% on day 2, and another 15% on day 3 of life. Hence a single scan on 3–4th day of life is likely to detect about 90% of all hemorrhages. However, in neonates with birth weight between 500 and 750 g, two thirds of IVH occur on day 1 and it may be reasonable to perform the first scan on day 1 itself. One third of hemorrhages increase in size and the maximum size is usually attained 3–5 days after the onset of hemorrhage. Hence serial ultrasounds are needed to follow the progression of bleed. Even when the initial ultrasounds are normal, it is necessary to repeat scan at around 3 weeks of postnatal age followed by another one closer to 36 weeks' PMA to detect cystic lesions of PVL or ventriculomegaly. Although cranial ultrasounds have a sensitivity of 100% and specificity of 91% for detecting hemorrhages larger than 5 mm, it has limited sensitivity (50%) and specificity (87%) for the diagnosis of PVL lesions.[4]

Complications

1. **PVHI:** The most common sequelae of PVHI is a large porencephalic cyst at the site of the lesion. This lesion is particularly common in preterm neonates with birth weight <750 g, and it accounts for most of the morbidity attributable to IVH. It is usually a single large cyst, often unilateral, on the same side as the large IVH and communicating with the lateral ventricle. In one third of cases, PVHI can be bilateral—the lesion is often asymmetric depending on the size of IVH on the same side. In contrast to PVHI, periventricular leukomalacia (PVL) is due to ischemia of periventricular white matter, is nonhemorrhagic, and results in multiple small or large cysts symmetrically distributed in periventricular area.
2. **Post hemorrhagic hydrocephalus (PHH):** Among all VLBW neonates with IVH, approximately 25% develop ventricular dilatation or hydrocephalus.[5] The exact incidence of PHH depends on the severity of IVH; the incidence being 4% with grade 1 IVH, 12% with grade 2 IVH, and 70% with severe grades.[5] The injury

to the periventricular white matter accompanying hydrocephalus is due to excessive pressure and distortion of nerve fiber tracts, free radical injury, and inflammation from iron and cytokines.

Management

Intraventricular Hemorrhage

The focus should be on preventing IVH in the first place (discussed below), management during acute phase, and management of complications. During acute phase, ensure airway patency, breathing and circulation. Maintain blood pressure in normal range, avoid hypercarbia, acidosis, hypoxia, rapid fluid boluses, pneumothorax, and seizures. Serial ultrasounds should be done to monitor progress of IVH and the development of complications.

Clinical monitoring in a neonate after IVH include biweekly or alternate day measurement of occipitofrontal circumference (OFC) and monitoring for clinical signs and symptoms of raised intracranial pressure (ICP). Serial ultrasounds are mandatory to monitor the progression of severe IVH and to measure the size of lateral ventricles because the classical signs of raised ICP and head enlargement are delayed for days to weeks after the onset of ventriculomegaly (Table 10.1). With a large IVH, there is a greater

Table 10.1: Criteria for diagnosis of hydrocephalus following IVH
Excessive head growth • Normal head growth between 26 and 32 weeks' gestation is approximately 1 mm/day and between 32 and 40 weeks is 0.7 mm/day. • A persistent increase of >2 mm/day should raise the suspicion of hydrocephalus. • It is recommended to measure head circumference on alternate days: increments of >4 mm in 2 days or >14 mm/week is labeled as hydrocephalus.
Signs and symptoms of raised ICP • Bulging fontanelle, splayed sutures, symptoms like lethargy, poor feeding, vomiting. • Neurological signs include changes in muscle tone, down set eyes and seizures.
Cranial ultrasound • 2D ultrasound to measure ventricular sizes; Levene's index provides guidance on intervention for various gestational ages. • Doppler ultrasound of anterior or middle cerebral artery to measure resistive index (RI). – RI > 0.85 suggests raised intracranial pressure. – RI = 1 (absent diastolic flow-impaired perfusion).

likelihood of rapid ventricular enlargement within days and need for intervention.

Levene's index[6] is measured from the falx to the lateral wall of the body of the ventricle. Reference ranges have been published according to gestational ages and measurement exceeding 4 mm above the 97th centile for ventricular index ('action line') indicates the need for therapeutic intervention. There is no role of ICP measurement in the management of PHH as progressive ventricular dilatation and head enlargement occurs first before an increase in CSF pressure.

Post-hemorrhagic Hydrocephalus

Among infants with PHH, spontaneous arrest of ventriculomegaly without any treatment occurs in one third; the remaining two-thirds require intervention (serial lumbar punctures in 14%, surgical treatment with insertion of a ventricular reservoir or ventriculo-peritoneal shunt in 34%, while 18% die).[5] The available interventions include temporary measures like serial lumbar punctures (LP), repeated aspiration of CSF through a ventricular access device, and permanent insertion of a ventriculoperitoneal (VP) shunt. Use of diuretic agents like acetazolamide and furosemide to decrease CSF production is associated with a higher risk of neurological complications, morbidity, and mortality, and hence is not recommended.[7]

While the optimal time for CSF tap is not clear, we follow a combination of clinical and objective evidence of ventriculomegaly to decide when to do therapeutic LP. Presence of two or more of the following features is taken as indication for performing therapeutic CSF tap:

- Head circumference increase >14 mm/week or >2 mm/day for *2 weeks*.
- Ventriculomegaly: Levene index greater than 'action line' (>97th centile + 4 mm).
- Features of raised ICP like bulging fontanelle, splayed sutures or neurological signs (lethargy, poor feeding, tone abnormalities or seizures).
- Resistive index >0.85 on Doppler of intracranial vessels.

Serial LP is effective only if communication exists between lateral ventricles and lumbar subarachnoid space. A minimum of 10 ml/kg of CSF and maximum of 20 ml/kg needs to be removed. The rate of removal should not be faster than 1 ml/kg/min to avoid complications like apnea, bradycardia and desaturation.[8] If LP is not successful in removing CSF or if the hydrocephalus is obstructive, ventricular tap is required. Ventricular puncture is, however, associated higher risk of CSF infection and development of loculated hydrocephalus.

Therapeutic LP produces an immediate improvement in symptoms of raised ICP but if symptoms persist or recur, a repeat LP can be performed based on the criteria described above. However, routine use of serial LP is not recommended to delay or avoid permanent shunt placement.[9] When the need for CSF removal exceeds 2 lumbar punctures or more than one ventricular tap, surgical placement of a ventricular access device (VAD) or ventriculo-subgaleal (VSG) shunt should be considered. Due to high rate of primary shunt failure (17% within 3 months of insertion)[10] and shunt infections (15.5%), VAD or VSG is often the first choice rather than a ventriculo-peritoneal shunt in infants.[11]

CSF tapping from the ventricular reservoir (ventriculosubgaleal shunts are self-draining) can continue as long as the following criteria are met—normal head growth and CSF protein <150 mg/dL and free of infection. Once these criteria are met and the infant has reached at least 2.5 kg weight, one can temporarily stop the reservoir taps and monitor head size. Approximately half of the infants respond to temporary surgical measures and may not need a permanent VP shunt placement. However, if the head growth is excessive despite these measures and the above criteria are met (infant weight of 2.5 kg and CSF protein has decreased to less than 150–200 mg/dl and is free of infection), VP shunt insertion is planned. The interval between VAD insertion and the decision to do VP shunt may be 4 weeks or more. Shunt infection and shunt malfunction are two important complications that require monitoring after shunt insertion.

Outcome and Prognosis

The severity of IVH is the major predictor of adverse short-term outcome (mortality and need for surgery). While the risk of mortality is only 4% with grade 3 IVH, almost 75% neonates with a parenchymal hemorrhage or grade 4 IVH die. The risk of neuromotor and cognitive impairment is more related to the presence of parenchymal hemorrhage than the presence or management of hydrocephalus.[12] Motor deficits and abnormal DQ occurred in 54% and 8%, respectively among neonates with grade 3 hemorrhage, while the same were 100% and 78%, respectively with grade 4 IVH.

PERIVENTRICULAR LEUKOMALACIA

Periventricular leukomalacia (PVL) refers to focal and diffuse white matter injury (WMI) that occur in the periventricular region of the brain.[1] The focal component involves loss of all cellular elements (premyelinating oligodendrocyte, axons and inter-neurons) deep in periventricular white matter. The injury evolves over several weeks into small macroscopic cystic lesions readily visualized by cranial ultrasound (cystic PVL) or as multiple microcystic lesions that evolve into glial scars and not readily seen by neuroimaging (non-cystic PVL). Cystic PVL (c-PVL) is rare in the current era and the majority of cases (up to 70% of preterm neonates) are constituted by non-cystic and diffuse PVL.

c-PVL, classified according to the grading system of deVries *et al.*[13] generally take 4 weeks to appear and sometimes disappear altogether leaving behind only ventriculomegaly. In diffuse PVL (d-PVL), the main target of injury is premyelinating oligodendrocyte that finally results in impaired myelination in various regions of the brain including cerebral white matter, thalamus, basal ganglia, cerebral cortex, brainstem, and cerebellum. Diffuse PVL is recognized in MRI as signal abnormalities, disturbances in diffusion parameters (diffusion tensor imaging) and decreased volume of neuronal structures (volumetric MRI) as early as at term equivalent age (40 weeks' PMA).

The risk factors for development of PVL include prematurity, multiple pregnancy (monochorionic twins), chorioamnionitis, intrauterine growth restriction, fetal distress, hypotension in postnatal period, hypocarbia, sepsis, and use of postnatal corticosteroids. The pathogenesis is mediated through an interplay between hypoxia, ischemia and inflammation of the oligodendrocyte progenitor cells present in the periventricular area of infants born at 23–32 weeks of gestation.

The clinical correlate of cystic PVL is spastic diplegia, while non-cystic PVL and diffuse PVL correlate with the cognitive, attention, and behavioral deficits observed later in childhood usually in the absence of major motor deficits. Among VLBW infants, 5–10% develop cerebral palsy and 25–50% develop significant cognitive and behavioral deficits. Given that cranial ultrasound lacks sensitivity to diagnose diffuse white matter injury and structured evaluation using a MRI at term equivalent age (40 weeks' PMA) predicts neurodevelopmental outcome in childhood,[14] there has been an increase in use of MRI in preterm neonates before discharge.

However, MRI cannot be recommended as a routine diagnostic or prognostic tool for evaluating all high-risk neonates at present.[15]

Prevention of Preterm Brain Injury

Table 10.2 enlists the evidence based interventions[16] for preventing preterm brain injury.

Table 10.2: Potential strategies to decrease risk of brain injury in preterm Infants[16]

Period	*Intervention*
Antenatal	• Prevent preterm delivery • Regionalization of care: Lesser odds of mortality if delivery occurs in well-equipped centers compared with less specialist centers. • *In-utero* transfer: Transport of preterm neonates after birth (the first 48 hours of life) is associated with increased rates of severe IVH; ideal strategy is to transfer the pregnant woman. • Antenatal steroids: Reduces IVH (all grades) by 46%. • Antenatal magnesium sulfate in women at risk of preterm birth <32 weeks' gestation decreases the risk of CP, the risk of severe and moderate CP, and the incidence of gross motor dysfunction. • Antibiotics for PPROM: Prolongs pregnancy, decreases EONS by 30%, fewer abnormal cranial ultrasound scans by 20%.
Postnatal	• Delayed cord clamping: Early benefits—Hemodynamic stability, less inotropes, less need for blood transfusion; Later benefits - Recent studies have shown improved motor function at 18–22 months. • Caffeine for apnea of prematurity: CAP trial showed that caffeine in the first 10 days decreased the incidence of CP and cognitive impairment at 18–21 months in at-risk LBW infants. • Indomethacin prophylaxis: Significantly reduces the incidence of severe IVH but no difference in developmental outcomes at 18–24 months was noted. We do not use Indomethacin prophylaxis in our unit. • Ventilator strategies: – Volume targeted ventilation produces a significant reduction in hypocarbia compared with pressure-limited ventilation. This translates into 30% reduction in the combined outcome of PVL or grades 3–4 IVH. – Synchronized mechanical ventilation. – Early surfactant administration. – Minimizing complications like pneumothorax. – Minimize mean airway pressure, extremes of $PaCO_2$. – Minimize use of postnatal steroids. • Prevent late onset sepsis, NEC and postnatal growth restriction.

REFERENCES

1. Volpe JJ. Brain injury in premature infants: a complex amalgam of destructive and developmental disturbances. Lancet Neurol. 2009;8(1):110–24.
2. Fanaroff AA, Stoll BJ, Wright LL, et al. Trends in neonatal morbidity and mortality for very low birthweight infants. Am J Obstet Gynecol. 2007;196(2):147 e141–8.
3. Volpe JJ. Intracranial Hemorrhage: Germinal Matrix–Intraventricular Hemorrhage of the Premature Infant. 5th ed. Philadelphia: Saunders Elsevier; 2008.
4. Carson SC, Hertzberg BS, Bowie JD, Burger PC. Value of sonography in the diagnosis of intracranial hemorrhage and periventricular leukomalacia: a postmortem study of 35 cases. AJR Am J Roentgenol. 1990;155(3):595–601.
5. Murphy BP, Inder TE, Rooks V, et al. Posthaemorrhagic ventricular dilatation in the premature infant: natural history and predictors of outcome. Arch Dis Child Fetal Neonatal Ed. 2002;87(1):F37–41.
6. Levene MI. Measurement of the growth of the lateral ventricles in preterm infants with real-time ultrasound. Arch Dis Child. 1981;56(12):900–4.
7. Whitelaw A, Kennedy CR, Brion LP. Diuretic therapy for newborn infants with posthemorrhagic ventricular dilatation. Cochrane Database Syst Rev. 2001(2):CD002270.
8. Whitelaw A, Aquilina K. Management of posthaemorrhagic ventricular dilatation. Arch Dis Child Fetal Neonatal Ed. 2012;97(3):F229.
9. Shooman D, Portess H, Sparrow O. A review of the current treatment methods for posthaemorrhagic hydrocephalus of infants. Cerebrospinal Fluid Res. 2009;6:1.
10. Fulkerson DH, Vachhrajani S, Bohnstedt BN, et al. Analysis of the risk of shunt failure or infection related to cerebrospinal fluid cell count, protein level, and glucose levels in low-birth-weight premature infants with posthemorrhagic hydrocephalus. J Neurosurg Pediatr. 2011;7(2):147–51.
11. Willis B, Javalkar V, Vannemreddy P, et al. Ventricular reservoirs and ventriculoperitoneal shunts for premature infants with posthemorrhagic hydrocephalus: an institutional experience. J Neurosurg Pediatr. 2009;3(2):94–100.
12. Levy ML, Masri LS, McComb JG. Outcome for preterm infants with germinal matrix hemorrhage and progressive hydrocephalus. Neurosurgery. 1997;41(5):1111–1117; discussion 1117–8.
13. de Vries LS, Eken P, Dubowitz LM. The spectrum of leukomalacia using cranial ultrasound. Behav Brain Res. 1992;49(1):1–6.
14. Anderson PJ, Treyvaud K, Neil JJ, et al. Associations of Newborn Brain Magnetic Resonance Imaging with Long-Term Neurodevelopmental Impairments in Very Preterm Children. J Pediatr. 2017;187:58-65 e51.
15. Pierrat V, Duquennoy C, van Haastert IC, Ernst M, Guilley N, de Vries LS. Ultrasound diagnosis and neurodevelopmental outcome of localised and extensive cystic periventricular leucomalacia. Arch Dis Child Fetal Neonatal Ed. 2001;84(3):F151–6.
16. Lea CL, Smith-Collins A, Luyt K. Protecting the premature brain: current evidence-based strategies for minimising perinatal brain injury in preterm infants. Arch Dis Child Fetal Neonatal Ed. 2017;102(2):F176–82.

Section

4

Cardiovascular System

CHAPTER

11

Patent Ductus Arteriosus in a Preterm Neonate

The ductus arteriosus that connects the pulmonary artery to the descending aorta is an essential conduit of fetal circulation and diverts a large portion of combined ventricular output away from the lungs. After birth at term, the ductus constricts within the first 24–48 hours of life, aided by the expansion of the lungs, an increase in oxygenation, and a fall in vasodilatory prostaglandins (*functional closure*). Subsequently, medial and intimal connective tissue proliferation and muscle atrophy convert this muscular structure into a thin ligamentum arteriosum, typically over the next three weeks (*anatomical closure*). In a preterm infant, the ductus tissue has a lower intrinsic tone, less smooth muscle fiber, fewer sub-endothelial cushions, and a high concentration of vasodilatory prostaglandins that predispose to a delay or failure of the ductus to close postnatally.

The incidence of patent ductus arteriosus (PDA) varies inversely with gestation. About 15–40% of very low birth weight infants (<1500 g) have a PDA. In extremely preterm infants (<28 weeks), the incidence is as high as 70–80%.[1–3]

HEMODYNAMIC CONSEQUENCES AND CLINICAL SIGNS

Significant shunting of blood from left-to-right circulation through the ductus can lead to complications related to pulmonary over circulation and systemic hypoperfusion. The clinical signs and complications associated with PDA depend on the magnitude of the left-to-right shunt, the ability of the neonate to initiate compensatory mechanisms, and the presence of co-morbid conditions, such as sepsis and respiratory distress syndrome.

Pulmonary over circulation can cause a reduction in lung compliance and ineffective gas exchange, leading to a prolonged need for respiratory support. Alveolar flooding can lead to protein leakage and surfactant inactivation, further accelerating the development of bronchopulmonary dysplasia (BPD).[4] An increased volume load to the left ventricular (LV) is also poorly tolerated, as preterm neonates have a poorly compliant LV with a limited capacity to increase stroke volume. Therefore, they compensate by increasing the heart rate. LV remodels in response to volume overload and assumes a larger, spherical shape.

Ductal 'steal' implies significant retrograde blood flow from the thoracic and abdominal aorta to the pulmonary circulation. A large ductus can steal up to 50% of the total aortic flow in neonates resulting in *systemic hypoperfusion*, especially in the 'non-vital' renal and mesenteric circulation. Contrary to the belief, ductal steal is present throughout the cardiac cycle but is best demonstrated during diastole on an echocardiogram as a retrograde flow in the descending aorta. Low diastolic aortic pressure can compromise coronary perfusion and aggravate myocardial dysfunction. Thus, a large PDA can contribute to significant morbidities, including renal insufficiency, necrotizing enterocolitis, intraventricular hemorrhage, myocardial ischemia, BPD, and mortality.[4,5]

DIAGNOSIS

A. Clinical

As outlined above, the clinical signs of a hemodynamically significant PDA (hsPDA) are due to hyperdynamic circulation resulting in bounding pulses (easily palpable dorsalis pedis), wide pulse pressure (>25 mm of Hg), a hyperactive precordium (visible pulsations in more than two rib spaces), systolic murmur (ejection systolic; rarely pansystolic or continuous), and persistent tachycardia, and are generally noted on day 3 or 4 of life. In a ventilated neonate, PDA can present with increased ventilatory settings, higher FiO_2 requirement, hypercarbia, metabolic acidosis, and recurrent apnea. Although these signs are reasonably specific, they lack sensitivity; a large hemodynamically significant PDA can remain clinically silent, causing a delay of 1–4 days in diagnosis if one were to rely on clinical signs alone.[6] A high index of suspicion is therefore required, particularly in extremely preterm neonates, to aid in early diagnosis and treatment.

B. Role of Echocardiography

Echocardiography is the gold standard for the diagnosis of PDA. It can assist in the evaluation of the presence of PDA; the direction and velocity of the ductal shunt ductal steal; and to rule out duct-dependent systemic or pulmonary circulation, where the closure of ductus is contraindicated (Table 11.1).[7,8]

These echocardiographic parameters are not specific for PDA in isolation, but their presence as a constellation, especially with clinical signs, significantly increases the likelihood of a hsPDA. The most common parameter used is the La/Ao ratio, where a value >1.5 has a sensitivity of 79% and a specificity of 95% after 24 hours of birth.[9] Presence of atrial shunting at the foramen ovale decreases the performance of La/Ao, E/A, and IVRT to detect a PDA. Diastolic reversal at the descending aorta and increased LPA diastolic velocity are more specific markers.[10]

While echocardiography is indicated in all preterm infants with suspected PDA, its role as a routine screening tool in all preterm neonates is being questioned as it does not offer clear benefits in terms of diagnosis or management. In extremely preterm neonates, however, routine screening for hsPDA is advisable to ensure early targeted treatment. Echocardiography can also be used to follow up spontaneous or therapeutic closure of a PDA. A practical approach for the timing of screening echocardiography can be found in Table 11.2.

Limitations of echocardiography: Although the criteria for assessment of hsPDA are established, there is no uniform agreement on the threshold to initiate treatment. Many neonatal units lack ready access to echocardiography, and it is still a consultative tool, making initial and serial assessments practically challenging. Moreover, echocardiography is highly operator dependent, and the findings should always be supplemented with clinical information.

C. Other Diagnostic Tests

Chest radiograph findings are nonspecific. Features like cardiomegaly, pulmonary plethora, and left atrial enlargement to appear late on a radiograph when significant PDA leads to congestive heart failure.

D. Role of Biomarkers

Three biomarkers [atrial natriuretic peptide (ANP), cardiac troponin T (TnT), and brain natriuretic peptide (BNP)] have been investigated as predictive and diagnostic tools for PDA. BNP, the most widely studied biomarker, correlates well with echocardiographic markers

Table 11.1: Echocardiographic findings used to evaluate ductus arteriosus and its hemodynamic significance

Parameter	*Echo view and mode*	*Echocardiographic findings*	*Parameters indicating the hemodynamic significance of DA8*
Ductal patency and size	High parasternal ductal view, 2D mode	**Ductal patency:** Two-dimensional (2D) imaging of the ductus in the high parasternal view can reveal a widely open ductus, but confirmation of its patency requires a color Doppler to indicate the direction of the shunt. A duct shunting blood from left to right produces a red signal which appears strongly contrasted against the blue signal in the left pulmonary artery (LPA) and descending aorta (DA). (Fig. 11.1a) However, a pure right-to-left shunting ductus (blue color on Doppler) will likely be missed. **Ductal size:** Measure the duct diameter at the narrowest portion of the ductal length (isthmus) in mm. (Fig. 11.1b)	Transductal diameter of >1.5 mm
Direction, velocity, and flow pattern shunt	High parasternal ductal view, color/ PW mode	The direction and velocity of the shunt depend on the pressure difference between pulmonary and systemic circulation; the shunt will be left-to-right if the pulmonary pressure is lower and vice versa. In almost equal pressures, the shunt can occur in both directions.	• Ductal velocity <2 meters/sec • Pulsatile left-to-right flow • Right to left shunt less than 30% of total time of cardiac cycle.

(Contd.)

Table 11.1: Echocardiographic findings used to evaluate ductus arteriosus and its hemodynamic significance (*Contd.*)

Parameter	*Echo view and mode*	*Echocardiographic findings*	*Parameters indicating the hemodynamic significance of DA8*
Assessing the hemodynamic significance of a shunt	Parasternal long axis view (PLAX)/Ductal view/Suprasternal aortic arch view	**Signs of pulmonary overcirculation:** A significant left-to-right shunt causes LV volume overload. This leads to an increase in left atrial and left ventricular size. **Signs of systemic hypoperfusion:** With increasing ductal shunt size, the normal low-velocity antegrade diastolic flow in the descending aorta decreases progressively and becomes absent, followed by retrograde in direction.	• LA: Ao root diameter ratio ≥1.4 (PLAX, M mode) • Left ventricular/ aortic root width ratio >2.2 (PLAX, M mode) • Antegrade left pulmonary artery diastolic flow >40 cm/sec (Ductal view, PW) • Descending aorta diastolic flow absence or reversal (subcostal view for flow in celiac or superior mesenteric artery, PW)
		Myocardial performance: Due to an increased left-to-right shunt and LV overload, the left ventricular stroke volume and left ventricular output also increase.	• LV output >320 ml/kg/min • E/A ratio >1 • Isovolumetric relaxation time (IVRT) <45 msec • Myocardial performance index (MPI)

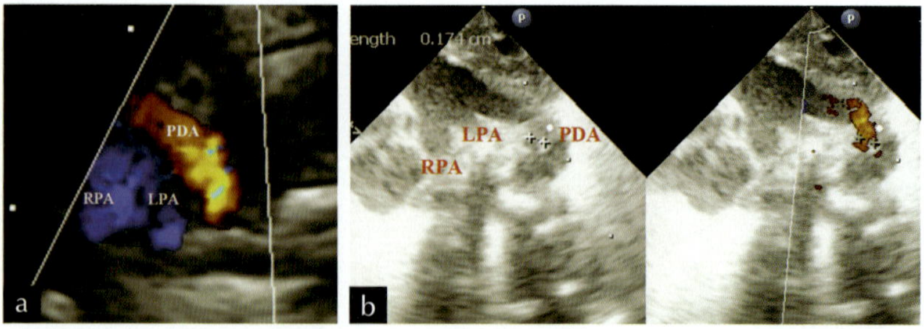

Fig. 11.1: Echocardiographic diagnosis of a PDA on the ductal view ('three-legged stool' appearance)

Table 11.2: Recommended timing of echocardiographic screening for PDA in preterm neonates[11]

Type of screening	*Gestation*	*Timing of screening for hsPDA*
Early targeted (Asymptomatic)	≤28 weeks	36 ± 6 hours, 72 ± 6 hours, and day 7
	29–30 weeks	36 ± 6 hours and 72 ± 6 hours
Symptomatic	<32 weeks	At the onset of symptoms

of PDA and can be assayed at the bedside using commercially available kits. BNP levels are higher in significant PDA and decline after therapeutic closure. The good sensitivity and specificity of BNP assay (88% and 92%, respectively), the easy availability of bedside kits, the lesser cost compared to echocardiography, and its decline in treatment response makes it an attractive biomarker.[11] However, BNP levels in preterm neonates vary with gestational age (higher in preterm), postnatal age (highest in the first three days and gradually declines with age), renal function, and the type of kit used. The test becomes accurate from day 3 of life and hence cannot be used within the first 48 hours of life. Therefore, BNP can be used only as an add-on test and cannot replace echocardiography for diagnosis or management. Due to the variability of assays across various settings, universal recommendations for standard thresholds of the biomarkers remain challenging.

MANAGEMENT

Despite a large number of studies done to ascertain the optimal treatment strategy for PDA, the management remains controversial. There has yet to be a clear consensus on whether PDA should be closed and, if so, when, how, and in whom? A lack of proven benefit after PDA closure can possibly be explained by the following reasons:[12]

1. There is no causal association between hsPDA and short- and long-term morbidities. Most PDAs in preterm neonates are known to close spontaneously with time; up to 90% of PDA close spontaneously among 30 weeks gestation, while it is around 65% among those <30 weeks' gestation.[13]
2. Studies have used variable definitions of 'hemodynamic significance,' The overall results have been diluted by some 'non-hemodynamically significant' PDAs.
3. In randomized trials focused on medical or surgical treatment of PDA in the intervention arm, up to one-third of the controls receiving rescue treatment to close a PDA. This overlap introduces bias in our ability to interpret the studies.[1,2] The frequent need for rescue treatment in placebo groups has led to contamination of the intervention, introducing bias.[2,14] Emerging evidence suggests that treatments that close the patent ductus may be detrimental. Neither individual trials, pooled data from groups of randomized-controlled trials, nor critical examination of the immediate consequences of treatment provide evidence that medical or surgical closure of the ductus is beneficial in preterm infants. These conclusions are supported by sufficient evidence. Neither continued routine use of these treatments nor additional clinical trials using similar designs seems to be justified. A definitive trial, comparing current standard management with novel strategies not primarily intended to achieve ductal closure, may be necessary to resolve doubts regarding the quality or conduct of prior studies.
4. Although hsPDA has been associated with significant neonatal morbidities such as BPD and necrotizing enterocolitis, the evidence that treatment improves either short-term or long-term outcomes is bleak.[15,16] Moreover, PDA closure alone might be insufficient to improve the associated morbidities or mortality.

Further, non-steroidal anti-inflammatory agents, the mainstay of PDA's pharmacological closure, are associated with significant side effects. Conversely, observational studies have also pointed out that persistent exposure to a PDA is not without harm and can be associated with a higher risk of mortality in preterm neonates <29 weeks' gestation.[2,17]

While considering these nuances in the existing literature, the clinician often must decide which neonates one can await spontaneous closure of PDA. Such a 'wait and watch' strategy seems reasonable in a more mature infant (>28 weeks' GA) who is stable, tolerating feeds, and on minimal or noninvasive respiratory support.[2] In such cases, fluid restriction and appropriate ventilatory titration can be coupled with watchful waiting. Although recent evidence in extremely preterm neonates reveals expectant management as a non-inferior approach to early treatment in terms of BPD, NEC, and mortality,[18] it may be unadvisable to wait watchfully, and early treatment is usually recommended.

A. Nonpharmacological Strategies

1. **Fluid restriction:** Although evidence for this approach is lacking, a careful attention to fluid balance is recommended for management of PDA. In a restricted regime, fluid intake is at most 120 to 130 mL/kg beyond day 3 of life. Ensuring adequate urine output and monitoring serum sodium levels during fluid restriction is important. Fluid restriction should be discontinued if serum sodium exceeds 147 mEq/L or increases by >4 mEq/L every 8 hours.[13] In neonates beyond the first week and on full enteral feeds, a fluid intake of up to 150 ml/kg/day may be permitted, with calorie-dense feeds to ensure optimal weight gain.
2. **Ventilatory strategies:** If neonates require invasive ventilation, higher PEEP (at least 4.5–5 cm H_2O) and lower Ti (0.35 s) may be helpful, though data is limited.[13,19] Conservative treatment may result in similar outcome, but without exposure to the harmful side effects of medication. A retrospective analysis revealed a ductal closure rate of 94% after conservative treatment with adjustment of ventilation. There is no role for the use of diuretics in the management of PDA.[20]

Observational studies have noted that conservative therapy is a feasible option with closure rates as reasonable as pharmacological therapy and may decrease the need for pharmacotherapy and ligation. However, if the neonate does not show clinical improvement or worsens, one should consider therapeutic closure.

B. Pharmacological Closure of PDA

Pharmacotherapy should be used in a select group of neonates in whom PDA might be actively contributing to hemodynamic compromise, and the risk of non-closure may be associated with morbidities. Examples include:

- Extreme preterm neonate with echocardiographically proven hemodynamically significant ductus arteriosus. We define hsPDA as a PDA with ductal diameter >1.5 mm with one of the following: LA/Ao ratio >1.5, LV/Ao ratio >2.2, a retrograde diastolic flow in descending aorta, celiac or cerebral arteries (>30% of antegrade flow), and left ventricular output >320 mL/kg/min.
- Preterm neonates with severe symptoms related to PDA like congestive cardiac failure, pulmonary hemorrhage, pulmonary edema, and inability to be weaned from mechanical ventilation.

The most widely studied and used drugs in the closure of PDA are the non-steroidal anti-inflammatory agents, namely indomethacin and ibuprofen, which are non-selective cyclo-oxygenase inhibitors. Both indomethacin and ibuprofen are equally efficacious, with a closure rate of 70–80%. However, there are concerns regarding their safety in neonates, especially in necrotizing enterocolitis, intestinal perforation, active bleeding, and concomitant use of corticosteroids, where they are contraindicated. The publication of case reports and further randomized trials has created increased interest in paracetamol as a lucrative and efficacious agent for ductal closure. Paracetamol inhibits prostaglandin production through inhibition of the peroxidase enzyme. Moreover, paracetamol has been shown efficacious in various situations where NSAIDs are either contraindicated or have failed to achieve PDA closure. A comparison of the three commonly used drugs, dosage, and regimens are shown in Table 11.3.

Monitoring during drug therapy: Monitor for side effects of therapy (Table 11.4) during medical closure of PDA, mainly if an NSAID is used.

Essential Considerations when Treating a PDA

1. **Choice of medication:** A recent network meta-analysis in 2018 revealed that high-dose oral ibuprofen had the highest efficacy regarding PDA closure and need for surgical ligation, with 3.6 times higher odds of closure than intravenous ibuprofen.[21] Another metanalysis in 2022, which included 70 trials, concluded that high-dose ibuprofen had the highest net clinical benefit in terms of closure and adverse events, followed by standard

Table 11.3: Drugs for medical management of PDA

	Indomethacin	*Ibuprofen*	*Paracetamol (PCM)*
Preparation	Intravenous preparation requires reconstitution. Oral suspension is not available but can be prepared by dissolving the powder content of a 25 mg indomethacin capsule in 25 ml of distilled water.	IV Ibuprofen is not available in India. The oral formulation is the most common and readily available form in India.	Available both as an injection (10 mg/ml) and oral suspension
Dosage (same for intravenous and oral formulation)	Loading dose: 0.2 mg/kg/dose Subsequent dose (adjusted as per postnatal age): • <2 days: 0.1 mg/kg/dose 12 hourly × 2 doses • 2–7 days: 0.2 mg/kg/dose 12 hourly × 2 doses • >7 days: 0.25 mg/kg/dose 12 hourly × 2 doses	Loading dose: 10 mg/kg/dose Subsequent dose: 5 mg/kg/dose 24 hourly × 2 doses (High dose Ibuprofen: 20 mg/kg/dose followed by 10 mg/kg/dose 24 hourly for two doses)[21]	• 15 mg/kg every 6 hours for three days
Drug administration	Administered as an infusion over 30 minutes or as a continuous infusion over 36 hours	Administered as an infusion over 30 minutes	• Administered as an infusion over 15–30 min
Contraindications	Thrombocytopenia (< 60 000/mm^3), the clinical bleeding tendency (bloody gastric aspirates, bloody stools, pulmonary hemorrhage, oozing from puncture sites), raised serum creatinine >1.6 mg/dl, urine output <1 ml/kg/h during the preceding 8 hours, severe IVH, and NEC.	Same as Indomethacin	• Elevated liver enzymes or hepatic failure.

(Contd.)

Table 11.3: Drugs for medical management of PDA *(Contd.)*

Side effects	Transient or permanent renal impairment, NEC, gastrointestinal hemorrhage or perforation, alteration of platelet function, and impairment of cerebral blood flow or cerebral blood flow velocity	Lesser risk of NEC and transient renal insufficiency	• No known renal adverse effects. Lower antiplatelet activity.
Persistence of a hemodynamically significant ductus at the end of 1st course	A repeat course (3 doses) of indomethacin can be considered (maximum of 2 courses). The first course can be prolonged by giving two more doses of 0.1 mg/kg Q 24 hourly. However, if the ductus fails to respond, it is unlikely to respond to further courses.	A repeat course (3 doses) for a maximum of 2 courses can be considered. Extension of the initial course by giving two more doses of 5 mg/kg Q 24 hourly can be considered. However, if the ductus fails to respond, it is unlikely to respond to further courses.	• A longer course of 15 mg/kg 6 hourly for 6–7 days can be considered based on echocardiography to guide treatment.

Table 11.4: Parameters to be monitored during therapeutic closure of PDA with NSAIDs

Baseline	Urine output, RFT, platelet count
Monitoring during therapy	
Daily	Urine output
Alternate day	RFT, platelet counts (daily if baseline counts are <150,000/mm^3)

dose oral PCM in neonates >28 weeks. Although the evidence is lacking in those less than 28 weeks, the best option was deemed to be oral PCM in terms of net clinical benefit.[22] IV Ibuprofen is not available in India.

Indomethacin versus ibuprofen: Both indomethacin and ibuprofen are equally efficacious, with a PDA closure rate of 70–80% in preterm babies 32 weeks. No difference was noted in treatment failure rates when ibuprofen (oral or IV) was compared with indomethacin (oral or IV). However, ibuprofen has a better safety profile (lesser renal impairment and NEC) and may be preferred.[23]

Oral paracetamol (PCM) versus ibuprofen/indomethacin: In several case reports, the efficacy of paracetamol for PDA closure was around 70–80%. Paracetamol is now preferred because it lacks the significant side effects of other NSAIDs and its applicability when contraindicated. In a Cochrane review including 27 trials and 2278 neonates, there was low- to moderate-quality evidence that there is little or no difference in the effectiveness of PCM compared to indomethacin or ibuprofen.[24] There are a few concerns with PCM, including its adverse effects on the developing brain in neonatal mice and the later development of autism in human children after prenatal exposure been reported. Hence, further studies are needed before paracetamol can be recommended as the universal drug of choice for medical closure.

2. **Route of medication:** Randomized studies comparing oral versus IV ibuprofen showed a higher closure rate with oral than IV formulation.[25] One can use IV formulation if the neonate is not on oral feeds.
3. **Feeding during medical closure:** Most neonatologists refrain from feed advancement and often withhold enteral feeds while using ibuprofen or indomethacin for PDA. A randomized trial showed that a neonate in whom feeds have just been initiated will achieve full enteral feeds earlier if they continue receiving trophic feedings rather than kept nil orally. Continued enteral feeding did not increase the risk of infection, necrotizing enterocolitis, or spontaneous intestinal perforation.[26] In our unit, we continue the same volume of feeds if the neonate is already on oral feeds and advance once the course is completed or allow trophic feeds unless there is feed intolerance or other contraindications of feeding.

4. **Timing of therapy:** The timing of treatment can be prophylactic, early targeted, and symptomatic (early and late).[8]
   a. **Prophylactic therapy** refers to the closure of PDA in high-risk preterm neonates even before it produces any symptoms. While prophylactic ibuprofen decreases the incidence of symptomatic PDA, the need for surgical ligation, and the incidence of pulmonary hemorrhage, it does not alter long-term outcomes. There is a trend toward decreased risk of IVH with an increased incidence of oliguria, questioning its overall benefit.[25] prophylactic indomethacin significantly reduced the incidence of severe grades of IVH with no translation of the effect to improved long-term neurodevelopment.[27] Prophylactic therapy is not recommended due to an unclear risk versus benefit.
   b. **Symptomatic treatment** is when signs of PDA first appear between 2–5 days of age (**early**) or until the second week of life (days 10–14, **late**). Whether to close early vs. late depends on the severity of symptoms and the neonate's gestational age. Late treatment may be justified in mature neonates with mild signs of PDA (metabolic acidosis, murmur, bounding pulses). Still, an early closure would be reasonable in very preterm neonates with symptomatic ductus and those with life-threatening manifestations like pulmonary hemorrhage, hypotension, or rapid respiratory deterioration. Ductus that remains patent beyond two weeks of age may not respond to drug therapy well, and adverse hemodynamic consequences might have already occurred.
   c. In extremely preterm neonates, Kluckow et al. showed that an **early-targeted therapy** based on echocardiographic parameters between 3–12 hours of life reduces the incidence of pulmonary hemorrhage and the need for later pharmacological closure.[28] However, the investigators stopped enrollment early due to the non-availability of Indomethacin. However, a recent trial of 273 extreme preterm neonates failed to demonstrate any benefit of early targeted treatment with Ibuprofen in terms of mortality or major complications (severe NEC or moderate to severe BPD).[29] Authors speculated that it may be due to adverse effects of Ibuprofen negating any benefit achieved with PDA treatment. Despite this many advanced centers hold the view that in neonates <26 weeks, the early targeted treatment is beneficial, especially in those with large shunts and needing respiratory support.[30]

5. **Surgical ligation:** Surgery should be considered if medical management fails (after two courses of pharmacotherapy) or if there are contraindications to medical therapy like NEC, gastrointestinal perforation, or renal impairment. Meta-analyses of studies comparing surgical vs. medical treatment noted that neonates undergoing surgery are at an increased risk of neurodevelopmental impairment, chronic lung disease, and ROP but lesser mortality risk.[31] However, surgery is more likely to have been performed on a sicker ventilator-dependent infant with other comorbidities.

   Surgical closure, although definite, is associated with complications like pneumothorax, chylothorax, infection, and vocal cord palsy. A peculiar hemodynamic complication of surgical ligation called the post ligation cardiac syndrome (PLCS) appears in one-third of the extremely low birth weight neonates undergoing surgery for PDA. Typically starting 4–12 hours post-operative, profound hypotension ensues due to a sudden increase in afterload (increased peripheral vascular resistance) to the left ventricle and decreased preload (less blood return from a pulmonary vein), leading to ventricular dysfunction.[13,32] The neonate presents with an increasing need for inotropes, oxygen lability, and worsening ventilatory requirements. Risk factors for post-ligation syndrome include surgery before four weeks of age, gestational age <26 weeks, birth weight <1000 grams, and need for inotropes before ligation. Management is supportive, including inotropes, optimal ventilation, and hydrocortisone for refractory cases.

6. **Transcatheter device closure:** Device closure is increasingly used for PDA closure. The device is delivered inside the PDA through a venous approach. It can be done bedside or in a catheterization laboratory. The success rate was >95% in a recent trial on 200 infants and more than 99% in 700–2000 g, with an effect sustained till six months.[33] Emerging evidence reveals a lower risk of hemodynamic complications compared to surgical ligation, with a high success rate. However, concerns still need to be addressed regarding long-term outcomes, optimal timing, and the type of device.

OUTCOMES

Many infants discharged with a PDA will have spontaneous closure by one year of age. It, therefore, appears safe to leave a small PDA open at discharge but with regular follow-up. The exact timing of post-discharge closure rates and their association with coexisting severe BPD requires further exploration.

REFERENCES

1. Clyman RI, Couto J, Murphy GM. Patent ductus arteriosus: are current neonatal treatment options better or worse than no treatment? Seminars in Perinatology. 2012 Apr;36(2):123.
2. Heuchan AM, Clyman RI. Managing the patent ductus arteriosus: current treatment options. Arch Dis Child Fetal Neonatal Ed. 2014 Sep;99(5):F431–6.
3. Rolland A, Shankar-Aguilera S, Diomandé D, Zupan-Simunek V, Boileau P. Natural evolution of patent ductus arteriosus in the extremely preterm infant. Arch Dis Child Fetal Neonatal Ed. 2015 Jan;100(1):F55–8.
4. Noori S, McCoy M, Friedlich P, Bright B, Gottipati V, Seri I, et al. Failure of ductus arteriosus closure is associated with increased mortality in preterm infants. Pediatrics. 2009 Jan;123(1):e138–44.
5. Groves AM, Kuschel CA, Knight DB, Skinner JR. Does retrograde diastolic flow in the descending aorta signify impaired systemic perfusion in preterm infants? Pediatr Res. 2008 Jan;63(1):89–94.
6. Hammerman C. Patent ductus arteriosus. Clinical relevance of prostaglandins and prostaglandin inhibitors in PDA pathophysiology and treatment. Clin Perinatol. 1995 Jun;22(2):457–79.
7. Evans N. Diagnosis of the preterm patent ductus arteriosus: clinical signs, biomarkers, or ultrasound? Semin Perinatol. 2012 Apr;36(2):114–22.
8. Hamrick SEG, Sallmon H, Rose AT, Porras D, Shelton EL, Reese J, et al. Patent Ductus Arteriosus of the Preterm Infant. Pediatrics [Internet]. 2020 Nov 1 [cited 2023 Apr 27];146(5). Available from: https://publications.aap.org/pediatrics/article/146/5/e20201209/75323/Patent-Ductus-Arteriosus-of-the-Preterm-Infant.
9. Iyer P, Evans N. Re-evaluation of the left atrial to aortic root ratio as a marker of patent ductus arteriosus. Arch Dis Child Fetal Neonatal Ed. 1994 Mar;70(2):F112–7.
10. Wyllie J. Neonatal echocardiography. Semin Fetal Neonatal Med. 2015 Jun;20(3):173–80.
11. El-Khuffash A, James AT, Corcoran JD, Dicker P, Franklin O, Elsayed YN, et al. A Patent Ductus Arteriosus Severity Score Predicts Chronic Lung Disease or Death before Discharge. J Pediatr. 2015 Dec;167(6):1354-1361.e2.
12. Kulkarni M, Gokulakrishnan G, Price J, Fernandes CJ, Leeflang M, Pammi M. Diagnosing significant PDA using natriuretic peptides in preterm neonates: a systematic review. Pediatrics. 2015 Feb;135(2):e510–25.
13. El-Khuffash A, Weisz DE, McNamara PJ. Reflections of the changes in patent ductus arteriosus management during the last ten years. Arch Dis Child Fetal Neonatal Ed. 2016 Sep;101(5):F474–8.
14. Vanhaesebrouck S, Zonnenberg I, Vandervoort P, Bruneel E, Van Hoestenberghe MR, Theyskens C. Conservative treatment for patent

ductus arteriosus in the preterm. Arch Dis Child Fetal Neonatal Ed. 2007 Jul;92(4):F244–7.

15. Benitz WE. Treatment of persistent patent ductus arteriosus in preterm infants: time to accept the null hypothesis? J Perinatol. 2010 Apr;30(4):241–52.
16. Clyman RI. Recommendations for the postnatal use of indomethacin: an analysis of four different treatment strategies. J Pediatr. 1996 May;128(5 Pt 1): 601–7.
17. Jones LJ, Craven PD, Attia J, Thakkinstian A, Wright I. Network meta-analysis of indomethacin versus ibuprofen versus placebo for PDA in preterm infants. Arch Dis Child Fetal Neonatal Ed. 2011 Jan;96(1):F45-52.
18. Heuchan AM, Young D. Early color Doppler duct diameter and symptomatic patent ductus arteriosus in a cyclo-oxygenase inhibitor naïve population. Acta Paediatr. 2013 Mar;102(3):254–7.
19. Letshwiti JB, Semberova J, Pichova K, Dempsey EM, Franklin OM, Miletin J. Conservative treatment of patent ductus arteriosus in very low birth weight infants. Early Hum Dev. 2017 Jan;104:45–9.
20. Green TP, Thompson TR, Johnson DE, Lock JE. Furosemide promotes patent ductus arteriosus in premature infants with respiratory-distress syndrome. N Engl J Med. 1983 Mar 31;308(13):743–8.
21. Mitra S, Florez ID, Tamayo ME, Mbuagbaw L, Vanniyasingam T, Veroniki AA, et al. Association of Placebo, Indomethacin, Ibuprofen, and Acetaminophen With Closure of Hemodynamically Significant Patent Ductus Arteriosus in Preterm Infants: A Systematic Review and Meta-analysis. JAMA. 2018 Mar 27;319(12):1221–38.
22. Eursiriwan S, Okascharoen C, Vallibhakara SAO, Pattanaprateep O, Numthavaj P, Attia J, et al. Comparison of Various Pharmacologic Agents in the Management of Hemodynamically Significant Patent Ductus Arteriosus in Preterm: A Network Meta-Analysis and Risk-Benefit Analysis. BMH. 2022;7(3):125–45.
23. Herrera C, Holberton J, Davis P. Prolonged versus short course of indomethacin for treating patent ductus arteriosus in preterm infants. Cochrane Database Syst Rev. 2007 Apr 18;2007(2):CD003480.
24. Jasani B, Mitra S, Shah PS. Paracetamol (acetaminophen) for patent ductus arteriosus in preterm or low birth weight infants. Cochrane Database of Systematic Reviews [Internet]. 2022 [cited 2022 Dec 16];(12). Available from: https://www.cochranelibrary.com/cdsr/doi/10.1002/14651858.CD010061.pub5/full
25. Ohlsson A, Walia R, Shah SS. Ibuprofen for the treatment of patent ductus arteriosus in preterm or low birth weight (or both) infants. Cochrane Database Syst Rev. 2020 Feb 11;2(2):CD003481.
26. Clyman R, Wickremasinghe A, Jhaveri N, Hassinger DC, Attridge JT, Sanocka U, et al. Enteral feeding during indomethacin and ibuprofen treatment of a patent ductus arteriosus. J Pediatr. 2013 Aug;163(2):406–11.
27. Schmidt B, Seshia M, Shankaran S, Mildenhall L, Tyson J, Lui K, et al. Effects of Prophylactic Indomethacin in Extremely Low-Birth-Weight Infants With

and Without Adequate Exposure to Antenatal Corticosteroids. Archives of Pediatrics & Adolescent Medicine. 2011 Jul 1;165(7):642–6.
28. Kluckow M, Jeffery M, Gill A, Evans N. A randomised placebo-controlled trial of early treatment of the patent ductus arteriosus. Arch Dis Child Fetal Neonatal Ed. 2014 Mar;99(2):F99–104.
29. Hundscheid T, Onland W, Kooi EMW, et al. Expectant management or early ibuprofen for patent ductus arteriosus. N Engl J Med 2022;388:980–90.
30. Clyman RI, Liebowitz M, Kaempf J, Erdeve O, Bulbul A, Håkansson S, et al. PDA-TOLERATE Trial: An Exploratory Randomized Controlled Trial of Treatment of Moderate-to-Large Patent Ductus Arteriosus at 1 Week of Age. J Pediatr. 2019 Feb;205:41–48.e6.
31. Weisz DE, More K, McNamara PJ, Shah PS. PDA ligation and health outcomes: a meta-analysis. Pediatrics. 2014 Apr;133(4):e1024–46.
32. Giesinger RE, Bischoff AR, McNamara PJ. Anticipatory perioperative management for patent ductus arteriosus surgery: Understanding postligation cardiac syndrome. Congenital Heart Disease. 2019 Mar;14(2):311–6.
33. Sathanandam SK, Gutfinger D, O'Brien L, Forbes TJ, Gillespie MJ, Berman DP, et al. Amplatzer Piccolo Occluder clinical trial for percutaneous closure of the patent ductus arteriosus in patients ≥700 grams. Catheter Cardiovasc Interv. 2020 Nov;96(6):1266–76.

CHAPTER

12

Approach to a Neonate with Shock

Shock is a physiologically compromised state of tissue hypoxia developing as a result of either inadequate delivery of oxygen to tissues and/or increased oxygen consumption or inability of the tissues to utilize oxygen to meet its metabolic demand. Hypotension (i.e. lower-than-expected blood pressure threshold) frequently, but not always, accompanies shock. A study reported 16–52% LBW neonates received volume expansion and 4–39% received vasopressors for shock.[1]

ETIOLOGY AND TYPES OF SHOCK

Table 12.1 describes major types of shock.

Most common mechanism of neonatal shock in preterm neonates is combination of poor myocardial contractility and loss of vasomotor tone.

Special considerations in preterm infants: Cardiovascular physiology of preterm neonates is different from those of term neonates. It continues to change as per gestational age and postnatal age. The hemodynamic changes during transition to extrauterine life affect BP in preterm neonates. Factors which contribute to higher incidence of hypotension in preterm neonates are myocardial immaturity (small contractile tissue and less amount of intracellular calcium) resulting in poor contractility, higher systemic vascular resistance (SVR) during transition period, perinatal asphyxia, left to right shunt at level of PDA (steal syndrome), reduction in venous return secondary to positive pressure ventilation, increased vascular permeability in sepsis and relative adrenal insufficiency.[3]

CLINICAL FEATURES

Although clinical presentation of neonatal shock varies by etiology, the cardinal features are common to most types such as:

Table 12.1: Types of neonatal shock		
Type of shock	*Main mechanism*	*Clinical example*
1. Distributive shock	Impaired peripheral vasomotor tone	Sepsis, Anaphylaxis
2. Hypovolemic shock	Reduction in circulating blood volume resulting in decrease in preload	Pure hypovolemia less common in neonates. Examples: twin to twin transfusion, abruption, intraventricular hemorrhage, pulmonary hemorrhage
3. Cardiogenic shock	Myocardial pump failure	Asphyxia, sepsis, congenital cardiac defects
4. Obstructive shock	Increased afterload	1. Obstruction in inflow tract—total anomalous pulmonary venous connection, tricuspid atresia, mitral atresia, pneumothorax 2. Obstruction in outflow tract—pulmonary stenosis, coarctation of aorta, aortic stenosis
5. Septic shock	Combination of hypovolemic, distributive and cardiogenic component	Fulminant gram-negative sepsis

1. **Signs of poor perfusion** such as cool extremities, acrocyanosis and pallor due to peripheral vasoconstriction. However, these signs are nonspecific.
2. **Prolonged capillary refill time** (>3–4 seconds). However, it has poor predictive value as a surrogate marker of low systemic blood fow.[4]
3. **Changes in heart rate:** In general, tachycardia is a nonspecific early sign of neonatal shock, while bradycardia is often regarded as preterminal finding. Unexplained increase in heart rate may be an early feature of septic shock.
4. **Neurological signs:** Nonspecific signs like lethargy, irritability and unresponsiveness to painful stimuli, generalized hypotonia, decreased deep tendon reflexes, etc.

5. **Hypotension:** Hypotension is regarded as a late sign of shock. However, there is a poor correlation between neonatal hypotension and systemic blood flow in preterm neonate. BP in neonate varies as per gestational age, weight and postnatal age. Hence, defining neonatal hypotension can be challenging.
6. **Oliguria:** Although there is a strong correlation between low urinary output (oliguria) and low systemic blood flow, it can be fallacious in initial 24 hours of life of neonate. Urine output of >1 ml/kg/hour has been defined as one of the therapeutic outcomes of neonatal shock.[10]

VARIOUS OPERATIONAL DEFINITIONS OF HYPOTENSION

There is no single universal definition of neonatal hypotension. Generally, mean blood pressure of less than 5th percentile for the gestational age as per different charts is considered as hypotension.

However, as a rule of thumb, hypotension in first 24 hours is defined as:

- Mean BP of <30 mm of Hg[6]
- Mean BP in mm of Hg is less than gestational age in week (Joint Working Group of the British Association of Perinatal Medicine; BAPM)[7]

However, these definitions do not take into account the increase in blood pressure seen beyond 24 hours of life. A practical BP threshold for 3rd centile as per post-menstrual age has been provided by McNamara et al.[8]

Some healthy ELBW neonates may have mean BP that qualifies for hypotension during first 24 hours, but their systemic perfusion is preserved. Treating hypotension in these infants may be associated with adverse outcome, hence low blood pressure in these babies may be tolerated *(permissive hypotension).*[9] *However, beyond initial 4–6 hours* permissive hypotension should be considered cautiously especially in extremely premature infants.[10]

For operational purpose, a neonate is considered to have shock if there are features of poor peripheral perfusion such as capillary refill time more than 3–4 seconds, poor peripheral pulse, oliguria (urine output <0.5 ml/kg/hour), base excess >5, arterial lactate >2 mmol/L along with or without presence of hypotension (less than 5th percentile for the gestational age as per Zubrow's charts) and superior vena cava flow <40 ml/kg/min. The common differential diagnosis of various clinical scenarios in neonatal shock has been described in Table 12.2.

Investigations

Although a battery of tests is available, it should be curtailed to the common causes suspected. The common tests that should be done in case of neonatal shock include:

1. **Complete blood count:** Hemoglobin, platelet count, total leucocyte count and differential count should be performed to determine degree of anemia and infection.
2. **Coagulation parameters:** Prothrombin time, activated partial thromboplastin time (interpret as per gestational age) should be done in cases where DIC, liver failure is suspected.
3. **Electrolytes, blood sugar, BUN/Creatinine and urinalysis** should be done if clinically oliguria or anuria is present. Hyperkalemia, both hypoglycemia and hyperglycemia can be a manifestation of neonatal shock.
4. **Chest X ray:** A neonate with respiratory distress and abnormal cardiopulmonary finding on examination should have a chest radiogram as early as possible.
5. **ECG:** Bedside electrocardiography should be requested for neonate presenting with sudden unexplained shock.
6. **Cranial ultrasound:** Preterm neonates with abnormal neurological signs and features of acute blood loss to rule out intracranial bleed.
7. **Arterial blood gas** (pH, PaO_2, $PaCO_2$, HCO_3) for adequacy of oxygenation and ventilation. Although a mixed venous oxygen saturation (SVO_2) of <70% is associated with poor outcomes in adult and children, studies in neonates are lacking at present.
8. **Serum lactate** for degree of tissue hypo perfusion. However, evidence for use of serum lactate in diagnosis of neonatal shock still lacking.
9. **Functional echocardiography** is one of the recommended methods to assess cardiac function. Left ventricular output (LVO) and right ventricular output (RVO) are equal in older children and adults. However, in neonate presence of shunts (at level of patent foramen ovale, patent ductus arteriosus) may result in unequal output from both ventricles. Hence, superior vena cava flow (SVC flow) is a better surrogate marker for systemic cardiac output in presence of shunt. SVC flow of <50 ml/kg/min and RVO of <150 ml/kg/min has been arbitrarily taken as

the lower limit of normal in preterm neonate for initiation of therapy.[12] Echocardiography also helps in assessing preload by measurement of IVC collapsibility (in spontaneously breathing babies) and IVC variability (in ventilated babies). Cardiac contractility can be assessed by fractional shortening (FS) measured in parasternal long axis view and measuring ejection fraction (EF) by Simpson's method in apical 4 chamber view. FS is preferred over EF in neonate. Normal value of FS ranges from 23–40% in preterm and 25–41% in term neonates.[12] It also helps to rule out structural cardiac diseases which may present with shock.

Table 12.2 depicts the various methods of assessment of hemodynamic status.

TREATMENT

Shock should be detected and managed before onset of hypotension. In management of neonatal hypotension, physiological variation with postnatal age and gestational age should be taken into account. Immediate management in any type of shock is to optimize perfusion and oxygen delivery to the tissues. Appropriate fluid resuscitation plays an important role in case of septic shock and hypovolemic shock. In case of fluid refractory shock, inotropes are to be initiated. Unlike in adults and children, dopamine continues to be the most used inotropic agent in neonatal shock. However, there is no consensus on the best first line drug. Increasingly, epinephrine is being preferred as first line inotropes especially in preterm neonates (Table 12.3).

Table 12.2: Assessment of hemodynamic status

Clinical parameters	*Laboratory parameters*	*Functional Echocardiography*
Heart rate Peripheral pulses Central pulses Capillary refill time Blood pressure-systolic, diastolic and mean BP Sensorium Urine output	Base deficit Arterial lactate	Preload: IVC variability, SVC flow Afterload: SVC flow Cardiac contractility: fractional shortening (FS), ejection fraction (EF) (Simpson's formula/just eyeballing)

*Trend is more important than a single value

Table 12.3: Pharmacotherapy in neonatal shock

Site of action, dose	*Clinical use and caution*
Dopamine	
Dose dependent stimulation of α and β adrenergic and dopaminergic receptors. • Lower doses (2–4 μg/kg/min): Renal and splanchnic vessel dilation through dopaminergic receptors • Moderate doses (5–10 μg/kg/min): Augmented cardiac contractility by stimulating β1, β2 receptors Higher doses (10–20 μg/kg/min): Elevated peripheral vascular resistance through α1 receptors. Thus, dose beyond 10 μg/kg/min is preferably avoided in VLBW as it leads to preferential increase in pulmonary venous resistance.	Dopamine is the most common used inotrope in neonatal septic shock. Caution in presence of PPHN and very preterm neonates.
Dobutamine	
Increases cardiac contractility and cardiac output through β1 receptor. Minimal effect on the systemic BP and afterload *Dose range:* 10–20 μg/kg/min	Preferred in perinatal asphyxia and myocardial dysfunction *Caution:* May cause hypotension

Evidence box: Dopamine vs dobutamine

1. Dopamine is more effective than dobutamine for the short-term treatment of hypotension in premature infants and does affect the incidence of severe periventricular hemorrhage, periventricular leukomalacia, or tachycardia[16]
2. In hypotension due to myocardial dysfunction, impaired SVR, and relative or absolute hypovolemia combination therapy of dobutamine and dopamine is preferred[17]

(Contd.)

Table 12.3: Pharmacotherapy in neonatal shock *(Contd.)*

Site of action, dose	*Clinical use and caution*
Epinephrine	
1. Nonselective α receptor and β1, β2 adrenergic receptor agonist: increases BP and systemic blood flow by increasing SVR and cardiac output 3. Dose: *Lower dose (0.01–0.1 μg/kg/min):* Action on β1 receptor increases myocardial contractility and peripheral vasodilatation. *Higher dose(>0.1 μg/kg/min):* Stimulation of α1 receptors increases peripheral vasoconstriction and PVR Recommended dose 0.1–0.3 μg/kg/min.	1. Low dose preferred as first line in preterm with/ without PPHN. 2. Used in dopamine resistant septic shock. 3. Causes hyperglycemia and lactic acidosis.

Evidence box:

Epinephrine vs dopamine:A randomized controlled trial (RCT) concluded both drugs were equally effective in preterm infants with hypotension. However, hyperglycemia and lactatic acidosis were more common with case of epinephrine.[18] Dopamine is being less preferred than epinephrine especially in preterm neonates due to:

1. About half of dopamine inotropic effects are due to norepinephrine release, and preterm neonates have decreased myocardial norepinephrine stores, thus it is a lesser effective positive inotrope in long run.[15]
2. The pattern of receptor stimulation is first dopaminergic, then α-adrenergic, and finally β-adrenergic, thus in preterm infants, higher doses of dopamine may result in excessive increases in SVR, potentially decreasing cardiac output.
3. Also, at higher doses (10–20 μg/kg/min) it might increase pulmonary vascular resistance significantly which is a major problem in preterms.

(Contd.)

Table 12.3: Pharmacotherapy in neonatal shock *(Contd.)*

Site of action, dose	*Clinical use and caution*
Norepinephrine	
1. Potent nonselective α agonist with some effect at β1 receptor 2. Dose: 0.1–0.3 μg/kg/min	Norepinephrine use may be associated with lower mortality and morbidity than dopamine in preterm infants with sepsis. Further clinical evidence is still required.[19]
Vasopressin	
1. An antidiuretic hormone that is formed in the hypothalamus and secreted from the posterior pituitary gland. 2. Vascular effects of vasopressin occur by vasoconstriction mediated by stimulation G protein–coupled V1a receptor. 3. Usual dose: 0.0002–0.006 μg/kg/min.	Indicated in vasopressor resistant shock. Useful in PPHN cases (decreases PVR) Caution in presence of myocardial dysfunction.
Evidence box: vasopressin: A recent RCT compared efficacy of vasopressin vs dopamine as initial therapy in ELBW infants with hypotension after birth and there was no difference between the 2 groups. However, infants who received vasopressin had some respiratory benefits and lesser tachycardia[20]	
Milrinone	
1. A selective phosphodiesterase III inhibitor 2. It enhances myocardial contractility without raising myocardial oxygen consumption or increasing afterload, and decreases vascular tone in the systemic and pulmonary vascular beds 3. Dose: 0.5–1 μg/kg/min (without loading dose)	1. Useful for treating low cardiac output state after corrective surgery for congenital heart defects 2. Persistent pulmonary hypertension as an adjunct to inhaled nitric oxide 3. It can cause hypotension, thrombocytopenia

(Contd.)

Table 12.3: Pharmacotherapy in neonatal shock *(Contd.)*

Site of action, dose	*Clinical use and caution*
Evidence box: Milrinone 1. Retrospective study on use of milrinone in neonatal population reported thrombocytopenia and hypotension are the most common adverse effects[21] 2. An RCT compared early prophylactic milrinone with placebo to prevent low systemic blood flow in high-risk pre-term infants. It failed to demonstrate any benefit[22]	
Steroids	
1. Hydrocortisone causes upgradation of cardiovascular adrenergic receptors (vasoconstriction and increased cardiac output), angiotensin II receptors and inhibits expression of inducible nitric oxide synthetase and vasodilatory prostaglandin action.[23,24] 2. Dose of hydrocortisone: 1–2 mg/kg/dose 6–12 hourly IV and gradually tapered after clinical improvement. (If the duration of treatment is 3 days or less, hydrocortisone can be discontinued without tapering)	1. In view of lack of evidence on effect of long term neurodevelopment, currently restricted to fluid refractory, dopamine resistant shock. 2. Used in Late onset glucocorticoid responsive circulatory collapse 3. Prior to steroid therapy measure base line serum cortisol level
Evidence box: Steroids 1. A Cochrane review of corticosteroid use for treating hypotension in preterm infants did not find sufficient evidence to support its use in primary treatment of hypotension. However, authors suggested to treat preterm infants with inotropic refractory shock with steroids[25]	

1. **Volume expansion:** has been used as first line management in neonatal shock although evidence is sparse in preterm neonate where excessive volume resuscitation may result in poor cardiorespiratory outcome. Cautious use of 10–20 ml/kg fluid (isotonic normal saline) can be useful in cases of hypotensive and septic shock. Same amount of PRBC can be used in case of severe anemia and acute blood loss.[11]
2. **Supportive management**
   - **Early support of airway and breathing** in form of either noninvasive ventilation or invasive ventilation to alleviate work of breathing (decision is to be taken at bedside by treating physician).
   - **Umbilical venous catheterization (UVC)** is a feasible, less time consuming during initial 7–14 days of life and hence efforts for UVC should be done as early as possible to provide fluid resuscitation and inotropic support.
   - **Correction of metabolic derangements like** hypoglycemia, hypocalcemia, hypokalemia.
   - **Antibiotics:** Administration of first line antibiotics as per unit policy in first hour of suspected septic shock.
   - **Blood product transfusion** where shock is due to acute blood loss (placenta previa, intraventricular hemorrhage). In emergency situation O-ve PRBC/whole blood can be given.
3. **Pharmacological management:**[15] It is provided in Table 12.3.
4. **Management of underlying cause:**
   - In case of suspected duct dependent lesion (e.g. any term healthy infant in shock beyond day 1: PGE1 infusion should be started empirically (dose 50–200 ng/kg/min) unless proven otherwise.
   - In case of tension pneumothorax urgent bedside thoracotomy (by insertion of a butterfly needle in 4th intercoastal space in midaxillary line) should be performed.
   - Arrhythmias: for supraventricular tachycardia emergency reversion by use of IV adenosine and synchronized cardioversion should be considered.

Late Onset Glucocorticoid Responsive Circulatory Collapse (LCC) in Premature Infants

This entity is seen in relatively stable very low birth weight (VLBW) neonates characterized by sudden onset of hypotension and/or oliguria, which is resistant to fluids and inotropes but responds rapidly to intravenous glucocorticoids. LCC occurs after the first week of life (mean 16–23 days). The causes for this is still not clearly established but attributed to relative adrenal insufficiency. An arbitrary cutoff of value of cortisol levels less than 200 nmol/L along with the clinical response points towards relative adrenal insufficiency.[26]

Pathophysiology-based Management of Shock

Management of shock needs to be individualized as per the underlying clinical condition. An approach based upon systolic, diastolic and combined systolic-diastolic categories is shared below.[8]

1. **Systolic hypotension:** it is defined as systolic arterial pressure less than third centile. The pathophysiology behind it is decrease in left ventricular stroke output. The common causes and treatment is given below.
   a. Cardiogenic shock:
      i. Arrythmia needs to be ruled out.
      ii. Start dobutamine, epinephrine to improve the myocardial systolic performance.
   b. Septic shock:
      i. Optimize the sepsis treatment.
      ii. Start dobutamine, epinephrine to improve myocardial systolic performance.
   c. PPHN: It should be considered when there is associated hypoxemia.
      i. Optimize alveolar ventilation, sedation, +/– muscle relaxant.
      ii. Pulmonary vasodilators like iNO, milrinone to be considered (Milrinone to be avoided with low or borderline mean/diastolic BP).
      iii. Increase preload by fluid bolus, vasopressin to increase SVR and pulmonary vasodilation
      iv. Dobutamine/epinephrine to improve the myocardial systolic performance.
2. **Diastolic hypotension:** it is defined as diastolic arterial pressure less than third centile. The pathophysiology behind it is decrease in systemic vascular resistance. The common causes and treatment is given below.

a. Systemic hypovolemia:
   i. Optimize preload: fluid boluses (max 2 of 10 ml/kg each)
   ii. Start vasopressin, dopamine: to increase SVR, once fluid is optimized
b. Warm shock:
   i. Optimize preload: fluid boluses (max 2 of 10 ml/kg each)
   ii. Start dopamine, norepinephrine, vasopressin: to increase SVR, once fluid is optimized
c. PDA:
   i. Close duct- NSAIDs, acetaminophen, surgery.
   ii. Start dobutamine to improve LV systolic function.

3. **Combined systolic-diastolic hypotension:** it is defined as both systolic and diastolic arterial pressure less than third centile. The pathophysiology behind it is cardiac systolic dysfunction. Based upon which component of blood pressure drops at the time of presentation the approach is given below:
   a. Low systolic arterial pressure at presentation
      i. Cardiogenic shock:
         - Start dobutamine, epinephrine to improve the myocardial systolic performance.
      ii. PPHN:
         - Increase preload by fluid bolus, vasopressin to increase SVR.
         - Start dobutamine, epinephrine to improve the myocardial systolic performance.
   b. Low diastolic arterial pressure at presentation
      i. Hypovolemia/Warm shock:
         - Optimize preload: fluid boluses (max 2 of 10 ml/kg each).
         - Start dopamine, norepinephrine, vasopressin: to increase SVR, once fluid is optimized.
      ii. PDA:
         - Start dobutamine to improve LV systolic function.
   c. Both systolic and diastolic arterial pressure low at presentation
      i. Severe warm shock with LV dysfunction
         - Optimize preload: fluid boluses (max 2 of 10 ml/kg each).
         - Start dopamine, norepinephrine, vasopressin: to increase SVR, once fluid is optimized.
         - Consider giving early hydrocortisone.

   Table 12.4 describes common case scenarios based management.

Table 12.4: Common clinical scenario-based management

Clinical scenario	*Common causes*	*Management*
ELBW <24 hours, hypotension, but other parameters stable (isolated hypotension)	Stable ELBW	Close clinical monitoring
Sick preterm baby (hemodynamic instability)	Low systemic blood flow, IVH, large PDA, adrenal insufficiency	General management: 10 ml/kg normal saline bolus, repeat if required 1st: Adrenaline 0.05–0.3 μg/kg/min 2nd: Dopamine <10 μg/kg/min and/or hydrocortisone 1–2 mg/kg 3rd line Noradrenaline: 0.1–0.5 μg/kg/min if suspected sepsis or predominantly diastolic hypotension. Consider treating PDA, administer blood product if IVH. Consider early antibiotics if suspicion of sepsis.
Term baby <24 hours with birth asphyxia, history of meconium aspiration	HIE, MAS, PPHN	Supportive: sedation, normal metabolic parameters General: normal saline 10 ml/kg bolus, repeat if required Inotropes: With normal BP: Dobutamine 10–20 μg/kg/min, ionodilators-milrinone, inhaled nitric oxide may be considered if features of PPHN are there 2nd line: low dose adrenaline 0.05–0.1 μg/kg/min 3rd line: dopamine <10 μg/kg/min Consider vasopressin as 2nd line if diastolic hypotension and PPHN with normal LV function With low BP: 1st line:adrenaline 0.05–0.3 μg/kg/min (start with low dose)

(Contd.)

Table 12.4: Common clinical scenario-based management (*Contd.*)

Clinical scenario	*Common causes*	*Management*
Term baby >24 hours with shock (gradual onset), sick looking	Sepsis	General: normal saline 10 ml/kg bolus (up to 40 ml/kg in septic shock), early blood product transfusion Inotropes: 1st line: dopamine 10–20 μg/kg/min 2nd line: adrenaline 0.1–0.5 μg/kg/min and/or hydrocortisone 1–2 mg/kg 3rd line: Noradrenaline 0.1-0.5 μg/kg/min suspected sepsis or predominantly diastolic hypotension Add early antibiotics
Term baby >24 hours with sudden onset circulatory collapse, previously well baby	Suspected duct dependent structural cardiac disease	General management: a trial bolus 10 ml/kg, be cautious for further fluid therapy Inotropes: first line: dopamine 10–20 μg/kg/min 2nd line: dobutamine Urgent bedside echocardiography to rule out duct dependent cardiac lesions If ECHO facility not available: consider empirical PGE1 infusion (50–200 ng/kg/min)

REFERENCES

1. Al-Aweel I, Pursley DM, Rubin LP, Shah B, Weisberger S, Richardson DK. Variations in prevalence of hypotension, hypertension, and vasopressor use in NICUs. J Perinatol Off J Calif Perinat Assoc. 2001 Aug;21(5):272–8.
2. Polin RA, Abman SH, Rowitch DH, Benitz WE, Fox WW. Fetal and neonatal physiology [Internet]. 2017 [cited 2017 Jun 8]. Available from: http://public.eblib.com/choice/PublicFullRecord.aspx?p=4558070.
3. Sahni M, Jain S. Hypotension in Neonates. NeoReviews. 2016;17(10):e579–e589.
4. Osborn DA, Evans N, Kluckow M. Clinical detection of low upper body blood flow in very premature infants using blood pressure, capillary refill time, and central-peripheral temperature difference. Arch Dis Child Fetal Neonatal Ed. 2004 Mar;89(2):F168–73.
5. Zubrow AB, Hulman S, Kushner H, Falkner B. Determinants of blood pressure in infants admitted to neonatal intensive care units: a prospective multicenter study. Philadelphia Neonatal Blood Pressure Study Group. J Perinatol Off J Calif Perinat Assoc. 1995 Dec;15(6):470–9.
6. Brierley J, Carcillo JA, Choong K, Cornell T, Decaen A, Deymann A, et al. Clinical practice parameters for hemodynamic support of pediatric and neonatal septic shock: 2007 update from the American College of Critical Care Medicine. Crit Care Med. 2009 Feb;37(2):666–88.
7. Report of working group of the British Association of Perinatal Medicine and Neonatal Nurses Association on categories of babies requiring neonatal care. Arch Dis Child. 1992 Jul;67(7 Spec No):868–9.
8. Giesinger RE, McNamara PJ. Hemodynamic instability in the critically ill neonate: An approach to cardiovascular support based on disease pathophysiology. Semin Perinatol. 2016 Apr;40(3):174–88.
9. Dempsey EM, Al Hazzani F, Barrington KJ. Permissive hypotension in the extremely low birthweight infant with signs of good perfusion. Arch Dis Child - Fetal Neonatal Ed. 2009 Jul 1;94(4):F241–4.
10. Durrmeyer X, Marchand-Martin L, et al; Hemodynamic EPIPAGE 2 Study Group. Abstention or intervention for isolated hypotension in the first 3 days of life in extremely preterm infants: association with short-term outcomes in the EPIPAGE 2 cohort study. Arch Dis Child Fetal Neonatal Ed. 2017 Nov;102(6):490–6.
11. Davis AL, Carcillo JA, Aneja RK, Deymann AJ, Lin JC, Nguyen TC, et al. American College of Critical Care Medicine Clinical Practice Parameters for Hemodynamic Support of Pediatric and Neonatal Septic Shock: Crit Care Med. 2017 Jun;45(6):1061–93.
12. Evans N. Which inotrope for which baby? Arch Dis Child - Fetal Neonatal Ed. 2005 Oct 13;91(3):F213–20.
13. Skinner J, Alverson D, Hunter S. Hemodynamic assessment. In: Echocardiography for the Neonatologist. 1st edition. London: Churchill Livingstone; 2000. p. 101–70.

14. Seri I. Circulatory support of the sick preterm infant. Semin Neonatol. 2001 Feb;6(1):85–95.
15. Noori S, Seri I. Neonatal Blood Pressure Support: The Use of Inotropes, Lusitropes, and Other Vasopressor Agents. Clin Perinatol. 2012 Mar;39(1):221–38.
16. Subhedar NV, Shaw NJ. Dopamine versus dobutamine for hypotensive preterm infants. Cochrane Database Syst Rev. 2003;(3):CD001242.
17. Noori S, Friedlich P, Seri I. The use of dobutamine in the treatment of neonatal cardiovascular compromise. NeoReviews. 2004;5(1):e22–e26.
18. Valverde E, Pellicer A, Madero R, Elorza D, Quero J, Cabañas F. Dopamine versus epinephrine for cardiovascular support in low birth weight infants: analysis of systemic effects and neonatal clinical outcomes. Pediatrics. 2006 Jun;117(6):e1213–22.
19. Nissimov, S., Joye, S., Kharrat, A. *et al.* Dopamine or norepinephrine for sepsis-related hypotension in preterm infants: a retrospective cohort study. *Eur J Pediatr*(2022). https://doi.org/10.1007/s00431-022-04758-4
20. Rios DR, Kaiser JR. Vasopressin versus dopamine for treatment of hypotension in extremely low birth weight infants: a randomized, blinded pilot study. J Pediatr. 2015 Apr;166(4):850–5.
21. Samiee-Zafarghandy S, Raman SR, van den Anker JN, McHutchison K, Hornik CP, Clark RH, et al. Safety of milrinone use in neonatal intensive care units. Early Hum Dev. 2015 Jan;91(1):31–5.
22. Paradisis M, Evans N, Kluckow M, Osborn D. Randomized trial of milrinone versus placebo for prevention of low systemic blood flow in very preterm infants. J Pediatr. 2009 Feb;154(2):189–95.
23. Noori S, Seri I. Evidence-based versus pathophysiology-based approach to diagnosis and treatment of neonatal cardiovascular compromise. Semin Fetal Neonatal Med. 2015 Aug;20(4):238–45.
24. Rios DR, Moffett BS, Kaiser JR. Trends in pharmacotherapy for neonatal hypotension. J Pediatr. 2014 Oct;165(4):697–701.e1.
25. Ibrahim H, Sinha IP, Subhedar NV. Corticosteroids for treating hypotension in preterm infants. Cochrane Database Syst Rev. 2011 Dec 7;(12):CD003662.
26. Kawai, M. Late-onset circulatory collapse of prematurity. Pediatr.Int.2017 Apr; 59, 391–6.

CHAPTER

13

Approach to a Neonate with Suspected Congenital Heart Disease

Congenital heart disease (CHD) occurs in approximately 8 neonates per 1000 live births. The incidence of CHD is fairly constant across the globe and has not changed over time.[1–2] An apparent increase in recent reports is the result of the easy availability of echocardiography and the inclusion of minor forms of CHDs.[3]

Critical CHD, defined as cardiac lesions requiring surgical or catheter-based intervention in infancy, accounts for approximately 25% of all CHDs.[4] While the majority of neonates with critical CHD are symptomatic and are identified soon after birth, a significant proportion remains undetected until after discharge. Understandably, delay in the diagnosis of critical CHD increases morbidity and mortality.[5] Therefore, an attempt must be made to diagnose CHDs before discharge particularly if they are critical. An accurate structural diagnosis, however, is seldom required for initial management and in the majority, a clinical hemodynamic classification of CHD is sufficient (Table 13.1).[6]

Table 13.1: Clinical presentation, pathophysiology and likely CHD

		Pathophysiology	*CHDs*
1.	Hypotension/ shock	Reduced cardiac output Obstructive lesions	Critical AS Severe CoA Interrupted aortic arch Hypoplastic left heart syndrome Obstructed TAPVC Ventricular dysfunction
2.	Cyanosis	Decreased PBF with low PA pressure Increased PBF with high PA pressure	TOF physiology Critical PS with atrial septal defect Transposition physiology Admixture physiology TAPVC

(*Contd.*)

Table 13.1: Clinical presentation, pathophysiology and likely CHD *(Contd.)*

		Pathophysiology	*CHDs*
			Single or common atrium Tricuspid atresia Single ventricle Truncus arteriosus
		No PS with normal PA pressure	Ebstein's anomaly Anomalous systemic venous connection
3.	Heart failure	Pulmonary plethora	Left-to-right shunt Cyanotic CHD with increased PBF
		Pulmonary venous hypertension	Obstructed TAPVC HLHS Ventricular dysfunction

AS: Aortic stenosis; *CHD:* Congenital heart disease; *CoA:* Coarctation of aorta; *HLHS:* Hypoplastic left heart syndrome; *PBF:* Pulmonary blood flow; *PS:* pulmonary stenosis; *TAPVC:* Total anomalous pulmonary venous connection; *TOF:* Tetralogy of Fallot

CLINICAL PRESENTATION

Risk Factors

The exact cause of CHDs is not known with many environmental and genetic factors playing a role in abnormal cardiac development. A positive family history of CHD in first-degree relatives, genetic syndromes, maternal illness such as diabetes mellitus, phenylketonuria and exposure to teratogenic drugs, and in-utero infections predispose to CHD.[7]

Timing and Mode of Presentation

The timing and type of presentation depend on:

i. The impact of CHD on fetal circulation.
ii. Transitional circulation—closing ductus arteriosus and falling pulmonary vascular resistance (PVR), and
iii. The nature and severity of the cardiac lesion.[7]

While most of the cardiac anomalies are tolerated well during fetal life, CHDs with ventricular dysfunction, atrioventricular valve regurgitation and severe obstruction to circulation result in fetal compromise. Other cardiac lesions manifest during or after the transition from fetal to neonatal circulation.

Hypotension and Shock

Unexplained hypotension and shock in the neonatal period are commonly due to cardiac malformation and warrant urgent evaluation by a pediatric cardiologist. In the majority, low cardiac output results from critical obstruction to the circulation of blood. Neonates with severe aortic stenosis (AS) and obstructed total anomalous pulmonary venous connection (TAPVC) present early as cardiac output is limited by the obstruction. Neonates with critical AS and hypoplastic left heart syndrome (HLHS) have insufficient forward flow across the aortic valve and the systemic circulation depends on patent ductus arteriosus (PDA) for blood supply to the upper as well as lower part of the body. On the other hand, in neonates with coarctation of aorta (CoA) and interrupted aortic arch (IAA), cardiac output to the upper half of the body is not affected while flow to the lower half of the body relies on PDA. Neonates with PDA-dependent systemic circulation become symptomatic once the PDA constricts a few days after birth. This delayed closure poses a substantial diagnostic challenge in the early neonatal period. A discrepancy in upper and lower limb pulse and SpO_2 provides an important clue towards PDA being part of cardiac malformation.

Heart Failure and Failure to Thrive

Hemodynamic effects of left-to-right shunt lesions depend upon age-related reduction in PVR. In a term neonate, a hemodynamically significant shunt coincides with lowered PVR approximately at 4–6 weeks of life. Preterm neonates, on the other hand, become symptomatic much earlier due to limited contractile reserve of immature myocardium. The myocardium of neonates being less distensible result in higher left ventricular (LV) end-diastolic pressure which in turn manifest with pulmonary venous hypertension causing respiratory distress. In addition, the reduced ability of preterm neonates to maintain pulmonary vasoconstriction may contribute to the early onset of hemodynamically significant left-to-right shunt.[7] Before the shunt is established, neonates remain asymptomatic while a neonate with an established shunt presents with poor feeding, feed intolerance, failure to thrive, tachypnea, tachycardia and hepatomegaly. Cardiomegaly and pulmonary plethora on CXR also indicate the presence of increased PBF.

An absence of murmur does not exclude left-to-right shunt. Instead, in neonates with large, non-restrictive ventricular septal defect (VSD) or PDA, the murmur is inaudible due to low-pressure gradients across the defect. It is therefore mandatory to look for heart failure, poor feeding and failure to thrive during follow-up visits at 4–6 weeks even if there is no murmur on auscultation. Ventricular contractile dysfunction is an uncommon cause of heart failure. This may result from profound birth asphyxia or is rarely due to congenital myocarditis.

Cardiac Murmur

Hemodynamically significant CHDs in neonates commonly present with heart failure, hypotension or shock and cyanosis. However, presentation with a murmur alone is not uncommon. An absence of cardiac murmur has very little discriminatory value in refuting or confirming the diagnosis of CHD.[9] Like cyanosis, an audible cardiac murmur has high specificity but lacks sensitivity (see later). A critical disease such as transposition of great arteries (TGA) and pulmonary atresia may not have any murmur while a loud murmur is audible in neonates with benign mild pulmonary stenosis (PS).[6,8]

Rhythm Abnormality

Rhythm abnormalities, both bradycardia and tachycardia, can present in the neonatal period irrespective of the presence or absence of CHD. A 12-lead electrocardiogram (ECG), particularly during the episode of abnormal rhythm is generally sufficient to diagnose and manage the rhythm abnormality. A detailed discussion of rhythm abnormality is beyond the scope of this chapter.

Cyanosis or Arterial Desaturation

Cyanosis, like other clinical signs, relies on many variables and therefore is an imprecise surrogate marker of hypoxemia.[6,10] Cyanosis is not apparent when hypoxemia is mild. The term arterial desaturation, therefore, should be preferred to cyanosis.[6,10]

Despite being the gold standard for hypoxemia, arterial blood gas (ABG) is not preferred due to its invasive nature and lack of easy availability. Further, the saturation reported in ABG (SaO_2) is not measured but is calculated from pH and PaO_2, assuming a normal oxygen dissociation curve, which may not be true in a sick neonate. Measurement of oxygen saturation by pulse oximetry (SpO_2), on the other hand, provides a much easier, non-invasive and reliable assessment of hypoxemia. Routine pulse oximetry has been shown to improve sensitivity in detecting cyanotic CHD in neonates and infants, especially with milder levels of hypoxemia.[10,11] Broadly,

SpO_2 less than 95% represents hypoxemia and at this cutoff value, pulse oximetry reaches high specificity of more than 99% and a sensitivity of 75% for detecting cyanotic CHD. All neonates with suspicion of hypoxemia should undergo 4-limb pulse oximetry before they are declared free of hypoxemia.[11–15]

Persistent arterial desaturation is always pathological and mandates evaluation. Age at the onset of cyanosis can give important clues towards structural pathology in the heart (Table 13.2). This timing-based suspicion of specific CHD, however, is less important once arterial desaturation is preferred over cyanosis.[10] Right-to-left shunt in CHDs diverts systemic venous blood away from the lungs, the destination for oxygenation, to the systemic circulation. More is the right-to-left shunt, lower is the arterial saturation and earlier it presents in the neonatal period. Arterial desaturation, however, is not synonymous with reduced pulmonary blood flow (PBF) and can exist in CHDs with increased PBF such as transposition

Table 13.2: Age of onset* of cyanosis in various CHDs

Onset of cyanosis	*Likely CHD*
1st week (day 1 to day 7)	1. TGA with IVS 2. Hypoplastic left heart syndrome 3. TOF with pulmonary atresia/ critical PS 4. Pulmonary atresia with IVS 5. Tricuspid atresia with VSD with PS 6. TAPVC 7. Common arterial trunk 8. Ebstein's anomaly
7 days to 1 month	1. Hypoplastic left heart syndrome 2. TGA with IVS or VSD 3. TOF 4. Severe PS 5. Truncus arteriosus
Late onset cyanosis	1. TOF 2. DORV with VSD with PS 3. TGA with VSD with PS 4. Tricuspid atresia with VSD with PS 5. Single ventricle with PS

*May vary depending on the extent of hemodynamic abnormality and arterial desaturation
CHD: Congenital heart disease; *DORV:* Double outlet right ventricle; *IVS:* Intact ventricular septum; *PS:* Pulmonary stenosis; *TAPVC:* Total anomalous pulmonary venous connection; *TGA:* Transposition of great arteries; *TOF:* Tetralogy of Fallot; *VSD:* Ventricular septal defect

and admixture physiology (see later). Thus, it is the amount of right-to-left shunt and not overall PBF that determines arterial oxygen saturation. Respiratory pathologies are an important cause of cyanosis in neonates. Although difficult sometimes, clinical assessment along with chest X-ray (CXR) allows this distinction in the majority.

Unlike other groups, cyanotic CHD is a heterogeneous group consisting of both increased and decreased PBF. Tetralogy of Fallot (TOF) is the most common cyanotic CHD. Cardiac malformations included in TOF are:

i. Mal-aligned subaortic VSD.
ii. Aortic override
iii. Right ventricular outflow tract (RVOT) (infundibular PS) and
iv. Right ventricular hypertrophy. RVOT obstruction impedes blood flow from RV to pulmonary arteries (PA).

A coexisting VSD provides a relatively low resistance path for RV blood with the resultant right-to-left shunt. This circulatory abnormality 'TOF physiology' is not unique to TOF and is seen in all CHDs with large VSD and PS. Hypoxemia in TOF physiology varies from minimal to severe and is proportionate to the severity of PS. Since PS is progressive, it is not uncommon to have late-onset cyanosis in neonates with TOF. A somewhat similar mechanism of hypoxemia exists in neonates with atrial septal defect (ASD) and PS albeit with a right-to-left shunt at the level of atrium.

The ventriculoarterial connection in neonates with TGA is inverted. As a result, desaturated systemic venous blood reaches the aorta despite reaching the physiologically correct right atrium and RV. Oxygenated blood from pulmonary veins, on the other hand, continues to circulate from the left atrium and LV to PA without contributing to tissue oxygenation. This unfavorable movement of blood, equivalent to a 'parallel circulation', in contrast to normal 'circulation in series' results in profound hypoxemia. The survival and oxygen saturation solely depends upon the amount of blood mixed in the 'systemic' and 'pulmonary' circuit and consequently, neonates with restrictive ASD present with severe hypoxemia. Other neonates with adequate ASD or a VSD and/or a PDA allow good mixing of blood and present with mild hypoxemia.

Admixture physiology is yet another form of cyanotic CHD wherein there is a near complete mixing of systemic (deoxygenated) and pulmonary (oxygenated) venous blood causing diversion of deoxygenated systemic venous blood to the aorta (right-to-left shunt). The presence of PS, by posing resistance to PBF, cause more right-to-let shunt and consequently more hypoxemia. Neonates with no or mild PS has mild hypoxemia. Admixture of 'systemic' and 'pulmonary' venous blood can occur at the level of systemic veins, atrium, ventricle or great arteries (Table 13.1).

Clinical signs lack specificity and may be present in more than one CHD. Likewise, a single CHD may have more than one presentation. Knowledge of pathophysiologic alteration helps in understanding the overlap and anticipating the type of CHD, making management much easier.

CLINICAL EVALUATION

Suspecting CHD in a Neonate

Universal Screening

CHD is multifactorial with a well-known occurrence in neonates without risk factors. The implications of missing critical CHD are enormous and therefore, all neonates irrespective of risk profile and clinical presentation should have a thoughtful screening for CHD, before discharge and on follow-up. The presence of one major or two minor Nada's criteria suggestsa high likelihood of CHD (Table 13.3).[6–8]

Pulse Oximetry Screening (POxS)

POxS is an excellent noninvasive tool for monitoring SpO_2 and should be part of standard neonatal care. SpO_2 measurement has a

Table 13.3: Nada's criteria for suspecting CHD

Presence of one major or two minor criteria suggests a high likelihood of structural heart disease	
Major criteria	1. Systolic murmur grade 3 or more especially when associated with a thrill 2. Diastolic murmur 3. Cyanosis 4. Congestive heart failure
Minor criteria	1. Systolic murmur <grade 3 2. Abnormal second heart sound 3. Abnormal ECG 4. Abnormal Chest X ray 5. Abnormal BP

high sensitivity for the detection of hypoxemia. Current generation pulse oximeters work well even in the setting of poor peripheral perfusion and at low saturation levels. Pulse oximetry screening (PoxS) should include measurement of saturation in both preductal (right hand) and postductal (foot) locations. The left subclavian artery may arise before or after the PDA and therefore left hand is not an appropriate site for pre-ductal measurement of SpO_2. The right subclavian artery on the other hand is rarely postductal and right arm SpO_2 almost always indicates pre-ductal location. Similarly, the post-ductal origin of the umbilical artery must be kept in mind.

POxS has established itself as a useful screening tool for CHDs, particularly for critical cyanotic CHDs[11–16] (Flowchart 13.1). As per the recent recommendations from the American Association of Pediatrics (AAP), all newborns should undergo POxS.[12-16]POxS should be done after 24 hours of age or shortly before discharge if the baby is less than 24 hours of age. Waiting until 24 hours of life decreases false-positive results due to respiratory ailments. This screening should include measurement of saturation in the right hand and either of the feet.[16]The updated guidelines-based interpretation of POxS is as follows:[16]

- The screening is considered 'negative' and the baby is declared 'pass' if the oxygen saturation is 95% or greater in both the right hand and foot and the difference is 3% between the right hand and foot.
- The screening is 'positive' and the baby is declared 'fail' if the saturation is 89% in either the right hand or foot.
- The screening mandates a 'retest' if the saturation is 90–94% in either the right hand or foot or if the difference in saturation is ≥4%. On the second measurement after 1 hour of the first one, neonates having a saturation 94% or a difference of ≥4% between the right hand and foot are declared 'fail' while others with a saturation ≥95% and a difference 3% are considered 'pass'.
- All neonates with'fail' in POxS should be managed as having CHD until proved otherwise.[13,16]

Evidence for pulse-oximetry screening[11]

The pulse oximetry can detect critical congenital heart disease with a sensitivity of 76.5% (95% CI 67.7–83.5%) and a specificity of 99.9% (99.7–99.9%). The false-positive rate for detection of critical congenital heart defects is lower when pulse oximetry is done after 24 hours from birth.

Flowchart 13.1: Pulse oximetry screening protocol and interpretation[16]

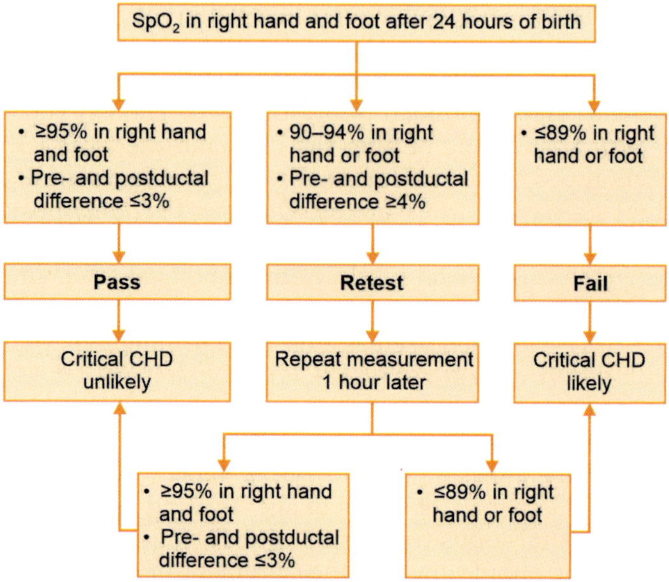

Hyperoxia Test

The hyperoxia test was once considered an important tool to differentiate cyanosis from a respiratory pathology. The easy availability of echocardiography in addition to the difficult performance and complex interpretation of the hyperoxia test has made this test irrelevant in contemporary clinical practice. A careful assessment of response to oxygen administration remains helpful in making this important distinction.

Practice tip

Near normal SpO_2 with oxygen supplementation by nasal prongs, mask or hood practically rules out significant cyanotic CHD necessitating urgent pediatric cardiology evaluation.[6,7]

Cardiac Murmur

Unlike children with a high occurrence of innocent murmur, any murmur in neonates is significant. Approximately 1% of neonates have murmurs, and of these 31–86% have CHD. Therefore, all neonates with audible murmur should be evaluated by a pediatric cardiologist.[9] The likelihood of CHD further increases if the murmur is diastolic, harsh systolic and or exists with other signs of cardiac involvement.

Evaluation for Suspected CHD

In neonates with risk factors and clinical signs suggestive of CHD, a detailed examination including the assessment of CXR and ECG must be performed (Table 13.4). The aim is to simply classify CHD as the initial management seldom requires lesion-specific diagnosis. Although this management-centric approach delays the accurate diagnosis of CHD it helps in early stabilization of the baby. Hemodynamic instability and or profound cyanosis (SpO_2 <70%) nevertheless mandate an urgent evaluation by a pediatric cardiologist.

Clinical Examination

Physical examination should preferably be performed in a warm and quiet environment. An absence of respiratory distress in a cyanosed neonate generally indicates CHD. A neonate with CHD and increased PBF and heart failure have tachypnea but with mild or no respiratory distress (retractions, grunting, etc.). The cardiac examination includes an assessment of heart rate, peripheral pulses, perfusion and evidence of heart failure. Blood pressure measurement in both upper and lower limbs is mandatory. A discrepancy in brachial and femoral pulses or blood pressure should indicate either severe obstruction or interruption of the aortic arch with lower body circulation dependent on PDA. Similarly, the presence of differential SpO_2 in the upper and lower limb implicates a role of PDA.

The diagnostic ability of cardiac examination in neonates is limited by small chest size and high heart rates. The location of the

Table 13.4: Physical examination for screening and detection of CHD
1. Evaluate ABC-airway, breathing, and circulation.
2. Presence and pattern of respiratory distress.
3. Examine pulse, capillary refill, SpO_2 and blood pressure in both pre- and postductal location.
4. Heart rate and rhythm.
5. Dysmorphism or anomalies that are known to have a higher incidence of CHD.
6. Evidence of heart failure–poor weight gain, tachycardia, tachypnea.
7. Abdomen for liver-sidedness (to assess situs) and hepatomegaly.
8. Precordial impulse to assess sidedness of the heart, heart sounds, mainly S_2.
9. Murmur and thrill–timing, site, intensity and radiation.

Adapted with permission from Clinical Approach to a Neonate with Cyanosis by Gupta SK[6]

spleen, liver and cardiac apex provides clues to situs and cardiac position. Hepatomegaly provides a much-needed clue to the presence of heart failure. This is particularly important as jugular venous pulse (JVP) is not useful in children and pedal edema is rare.

Chest X-ray and Electrocardiogram

CXR and ECG are complementary to clinical examination. In general, the presence of cardiomegaly, pulmonary oligemia or plethora in addition to abnormalities of situs and cardiac position strongly suggest underlying CHD. CXR is particularly useful in categorizing cyanotic CHD in decreased and increased PBF situations. Cardiomegaly and pulmonary plethora indicate high PBF while the presence of small heart and oligemia suggest possible CHD with decreased PBF. An algorithmic approach to CXR interpretation in classifying cyanotic CHD (Flowchart 13.2). Typical appearances of cardiac shadow in CHD, such as 'egg-on-side' in TGA, 'figure-of-eight' in TAPVC, 'boot-shaped heart (cor-en-sabot)'

Flowchart 13.2: Algorithm for interpretation of CXR to classify CHD

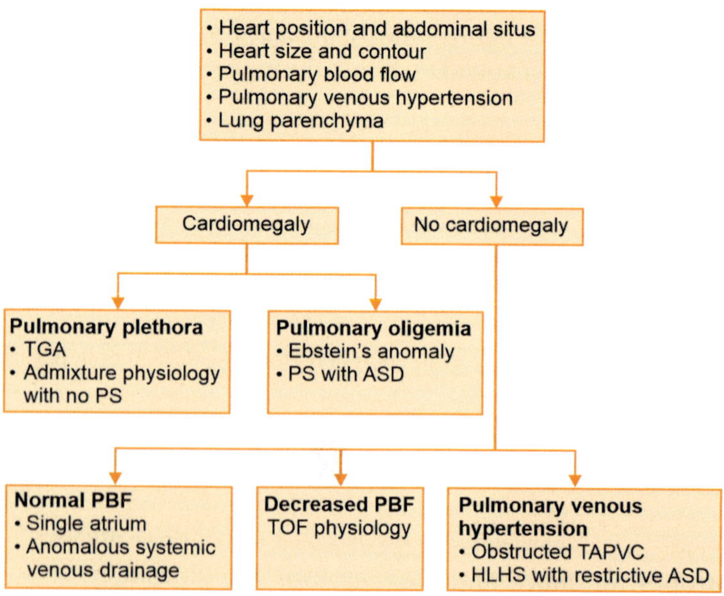

ASD: Atrial septal defect; *HLHS:* Hypoplastic left heart syndrome; *PS:* Pulmonary stenosis; *TAPVC:* Total anomalous pulmonary venous connection; *TGA:* Transposition of great arteries; *TOF:* Tetralogy of Fallot

Adapted with permission from Clinical approach to a neonate with cyanosis by Gupta SK[6]

in TOF etc. are consequent to postnatal hemodynamic changes and, therefore, are rarely seen in the neonatal period. Further, similar to cyanosis and cardiac murmur, these typical appearances have high specificity but lack sensitivity.[6,9,10]

Right ventricular dominance is characteristic of a normal neonatal ECG. Many common CHDs also have a similar pattern of right axis deviation (RAD) and right ventricular hypertrophy (RVH). This overlap interferes with the interpretation of ECG and makes it an unreliable tool if used in isolation. ECG, however, remains the cornerstone for the diagnosis of rhythm abnormalities. In addition, characteristic ECG patterns point to specific cardiac malformation. For example, left axis deviation (LAD) in the presence of left ventricular hypertrophy (LVH) indicates tricuspid atresia while LAD with RVH indicates atrioventricular septal defect (AVSD). An appearance of polyphasic QRS complexes with tall 'Himalayan' P wave is well known to indicate Ebstein's anomaly of the tricuspid valve.[6]

Echocardiography

Echocardiography is the gold standard for the diagnosis of CHD. In addition to providing structural details, an echocardiogram allows the detection of all physiologic alterations necessary for early and definitive management. While an accurate diagnosis is desirable it is not essential for initial stabilization. Optimal performance and interpretation of echocardiography mandate careful examination by an experienced operator failing which diagnostic errors are unacceptably high. This is an important consideration while scheduling an echocardiogram. In general, urgent echocardiograms should be limited to neonates with hemodynamic instability, profound hypoxemia and rapidly worsening clinical status.

MANAGEMENT

Medical management is the key to initial stabilization. Critically sick neonates must be treated in consultation with a pediatric cardiologist. Other neonates must receive care and drug therapy according to the hemodynamic subtype of CHD (Table 13.1). Judicious use of diuretics and fluid restriction for heart failure, inotropes for shock and beta blockers for cyanotic CHD with decreased PBF allows prompt stabilization. All neonates with cyanosis should also be advised iron supplementation to support compensatory erythrocytosis. There is no definite SpO_2 cutoff that defines adequate oxygenation in a neonate with CHD. For practical purposes, SpO_2<70% or the presence of tissue hypoxia and lactic acidosis warrants an urgent evaluation for possible percutaneous or surgical intervention. In the interim, neonates should receive oxygen supplementation and PGE1 infusion. An algorithmic approach for screening and managing neonates with CHD is presented in Flowchart 13.3.

PGE1 Infusion

Intravenous PGE1 has revolutionized the management of neonates with CHD. By promoting recanalization of closed ductus arteriosus or maintaining its patency allows rapid stabilization of neonates with PDA-dependent systemic or pulmonary blood flow. PGE1 infusion by re-establishing patency of arterial duct results in rapid normalization of shock and hypoxemia. Neonates with hemodynamic instability and or profound hypoxemia should promptly be started on PGE1 infusion even before echocardiographic confirmation. PGE1 infusion can lead to clinical worsening, by promoting pulmonary venous hypertension if the ASD is restrictive in obstructed TAPVC, HLHS, mitral atresia and TGA with intact ventricular septum. Fortunately, this is rare and provides a clue towards the existence of one of these malformations. As a caution, pulmonary venous hypertension on CXR should prompt echocardiographic confirmation before considering PGE1 infusion. Approximately 10–12% of neonates receiving PGE1 infusion have side effects, the most serious being apnea, which is, dose-dependent and may need mechanical ventilation.

Percutaneous or Surgical Interventions for Immediate Stabilization

It is not uncommon to encounter a neonate in whom severe hypoxemia or heart failure persists despite medical stabilization. These neonates require percutaneous or surgical intervention for stabilization. Critical stenosis of the aortic valve and pulmonary valve must be dealt with urgently by percutaneous balloon dilatation. Percutaneous balloon atrial septostomy improves saturation in neonates with TGA by enlarging ASD. A surgical aortopulmonary shunt (Blalock Taussig Thomas shunt) or percutaneous PDA stenting improves saturation in patients with TOF physiology and other CHDs with PDA-dependent pulmonary circulation. Patients with critical lesions such as obstructive TAPVC must be operated upon urgently.

Flowchart 13.3: Algorithm for screening and management of CHD in neonates

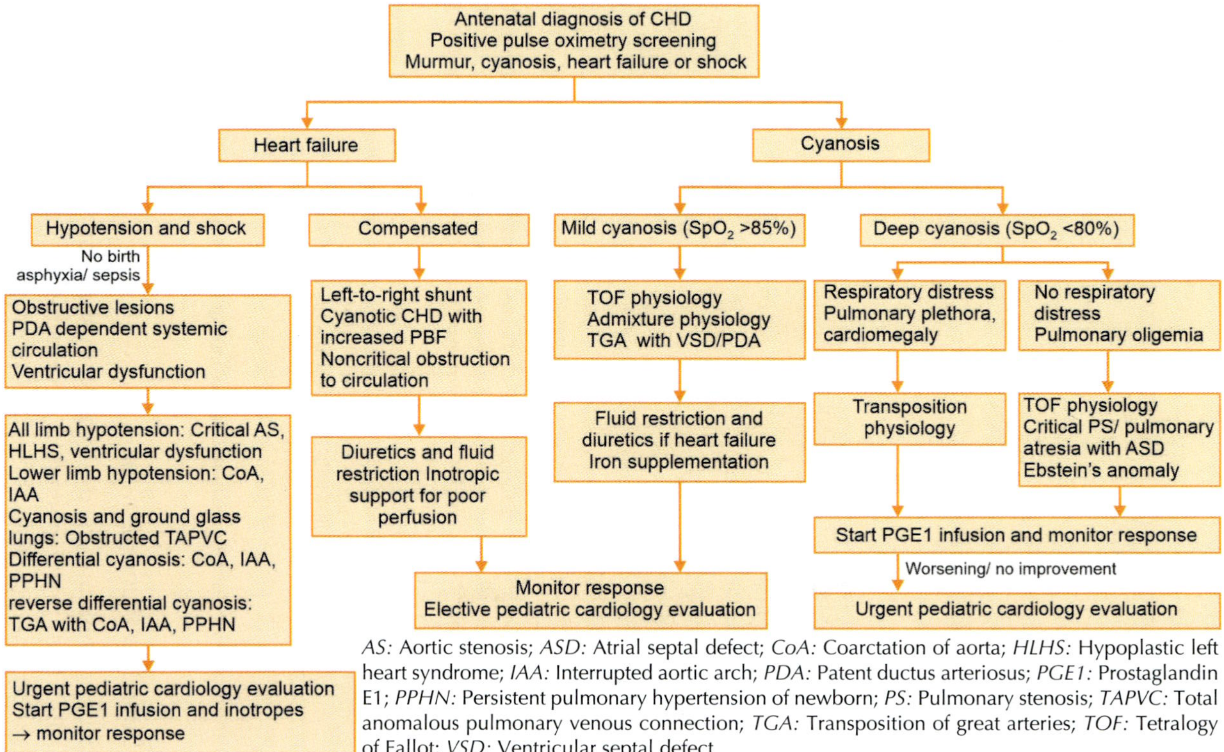

AS: Aortic stenosis; *ASD:* Atrial septal defect; *CoA:* Coarctation of aorta; *HLHS:* Hypoplastic left heart syndrome; *IAA:* Interrupted aortic arch; *PDA:* Patent ductus arteriosus; *PGE1:* Prostaglandin E1; *PPHN:* Persistent pulmonary hypertension of newborn; *PS:* Pulmonary stenosis; *TAPVC:* Total anomalous pulmonary venous connection; *TGA:* Transposition of great arteries; *TOF:* Tetralogy of Fallot; *VSD:* Ventricular septal defect

Table 13.5: Definitive management of common CHDs

Correction possible	*Only multistage surgical palliation possible*[4]
Neonatal intervention • AVBD for critical AS • PVBD for critical PS with IVS • PDA stenting for PDA-dependent PBF[1] • BAS for TGA with intact ventricular septum Neonatal surgical repair • Severe CoA • TAPVC • TGA Surgery/intervention during infancy • Truncus arteriosus • Left-to-right shunt[2] • TOF and TOF physiology[3] Surgery during childhood • Atrial septal defect[2] • Single atrium • Ebstein's anomaly	• Single ventricle physiology • DORV, non-routable VSD • Tricuspid atresia, VSD • HLHS and mitral atresia

1. Final surgical treatment based on cardiac morphology.
2. Percutaneous device closure of PDA and VSD in select cases.
3. Severe hypoxia warrants surgical Blalock–Taussig shunt or percutaneous stenting of the right ventricular outflow tract (RVOT) to improve saturation.
4. Early BT shunt/ PDA stent for severe hypoxemia and early PA band for non-resolving heart failure to prepare for future cavopulmonary connection.

AS: Aortic stenosis; *AVBD:* Aortic valve balloon dilatation; *BAS:* Balloon atrial septostomy; *CHD:* Congenital heart disease; *CoA:* Coarctation of aorta; *DORV:* Double outlet right ventricle; *HLHS:* Hypoplastic left heart syndrome; *IVS:* Intact ventricular septum; *PBF:* Pulmonary blood flow; *PDA:* Patent ductus arteriosus; *PS:* Pulmonary stenosis; *PVBD:* Pulmonary valve balloon dilatation; *TAPVC:* Total anomalous pulmonary venous connection; *TGA:* Transposition of great arteries; *TOF:* Tetralogy of Fallot; *VSD:* Ventricular septal defect.

Adapted with permission from Clinical approach to a neonate with cyanosis by Gupta SK[6]

Definitive Management

Surgery remains the destination therapy for the majority of CHDs. All CHDs are not amenable to corrective surgery and only palliative surgery is possible. Brief knowledge of surgical management for various CHDs is important for preliminary counselling and planning timely referrals (Table 13.5).

SUMMARY

1. All neonates should be screened for CHD.
2. All neonates with cardiac murmur must be evaluated for CHD.
3. All neonates should have pulse oximetry screening before discharge.
4. Initial assessment should be aimed at the hemodynamic classification of CHD.
5. Echocardiographic accurate diagnosis is seldom essential for initial stabilization.
6. PGE1 infusion can be started without echocardiographic confirmation in the majority.
7. Hemodynamic instability and or profound hypoxemia mandates urgent evaluation by a pediatric cardiologist.

REFERENCES

1. Gupta SK, Kothari SS. Prevalence of congenital heart disease. Indian J Pediatr 2013;80:337–9.
2. Hoffman JI, Kaplan S. The incidence of congenital heart disease. J Am Coll Cardiol 2002;39:1890–900.
3. Van der Linde D, Konings EM, Slager MA, Witsenburg M, Helbing WA, Takkeberg JJ, et al. Birth prevalence of congenital heart disease worldwide: a systematic review and meta-analysis. J Am Coll Cardiol 2011;58:2241–7.
4. Oster M, Lee K, Honein M, Colarusso T, Shin M, Correa A. Temporal trends in survival for infants with critical congenital heart defects. *Pediatrics*. 2013;131(5):e1502–8.
5. Kuehl KS, Loffredo CA, Ferencz C. Failure to diagnose congenital heart disease in infancy. Pediatrics 1999;103:743.
6. Gupta SK. Clinical approach to a neonate with cyanosis. Indian J Pediatr 2015;82:1050–60.
7. Ronald I Clyman. Mechanism regulating closure of ductus arteriosus. In: Fetal and neonatal physiology E-book. Polin RA, Abman SH, Rowitch D, Benitz WE (editors).5th edition. Philadelphia Elsevier 2017. Pg 592–99.
8. Wechsler SB, Wernovsky G. Cardiac disorders. In: Manual of neonatal care. Cloherty JP, Eichenwald EC, Stark AR (editors). 6th edition, Lippincott Williams & Wilkins. 2008;388–435.
9. Frank JE, Jacobe KM. Evaluation and management of heart murmurs in children. Am Fam Physician 2011;84:793–800.
10. Gupta SK. Cyanotic congenital heart disease – not always blue to provide a clue: time to replace cyanosis with arterial desaturation! Ann PediatrCardiol 2022;15:511–4.
11. Ewer AK, Middleton LJ, Furmston AT, Bhoyar A, Daniels JP, Thangaratinam S, Deeks JJ, Khan KS, PulseOx study group. Pulse oximetry screening for

congenital heart defects in newborn infants (PulseOx): a test accuracy study. Lancet 2011;378:785–94.

12. Ewer AK. Pulse oximetry screening for critical congenital heart defects in newborn infants: should it be routine? Arch Dis Child Fetal Neonatal 2014;99:F93–5.
13. Thangaratinam S, Brown K, Zamora J, Khan KS, Ewer AK. Pulse oximetry screening for critical congenital heart defects in asymptomatic newborn babies: a systemic review and meta-analysis. Lancet 2012;379:2459–64.
14. Mahle WT, Martin GR, Beekman RH III, Morrow WR; Section on Cardiology and Cardiac Surgery Executive Committee. Endorsement of Health and Human Services recommendation for pulse oximetry screening for critical congenital heart disease. *Pediatrics*. 2012;129(1):190–192.
15. Kemper AR, Mahle WT, Martin GR, Cooley WC, Kumar P, Morrow WR, Kelm K, Pearson GD, Glidewell J, Grosse SD, Lloyd-Puryear M, Howell RR. Strategies for implementing screening for critical congenital heart disease. *Pediatrics*. 2011; 128:e1–8.
16. Martin GR, Ewer AK, Gaviglio A, Hom LA, Saarinen A, Sontag M, Burns KM, Kemper AR, Oster ME. Updated strategies for pulse oximetry screening for critical congenital heart disease. Pediatrics 2020;146:e20191650.

SUGGESTED READING

1. Allen HD, Driscoll DJ, Shaddy RE, Feltes TF (Ed). Moss & Adams' heart disease in infants, children and adolescents – including the fetus and young adult.
2. Tandon R. Bedside approach. In: Tandon R (Ed). The diagnosis of congenital heart disease. 2nd edition, New Delhi, Sitaram Bhartia Institute of Science and Research Publishers; 2011.

Section

5

Respiratory System

CHAPTER

14

Approach to Respiratory Distress in the Newborn

Respiratory distress occurs in 4–7% of all neonates[1,2] and is the reason for 30–40% of all admissions to the NICU. It is more common among preterm (30%) and post-term (21%) than among term neonates (4.2%).[2] A neonate can develop respiratory distress due to various conditions, which are not limited to respiratory or cardiovascular causes alone. Appropriate management includes evaluating the neonate for the severity and cause of respiratory distress and initiating respiratory support when appropriate.

DEFINITION

The National Neonatal Perinatal Database of India (NNPD)[3] defines respiratory distress as the presence of any two of the following features:

1. Respiratory rate >60/minute
2. Subcostal/intercostal recessions
3. Expiratory grunt/groaning

In addition to the above features, the presence of nasal flaring, suprasternal retractions, and decreased air entry on auscultation of the chest also indicates the presence of respiratory distress. Gasping, choking, or stridor (signs of upper airway obstruction), apnea or poor respiratory effort or bradycardia, poor perfusion, and cyanosis are life-threatening signs that require prompt intervention.[4]

CAUSES

Respiratory distress can occur due to various conditions (Table 14.1), and the frequency of a given disease depends on multiple factors, of which gestation is the most important. In preterm neonates, respiratory distress syndrome (RDS) is the most common cause, while in late preterm and term neonates, transient tachypnea of the newborn (TTN) is the predominant cause.[2]

Table 14.1: Common causes of respiratory distress in the newborn

Table 14.1: Common causes of respiratory distress in the newborn
Airway • Choanal atresia • Pierre Robin sequence • Tracheoesophageal fistula • Laryngotracheomalacia • Vocal cord paralysis
Pulmonary diseases • Transient tachypnea of the newborn (TTN) • Respiratory distress syndrome (RDS) • Meconium aspiration syndrome • Pneumothorax and other air-leak syndromes • Persistent pulmonary hypertension of the newborn • Pulmonary hypoplasia • Lung malformations • Congenital diaphragmatic hernia
Cardiac diseases • Congenital heart disease • Arrhythmia • Congestive cardiac failure • Cardiomyopathy
Thoracic causes Chest wall deformity Skeletal dysplasia
Neuromuscular diseases • Central nervous system damage (birth trauma, hemorrhage), meningitis, asphyxia • Medication (maternal sedation, narcotic withdrawal) • Muscular disease (myasthenia gravis) • Spinal cord injury
Others • Sepsis • Anemia • Polycythemia • Hypo- and hyperthermia

INVESTIGATION AND MANAGEMENT

Initial Assessment

An initial assessment of respiratory distress is done to rule out life-threatening conditions which require immediate management, such as inadequate respiratory efforts or obstructed airway (gasping, choking, stridor or apnea) or circulatory collapse (bradycardia, hypotension, and poor perfusion). If such features are present, emergency measures such as oxygen administration, bag and mask ventilation, or intubation should be initiated as necessary.

General Examination

Look for dysmorphic features, craniofacial malformations, features of intrauterine growth restriction, scaphoid abdomen, and drooling of saliva. Note the color of the neonate (pink vs. *cyanosed*) and use a pulse oximeter to determine the oxygen saturation.

Assessment of Respiratory Distress

Inspection: Observe whether the neonate is breathing comfortably or if signs of respiratory distress are present. Some respiratory sounds are audible to the ears without a stethoscope. **Stridor** is a harsh "crowing" sound produced due to narrowing the upper airway at the level of the larynx or extrathoracic trachea. It is often inspiratory but can be expiratory or biphasic. Stridor can occur in newborns due to laryngomalacia, Pierre Robin sequence, vocal cord palsy, laryngeal or subglottic narrowing due to edema, web, or stenosis.[5] **Grunting** is an expiratory noise due to the closure of the glottis during expiration. By this mechanism, neonates can increase their functional residual capacity (FRC). **Stertor or snoring** is a low-pitched inspiratory noise produced due to obstruction at the level of the nasopharynx (adenoid hypertrophy) or oropharynx (micrognathia, macroglossia). This sound can be inspiratory, expiratory, or both.

Note the symmetry of chest excursions and synchrony with abdominal wall movement. A rounded chest wall with increased anteroposterior diameter is a marker of hyperinflation. Pectus carinatum or pigeon chest deformity may be noted in chronic conditions with an increased respiratory effort that causes the sternum to protrude. On the other hand, the pectus excavatum or funnel chest is a developmental deformity wherein the sternum and costal cartilage are depressed.

Palpation and percussion: While palpation and percussion are done sparingly in neonates, one can get valuable information by feeling the tracheal position, locating the apex beat, palpating for crepitus or murmurs, and percussing for normal resonance. Dullness on percussion may be noted over areas of consolidation or collapse, stony dullness over pleural effusion, and hyper-resonance over pneumothorax or bulla.

Auscultation: Assess whether the breath sounds are heard equally and symmetrically in all areas, whether there is a prolongation of the inspiratory or expiratory phase, and presence of added sounds like rales, rhonchi, wheeze, and stridor.

Respiratory distress score: The severity of respiratory distress can be objectively graded using respiratory distress scores. The two commonly used scores are the Silverman–Anderson Score[5] (Table 14.2) and Downes' Vidyasagar Score[6] (Table 14.3). The signs of respiratory distress are assigned a numerical value (0 indicating normal and 2 indicating the worst). The final summary score grades the severity of distress into none (score = 0) or mild (<3), moderate (4–6), and severe (≥7). Using these scores, nurses and clinicians can monitor the progression of respiratory distress and initiate optimal treatment. Neonates with mild to moderate distress can be managed using positive distending pressure like CPAP, while those with severe distress may need intubation and mechanical ventilation.

Respiratory distress score: Evidence

Silverman score does not include assessment of skin color, breath sounds, or tachypnea but correlates well with mortality.

The Downe's score shows a good correlation with physiological parameters such as pH, A-a DO_2 and PaO_2.

A score of 7 or more at age 24–30 hours, when the score is usually at its peak is associated with higher mortality compared to no mortality when the score is less than 6.

Serial monitoring is more important than one-time assessment. In impending respiratory failure, the score can be falsely low due to apnea, poor perfusion, and failure to maintain body temperature. The choice of one score over the other is often based on the unit's preference and training received by health care professionals.

Oxygen Saturation

Oxygen saturation measured using pulse oximetry is considered the sixth vital sign. Saturation below 90% indicates hypoxia.[9] It should be checked in preductal (right hand) and postductal sites (right/left leg). A pre-postductal difference of more than 5–10% indicates probable right-to-left shunt through patent ductus arteriosus (PDA) in the setting of persistent pulmonary hypertension of the newborn (PPHN). Central cyanosis is bluish discoloration of the

Table 14.2: Silverman–Anderson score for grading the severity of respiratory distress

Component	*Upper chest retractions*	*Lower chest retractions*	*Xiphoid retractions*	*Alar nasi flaring*	*Expiratory grunt*
Observation	Observe the synchrony of the upper chest with abdomen movement during inspiration	Observe the retractions between the ribs below the mid-axillary line	Retraction below the xiphoid process	Observe the nasal flaring before application of nasal interface	
Score 0	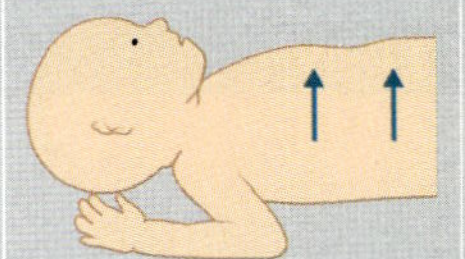 Upper chest synchronized with abdomen	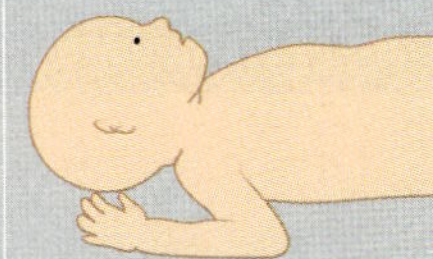 None	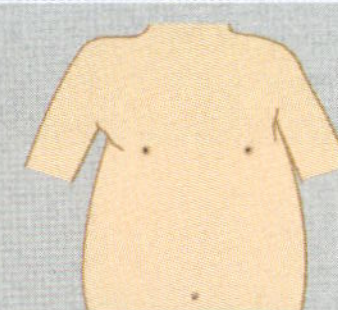 None	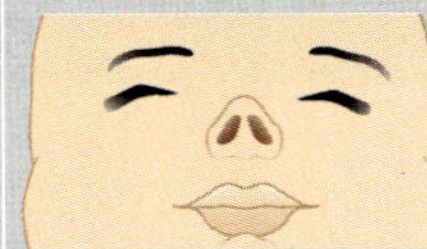 None	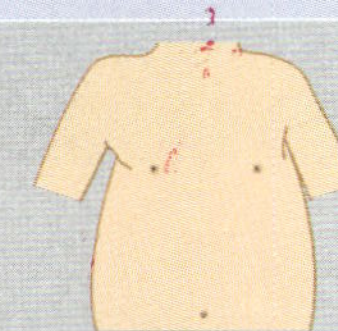 None
Score 1	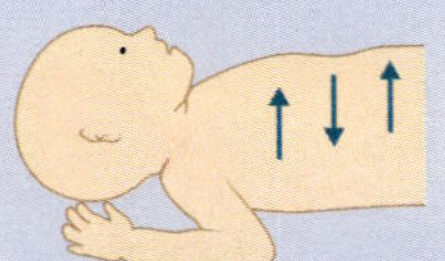 Upper chest lags compared to abdomen	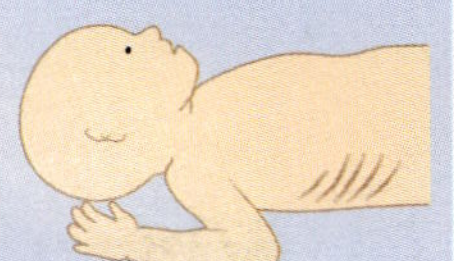 Just visible	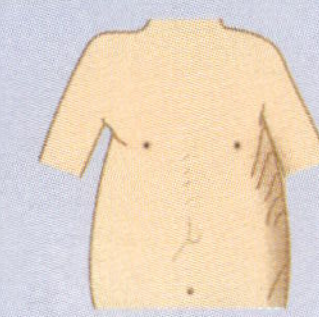 Just visible	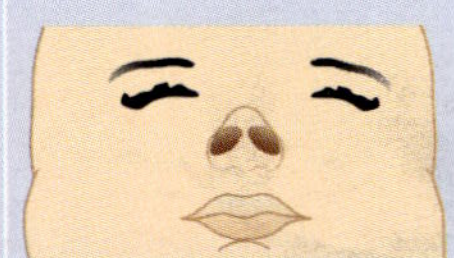 Just visible	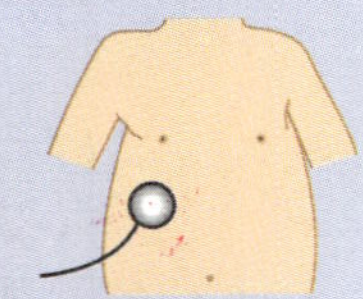 Audible with stethoscope

(Contd.)

Table 14.2: Silverman–Anderson score for grading the severity of respiratory distress (*Contd.*)					
Component	*Upper chest retractions*	*Lower chest retractions*	*Xiphoid retractions*	*Alar nasi flaring*	*Expiratory grunt*
Score 2	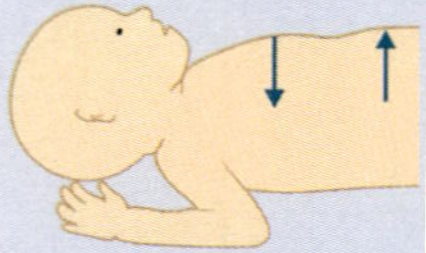 See-saw movement of the chest and abdomen	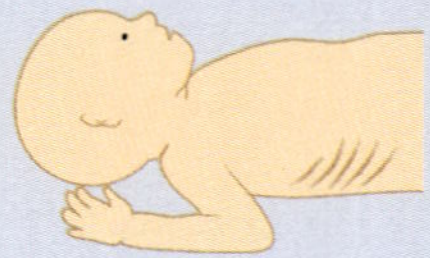 Marked	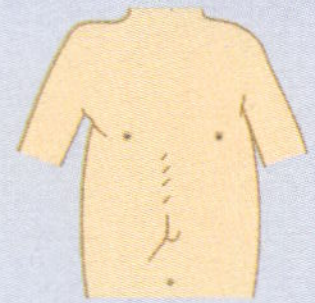 Marked	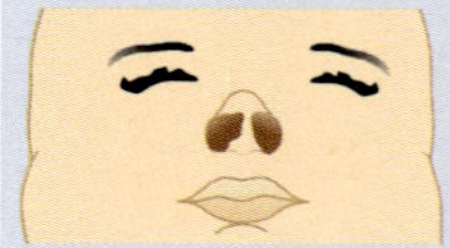 Marked	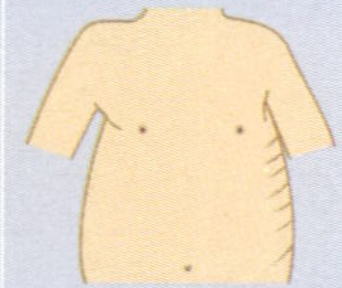 Audible without stethoscope

Table 14.3: Downe's score for grading severity of respiratory distress			
Feature	*Score 0*	*Score 1*	*Score 2*
Cyanosis of lips and oral mucosa	None	In-room air	In 40% FiO_2
Retractions (intercostal, subcostal and suprasternal)	None	Mild	Severe
Expiratory grunt	None	Audible with stethoscope	Audible without stethoscope
Air entry	Normal	Decreased	Barely audible
Respiratory rate	<60	60–80	>80 or apnea

entire body, including the skin, mucous membranes, and tongue. It is an important indicator of hypoxia. The deoxyhemoglobin level should be at least 2.5 g/dl in the blood for cyanosis to manifest. Polycythemic neonates with high hemoglobin may manifest cyanosis when oxygen saturation is 88%, while anemic neonates may not appear cyanosed until saturation drops below 65%.[8] Hence pulse oximeter is an essential tool to identify hypoxia. Peripheral cyanosis can be due to cold exposure, polycythemia, or potentially serious conditions like hypoglycemia, sepsis, or decreased left ventricular output like hypoplastic left heart syndrome or coarctation of aorta. The uses and limitations of pulse-oximetry are listed below:

- **Diagnosis:** Pulse-oximetry is the best tool for the continuous and noninvasive diagnosis of hypoxia. The normal range of SpO_2 at sea level is 97–99%, with a lower limit of 94%. Hypoxia is considered in neonates if SpO_2 is less than 90%.
- **Grading the severity of hypoxic respiratory failure:** The oxygen saturation index provides non-invasive and continuous monitoring of oxygenation status. It is calculated as MAP X FiO_2 divided by SpO_2. OSI correlates well with oxygenation index (OI = 2 × OSI for OI between 5 and 25).
- **Diagnosis of PPHN:** Preductal–postductal oxygen saturation difference >5% and labile oxygen saturation should raise the suspicion of PPHN.
- **Screening of critical congenital heart disease in neonates:** Universal predischarge pulse oximetry screening reduces early cardiac deaths due to critical congenital heart disease by one-third. The screening is done at 24 hours of age or before hospital discharge. Saturations are recorded in the right hand (preductal) and either leg (postductal). Saturation of at least 95% on both sites and a difference of 3% or less between the two readings is considered a PASS. A saturation of less than 90% on any site mandates immediate assessment, while intermediate values need re-testing.

Limitations of Pulse-oximetry

- Not a good tool to detect hyperoxia, as SpO_2 readings above 95% may occur with PaO_2 values of 80–300 mm Hg (sigmoidal oxygen dissociation curve).
- Not reliable below SpO_2 <70%.
- Ambient light, dyshemoglobinemia (methemoglobin and carboxyhemoglobin), low peripheral perfusion states, and movement of limbs interfere with the measurement.

Cardiac examination: Examination of the respiratory system is incomplete without simultaneous assessment of the cardiac system. Neonates with cardiac disease who manifest tachypnea without significant retractions may have poor perfusion, cyanosis, and abnormal heart sounds or murmurs on auscultation. Table 14.4 shows the differences in manifestation between respiratory and cardiac disorders. Monitor pulse rate, blood pressure, and capillary refill time to identify hypoperfusion secondary to prolonged hypoxemia. Hyperoxia test (Flowchart 14.1) is a simple bedside test used to distinguish cyanotic heart disease from pulmonary disease. The arterial blood gas is obtained when the neonate receives room

Table 14.4: Differences in respiratory and cardiac disorders in the newborn

	Respiratory disorders	*Cardiac disorders*
Clinical findings	• Cyanosis • Severe retractions • Normally split second heart sound • Liver may be pushed down with lung hyper-expansion but liver span will be normal	• Cyanosis, gallop rhythm, or murmur • Effortless tachypnea or mild distress • Single second heart sound • Large liver when associated with cardiac failure
Chest X-ray	• Normal heart size • Abnormal pulmonary parenchyma, such as total whiteout or patches of consolidation in pneumonia, fluid in the fissures in TTN or ground glass • Appearance in RDS	• Cardiomegaly • Decreased pulmonary vascularity and normal cardiac size—pulmonary oligemia. The blood flow to the pulmonary circulation is decreased due to right ventricular outflow obstruction with an associated right-to-left shunt • Increased pulmonary vascularity due to left-to-right shunt lesions and in cyanotic lesions such as transposition of the great vessels or total anomalous pulmonary venous return
Blood gas analysis	Increased $PaCO_2$ and decreased PaO_2	Normal $PaCO_2$ and decreased PaO_2. However, $PaCO_2$ may be raised with pulmonary congestion or an associated lung infection
Hyperoxia test	PaO_2 >150 mm Hg (except in severe PPHN)	PaO_2 <150 mm Hg

Flowchart 14.1: Hyperoxia test and its interpretation

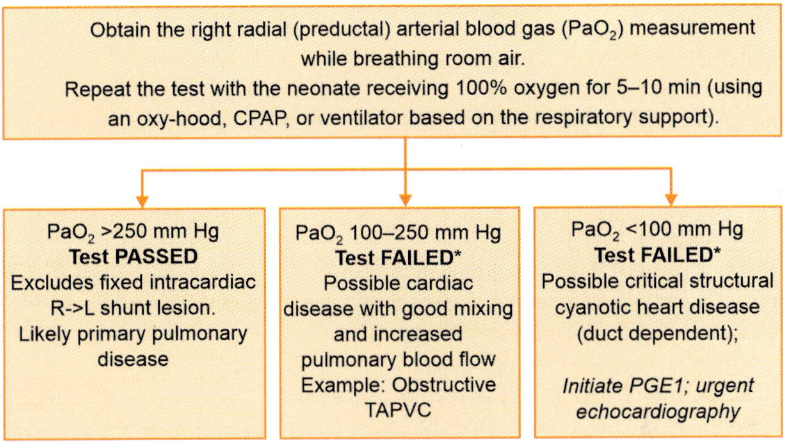

*Persistent Pulmonary hypertension of the newborn (PPHN) can also result in a failed hyperoxia test. Unlike infants with a duct-dependent cardiac disease, those with PPHN show a pre-to-post ductal saturation difference greater than 10% on pulse- oximetry (where shunting is at ductal level) and labile saturations with agitation or clinical interventions (e.g. suctioning). Infants with cyanotic heart disease have fixed low oxygen saturations.

air (FiO_2 = 21%) and while on 100% FiO_2 for 10 minutes. Neonates with cyanotic heart disease do not have an increase in PaO_2 above 100 mm Hg after 100% oxygen administration.

Approach to Management

Specific management depends on the underlying condition. History, clinical examination, and necessary investigations help establish the diagnosis.

History

A detailed history is essential in assigning a cause of respiratory distress (Table 14.5).

Evolution of Respiratory Distress

The risk factors and evolution of respiratory distress can give a clue to diagnosis (Table 14.6).

Investigations

The common investigations performed on a neonate with respiratory distress are provided below. The selection of tests depends on the clinical condition, availability, and whether a particular test would

Table 14.5: Relevant history in a neonate with respiratory distress
Antenatal
Maternal history of
Diabetes mellitus: TTN, RDS
Pregnancy-induced hypertension or Intrauterine growth retardation: Polycythemia, hypoglycemia
Asthma: TTN
Fever or urinary tract infection in the preceding two weeks of delivery: neonatal early onset sepsis
Substance abuse: Narcotic drug withdrawal
Polyhydramnios: Tracheoesophageal fistula, neuromuscular disorders
Oligohydramnios: Pulmonary hypoplasia
Rh isoimmunization: Hydrops fetalis
Antenatal steroids: non-receipt predisposes to RDS
Previous sibling with respiratory distress: Surfactant protein B deficiency
Intranatal
Prolonged rupture of membranes, intrapartum fever, or chorioamnionitis: Sepsis
Meconium-stained liquor: Meconium aspiration syndrome, asphyxia
Fetal distress: Asphyxia
C-section without labor: TTN, RDS, PPHN
Breech presentation, instrumental delivery: Trauma, Erb's with phrenic nerve palsy
Postnatal
Onset of respiratory distress: Onset at birth: TTN, RDS, pneumothorax or air leak, MAS, congenital malformations
Onset hours or days later: Congenital heart disease, sepsis

TTN: Transient tachypnea of the newborn; *RDS:* Respiratory distress syndrome; *UTI:* Urinary tract infection; *Rh:* Rhesus; *PPHN:* Persistent pulmonary hypertension of the newborn; *MAS:* Meconium aspiration syndrome.

Table 14.6: Risk factors and evolution of respiratory distress in common neonatal conditions

Disorder	*Evolution of the condition*
Respiratory distress syndrome	Infants with RDS are preterm and typically present within the first several hours of life, mostly immediately after delivery. The distress is marked by tachypnea, nasal flaring, grunting, and subcostal and intercostal retractions. In infants who do not receive exogenous surfactant therapy, the endogenous surfactant synthesis results in recovery of the distress in the first week.
TTNB	Risk factors include cesarean section without labor, precipitous delivery, late preterm or early term births, and gestational diabetes. Respiratory distress has onset immediately after birth, but it is mild and self-limited, with resolution in 72 hours.

(*Contd.*)

Table 14.6: Risk factors and evolution of respiratory distress in common neonatal conditions (*Contd.*)

Disorder	*Evolution of the condition*
Pneumonia	Risk factors for early onset sepsis include group *B Streptococcus* carriage in pregnant mothers, chorioamnionitis, maternal fever, prolonged rupture of membranes, preterm premature rupture of membranes, and spontaneous onset of preterm labor. Neonatal pneumonia presents as a generalized sepsis illness. Onset can be delayed by a few hours and is generally indistinguishable from RDS.
Meconium aspiration	Risk factors include meconium-stained amniotic fluid, post-term gestation, fetal distress, or perinatal depression. Onset is at birth with progressive worsening.
Pulmonary hypoplasia	Risk factors include severe oligohydramnios, renal dysplasia or agenesis, lower urinary tract obstruction, premature rupture of membranes in early gestation, diaphragmatic hernia, neuromuscular disorder. Respiratory distress has onset at birth and is severe.

be helpful in the given scenario. For example, in a neonate with suspected tension pneumothorax, it would be wise to do a transillumination of the thorax and proceed with treatment rather than wait for a chest X-ray.

1. **Gastric aspirate shake test:** The gastric aspirate shake test is a simple bedside test to predict the risk of RDS. It is advantageous in areas where radiography is unavailable. The test involves mixing 0.5 mL of gastric aspirate obtained within one hour of birth and an equal volume of 95% ethyl alcohol in a clean glass test tube (size 10 mm × 110 mm). Cork the test tube, shake it vigorously for 15 seconds, and allow it to stand for 15 minutes before examining the liquid-air interface for the stability of bubbles.[9] The presence of an entire rim of bubbles is considered a positive test, the absence of bubbles is considered negative, and the incomplete rim of bubbles is an intermediate test. The test is highly specific but has a sensitivity of only 70%. In one study, no infant with a positive test developed RDS, while 66% of those with a negative test result had RDS.
2. **Transillumination:** A fiber-optic bright light source applied to the chest wall can be used to promptly identify air leaks like pneumothorax, pneumomediastinum, pneumopericardium, and pneumoperitoneum. Severe pulmonary interstitial emphysema

(PIE) and emphysematous bullae may also transilluminate. The room must be dark while performing this test, and one must also differentiate the slight normal halo of light around the probe from increased transillumination noted from air collection. When used in small neonates, care must be exercised to avoid skin burning from the light source.

3. **Chest radiography:** Radiography is the primary diagnostic tool for respiratory distress in neonates. The commonly taken view is anteroposterior, while lateral and cross-table lateral views can be used to evaluate air leaks, pleural effusions, and placement of tubes or catheters (*see* Chapter 38: Neonatal Chest X-ray).
4. **Ultrasound:** Point of care lung ultrasonography can be used to diagnose various pulmonary conditions like RDS, TTN, pleural and pericardial effusions, detection of pneumothorax, evaluation of mediastinal and thoracic masses, assess the position and movement of the diaphragm as in eventration and diaphragmatic palsy, and confirm the position of intravascular catheters.
5. **Fluoroscopy:** Fluoroscopy is like a continuous X-ray study and can be used to evaluate vascular, tracheal, and esophageal anomalies, tracheoesophageal fistula, diaphragmatic activity, and swallowing studies.
6. **Arterial blood gas analysis (ABG):** ABG provides a snapshot of the patient's respiratory condition and must always be interpreted in the clinical context.
   a. Normal values are pH 7.35–7.45, PaO_2 50–70 mm Hg, PCO_2 35–45 mm Hg, bicarbonate 20–24 mEq/L, and base deficit of 3–5.
   b. Respiratory failure is present when there is hypoxemia (PaO_2 <50), hypercarbia ($PaCO_2$ >60), and acidosis (pH <7.2).
   c. Hypoxemia may result from both cardiac and respiratory causes.
   d. Hypercarbia is a better indicator of respiratory failure. Rising $PaCO_2$ ($PaCO_2$ >45) in the presence of falling pH (pH <7.25) denotes failure of gas exchange.
   e. The goal of ventilation is not to make the blood gases entirely normal but to keep them within acceptable target ranges.
7. **Oxygenation indices:** These indices give an idea about the severity of respiratory illness and help institute appropriate therapy and predict death and adverse respiratory outcomes. The three commonly used oxygenation indices are:

a. **Alveolar-arterial oxygen pressure difference (A–a DO_2):** This can be calculated using the formula: $AaDO_2$ = (713 × FiO_2) – ($PaCO_2$/0.8) – (PaO_2), where 0.8 indicates respiratory quotient on a mixed diet and 713 is derived from 760 mm Hg (atmospheric pressure at sea level)- 47 mmHg (alveolar water vapor pressure). In healthy infants, $AaDO_2$ is less than 20 in room air. In the face of hypoxia, normal $AaDO_2$ indicates alveolar hypoventilation or a low FiO_2. A high $AaDO_2$ may result from ventilation-perfusion (V/Q) mismatch or shunt. If one were to increase the FiO_2 to 100% and observe an increase in PaO_2, then V/Q mismatch might be operating, while no change in PaO_2 means shunt. The normal $AaDO_2$ is highly dependent on FiO_2 (for each 10% increase in FiO_2, the $AaDO_2$ value increases by 5–7 points), so the value should not be interpreted without FiO_2.

b. **Arterial-to-alveolar oxygen tension ratio (a/A ratio):** The a/A ratio should be close to 1 in a healthy infant. A ratio of less than 0.3 indicates disturbances in oxygen transfer.

c. **Oxygenation index:** OI = [mean airway pressure × FiO_2/PaO_2 (mm Hg)] × 100. OI is a very sensitive indicator of the severity of respiratory illness as it factors in the pressure cost of achieving oxygenation, namely MAP. It indicates the severity of hypoxemic respiratory failure (HRF) in neonates. An OI >15 indicates a ventilation-perfusion mismatch, and OI ≥40 is associated with a poor prognosis with mortality approaching 80%. Infants with hypoxic respiratory failure and OI >25 may benefit from inhaled nitric oxide (iNO); when OI exceeds 40, ECMO therapy is indicated. Limitations include the need for an indwelling arterial catheter for frequent sampling. OI provides only an intermittent measurement of oxygenation status.

8. **Other investigations:** Send sepsis screen, blood culture, and CSF examination as indicated. Monitor blood sugars and electrolytes. Consider echocardiography to rule out congenital heart disease and to evaluate PPHN.

Treatment of Respiratory Conditions

The management of individual conditions is discussed in subsequent chapters. The basic principles of treatment include:

- **Supportive care:** Assess temperature, airway, breathing, and circulation.

- Correct hypothermia
- **Airway:** Assess the airway for the presence of secretions. Suction the airway, if needed, and place a shoulder roll.
- **Breathing:** Assess for respiratory distress using an objective scoring system. Check SpO_2. Intubate if respiratory distress is severe or infant apneic.
- **Circulation:** Assess heart rate, blood pressure, and urine output. Check blood glucose level, and initiate intravenous fluids if distress is severe.

- **Respiratory support:** Respiratory support provided to the infant depends on the severity of respiratory distress, hemodynamic stability, the presence of spontaneous efforts, the underlying condition, and the presence of complications. The objective is to ensure adequate oxygenation and ventilation and thereby decrease the work of breathing.
- **Monitoring for and management of complications:** Monitor for worsening distress using Silverman's score, watch for hemodynamic instability, features of PPHN, acute kidney injury due to hypoxia and complications due to mechanical ventilation, etc.

REFERENCES

1. Misra PK. Respiratory distress in newborn. A prospective study. *Indian Pediatr*. 1987;24(1):77–80.
2. Kumar A, Bhat BV. Epidemiology of respiratory distress of newborns. Indian J Pediatr. 1996;63(1):93–8.
3. South East Asia Regional Neonatal Perinatal Database. www.newbornwhocc.org/pdf/nnpd_report_2002-03.PDF.
4. Aly H. Respiratory disorders in the newborn: Identification and diagnosis. *Pediatr Rev*. 2004;25(6):201–8.
5. Silverman WA, Andersen DH. A controlled clinical trial of effects of water mist on obstructive respiratory signs, death rate and necropsy findings among premature infants. *Pediatrics*. 1956;17(1):1–10.
6. Downes JJ, Vidyasagar D, Boggs TR, Jr., Morrow GM. Respiratory distress syndrome of newborn infants. A new clinical scoring system (RDS score) with acid-base and blood-gas correlations. *Clin Pediat*.1970;9(6):325–31.
7. Organization WH. Oxygen therapy for children: a manual for health workers. 2016; http://www.who.int/maternal_child_adolescent/documents/child-oxygen-therapy/en/. Accessed 25/12/2017, 2017.
8. Sasidharan P. An approach to diagnosis and management of cyanosis and tachypnea in term infants. *Pediatr Clin North Am*. 2004;51(4):999–1021, ix.
9. Evans JJ. Prediction of respiratory-distress syndrome by shake test on newborn gastric aspirate. N Engl J Med. 1975;292(21):1113–5.

CHAPTER

15

Respiratory Distress in Term Neonates

Respiratory distress (RD) is noted in 4–7% of neonates and is a significant cause of morbidity and mortality.[1–3] The typical cause of distress in preterm neonates is respiratory distress syndrome (RDS), but the causes are more varied in term neonates.[1–3]

ETIOLOGY

The etiology of respiratory distress among term neonates is more diverse (Table 15.1). According to the 2002–03 NNPD, the incidence of RD among inborn term neonates was 4.4%, and the common etiologies were transient tachypnea of the newborn (46.7%), followed by meconium aspiration syndrome (MAS; 29%), RDS (3.7%), pneumothorax (3.4%), and pneumonia (2.1%). About 19% of these neonates needed invasive ventilation, and the overall case fatality rate (CFR) was 25%. Among outborn term neonates, 31% had RD, and the two common etiologies were pneumonia (40%) and MAS (33%); two-thirds of the neonates required invasive ventilation, and the CFR was even higher (38.5%).

TRANSIENT TACHYPNEA OF THE NEWBORN

Pathophysiology

Failure to effectively clear the fetal lung fluid immediately after birth. In utero, the type II alveolar cells actively secrete lung fluid by secreting chloride into the alveolus (sodium and water follow the chloride into the alveoli). With the onset of labor, epinephrine levels increase and stimulate the amiloride-sensitive epithelial sodium channels (ENaC), leading to lung fluid absorption into the interstitium.

Risk Factors

TTN occurs in fewer than 1% of infants born at term gestation. The incidence is higher among preterm infants (10% among

Table 15.1: Causes of respiratory distress in term neonates
Common causes
Transient tachypnea of the newborn (TTN)
Pneumonia
Meconium aspiration syndrome
Air leak (pneumothorax)
Persistent pulmonary hypertension of the newborn (PPHN; primary or secondary causes)
Non-pulmonary (congenital heart disease, hypoxic–ischemic encephalopathy)
Less common causes:
Pulmonary causes:
• Pulmonary hemorrhage
• Respiratory distress syndrome
• Pleural effusion (including chylothorax)
• Pulmonary hypoplasia
Airway and lung malformations:
• Choanal atresia
• Congenital diaphragmatic hernia
• Tracheoesophageal fistula
• Congenital pulmonary adenomatoid malformation (CPAM)
• Lobar emphysema
• Pulmonary sequestration
Neuromuscular disorders (e.g. congenital myotonic dystrophy)
Metabolic acidosis (secondary to inborn errors of metabolism and other causes)
Rarer causes
Surfactant protein deficiency syndromes
Alveolar capillary dysplasia

33–34 weeks of gestation and 5% among infants 35–36 weeks). Elective cesarean section performed before labor is associated with a higher risk (35/1000 births) compared to a c-section after the onset of labor (12/1000 births) or after vaginal birth (5/1000 births). Other risk factors include male sex, maternal or family history of asthma, macrosomia, and maternal diabetes.

Clinical Features

Symptoms start shortly after birth (generally within 6 hours) and include tachypnea, grunting, and mild respiratory distress. The condition resolves typically in 4–72 hours. Some neonates require supplementary oxygen (generally <40% FiO_2) or CPAP support. Lung hyperinflation may result in a barrel-shaped chest with pushed-down liver and spleen, making them palpable. Auscultation may reveal the presence of crackles. Kasap et al. noted that if the peak respiratory rate in the first 36 hours of life exceeds 90/min, the risk of TTN lasting beyond 72 hours is higher.[4]

Imaging

Chest X-ray: Chest radiograph shows retained fetal lung fluid in the fissures, perihilar streaking, relative cardiomegaly, and slightly hyperexpanded lungs. The findings improve within 48 hours as the clinical condition improves, but complete resolution of perihilar markings may require 3–7 days.

- **Lung ultrasound:** Ultrasound is simple and readily available at the bedside but requires appropriate equipment and trained staff. Ultrasound of a normal lung shows horizontal A-lines (reverberation artifact from the pleural line), parallel to the pleural line and equidistant from one another. Unlike RDS (refer to Chapter 16: Respiratory Distress in Preterm Neonates), lung ultrasound findings in TTN have both alveolar interstitial patterns (represented by B-lines) and normal areas (represented by A-lines). A characteristic finding in TTN is a sharp boundary between the relatively aerated superior lung fields and interstitial edema in the basal lung fields- called the double lung point (Fig. 15.1). In severe disease, the lung parenchyma may appear white-out, and pleural effusion may be noted.

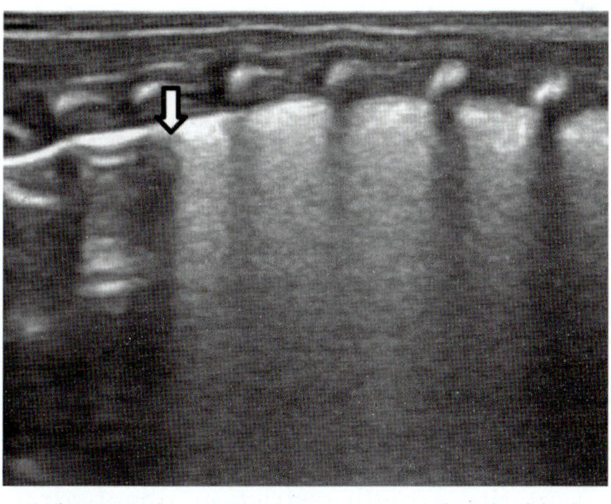

Fig. 15.1: Lung ultrasound in TTN demonstrating the double lung point sign- the sharp boundary between aerated superior lung field and alveolar interstitial edema in inferior areas

Management

- Neonates with respiratory distress should be transferred to SNCU/NICU for continued monitoring. A chest radiograph may be obtained if the distress persists beyond 6 hours after the onset. Silverman or Downe's scores should be continually monitored. Non-invasive respiratory support (CPAP) or oxygen administration (target SpO_2 between 90 and 95%) should be provided based on the degree of distress and oxygenation status.
- Neonates with persistent tachypnea (respiratory rate >80/min) or severe distress may be provided gavage feeding; a few neonates might even require intravenous fluids.
- Rarely neonates with TTN can have a severe disease requiring mechanical ventilation and manifest features of PPHN.
- An alternate diagnosis should be considered if:
  - Tachypnea persists beyond 5 or 6 days (rule out congenital heart disease)
  - Hemodynamic instability or risk factors for sepsis are present
  - Severe respiratory distress with the need for mechanical ventilation (rule out PPHN and alternate pulmonary diagnosis)
- Other therapies: Limited evidence shows that drugs such as inhaled beta-agonist (salbutamol), inhaled epinephrine, corticosteroids, diuretics, and fluid restriction do not impact clinical outcomes in neonates with TTN. They are not recommended in the management of TTN.
- Prevention: Given the increased respiratory morbidity, the American College of Obstetricians and Gynecologists and the AAP have recommended deferring elective delivery until 39 completed weeks of gestation.

MECONIUM ASPIRATION SYNDROME

Meconium aspiration syndrome (MAS) refers to varying degrees of respiratory distress in neonates born through the meconium-stained amniotic fluid (MSAF). About 12–14% of births are complicated with MSAF, and 5% of those exposed to MSAF develop MAS.[4,5] In India, the incidence of MAS is higher, and the disease morbidity and mortality are also higher. The risk factors include advanced gestation (the incidence of MSAF beyond 42 weeks of gestation is 25–50%), intrauterine growth restriction, oligohydramnios, fetal distress, perinatal asphyxia, and thick meconium. However, MAS can also occur in vigorous neonates and with thin meconium.

Pathophysiology

In term neonates, fetal stress due to hypoxia and acidosis can cause a vagal response and increased peristalsis and anal sphincter relaxation and passage of meconium *in utero*. MSAF in a preterm neonate might indicate fetal diarrhea due to sepsis, particularly *Listeria*. Fetal gasping efforts *in utero* or after birth can lead to the aspiration of meconium and MAS. Inhaled meconium results in respiratory distress by the following mechanisms:

- **Airway obstruction:** Complete obstruction results in atelectasis, while partial obstruction produces a ball-valve effect resulting in localized emphysema. Air leaks, such as interstitial emphysema, pneumothorax, and pneumomediastinum, are common.
- **Surfactant inactivation:** Fatty acids in the meconium cause atelectasis and worsen ventilation-perfusion mismatch. Meconium also exerts toxic effects on type II pneumocytes, reduces the levels of surfactant proteins A and B, and causes damage to the alveolar-capillary membrane.
- **Inflammation:** Meconium causes the release of cytokines and complement activation. The inflammation can begin antenatally and continue after birth.
- **Worsening of persistent pulmonary hypertension:** PPHN can occur in 15–20% of neonates with MAS and is proposed to be due to pulmonary vasoconstriction secondary to hypoxia, hypercapnia, acidosis, and hypertrophic media of pulmonary vessels due to intrauterine hypoxia. PPHN worsens the hypoxia leading to a vicious cycle.

Diagnosis

The diagnosis of MAS is based on the clinical history and supportive chest X-ray findings of bilateral diffuse patchy infiltrates (representing atelectasis) alternating with areas of hyperinflation (representing air-trapping). Air leaks, including pneumothorax, pneumomediastinum, and interstitial emphysema, are common in MAS.

The diagnosis of MAS is based on

- Respiratory distress in a neonate born through MSAF.
- Onset within the first 2 hours of life and lasting for at least 12 hours.
- Need for supplemental oxygen to maintain oxygen saturation 92%.
- Absence of alternate etiologies such as congenital malformations of the lung or cardiac disease and the presence of characteristic chest X-ray findings.

Cleary and Wiswell classified MAS based on the severity of illness as mild MAS as a disease requiring less than 40% oxygen for fewer than 48 hours, moderate MAS as needing more than 40% oxygen for more than 48 hours with no air leak, and severe MAS as a disease requiring assisted ventilation for more than 48 hours. Severe MAS is associated with persistent pulmonary hypertension (PPHN). Thus, the spectrum of MAS can range from mild respiratory distress with minimal oxygen requirement to severe distress with hypoxemic respiratory failure requiring high-frequency ventilation, inhaled nitric oxide (iNO), and or extracorporeal membrane oxygenation (ECMO). One-third of neonates with MAS require intubation and mechanical ventilation. The severity of the disease in the chest X-ray may not always correlate with the clinical picture. The oxygenation index provides an objective measure of hypoxemia: mild hypoxemia (OI <15), moderate (OI 15–25), and severe (OI 25–40). An OI over 25 for more than 4 hours is an indication for initiating inhaled nitric oxide therapy, and OI >40 indicates the need for ECMO.

Management

Neonates born through MSAF and manifesting respiratory distress should be transferred to NICU for close monitoring and respiratory management. Initial investigations include a chest X-ray and sepsis screen if risk factors are identified.

1. **General measures:** Maintain normal body temperature and provide nutrition to maintain normal blood sugar levels. Avoid precipitators of PPHN such as hypothermia, hypoxia, acidosis, pain, and excessive handling/stimulation. Neonates with MAS can have additional morbidities such as sepsis, hypotensive shock, myocardial dysfunction, hypoxic-ischemic encephalopathy, and renal dysfunction that require appropriate management.
2. **Oxygen saturation:** The goal is to maintain preductal saturation between 92 and 95%. Supplemental oxygen via nasal prongs or HFNC should be provided.
3. **Noninvasive support:** Neonates with respiratory distress (Downe score >4 and requiring supplemental oxygen) should be offered nasal CPAP. Initial CPAP pressure can be 5 cm of H_2O, and FiO_2 is adjusted to maintain target saturations. Pneumothorax should be ruled out before initiating CPAP in MAS, and CPAP pressures should be cautiously increased due to the risk of air leaks. Nasal CPAP is superior to oxygen therapy in reducing the need for mechanical ventilation in neonates with MAS.[6] Neonates can be

weaned from CPAP when the SpO_2 is consistently greater than 90%, FiO_2 is less than 30%, and respiratory distress resolves (respiratory rate <60 breaths/min, no or mild retractions, and no grunting). Mechanical ventilation should be considered if the neonate fails to maintain SpO_2 on a CPAP pressure of 6–7 cm and FiO_2 of >60%.

4. **Mechanical ventilation:** About 30–40% of infants with MAS require mechanical ventilation. Indications for intubation are CPAP failure or respiratory acidosis (pH <7.25 and $PaCO_2$ >60 mmHg). Ventilatory settings depend on the underlying pathology. Predominantly atelectatic lungs require higher mean airway pressure, whereas predominantly hyperinflated lungs pose a higher risk of air trapping and air leaks and require lower PEEP. Lower rates and adequate expiratory time must be provided to avoid air trapping. High-frequency ventilation may be considered if the MAP is >12 cm H_2O or peak inspiratory pressure >25 cm H_2O or before initiating iNO.
5. **Surfactant:** Surfactant therapy in severe MAS improves oxygenation and reduces the need for extracorporeal membrane oxygenation (ECMO). But there is no effect on mortality, air leak, duration of ventilation, or chronic lung disease. Surfactant therapy may be considered in neonates with severe MAS requiring invasive ventilation and OI >15. Bolus administration of the natural surfactant preparation in the usual dose (100 mg/kg) is preferred.
6. **Inhaled nitric oxide (iNO):** iNO should be considered in neonates with PPHN when OI reaches 15–25. Lung recruitment should be optimized with high-frequency ventilation, and iNO therapy should be started at an initial dose of 20 parts per million (ppm) to improve PaO_2 by at least 20 mm Hg. Once the FiO_2 requirement falls to 60% or less, iNO can be weaned in decrements of 5 ppm every 4 h until 5 ppm and then by 1 ppm. Inhaled nitric oxide therapy reduces the need for ECMO and mortality in term or near-term neonates with hypoxemic respiratory failure and PPHN.
7. **Other therapies:** Routine use of antibiotics or steroids has no role. Antibiotics should be considered only in the presence of risk factors for sepsis or if the clinical course is consistent with sepsis.

Outcome

Case fatality rate due to MAS varies from 13–32%. In a study of 170 neonates with MAS[7], one-third required mechanical ventilation, and a significant percentage had complications such as PPHN, hypotensive shock, HIE, and myocardial dysfunction. A study from South India reported that 18% of infants with MAS had severe developmental delays as assessed by using DASII at 9 months of age.[8]

PNEUMONIA

Pneumonia accounts for 18–68% of neonates presenting with respiratory distress in the neonatal period, and the case fatality rate varies from 11–18%. Pneumonia is a part of systemic sepsis in neonates and can be associated with bloodstream infections and meningitis. Pneumonia can be classified as congenital, early-, and late-onset based on the timing of the onset of symptoms. Congenital pneumonia can lead to stillbirth or manifest immediately after birth as it is associated with chorioamnionitis, maternal *Toxoplasma*, cytomegalovirus infection, or syphilis. Early-onset pneumonia manifests within the first 72 hours and generally results from *in utero* ascending infection or transmission during birth or shortly afterward. Late-onset pneumonia (nosocomial or community-acquired) is usually caused by environmental pathogens transmitted through the hands of the caregiver.

Clinical Presentation and Management

Clinical features and radiological manifestations of early-onset pneumonia overlap with RDS. The presence of risk factors such as maternal fever (>38°C), foul-smelling liquor, prolonged rupture of membranes (>24 hours), clinical findings such as poor feeding, lethargy, hypotension, multiple organ dysfunction can be suggestive of sepsis/ pneumonia. Chest X-ray may show coarse patchy infiltrates, diffuse haziness or granularity, air bronchogram, or consolidation. However, radiological changes take longer to resolve than RDS. In addition, the pathogen may be isolated in a blood culture. Management includes general measures, respiratory support, and appropriate antibiotic therapy.

RESPIRATORY DISTRESS SYNDROME

Surfactant deficiency leading to RDS can occur in 0.3% of term neonates compared to 10.5% among preterm infants <34 weeks' gestation. Clinical manifestations in the former group are similar, with symptom onset within minutes to hours after birth. Chest X-ray shows bilateral diffuse opacities and loss of lung volume. Pathologies such as meconium aspiration, hypothermia, sepsis, pulmonary edema, and maternal diabetes can contribute to surfactant inactivation or diminished synthesis in term neonates. Surfactant replacement therapy results in an immediate improvement in lung compliance and oxygen requirement. If respiratory distress is out of proportion to the gestational age, or the response to surfactant therapy is poor or temporary, one should consider the possibility of disorders of surfactant protein synthesis.

DISORDERS OF SURFACTANT PROTEIN SYNTHESIS

Surfactant is synthesized by type II alveolar cells in the endoplasmic reticulum, further processed in the Golgi bodies, and stored in lamellar bodies until secreted into the alveoli. The secreted surfactant spreads as a lipid in the alveoli and is recycled again by the type II cells. Surfactant proteins B and C facilitate the adsorption of the surfactant film in the alveolar air-liquid interface, and SP-B also contributes to the formation of tubular myelin. ABCA3 protein helps import surfactant phospholipids from the cytosol into the lamellar body and is essential for synthesizing the lamellar body.

Mutations in surfactant proteins B and C (SFTPB and SFTPC) primarily affect surfactant folding, leading to its accumulation in the Golgi bodies and impaired formation of tubular myelin. Mutations in ABCA3 lead to abnormal lamellar body formation. Mutations in the SFTPB gene and ABCA3 gene are inherited as an autosomal recessive disorder. In contrast, SFTPC mutations are inherited as an autosomal dominant trait with variable penetrance and severity (45%) or as a sporadic disease due to *de novo* mutations.

Clinical Presentation[9]

- **Surfactant protein B deficiency:** Classic deficiency results in severe respiratory failure in term neonates and death in a few months unless lung transplantation is performed. Cases with partial deficiencies are also identified where the clinical course is less severe.
- **Surfactant protein C deficiency:** Presents with chronic interstitial lung disease in infancy and childhood. Generally, symptoms manifest by 2–3 months of age, with only 10% presenting in the neonatal period. Older infants present with tachypnea, retractions, hypoxemia, digital clubbing, and failure to thrive. Chest X-ray shows hyperinflation with increased interstitial markings.

- **ABCA3 protein deficiency:** Presents with variable severity, with onset in the neonatal period being more common (80% of cases). Neonates have respiratory distress and failure with high mortality unless a lung transplant is performed.

Management

Respiratory failure is managed with conventional or high-frequency ventilation, inhaled nitric oxide, and extracorporeal membrane oxygenation (ECMO). Surfactant replacement therapy results in only transient improvement. The presence of family history should prompt an earlier diagnosis.

The initial investigations include the analysis of common mutation of surfactant protein genes in blood and examination of bronchoalveolar lavage (BAL) fluid for SP-B protein and aberrant SP-C peptide by immune-histochemistry. If surfactant had been administered exogenously, SP-B might be detected in the lavage fluid for 24–48 hours. The absence of SP-B and isolation of aberrant SP-C indicates the need for a lung biopsy. In addition, electron microscopy analysis of lung biopsy specimens may reveal aberrant lamellar body formation in SP-B and ABCA3 mutations. If SP-B is undetectable or significantly reduced in lung tissue obtained by biopsy or if a homozygous mutation is identified in gene testing, compassionate care or lung transplantation are the only options. The presence of SP-B in biopsy and the absence of the known mutations suggest that the infant is not SP-B deficient and supportive care should be continued.

The 5-year survival rate for SP-B deficient infants who received a lung transplant is approximately 50%. In case of death of the neonate before a definitive diagnosis, the family should be offered a post-mortem examination along with immunologic staining of the lung for surfactant proteins.

REFERENCES

1. Gnanaratnem J, Finer NN. Neonatal acute respiratory failure. Curr Opin Pediatr. Jun 2000;12(3):227–32.
2. Edwards MO, Kotecha SJ, Kotecha S. Respiratory distress of the term newborn infant. Paediatr Respir Rev. Mar 2013;14(1):29-36; quiz 36–7. doi:10.1016/j.prrv.2012.02.002.
3. Reuter S, Moser C, Baack M. Respiratory distress in the newborn. Pediatr Rev. Oct 2014;35(10):417–28; quiz 429. doi:10.1542/pir.35–10–417.
4. Wiswell TE, Tuggle JM, Turner BS. Meconium aspiration syndrome: have we made a difference? Pediatrics. May 1990;85(5):715–21.

5. Wiswell TE, Knight GR, Finer NN, et al. A multicenter, randomized, controlled trial comparing Surfaxin (Lucinactant) lavage with standard care for treatment of meconium aspiration syndrome. Pediatrics. Jun 2002;109(6):1081–7.
6. Pandita A, Murki S, Oleti TP, et al. Effect of Nasal Continuous Positive Airway Pressure on Infants With Meconium Aspiration Syndrome: A Randomized Clinical Trial. JAMA Pediatr. Feb 1 2018;172(2):161–5. doi:10.1001/jamapediatrics.2017.3873.
7. Louis D, Sundaram V, Mukhopadhyay K, Dutta S, Kumar P. Predictors of mortality in neonates with meconium aspiration syndrome. Indian Pediatr. Aug 2014;51(8):637–40.
8. Chettri S, Bhat BV, Adhisivam B. Current Concepts in the Management of Meconium Aspiration Syndrome. Indian J Pediatr. Oct 2016;83(10):1125–30. doi:10.1007/s12098–016–2128–9.
9. Magnani JE, Donn SM. Persistent Respiratory Distress in the Term Neonate: Genetic Surfactant Deficiency Diseases. Current pediatric reviews. 2020;16(1):17–25. doi:10.2174/1573396315666190723112916.

CHAPTER

16

Respiratory Distress in Preterm Neonates

Respiratory distress occurs in 6–7% of all neonates in India, with preterm neonates having the highest incidence (30%).[1,2] Among very low birth weight neonates (VLBW), respiratory distress syndrome (RDS) is the most common cause of respiratory distress (36%), followed by pneumonia (28%) and transient tachypnoea of the newborn (27%). VLBW neonates with respiratory distress have a higher case fatality rate than those without respiratory distress.[2]

RESPIRATORY DISTRESS SYNDROME (RDS)

A preterm neonate is said to have RDS if respiratory distress occurs in the first 6 hours of life and chest X-ray shows poor lung expansion with air bronchogram/reticulogranular pattern/ground-glass opacity or there is a negative gastric aspirate shake test.

Pathophysiology

Neonates born before the alveolarization stage of lung development (32 weeks) have underdeveloped alveolar sacs and delayed production and secretion of functional surfactant. Neonates with RDS have a surfactant pool of only 10 mg/kg compared to 100 mg/kg in term infants. The surfactant deficiency results in increased surface tension, causing alveolar collapse in preterm neonates. These preterm neonates thus manifest with increased work of breathing to keep the alveoli distended. Gradually, diffuse atelectasis ensues, which leads to lung injury, causing accumulation of protein exudate and edema fluid (forming the hyaline membrane in the alveoli) that further inactivates surfactant.

Epidemiology

The incidence of RDS is 1.2% among all neonates in India.[3] The incidence increases with decreasing gestational age—from 55% at 27–28 weeks to 35% at 31–32 weeks to 2% at 35–36 weeks.[4]

Antenatal corticosteroids administered to pregnant women at risk of preterm delivery significantly reduce RDS risk (RR 0.71, 95% CI 0.65–0.78).[5] Besides prematurity, other risk factors like male gender, white race, cesarean delivery, maternal diabetes, and chorioamnionitis predispose a neonate to RDS.

Clinical Presentation

Neonates with RDS present with respiratory distress in the first 6 hours of life in the form of tachypnea, increased xiphoid, upper chest and lower chest retractions, grunt, and nasal flaring. In addition, the neonate may require supplemental oxygen to maintain a target saturation of 90–95%. In the absence of surfactant replacement therapy (SRT), respiratory distress worsens, with the peak severity at 24–48 hours. In neonates who survive without SRT, the disease resolves in 3–5 days. This clinical course differentiates it from transient tachypnea, which has an improving clinical course and does not worsen, and the condition resolves in 24–72 hours.

Management

The basic principles of management are to provide appropriate respiratory support to maintain adequate oxygen saturation and decrease the work of breathing.

Investigations

1. **Shake test:** It is a simple bedside test done on the gastric aspirate, reflecting the adequacy of pulmonary surfactant in the neonate (*see* Chapter 14: Approach to Respiratory Distress in the Newborn, for further details).
2. **Chest radiograph:** Neonates with mild RDS will have low volume lungs along with reticulogranularity, which occurs due to the presence of air in terminal bronchioles juxtaposed with the collapsed alveoli with no air. Moderate RDS shall have air bronchograms that happen when more distal airways collapse, thus making the air in proximal bronchi prominent. Severe RDS presents as white-out lung fields due to diffuse alveolar atelectasis.
3. **Ultrasound:** A high-resolution linear probe of 10 MHz is preferred for neonatal lung USG. Normal pleura appears as a regular echogenic line known as a 'pleural line,' which moves continuously during respiration. 'A-lines' in a normal lung appear as a series of regular echogenic lines parallel to the pleural line and equidistant to each other (Fig. 16.1a). A few vertically

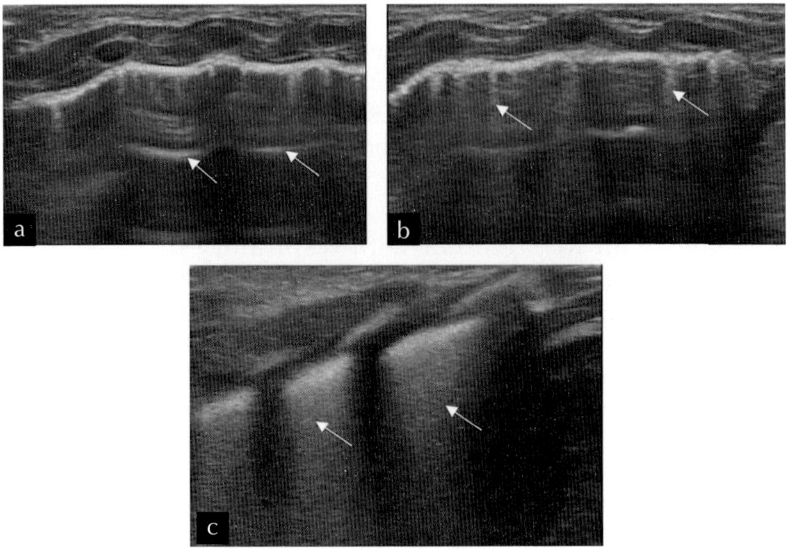

Fig. 16.1: Ultrasound images showing (a) A-lines and (b) B lines seen in normal newborn lungs and (c) confluent B lines seen in RDS (white arrows).

oriented lines running from the pleural line to the edge of the screen, known as 'B lines,' can be present in a normal newborn with fluid-rich lungs, which disappear completely in 24–36 hours (Fig. 16.1b). Confluent B lines that give the appearance of the white lung (Fig. 16.1c), pleural line abnormalities such as thickening, irregularities, and coarse appearance, small subpleural hypoechoic areas signifying consolidation, and absence of areas with the normal pattern are usually seen in neonates with RDS. Together, these signs have nearly 100% sensitivity and specificity in identifying RDS.[6]

Treatment

1. **Supportive care:** Maintaining a thermoneutral environment and normal blood glucose, initiating enteral or parenteral nutrition, and regular vital monitoring, including respiratory distress scoring and hemodynamic and saturation monitoring to identify impending respiratory failure or hemodynamic compromise, form the mainstay of supportive care.
2. **Respiratory support:** The main principle is to decrease the work of breathing:
   - *Continuous positive airway pressure (CPAP):* Preterm neonates (<35 weeks) with any sign of respiratory distress must be

initiated on CPAP. CPAP is usually started at 5 cm of H_2O, with 5 L/min flow and an adequate FiO_2 to maintain oxygen saturation of 91–95%. The CPAP pressure and FiO_2 should be subsequently titrated based on the retractions, chest expansion, and oxygen saturation.

- *Noninvasive positive pressure ventilation (NIPPV):* Early initiation of NIPPV compared to CPAP decreases the risk of respiratory failure and the need for invasive ventilation.[7] We reserve NIPPV for neonates with CPAP failure before initiating mechanical ventilation.
- *Mechanical ventilation:* Neonates with worsening respiratory distress scoring or hypoxemia/hypercarbia despite CPAP pressures of 7–8 cm H_2O and FiO_2 of 60% or more should be intubated and ventilated.
- When used as primary support in preterm neonates, the heated, humidified high-flow nasal cannula (HHHFNC) has a higher risk of treatment failure. Therefore, it is not recommended as the primary support in neonates with RDS.[8]

3. **Surfactant therapy:** Preterm neonates with increasing FiO_2 requirement and worsening respiratory distress on CPAP must be given intratracheal surfactant. Among animal-derived surfactant preparations, poractant alfa at a dose of 200 mg/kg reduces mortality and bronchopulmonary dysplasia (BPD) compared to low-dose poractant or beractant (bovine surfactant).[9] *See* Chapter 44: Surfactant Replacement Therapy in Neonates, for different techniques of surfactant administration.
4. **Monitoring and management of complications:** Respiratory distress scoring should be continually performed to identify neonates with hypoxic respiratory failure early. Neonates may develop pneumothorax while on noninvasive or invasive respiratory support or after surfactant administration. Air leaks must be suspected in any neonate with sudden deterioration. The neonates must also be monitored for pulmonary hemorrhage or patent ductus arteriosus (because of the sudden fall in pulmonary pressures following surfactant administration).

PULMONARY HEMORRHAGE

The incidence of pulmonary hemorrhage is up to 5–6% in preterm, very low birth weight neonates.[10] It used to be common in neonates who received intratracheal surfactant. Surfactant therapy causes a rapid lowering of intrapulmonary pressures, which causes left to right shunting of blood via patent ductus arteriosus, increasing pulmonary blood flow and making the immature lung prone to hemorrhage. It can be prevented by ensuring adequate CPAP/ PEEP following surfactant administration. Other risk factors of pulmonary hemorrhage include sepsis, PDA, hypothermia, and bleeding disorders.

Clinical Presentation

Pulmonary hemorrhage presents with rapid clinical deterioration in the form of cyanosis, apnea, worsening respiratory distress, bradycardia, and shock. Red or pink-tinged secretions can be seen on suctioning of the oropharynx or endotracheal tube.

Management

Investigation: Chest X-ray findings vary from mild haziness in bilateral lung fields to complete white-out, depending on the extent of hemorrhage. An echocardiogram should be done to rule out hemodynamically significant PDA and evaluate the left ventricular function. Sepsis screen and blood culture are to be performed if there is a strong clinical suspicion of sepsis. Platelet count and PT/ APTT may be indicated in the presence of a bleeding diathesis.

Treatment

1. **Supportive care:** The etiology of pulmonary hemorrhage should be identified and promptly corrected. Vitamin K 1 mg must be administered intravenously as a slow bolus. In case of shock, normal saline boluses and appropriate inotropes must be initiated. Thrombocytopenia and clotting abnormalities should be managed with platelet and FFP transfusion. PRBC transfusion might be required in the presence of significant anemia.
2. **Respiratory support:**
   - The trachea must be suctioned post endotracheal intubation, and the neonate must be mechanically ventilated with a higher positive end-expiratory pressure (PEEP) of 6–7 cm of H_2O. In case of persisting bleeding, consider increasing the mean airway pressure (MAP) or switching to high-frequency ventilation.
   - Surfactant therapy may improve lung compliance and oxygenation in neonates with severe pulmonary hemorrhage.

PNEUMOTHORAX

The incidence of pneumothorax among VLBW neonates is nearly 4%.[11] Pneumothorax occurs due to higher transpulmonary pressure generated in a neonate with respiratory distress. The most common cause of pneumothorax in preterm neonates is RDS. There is a male preponderance, probably due to the higher incidence of RDS and TTN among boys.

Clinical Presentation

Pneumothorax presents as a sudden deterioration in a neonate on noninvasive or invasive respiratory support in the form of an increase in respiratory distress or FiO_2 requirement with decreased air entry on the affected side. In tension pneumothorax, the accumulation of large volumes of air in the pleural space compresses the lungs. It reduces the venous return to the heart, causing hypotension, poor peripheral perfusion, apnea, and bradycardia.

Management

The primary management principles include early and accurate detection of pneumothorax, identifying signs of tension pneumothorax, and providing specific treatment.

Investigations

1. **Transillumination:** This bedside test is done ideally with a fiber-optic source of light placed firmly perpendicular to the neonatal chest in a darkened room. Typically, only 1 cm around the light will transilluminate and form a halo. If the illumination spreads beyond this 1 cm halo, it is taken as a positive transillumination test suggestive of pneumothorax (Fig. 16.2). Transillumination may be false-negative in neonates with skin edema and false-positive in neonates with lobar emphysema or pneumomediastinum.

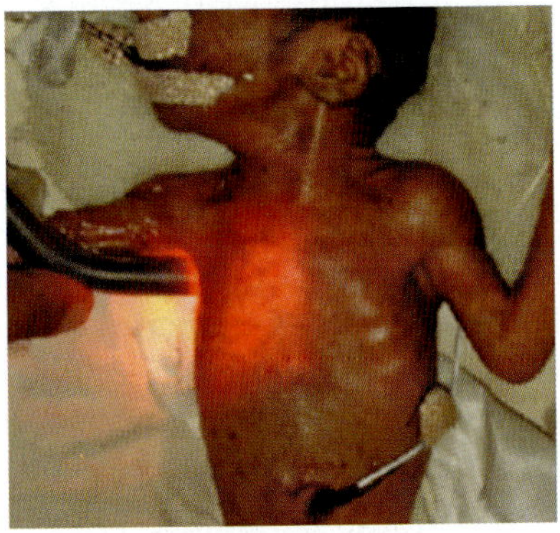

Fig. 16.2: Positive transillumination test in an infant with right-sided pneumothorax

2. **Chest X-ray:** Pneumothorax is evident as increased radiolucency of the ipsilateral side with sharp margins of a collapsed lung and no lung markings beyond that. The mediastinal shift may be apparent in cases with tension pneumothorax.
3. **Lung ultrasound:** Normal lung creates a sliding sign wherein two pleural layers slide along each other. Pneumothorax is evident as the absence of the lung sliding sign (due to the presence of air between the visceral and parietal pleura) and the lack of B lines in the affected area. The junction between the sliding lung and absent sliding is known as the lung point and is nearly 100% specific for pneumothorax.

Treatment

1. **Needle aspiration:** For emergency management of tension pneumothorax, needle aspiration is performed in the 2nd intercostal space in the midclavicular line using a butterfly needle of 21 G (green) or 23 G (blue) connected to a 10 ml syringe via a 3-way stopcock. Needle aspiration is usually followed by tube thoracostomy for complete resolution of pneumothorax. However, recent studies show that nearly half of the neonates with a pneumothorax who underwent needle aspiration do not require chest drain insertion.[12]
2. **Chest tube insertion:** This is performed in the 4th or 5th intercostal space in the mid-axillary line using an 8 or 10 Fr chest tube and connected to an underwater seal. Chest drains are kept in place until complete resolution of pneumothorax (stops bubbling or swinging) and removed after being clamped for several hours with no evidence of increased respiratory distress.

PULMONARY INTERSTITIAL EMPHYSEMA (PIE)

PIE results from alveolar rupture following overdistension of alveoli. This causes air to escape into the connective tissue sheath surrounding airways and into the interlobular septa. PIE occurred in nearly 32% of VLBW neonates in the pre-surfactant era, which has come down to almost 5–6% in recent studies.[13] Lower gestational age and birth weight, severe RDS, invasive mechanical ventilation, prolonged invasive ventilation, surfactant requirement, and higher peak inspiratory pressure are significant risk factors for PIE.

Clinical Presentation

PIE presents with gradually worsening respiratory distress, hypercarbia, and hypoxia, requiring increased respiratory support and FiO_2 requirement.

Management

Investigation

Chest X-ray: It is the diagnostic modality of choice for PIE which can be appreciated as tortuous wavy, linear radiolucencies (air in interstitium) radiating from hilum to periphery. Extensive PIE may give a honeycomb appearance on the chest X-ray.

Treatment

PIE is usually managed conservatively with gentle ventilation. Positioning the affected side down for localized PIE usually results in resolution in 48 hours. Selective intubation of the main stem bronchus of the uninvolved side has also been tried in some cases. More severe cases benefit from switching to high-frequency ventilation.

OTHER CAUSES OF RESPIRATORY DISTRESS

- **Pneumonia:** Pneumonia is the second most common cause of respiratory distress among preterm neonates and must be suspected in cases with maternal risk factors of early-onset neonatal sepsis or worsening respiratory distress in a neonate on invasive or non-invasive respiratory support. Further details on the management have been provided in Chapter 15: Respiratory Distress in Term Neonates.
- **Transient tachypnea of the newborn (TTN):** Though a disease of term neonates, late preterm neonates are also affected by TTN due to inadequate resorption of fetal lung fluid. Neonates suffering from TTN show maximum distress at birth with gradual improvement in respiratory distress with adequate respiratory support. The distress usually settles in 48–72 hours (refer to Chapter 15: Respiratory Distress in Term Neonates).
- **Rarer causes:**
  - *Patent ductus arteriosus (PDA):* A hemodynamically significant PDA presents with gradually increasing respiratory distress,

hypoxia, hypercarbia, and hyperdynamic precordium with or without a systolic murmur in the left parasternal area. The condition has been dealt with in Chapter 11: Patent Ductus Arteriosus in Preterm Neonates.

- *Pulmonary hypoplasia:* Pulmonary hypoplasia results from a variety of causes that result in inadequate development of lung parenchyma in utero, such as space-occupying lesions in the chest (congenital diaphragmatic hernia), chest wall malformations (skeletal dysplasia), neuromuscular disorders which prevent normal fetal breathing movement, and severe oligohydramnios (bilateral renal agenesis or prolonged rupture of membranes). A low volume lung ventilation according to lung size and not body size would be the optimal approach to ventilatory management of these neonates. Pulmonary hypoplasia is generally associated with raised pulmonary artery pressures. In severe cases, inhaled nitric oxide may be required to decrease the increased pulmonary pressure.
- *Surgical conditions* like tracheoesophageal fistula, congenital diaphragmatic hernia, choanal atresia, congenital lobar emphysema, and congenital cystic adenomatoid malformation can also lead to respiratory distress among preterm neonates and have been described elsewhere.

PROGNOSIS

The prognosis depends on the underlying cause of respiratory distress. Earlier stabilization of neonates with respiratory distress syndrome using delivery room CPAP and timely surfactant administration improves the prognosis. Volume-targeted ventilation help in decreasing the incidence of air leak syndromes (RR 0.52, 95% CI 0.31–0.87).[14] A longer duration of mechanical ventilation has a significantly increased risk of neurodevelopmental impairment. Pulmonary hemorrhage and pulmonary interstitial emphysema have been associated with high mortality of nearly 50% among preterm neonates,[15,16] with mortality being the highest among extremely low birth weight neonates and those presenting within 24 hours of life. Nearly 40–50% of survivors of pulmonary hemorrhage or PIE develop bronchopulmonary dysplasia.[16,17] The overall mortality in neonates with pneumothorax used to be high (up to 20%), with preterm neonates more predisposed to mortality and recurrence.[18]

REFERENCES

1. Kumar A, Bhat BV. Epidemiology of respiratory distress of newborns. Indian J Pediatr. 1996 Feb;63(1):93–8.
2. Bhakoo ON, Narang A, Karthikeyan G, Kumar P. Spectrum of respiratory distress in very low birthweight neonates. Indian J Pediatr. 2000 Nov;67(11):803–4.
3. South East Asia Regional Neonatal-Perinatal Database. www.newbornwhocc.org/pdf/nnpd_report_2002-03.PDF. Accessed 17 Feb 2022.
4. Rubaltelli FF, Bonafe L, Tangucci M, Spagnolo A, Dani C. Epidemiology of neonatal acute respiratory disorders. A multicenter study on incidence and fatality rates of neonatal acute respiratory disorders according to gestational age, maternal age, pregnancy complications, and type of delivery. Italian Group of Neonatal Pneumology. Biol Neonate. 1998;74(1):7–15.
5. McGoldrick E, Stewart F, Parker R, Dalziel S. Antenatal corticosteroids for accelerating fetal lung maturation for women at risk of preterm birth. Cochrane Database Syst Rev [Internet]. 2020;(12). Available from: https://doi.org//10.1002/14651858.CD004454.pub4.
6. Copetti R, Cattarossi L, Macagno F, Violino M, Furlan R. Lung Ultrasound in Respiratory Distress Syndrome: A Useful Tool for Early Diagnosis. Neonatology. 2008;94(1):52–9.
7. Lemyre B, Laughon M, Bose C, Davis PG. Early nasal intermittent positive pressure ventilation (NIPPV) versus early nasal continuous positive airway pressure (NCPAP) for preterm infants. Cochrane Database Syst Rev. 2016 Dec 15;12(12):CD005384.
8. Bruet S, Butin M, Dutheil F. Systematic review of high-flow nasal cannula versus continuous positive airway pressure for primary support in preterm infants. Arch Dis Child Fetal Neonatal Ed. 2022 Jan;107(1):56–9.
9. Singh N, Halliday HL, Stevens TP, Suresh G, Soll R, Rojas-Reyes MX. Comparison of animal-derived surfactants for the prevention and treatment of respiratory distress syndrome in preterm infants. Cochrane Database Syst Rev. 2015 Dec 21;(12):CD010249.
10. Tomaszewska M, Stork E, Minich NM, Friedman H, Berlin S, Hack M. Pulmonary Hemorrhage: Clinical Course and Outcomes Among Very Low-Birth-Weight Infants. Arch Pediatr Adolesc Med. 1999 Jul 1;153(7):715–21.
11. Vermont Oxford Network database summary for infants 501-1500 grams born in 2020. Burlington, VT: Vermont Oxford Network,2021. Available from: https://headless.vtoxford.org/wp-content/uploads/2021/06/2020-VLBW-Network-Summary.pdf (Accessed on 17/03/2022).
12. Murphy MC, Heiring C, Doglioni N, Trevisanuto D, Blennow M, Bohlin K, et al. Effect of Needle Aspiration of Pneumothorax on Subsequent Chest Drain Insertion in Newborns: A Randomized Clinical Trial. JAMA Pediatr. 2018 Jul 1;172(7):664–9.
13. Morley CJ, Davis PG, Doyle LW, Brion LP, Hascoet JM, Carlin JB. Nasal CPAP or intubation at birth for very preterm infants. N Engl J Med. 2008 Feb 14;358(7):700–8.

14. Klingenberg C, Wheeler KI, McCallion N, Morley CJ, Davis PG. Volume-targeted versus pressure-limited ventilation in neonates. Cochrane Database Syst Rev. 2017 Oct 17;10(10):CD003666.
15. Ahmad KA, Bennett MM, Ahmad SF, Clark RH, Tolia VN. Morbidity and mortality with early pulmonary haemorrhage in preterm neonates. Arch Dis Child Fetal Neonatal Ed. 2019 Jan;104(1):F63–8.
16. Gaylord MS, Thieme RE, Woodall DL, Quissell BJ. Predicting mortality in low-birth-weight infants with pulmonary interstitial emphysema. Pediatrics. 1985 Aug;76(2):219–24.
17. Bozkaya A, Yurttutan S, Özkars MY, Doğaner A. Respiratory problems in preterm infants with pulmonary hemorrhage. J Matern Fetal Neonatal Med. 2021 Aug 12;1–6.
18. Miall L, Shore H, Salar S, Dunbavand G. G225(P) The incidence and outcomes of pneumothorax in neonates in the 21st century. Arch Dis Child. 2020 Oct 1;105(Suppl 1):A82.

CHAPTER

17

Apnea

About 30–45% of preterm neonates exhibit a periodic breathing pattern characterized by three or more respiratory pauses of greater than 3 seconds in duration. Periodic breathing is a regular event in preterm neonates, reflective of the immaturity of the respiratory control system, and does not merit any treatment. In contrast, apnea is a pathological cessation of breathing that results in hemodynamic disturbances and merits treatment.

DEFINITION

Apnea is defined as cessation of breathing for longer than 20 sec or a shorter duration in the presence of significant bradycardia (heart rate <80 bpm) or change in skin color (pallor or cyanosis).[1]

INCIDENCE

Apnea is a common manifestation of many neonatal diseases. It is usually related to the immaturity of the respiratory control system in preterm neonates and is referred to as the apnea of prematurity (AOP). Apnea can also be a manifestation of many other diseases.

The incidence of AOP is inversely proportional to the gestational age. While it occurs in almost all neonates born before 28 weeks of gestation, the incidence reduces to about 20% in neonates born at 34 weeks.

ETIOLOGY[2]

Apnea of Prematurity (AOP): It is related to the immaturity of the brainstem and peripheral chemoreceptors, resulting in abnormal ventilator response to hypercarbia and hypoxia, along with immature reflex responses. This condition usually presents after 1–2 days of life and mainly within the first seven days. The need for ventilatory support in the initial few days of life may delay its detection.

Apnea occurring in the first 24 hours and beyond 7 days of life is more likely to have a secondary cause.

Secondary Causes

These include:

a. **Temperature instability:** Hypothermia and hyperthermia, especially with frequent fluctuations in body temperature.
b. **Neurological:** Intracranial infections, intracranial hemorrhage, seizures, perinatal asphyxia, and placental transfer of drugs such as narcotics, magnesium sulfate, or general anesthetics.
c. **Pulmonary:** Respiratory distress syndrome (RDS), pneumonia, airway obstruction due to neck flexion or secretions, pulmonary hemorrhage, airway malformations, pneumothorax.
d. **Infections:** Sepsis, pneumonia, meningitis, necrotizing enterocolitis.
e. **Metabolic:** Acidosis, hypoglycemia, hypocalcemia, hyponatremia, hypernatremia.
f. **Hematological:** Anemia, polycythemia.
g. **Cardiac:** Congenital heart disease, hypo/hypertension, congestive heart failure, patent ductus arteriosus.
h. **Gastrointestinal:** Gastroesophageal reflux, NEC.
i. **Others:** Pain caused by nasal trauma following CPAP and screening for ROP.

Practice tip!

AOP is a diagnosis of exclusion. It should be considered after secondary causes have been excluded. Common causes of secondary apnea include temperature instability, airway obstruction, painful stimuli, hypoglycemia and hypocalcemia, respiratory distress syndrome, sepsis, polycythemia, and anemia.

TYPES

a. **Central apnea (40%):** This is characterized by cessation of inspiratory efforts due to reduced central nervous system drive.
b. **Obstructive apnea (10%):** The neonate cannot breathe because of obstructed airways. There is chest wall motion without any airflow.
c. **Mixed apnea (50%):** It has both components—reduced central drive and an obstructed airway.

The typical cause of obstruction in preterm neonates is abnormal neck position (excessive flexion or extension) or secretions. Other causes of obstruction are uncommon.

MONITORING

All neonates born before 34 weeks' gestation should be monitored for apnea in the first week of life. More mature neonates should be monitored for apnea if they are sick.

MANAGEMENT

Emergency Treatment: The neonate should be checked for bradycardia, cyanosis, and airway obstruction. Position the neck in neutral or slight extension and suction the airway if secretions are present. Most apneic spells respond to tactile stimulation. Oxygen by a headbox or nasal cannula is provided if the neonate is hypoxic (SpO_2 <90%). If the neonate does not respond to tactile stimulation, positive pressure ventilation (PPV) should be initiated.

Clinical examination: After stabilization, the neonate should be evaluated for the possible underlying cause. History should be reviewed for secondary causes such as perinatal asphyxia, maternal drugs, neonatal sepsis, and feed intolerance. The infant should be examined for temperature instability, hypotension, pallor, cardiac murmur for PDA, and poor perfusion.

Investigations: Neonates with apnea should be subjected to the following investigations, *on an individualized basis*, to exclude common secondary causes of apnea: blood glucose, hematocrit, electrolytes, sepsis workup, chest X-ray, ultrasound head, and other investigations depending on the history and physical examination (Table 17.1).

Table 17.1: Investigations to rule out secondary causes of apnea

Suspected cause for apnea	*Clinical features*	*Investigations*
Sepsis, pneumonia, meningitis	Lethargy, decreased feeding, fast breathing, retraction, brady/tachycardia, shock	Sepsis workup, chest X-ray
Patent ductus arteriosus	Tachycardia, bounding pulses, hyperkinetic precordium, cardiac murmur, increased requirement for respiratory support	Chest X-ray, echocardiography

(Contd.)

Table 17.1: Investigations to rule out secondary causes of apnea (*Contd.*)		
Suspected cause for apnea	*Clinical features*	*Investigations*
Periventricular-intraventricular hemorrhage	Sudden onset of pallor, shock, deranged sensorium	Cranial ultrasonography
Metabolic: hypoglycemia, hypocalcemia, hyponatremia	Jitteriness, poor feeding, seizures	Blood sugar, serum calcium and electrolytes
Anemia	Pallor, poor weight gain, history of increased blood letting	Packed cell volume (PCV)
Polycythemia	Plethora, lethargy, jitteriness, feed intolerance	Packed cell volume (PCV)

Prevention

- Nurse the infant in a servo-controlled radiant warmer or incubator to avoid fluctuation in body temperature.
- Maintain head and neck in a neutral/slightly extended position; use a shoulder roll if required.
- Maintain the patency of the upper airway by gently removing the secretions. Avoid vigorous suction. For feeding, an orogastric tube is preferred over a nasogastric one as the latter increases airway resistance.
- Maintain oxygen saturation between 90 and 95% by ensuring rational use of supplemental oxygen. Hyperoxia should be avoided. Saturation should be monitored by continuous pulse oximetry.

Treatment

General Measures

- Maintain airway, breathing, and circulation.
- Clear airway by suctioning, if required.
- Maintain the environmental temperature in the lower end of the thermo-neutral zone and avoid large swings.
- Oral feeding can be continued if the apnea is occasional and not severe. Avoid oral feeds in case of repeated episodes requiring positive pressure ventilation. Decreasing the volume of bolus feeding may be considered by giving feeds in small volumes more frequently (e.g. hourly feeding in place of 2- or 3-hourly feeds).

- Treat the underlying causes: sepsis, anemia, polycythemia, hypoglycemia, hypocalcemia, and RDS.
- Transfuse packed cells if required (refer to the chapter on 'Blood components')

Specific Measures

Methylxanthines

Methylxanthines have been the mainstay of pharmacotherapy for apnea of prematurity. The primary mechanism of action of methylxanthines is through the competitive antagonism of A1 and A2a adenosine receptors, which increases the minute ventilation, improves CO_2 sensitivity, stimulates the respiratory center in the medulla, decreases hypoxic depression of breathing, enhances diaphragmatic contractility, and decreases the periodic breathing. Adverse effects include tachycardia, jitteriness, irritability, feed intolerance, vomiting, and hyperglycemia.

There are two drugs in the methylxanthines group—caffeine and aminophylline (theophylline). The efficacy of both drugs is similar, but the former has fewer side effects and better dosage convenience, as it requires once-daily administration compared to thrice-daily dosing of aminophylline. However, it is pretty expensive (Table 17.2).

Methylxanthines for AOP are indicated in the following circumstances (Flowchart 17.1).

a. When apneic episodes are frequent, or
b. If the neonate requires PPV for apnea unresponsive to tactile stimulation.

Table 17.2: Comparison of caffeine citrate and theophylline

	Caffeine citrate	*Theophylline*
Half-life (hours)	25–371 (mean 101)	13–29
Dose	*Loading dose:* 20 mg/kg of caffeine citrate (i.e. 10 mg/kg of caffeine alkaloid) *Maintenance dose:* 5–10 mg/kg/d of caffeine citrate (2.5–5 mg/kg of caffeine alkaloid)	*Loading dose:* 5–6 mg/kg *Maintenance dose:* 1.5–3 mg/kg Q8–12 hours
Therapeutic drug level	8–20 μg/ml	5–10 μg/ml
Toxicity	Broad therapeutic window	Narrow therapeutic window

Evidence

A recent Cochrane review concluded that the methylxanthines are effective in reducing the number of apneic attacks and the need for mechanical ventilation two to seven days after starting treatment.[3]

The 'Caffeine therapy for Apnea of Prematurity (CAP)' trial[4] has shown that among infants <30 weeks of gestation, caffeine therapy:

- educed the need for supplemental oxygen at a postmenstrual age of 36 weeks, i.e. the risk of BPD (adjusted OR: 0.63; 95% CI 0.52–0.76).
- Results in earlier discontinuation of respiratory support by 1 week.
- Reduced the risk of cerebral palsy (aOR 0.58; 95% CI 0.39–0.87) and cognitive impairment at 18–21 months corrected age

Caffeine therapy also showed consistent benefits for motor development at 5 years and at 11 years of age.[5–7]

Flowchart 17.1: Algorithm for management of neonatal apnea

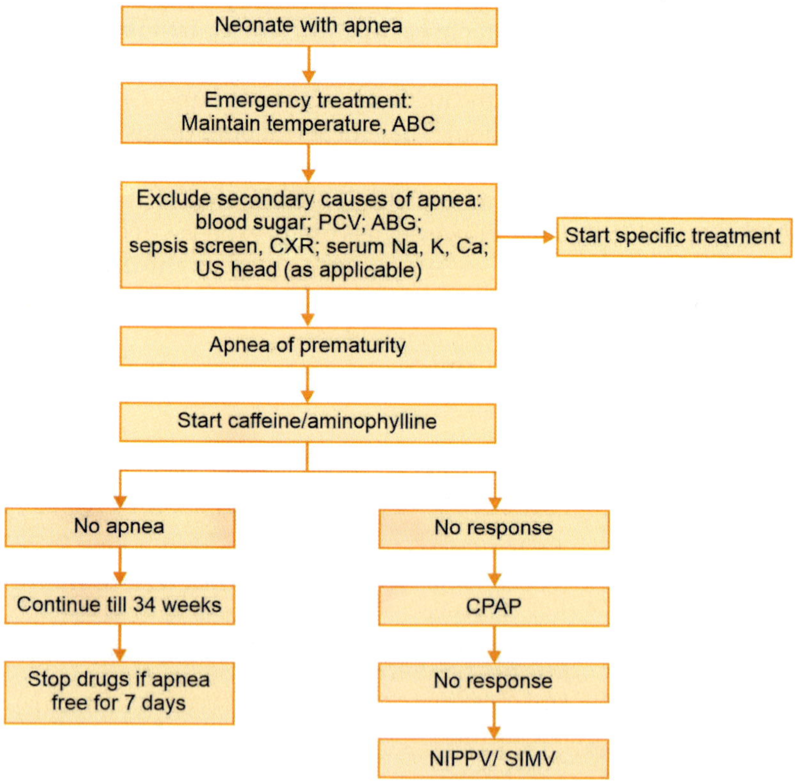

ABC: Airway, breathing, and circulation; *PCV:* Packed cell volume; *ABG:* Arterial blood gas; *Na:* sodium; *K:* potassium; *Ca:* Calcium; *US:* Ultrasound; *CPAP:* Continuous positive airway pressure; *SIMV:* Synchronized intermittent mandatory ventilation; *NIPPV:* Nasal intermittent positive pressure ventilation

Other indications include:

a. Prophylactic caffeine for neonates <28 weeks' gestation (for prevention of BPD).
b. Post-extubation in preterm neonates <32 weeks of gestation.

Methylxanthines are usually administered through the intravenous route. The oral route is preferred once the neonate is stable and tolerates oral feeds.

In extreme preterm neonates initiated on 5 mg/kg/day maintenance dose of caffeine, dose adjustments can be made by increasing caffeine citrate by 1 mg/kg/day every 1–2 weeks until it reaches 8 mg/kg/day by the fifth week of life to account for increasing clearance of caffeine with increasing postnatal age.

Methylxanthines should be continued until 34 weeks of postmenstrual age and stopped if no apnea episode has occurred in the last seven days. Caffeine or aminophylline initiated to facilitate extubation in very preterm neonates may be stopped after 5–7 days of therapy.[10] Methylxanthines should be discontinued at least 5–7 days before discharge. This is especially relevant for caffeine because of its longer half-life.

Continuous positive airway pressure (CPAP)

Nasal CPAP is usually administered when clinically significant apneic episodes persist despite optimal methylxanthine therapy.[11] CPAP results in a substantial reduction in obstructive and mixed apneas. The beneficial effect has been attributed to splinting of the upper airways by the positive airway pressure.

Nasal intermittent positive pressure ventilation

Infants with AOP and not responsive to CPAP can be given a trial of nasal intermittent positive pressure ventilation (NIPPV). NIPPV may improve the patency of the upper airway by creating intermittently elevated pharyngeal pressure. This periodic inflation of the pharynx may activate respiratory drive by the Head's paradoxical reflex, where lung inflation provokes an augmented inspiratory reflex.[12]

Evidence

A Cochrane review has shown the beneficial effect of NIPPV for treating preterm neonates with apnea that are frequent or severe. It showed a greater reduction in frequency of apneas (events/hr) compared to nCPAP.[13]

Mechanical ventilation

The neonate should be ventilated if significant apnea persists despite pharmacotherapy and CPAP/NIPPV. Given that there is no underlying lung disease in AOP, only minimal settings are required: PIP 12–14 cm H_2O; PEEP 4–5 cm H_2O; frequency 20–25 per minute; Ti 0.4–0.45 seconds; and FiO_2 of 0.21–0.3.

Persistent Apnea

Apneic episodes may persist beyond 37–40 weeks in some neonates, especially those born before 28 weeks. Up to 10% of neonates may require caffeine re-initiation for apnea recurrence after stopping caffeine at 34 weeks' PMA.[14] Methylxanthines should be continued if apneic episodes continue to occur beyond 34 weeks of PMA. The neonate should be re-evaluated for secondary causes of apnea, especially neurological problems and gastroesophageal reflux.

OUTCOMES[15]

The precise long-term effects of fluctuations in heart rate and saturation during apneic episodes have yet to be clearly defined. Retrospective studies have suggested that recurrent episodes are associated with worse neurodevelopment outcomes at 1–2 years. Prospective studies are required to examine the association of apnea with long-term neurodevelopment. AOP is not an independent risk factor for SIDS.

REFERENCES

1. American Academy of Pediatrics. Task Force on Prolonged Infantile Apnea. Prolonged infantile apnea. Pediatrics. 1985;76:129–31.
2. Zhao J, Gonzalez F, Mu D. Apnea of prematurity: from cause to treatment. Eur J Pediatr. 2011;170:1097–105.
3. Henderson-Smart DJ, De Paoli AG. Methylxanthine treatment for apnoea in preterm infants. Cochrane Database Syst Rev. 2010 Dec 8;(12):CD000140.
4. Schmidt B, Roberts RS, Davis P, Doyle LW, Barrington KJ, Ohlsson A, et al. Caffeine therapy for apnea of prematurity. N Engl J Med. 2006 8;354:2112–21.
5. Schmidt B, Roberts RS, Davis P, Doyle LW, Barrington KJ, Ohlsson A, et al. Long-term effects of caffeine therapy for apnea of prematurity. N Engl J Med. 2007;357:1893–902.
6. Schmidt B, Anderson PJ, Doyle LW, Dewey D, Grunau RE, Asztalos EV, et al. Survival without disability to age 5 years after neonatal caffeine therapy for apnea of prematurity. JAMA. 2012;307:275–82.
7. Schmidt B, Roberts RS, Anderson PJ, Asztalos EV, Costantini L, Davis PG, et al. Academic Performance, Motor Function, and Behavior 11 Years After Neonatal Caffeine Citrate Therapy for Apnea of Prematurity: An 11-Year Follow-up of the CAP Randomized Clinical Trial. JAMA Pediatr. 2017;171:564–72.

8. Henderson-Smart DJ, De Paoli AG. Prophylactic methylxanthine for prevention of apnoea in preterm infants. Cochrane Database Syst Rev. 2010 Dec 8;(12):CD000432.
9. Saroha V, Patel RM. Caffeine for preterm infants: Fixed standard dose, adjustments for age or high dose? Semin Fetal Neonatal Med. 2020;25:101178.
10. Miller MJ, Martin RJ. Apnea of prematurity. Clin Perinatol. 1992 Dec;19(4):789–808.
11. Henderson-Smart DJ, Subramaniam P, Davis PG. Continuous positive airway pressure versus theophylline for apnea in preterm infants. Cochrane Database Syst Rev. 2001;(4):CD001072.
12. Lin CH, Wang ST, Lin YJ, Yeh TF. Efficacy of nasal intermittent positive pressure ventilation in treating apnea of prematurity. Pediatr Pulmonol. 1998;26:349–53.
13. Lemyre B, Davis PG, de Paoli AG. Nasal intermittent positive pressure ventilation (NIPPV) versus nasal continuous positive airway pressure (NCPAP) for apnea of prematurity. Cochrane Database Syst Rev. 2002;(1):CD002272.
14. Haddad W, Sajous C, Hummel P, Guo R. Discontinuing caffeine in preterm infants at 33-35 weeks corrected gestational age: Failure rate and predictive factors. J Neonatal-Perinat Med. 2015 Mar 10;
15. Greene MM, Patra K, Khan S, Karst JS, Nelson MN, Silvestri JM. Cardiorespiratory events in extremely low birth weight infants: neurodevelopmental outcome at 1 and 2 years. J Perinatol Off J Calif Perinat Assoc. 2014 Jul;34(7):562–5.

CHAPTER

18

Congenital Diaphragmatic Hernia

Congenital diaphragmatic hernia (CDH) refers to herniation of abdominal contents into the thorax through a posterolateral defect (Bochdalek; 95%) or, less commonly, an anterior or central diaphragmatic defect. The defect is located more commonly on the left side (85%) than on the right side (10–15%) or bilaterally (<2%). Failure of pleuroperitoneal folds to fuse during the 4th–10th weeks of gestation causes compression of lungs by herniated abdominal viscera, which hampers bronchiolar and vascular branching and results in lung hypoplasia and pulmonary hypertension.

PRENATAL MANAGEMENT

Most cases of CDH (60%) are now detected antenatally during the routine anomaly scan by visualization of herniated abdominal contents in the thorax. After prenatal diagnosis, a more detailed evaluation is essential to assess certain prognostic factors, which help predict postnatal survival (Table 18.1).

Table 18.1: Prenatal prognostic factors for prediction of postnatal survival in CDH

S. No.	*Prognostic factors*	*Remarks*
1.	Syndromic association	Karyotypic abnormalities may be present in up to 20%, most commonly trisomy 18, 13, and 21. Syndromic associations (e.g. Fryns syndrome) can be found in 10–15% of cases of CDH who have additional malformations.
2.	Presence of additional malformations	These can be present in all major organ systems, with the occurrence of congenital heart diseases in 15% of the cases.
3.	Liver herniation	Presence of liver herniation in a left-sided CDH is a poor prognostic factor. Liver herniation is universally present in right-sided CDH and is not predictive.

(Contd.)

Table 18.1: Prenatal prognostic factors for prediction of postnatal survival in CDH *(Contd.)*

S. No.	*Prognostic factors*	*Remarks*
4.	Fetal lung volume	Low lung volume (<30% of the expected), estimated using MRI or 3D ultrasonography (USG), predicts poor postnatal survival. A surrogate measurement can be used instead on 2D USG which is known as observed/ expected lung area to head circumference ratio (O/E LHR). LHR is calculated for the contralateral (less affected) lung at the level of atria, divided by head circumference, which is normalized for gestational age to give O/E LHR. The parameter is classified as extreme (<15%), severe (15–25%), moderate (25–35%), and mild (35–45%), with improving survival with increasing O/E LHR.

Other factors like early gestation at diagnosis, stomach herniation, right-sided CDH, etc. have not proven to be reliable predictors of survival.

In utero fetal tracheal occlusion (FETO) has been found to improve survival in isolated severe left-sided CDH (O/E LHR <25%). However, FETO requires adequate expertise and experience in prenatal surgery, which may not be available at most centers.

Evidence: Fetal surgery in CDH

TOTAL trial was a multi-centric randomized trial conducted in centres with experience in FETO procedure, comparing FETO at 27–29 weeks gestation with expectant management, in fetuses with isolated severe left-sided CDH. There was significant improvement in survival to discharge among infants in FETO group (16/40; 40%), compared to expectant care group (6/40; 15%), albeit with a higher risk of preterm birth (75% vs. 29%) and preterm prelabour rupture of membranes (PPROM; 47% vs. 11%).

POSTNATAL MANAGEMENT (FIG. 18.1)

Delivery should be conducted at a tertiary care center with high volume (6 CDH cases in a year) at or beyond 39 weeks of gestation through a delivery mode guided by usual obstetric indications. Antenatal steroids and surfactant therapy are indicated for preterm neonates <34 weeks based on individual unit protocols.

Delivery

Respiratory care
- Intubation at birth* (avoid ventilation using mask)
- Use low peak pressure (<25 cm H_2O) to achieve ventilation (target preductal SpO_2 80–95%)

Supportive care
- Insert an intragastric tube to decompress bowel loops
- Chest compressions and medications as per NRP recommendations
- Avoid using paralytic agents

Shift to NICU

Respiratory care
- Targets:
  - Preductal SpO_2 80–95%
  - Postductal SpO_2 >70%
  - $PaCO_2$ 50–70 mm Hg
- Preferred ventilation mode: Conventional (assist control) ± volume target (initial VT at 4–4.5 ml/kg)
- Settings: PIP<25 cm H_2O, PEEP 4–6 cm H_2O, RR 40–60/min, FiO_2 based on SpO_2 (reduce if preductal SpO_2 >95%)
- Rescue mode: High frequency ventilation (inadequate ventilation despite maximal settings on CMV)

Hemodynamic care
- Targets:
  - Blood pressure normal for gestation
  - No signs of hypoperfusion (CFT>3 s, poor pulses, low urine output, lactate >5 mmol/L)
- If above targets not achieved:
  - Echocardiography# for functional assessment
  - Saline bolus at 10 ml/kg, repeat bolus if suboptimal fluid status on 2D-Echo
  - Vasoactive agents (dobutamine, milrinone, adrenaline, etc.) as needed
- Features of PPHN: Manage as per protocol (see the protocol on 'PPHN')

Supportive care
- Vascular access: Umbilical lines (UAC and UVC; if UVC malpositioned, manage with low lying UVC for first 24–48 hours and switch to PICC line later)
- Nutrition: Parenteral nutrition, restricted fluid (40–60 ml/kg/day on day 1, increase thereafter)
- Sedation: Avoid any noise/ light/ tactile stimuli; opioids (fentanyl 1–4 μg/kg/hour) ± midazolam (10–60 μg/kg/hr); avoid paralytic agents

Medical stabilization achieved?

Yes

Neonate meets criteria for medical stabilization:
- Preductal SpO_2 85–95% on FiO_2 <50%
- Blood pressure normal for gestation
- Lactate <3 mmol/L
- Urine output >1 ml/kg/hour

Surgical repair
- Closure of the diaphragmatic defect
  - Approach: open OR thoracoscopic (choice based on individual institution)
  - Repair: primary (sutures alone) OR using Gore-Tex patch/ split abdominal wall muscle flap (for large defects)
- No routine chest tube placement postoperatively

No

Does the neonate meet ECMO criteria?
- Despite maximal ventilator settings (PIP >28 cm H_2O or mean airway pressure >17 cm H_2O), the neonate continues to have
  - Inadequate oxygenation (preductal SpO_2 <85% or postductal SpO_2 <70% or oxygenation index ≥40 for at least 3 hours)
  - Inadequate ventilation (pH <7.15 due to increased pCO_2)
- Persistent metabolic acidosis (pH <7.15, lactate ≥5 mmol/L)
- Persistent shock (refractory to fluid and vasopressor therapy)

Follow ECMO protocol (surgical repair while on ECMO)

(Contd.)

(*Contd.*)

Postoperative period	
Acute postoperative care • Gradually wean off ventilation as tolerated (may require prolonged support) • Monitor for persistent pulmonary hypertension (follow PPHN protocol) • Look for hemorrhage, chylothorax, and infection • Introduce feeds when clinically stable and no gastric aspirates (usually after 3–5 postoperative days)	**Long-term care** Evaluate and manage late complications: • Gastrointestinal: GERD (most common cause of readmissions in the first year), CDH recurrence, poor growth, obstruction • Pulmonary: restrictive or obstructive lung disease, infections • Cardiac: persistent pulmonary hypertension • Neurodevelopment: cognitive defects, behaviour problems, ADHD • Hearing: Sensorineural hearing loss • Chest deformities and scoliosis

Fig. 18.1: Management algorithm of a neonate born with congenital diaphragmatic hernia after birth

(Adapted from CDH EURO Consortium. Standardized Postnatal Management of Infants with Congenital Diaphragmatic Hernia in Europe: The CDH EURO Consortium Consensus - 2015 Update. Neonatology. 2016;110(1):66–74.)

ADHD: Attention deficit hyperactivity disorder; *ECMO:* Extracorporeal membrane oxygenation; *GERD:* Gastro-esophageal reflex disease; *PPHN:* Persistent pulmonary hypertension of the newborn

*A trial of spontaneous breathing may be given in CDH neonates who are predicted to have favorable prognostic factors (O/E LHR >50%, absence of liver herniation, etc.)

#Echocardiography needs to be performed in all cases of CDH within 24 hours of birth to rule out structural heart defects.

BIBLIOGRAPHY

1. Cordier AG, Russo FM, Deprest J, Benachi A. Prenatal diagnosis, imaging, and prognosis in Congenital Diaphragmatic Hernia. Semin Perinatol. 2020;44(1):51163.
2. Deprest JA, Benachi A, Gratacos E, et al. Randomized Trial of Fetal Surgery for Moderate Left Diaphragmatic Hernia. N Engl J Med. 2021;385(2):119–29.
3. Deprest JA, Nicolaides KH, Benachi A, et al. Randomized Trial of Fetal Surgery for Severe Left Diaphragmatic Hernia. N Engl J Med. 2021;385(2):107–18.
4. De Bie FR, Avitabile CM, Joyeux L, et al. Neonatal and fetal therapy of congenital diaphragmatic hernia-related pulmonary hypertension. Arch Dis Child Fetal Neonatal Ed. 2022;107(5):458–66.
5. Horn-Oudshoorn EJJ, Knol R, Te Pas AB, et al. Perinatal stabilisation of infants born with congenital diaphragmatic hernia: a review of current concepts. Arch Dis Child Fetal Neonatal Ed. 2020;105(4):449–54.
6. Jancelewicz T, Brindle ME, Guner YS, et al. Toward Standardized Management of Congenital Diaphragmatic Hernia: An Analysis of Practice Guidelines. J Surg Res. 2019;243:229–35.

CHAPTER

19

Tracheoesophageal Fistula

The incidence of esophageal atresia (EA)/tracheoesophageal fistula (TEF) is reported to be 1.8/10000 live births, with survival up to 95%. The most common EA/TEF variant is Gross type C defect (proximal EA with distal TEF; Fig. 19.1). Over half of the affected infants have additional malformations (cardiovascular, gastrointestinal, genitourinary, etc.), and 10% have chromosomal abnormalities. Other well-known associations include VACTERL (vertebral, anorectal, cardiac, TEF, renal, and limb abnormalities) and CHARGE syndrome (coloboma, heart defects, atresia choanae, retarded growth, genital and ear anomalies).

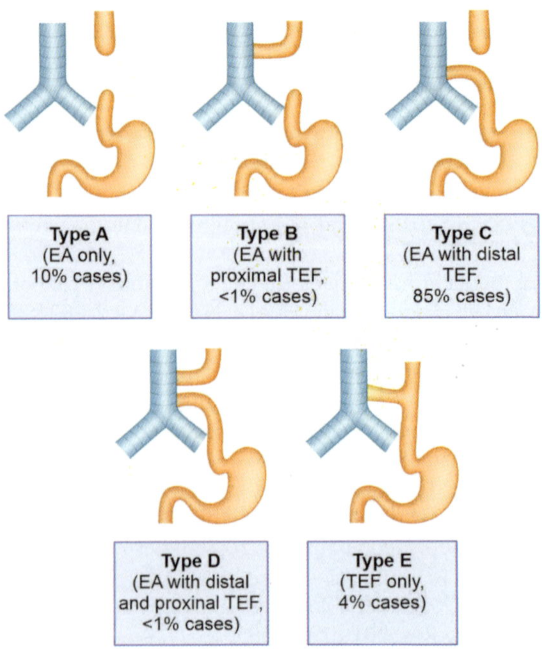

Fig. 19.1: Gross classification of esophageal atresia (EA)/tracheoesophageal fistula (TEF)

DIAGNOSIS

Although diagnosed postnatally in most cases, prenatal diagnosis is made in around one-third of the patients. Antenatal ultrasound (USG) findings that suggest EA/TEF include polyhydramnios, absent or small stomach shadow, and, more specifically, dilated proximal esophageal pouch and hypopharynx. A type C defect can be challenging to diagnose prenatally due to a normal appearing stomach filled with fluid via a distal TEF. Therefore, it may be prudent to pass an orogastric (OG) tube at birth in neonates with a history of unexplained polyhydramnios in the mother.

A neonate with EA/TEF presents soon after birth with excessive frothing from the mouth, drooling of secretions, choking, coughing and cyanosis during feeding, and respiratory distress resulting from chemical pneumonitis owing to aspiration of gastric contents through the TEF. The inability to pass an OG tube and its demonstration in the upper esophageal pouch on a chest radiograph is usually diagnostic. Further, the presence of bowel gas on the X-ray suggests a distal TEF (type C defect; Fig. 19.2a), while its absence indicates pure EA (type A defect; Fig. 19.2b).

MANAGEMENT

The goal of management is to stabilize the neonate, prevent aspiration-induced pneumonitis, and investigate for associated anomalies, while preparing for surgery (Fig. 19.3).

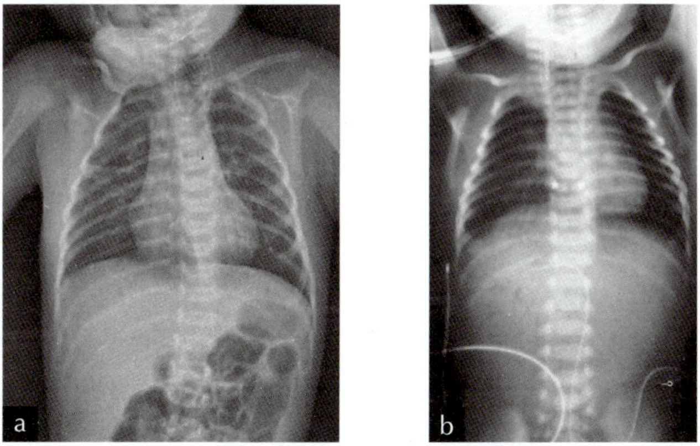

Fig. 19.2: X-ray of chest and abdomen showing esophageal atresia/ tracheoesophageal fistula spectrum: (a) Type C defect (EA with distal TEF) with intraluminal gas and (b) Type A defect (pure EA) with no intraluminal gas

Respiratory System

Preoperative

Stabilization
- Nil per oral (NPO)
- Head end elevation
- Upper pouch decompression (slow intermittent suction via replogle tube/ suction catheter at 3–5 cm H_2O pressure)
- Keeping the neonate calm (to avoid swallowing of air)

Investigations
- In all cases:
  - Echocardiogram to look for cardiac anomalies and aortic arch sidedness (must be performed before surgery)
  - Renal ultrasound
- In select cases[1]:
  - Infantogram, genetic studies etc.

Respiratory care
- Avoid positive pressure ventilation (including CPAP)
- When required, low mean airway pressures (MAP) should be used
- Rescue mode: High frequency ventilation (can be used with low MAP)
- Urgent gastric decompression or TEF ligation may be needed in difficult cases.

Preoperative preparation
- Broad-spectrum antibiotics[2]
- Vascular access: Umbilical lines (UAC and UVC; if UVC is malpositioned, manage with a low-lying UVC for the first 24–48 hours and switch to PICC line after surgery)
- Parenteral nutrition
- Rigid bronchoscopy (performed immediately before surgical repair) may be considered[3]

Surgery

- Immediate primary repair is preferred and feasible in most cases (TEF division followed by primary anastomosis of the esophageal segments). It can be done via:
  - Open approach (using right extrapleural thoracotomy)[4]
  - Thoracoscopic approach (in term neonates with normal pulmonary status): longer operative time but associated with shorter hospital stay, time to extubation, and time to first oral feed
- Long gap EA (any esophageal atresia that lacks intra-abdominal air or all other types that technically prove difficult to repair) may require:
  - Delayed primary repair (after Foker procedure, which involves lengthening of esophageal ends by placing them under traction with sutures for prolonged periods of up to 3 weeks)
  - Staged repair (usually in preterm neonates <1500 g; involves esophagostomy, gastrostomy and TEF division initially followed by late esophageal anastomosis)
  - Esophageal replacement (in cases where primary repair has failed or is not feasible)

Postoperative period

Acute postoperative care
- Meticulous care of the trans-anastomotic feeding tube, endotracheal tube (ETT) and neck movements
- Suction catheter length should be clearly marked for oral and ETT suctioning
- Elective ventilation and paralysis for 2–7 days (individualised based on tension in anastomosis)
- Extubation after stabilization of respiratory status (to minimize reintubations and excessive neck manipulation); may use CPAP post-extubation when necessary[5]
- Contrast esophagogram on 5th–7th postoperative day (for anastomotic leaks); if no leak, start oral feeds and remove chest tube.

(Contd.)

(*Contd.*)

Monitoring and follow-up
Immediate complications • Anastomotic leaks (15%): diagnosed on contrast esophagogram; most leaks (95%) heal spontaneously; and are managed conservatively with broad-spectrum antibiotics and existing chest tube drainage. **Short-term complications** • Anastomotic strictures (40%): diagnosed by contrast esophagogram and endoscopy; treated by endoscopic balloon dilatation, intralesional steroids, topical application of mitomycin C, stents and segmental resection in resistant cases. • TEF recurrence (5–10%): presents with choking, coughing and cyanosis while feeding; diagnosed by contrast esophagogram and bronchoscopy/endoscopy; and managed with surgical correction. **Long-term complications** • Gastrointestinal: Dysphagia (50%), GERD (50%; managed with acid suppression and in refractory cases, with fundoplication), Barrett esophagus (6%) and esophageal cancer (1%); requires follow-up with endoscopy at regular intervals to detect early esophagitis. • Airways: Tracheobronchomalacia (clinically significant in 15–20%; requires aortopexy in 3–5%), vocal cord dysfunction, coexisting laryngeal clefts. • Pulmonary (20–30%): Infections, asthma, bronchiectasis, restrictive lung disease. • Chest wall deformities: Scoliosis, shoulder girdle muscle weakness. • Growth and development: Poor growth, delayed psychomotor development (but lack of long-term data on these outcomes).

Fig. 19.3: Management algorithm of a neonate born with EA/TEF

EA: Esophageal atresia; *GERD:* gastroesophageal reflux disease; *TEF:* Tracheoe-sophageal fistula)

[1]Additional investigations may be required in presence of findings suggestive of syndromic associations like VACTERL, CHARGE, trisomy 21 or 18, etc.

[2]Preoperative antibiotics are indicated if there is suspicion of aspiration pneumonia or risk factors for early onset sepsis.

[3]Pre-repair bronchoscopy is a useful adjunct to confirm the diagnosis before thoracotomy, to assess any associated tracheobronchomalacia or additional TEFs, and to allow the positioning of a Fogarty catheter to occlude the fistula.

[4]A left-sided approach must be taken in the presence of a right-sided aortic arch. The extrapleural approach helps prevent a pleural empyema if an anastomotic leak develops.

[5]Post-extubation CPAP in operated EA/TEF cases has not been associated with an increased risk of anastomotic leak or fistula recurrence.

PROGNOSIS

Several groups have devised stratification systems to prognosticate neonates with EA/TEF. Most of these systems are based on birth weight and the presence of critical cardiac anomalies. Neonates with birth weight <1.5–2 kg and major cardiac defects have the poorest survival among neonates with EA/TEF. However, the prognosis has improved significantly (up to 95%) with refinements in surgical techniques and neonatal care.

BIBLIOGRAPHY

1. Mohammed S, Hamilton TE. Advances in Complex Congenital Tracheoesophageal Anomalies. Clin Perinatol. 2022;49(4):927–41.
2. Morini F, Conforti A, Bagolan P. Perioperative Complications of Esophageal Atresia. Eur J Pediatr Surg. 2018;28(2):133–40.
3. van der Zee DC, Tytgat SHA, van Herwaarden MYA. Esophageal atresia and tracheo-esophageal fistula. Semin Pediatr Surg. 2017;26(2):67–71.
4. van der Zee DC, van Herwaarden MYA, Hulsker CCC, Witvliet MJ, Tytgat SHA. Esophageal Atresia and Upper Airway Pathology. Clin Perinatol. 2017;44(4):753–62.
5. Walk RM. Esophageal Atresia and Tracheoesophageal Fistula: Overview and Considerations for the General Surgeon. Surg Clin North Am. 2022;102(5):759–78.

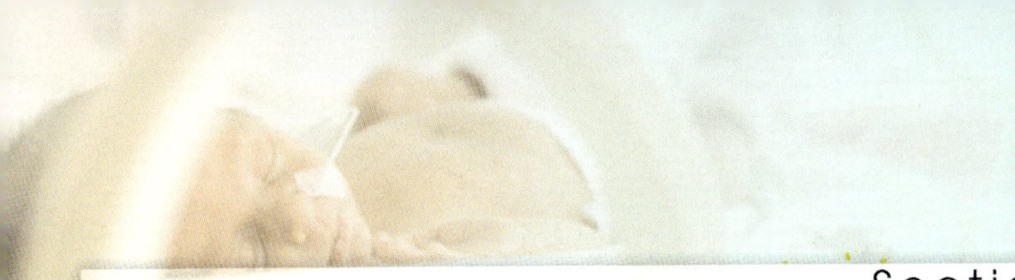

Section

6

Gastrointestinal and Hepatobiliary Tract and Nutrition

CHAPTER

20

Jaundice in the Newborn

Jaundice is the most common morbidity in the first week of life, occurring in about 60% of term and 80% of preterm newborns. Globally, it ranks 7th among all causes of mortality in the early neonatal period.[1] It is also the most common cause of readmission after discharge from the birth hospitalization. In neonates, jaundice appears when total serum bilirubin (TSB) concentration exceeds 5–7 mg/dl. In most cases, it is benign and does not require any intervention. The primary concern with neonatal jaundice is the risk of bilirubin-induced neurological dysfunction (BIND), which is, fortunately, rare. Nevertheless, a few neonates develop long-term sequelae of BIND that are entirely preventable in most of them.

PHYSIOLOGICAL JAUNDICE

Jaundice attributable to the physiological immaturity of neonates to handle a high burden of bilirubin is termed 'physiological jaundice.' Neonatal bilirubin production is 2–3-fold that of adults, owing to increased hematopoiesis and a shortened RBC lifespan. The enzymes for bilirubin conjugation (UGT1A1) have little activity in neonates. Enterohepatic circulation is also enhanced due to deficient intestinal flora and high intestinal beta-glucuronidase activity, causing the reabsorption of conjugated bilirubin.

In term neonates, physiological jaundice usually appears between 24 and 72 hours of life, rises to a peak level of 12–15 mg/dl by 3 days, and then starts falling. In preterm neonates, the peak level occurs between 3 and 7 days, and TSB can rise over 15 mg/dl. It may take weeks before the TSB falls under 2 mg/dl in both term and preterm neonates. Jaundice in most neonates is physiological and rarely requires treatment.

PATHOLOGICAL JAUNDICE

'Pathological jaundice' is an arbitrarily and loosely defined term for bilirubin levels beyond the normal physiological range that generally requires further investigation and treatment. It includes:

- Visible jaundice in the first 24 hours of life (however, slight jaundice appearing on the face by 18–24 hours is common and may be considered physiological).
- Presence of jaundice on arms and legs on day 2 of life
- Yellow palms and soles at any age
- Presence of jaundice on arms and legs on day 2 of life
- Yellow palms and soles at any age
- TSB more than 95th centile as per age-specific bilirubin nomogram
- Rise of TSB more than 0.3 mg/dl/hour on day 1 and 0.2 mg/dl/hour beyond 24 hours
- Any jaundice with features of BIND
- Clinical jaundice persisting beyond 2 weeks in term and 3 weeks in preterm neonates.

Causes

Increased production	• Polycythemia. • Extravasated blood (hematomas or internal hemorrhage-pulmonary/intracranial/gastrointestinal) • Hemolytic diseases (immune-mediated, red cell membrane enzymatic defects, hemoglobinopathies)
Decreased clearance	• Increased enterohepatic circulation (GI obstruction) • Cholestasis (due to anatomical causes like biliary atresia, or inborn errors of metabolism like tyrosinemia, galactosemia, etc.)

IDENTIFYING HIGH-RISK NEONATES

Approximately 5–10% of neonates develop clinically significant jaundice that requires treatment to lower the TSB levels. Factors that increase the risk of developing significant jaundice include:

- Lower gestational age (<40 weeks)
- Hemolytic disease
- History of phototherapy in parents or sibling
- Scalp hematoma or significant bruising
- Exclusively breastfed infant with suboptimal milk intake
- Down syndrome
- Macroscopic infant of a diabetic mother

All neonates should be visually inspected for jaundice at least every 12 hours during the initial 3–5 days of life. Those with the risk factors listed above should be identified and kept under close monitoring.

The new American Academy of Pediatrics (AAP) 2022 guidelines recommend that transcutaneous bilirubin (TcB) or TSB value be obtained for all neonates between 24 and 48 hours of life, and post-discharge surveillance be decided based on the difference between this value and the corresponding phototherapy (PT) cutoff. The suggested intervals also consider gestational age at discharge and hyperbilirubinemia neurotoxicity risk factors (listed below).[2]

Estimation of Serum Bilirubin

1. **Visual inspection:** Visual inspection of jaundice (Table 20.1) can help estimate the serum bilirubin levels using Kramer's rule, and if done diligently, has reasonable accuracy (comparable to TcB). The absence of jaundice on visual inspection reliably excludes jaundice. However, it cannot be relied upon at higher TSB levels and following phototherapy.
2. **Transcutaneous bilirubinometry:** TcB measures the reflected light spectra from bilirubin in the skin and subcutaneous tissues.

Table 20.1: Visual inspection of jaundice

1. Examine the baby in bright natural light or bright white fluorescent light.
2. The baby should be naked. Ensure there is no yellow or off-white background.
3. Examine blanched skin and gums or sclerae.
4. Note the extent of jaundice (Kramer's zone).
5. Note the depth of jaundice (Light staining as lemon yellow; deep staining as orange-yellow).

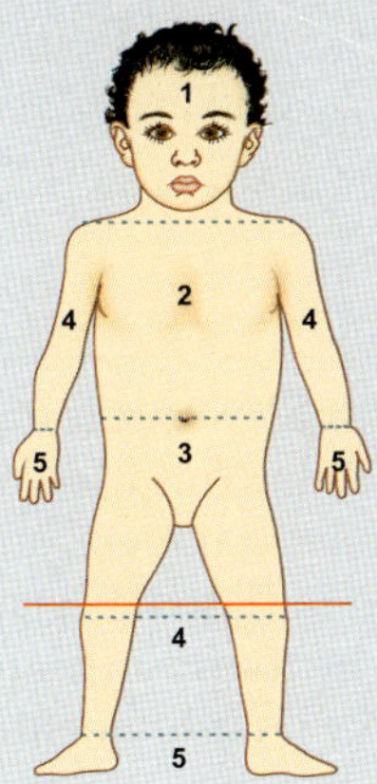

Kramer's zones	Approximate TSB level	
	Light staining jaundice	Deep staining jaundice
1. Face and neck	5–7 mg/dl	7–9 mg/dl
2. Chest and upper abdomen	7–9 mg/dl	9–11 mg/dl
3. Lower abdomen and thighs	9–11 mg/dl	11–13 mg/dl
4. Legs and arms/ forearms	11–13 mg/dl	14–16 mg/dl
5. Palms and soles	13–15 mg/dl	17 mg/dl or more

Although it cannot substitute TSB, it is a good screening tool to determine whether serum bilirubin level should be measured. It is quick and noninvasive and reduces painful sampling needs by almost 30%. TcB values correlate well with TSB (lie within 3 mg/dl) at levels below 15 mg/dl.[2] Above that, TcB tends to underestimate the TSB. TcB level above 15 mg/dl or lying within 3 mg/dl of the PT threshold warrants TSB measurement.

TcB can be used for neonates of all gestations[3] and in mixed racial populations. Measurements are affected by the skin's melanin content; depending on the instrument, it may overestimate or underestimate TSB in dark-skinned neonates. For the same reason, it is believed to be unreliable for skin bleached from PT; however, it can be used for rebound measurements taken 24 hours after stopping PT.

Measurement of Serum Bilirubin

High-performance liquid chromatography (HPLC) remains the gold standard for the estimation of TSB. However, this test is available for research purposes only. Laboratory estimation of TSB is usually performed by the van den Bergh reaction. It has marked inter-laboratory variability, with the coefficient of variation being up to 10–12%. Novel methods for bilirubin measurement include spectrophotometry, optical imaging of conjunctiva, and exhaled carbon monoxide (CO) spectroscopy. CO is produced in equimolar amounts when heme is degraded, and ETCO >2 ppm may help identify infants undergoing hemolysis.[4]

Indications of TSB measurement:

- Jaundice in the first 24 hours of life.
- Confirmation of high TcB levels before initiating therapy.
- Monitoring during and up to 24 hours after phototherapy.

APPROACH TO A JAUNDICED NEONATE

Thorough history taking and examination usually guide lab investigations in cases of pathological jaundice (detailed in Table 20.2). However, treatment should never be delayed, and phototherapy or exchange transfusion should be initiated as soon as possible when indicated. While no cause may be found in many cases, a cause for jaundice should be sought after in all neonates requiring phototherapy.[5]

Table 20.2: History, examination and laboratory tests

History	Examination	Laboratory tests
• Family history suggestive of hemolytic anemia/liver disease/sibling with jaundice • Antenatal history to indicate TORCH infections, gestational diabetes mellitus, intake of drugs that displace bilirubin or that trigger hemolysis in G6PD deficiency • Birth history suggestive of trauma or asphyxia • Feeding history (milk or formula, adequacy) and history suggestive of pyloric stenosis or intestinal obstruction	• Gestational assessment • Features suggestive of dehydration/ low caloric intake • Pallor/petechiae/ bruising/enclosed hemorrhage • Hepatosplenomegaly • Signs of infection (congenital/ acquired)	• Essential—Blood typing (mother and infant), direct Coombs' test, peripheral smear, G6PD levels • Optional—Direct bilirubin levels, TSH, sepsis screen, metabolic workup

THERAPEUTIC OPTIONS

Phototherapy

Phototherapy (PT) remains the mainstay of treating hyperbilirubinemia in neonates. It can be provided using compact fluorescent lamps (CFL), high-intensity light-emitting diodes (LED), fiber-optic units, and halogen lights. CFL is the most used device with its easy availability and low cost. However, the use of LEDs has increased recently. Although their efficacy in reducing TSB levels is similar compared to conventional sources as per 2 meta-analyses,[6,7] they have several advantages such as a longer life, narrow emission spectrum, less infrared radiation (thus less water loss), and less heat production (allowing the device to be placed closer to the infant thus increasing the irradiance). Halogen lights are unsafe to use as they produce much heat and may lead to thermal injury. Fiber-optic devices are designed to transmit light from LED or halogen sources to pads or blankets via flexible optic fibers. They provide higher irradiance than fluorescent lamps and produce minimal heat but would not cover adequate surface area for stand-alone use. Typically used to provide under-surface PT to increase the efficacy of the overhead source (e.g. Biliblanket), they may also be used for continuing PT in neonates undergoing ET.

Efficacy of PT mainly depends on the light source (irradiance of light, spectrum of wavelength), the exposed body surface area, and the underlying cause of jaundice. Effective PT requires at least 30 $\mu W/cm^2/nm$ irradiance, with a wavelength between 460 and 490 nm (matches the absorption spectrum of bilirubin). The PT unit should be kept as close to the baby as possible for greater irradiance.[5] Light rays should be perpendicular to the baby in an incubator to minimize reflectance. Moreover, the irradiance of PT units should be periodically measured, at several points on the unit, as it decays with time. Reflective white curtains have been shown to cause a greater decline in TSB and may even decrease the length of hospital stay.[8] Maximizing the exposed surface area by removing all clothes and minimizing the area covered by diapers is essential. Turning the infant to expose unbleached skin does not improve the efficacy of PT. The baby's eyes should be covered with a small patch, temperature monitored, and breastfeeding continued, minimizing interruptions to less than 30 minutes. Routine fluid or feed supplementation is not required.

The rate of decline of TSB with PT depends on the spectral power (average irradiance across the surface area) and the cause of jaundice. Effective PT causes a decrease in TSB by at least 2 mg/dl within 4–6 hours of initiation. Lack of fall in TSB or rising levels indicates ongoing hemolysis.

Indications

1. TSB levels at or above the phototherapy threshold.
2. Neonates with features of BIND while exchange transfusion is being arranged.
3. Home-based LED phototherapy is now considered a feasible option for discharged neonates whose TSB is not more than 1 mg/dl above PT cutoff and are otherwise well, with no risk factors for bilirubin neurotoxicity (only if daily monitoring of TSB can be ensured).[2]

The PT thresholds are based on AAP nomograms (2022), which have separate charts for neonates with and without hyperbilirubinemia neurotoxicity risk factors (gestation <38 weeks, serum albumin <3 g/dl, sepsis, isoimmune hemolytic disease, and significant clinical instability in last 24 hours). Each chart has separate cutoff lines for different gestations (>35 weeks), with higher cutoffs for lower gestational age neonates. Readers may refer to the AAP publication for the charts.[2]

The 2022 AAP guidelines have raised thresholds for each gestation compared to the 2004 guidelines, recognizing that neurotoxicity occurs way above the previous thresholds. However, using higher cut-offs also entails ensuring adherence to rigorous follow-up, which may not be possible in resource-limited settings.[2]

No evidence-based guidelines exist for neonates below 35 weeks of gestation for initiating PT or exchange transfusion. Consensus-based guidelines from NICE (2010), Norwegian guidelines, and the AAP Committee on Fetus and Newborn are available. *We follow the NICE guidelines for neonates below 35 weeks gestation in our unit*. NICE guidelines can be accessed at https://www.nice.org.uk/guidance/cg98/evidence/full-guideline-245411821.

Contraindications

Congenital porphyria (or a family history of porphyria) is an absolute contraindication to initiating PT. Severe blistering and agitation on exposure to PT should alert for the presence of this disease.

The presence of conjugated hyperbilirubinemia, especially in sick LBW babies, should not be considered a contraindication to starting PT.

Monitoring

Neonates undergoing PT should be assessed for hydration status, hypo/hyperthermia, deteriorating feeding pattern, and features of BIND. Hemoglobin or hematocrit levels should be measured for all neonates receiving PT. After initiation of PT, TSB levels should be measured every 4–6 hours initially and then every 6–12 hours once the TSB is stable or declining. PT may be discontinued once TSB falls 2 mg/dl below the PT threshold at which it was initiated, as per the 2022 AAP recommendations.[2]

Following discontinuation of PT, rebound hyperbilirubinemia may occur, and rebound TSB should be measured at least 12 hours after discontinuation of PT (preferably 24 hours, in which case TcB can be used). In neonates at higher risk for rebound hyperbilirubinemia (gestation below 38 weeks, PT initiated within 48 hours of life, hemolytic disease), TSB may be obtained after 6 hours.

Adverse Effects

PT is a remarkably safe therapy that has stood the test for decades. PT does not use UV light, and exposure is mostly harmless. It may cause transient diarrhea or an erythematous rash. In neonates with conjugated hyperbilirubinemia, it may lead to dark brown discoloration of the skin (bronze baby syndrome) due to the accumulation of photoproducts of bilirubin. Recent studies suggest PT may not be as harmless as it is thought to be and may be sub-clinically carcinogenic and genotoxic.[9] Oxidative injury to cell membranes and DNA may occur, especially in extremely LBW neonates. It thus becomes essential to minimize the duration of PT whenever possible and limit its use to evidence-based indications.

Exchange Transfusion

Double volume exchange transfusion (DVET) is the most effective method for rapidly removing bilirubin. It replaces 85% of circulating RBCs and causes a fall in TSB by about 50% immediately post-procedure.[10] After equilibration occurs with extravascular bilirubin, TSB usually would return to 2/3rd of the pretransfusion level. For infants with Rh isoimmunization, DVET has the added advantage of removing circulating and bound maternal antibodies from the baby's serum.

DVET is usually performed by a pull-and-push technique using the umbilical venous route. The umbilical catheter should be inserted just enough to get a free flow of blood. Individual aliquot volume should not exceed 10% of blood volume, with a maximum of 20 ml for a 3 kg term infant. A blood warmer is recommended to prevent hypothermia during the procedure. TSB levels should be measured at 2 and 6 hours after transfusion, and then 12 hourly until PT can be discontinued (Table 20.3).

Table 20.3: Type and volume of blood for exchange transfusion

S.No.	*Condition*	*Type of blood*
1.	Rh isoimmunization	Rh negative and blood group 'O' or that of baby Suspended in AB plasma Cross-matched with the baby's and mother's blood
2.	ABO incompatibility	Rh compatible and blood group 'O' *(not that of the baby)* Suspended in AB plasma Cross-matched with the baby's and mother's blood

(*Contd.*)

Table 20.3: Type and volume of blood for exchange transfusion (*Contd.*)

S.No.	*Condition*	*Type of blood*
3.	Other conditions (G6PD deficiency, non-hemolytic, other isoimmune hemolytic jaundice	Baby's group and Rh type Cross-matched with the baby's and mother's blood

- Volume of blood: Twice the blood volume of the baby (total volume: 160–180 ml/kg).
- To prepare blood for DVET, mix two-thirds of the total volume as packed red blood cells and one-third as plasma.

Indications

- Acute bilirubin encephalopathy (irrespective of TSB level).
- TSB levels above exchange cutoff (based on AAP nomograms, as described above)
- In Rh-isoimmunized neonates, if cord bilirubin is 5 mg/dl or cord Hb is 10 g/dl. (However, if the baby shows signs of hydrops or cardiac decompensation in the presence of low PCV (<35%), partial exchange transfusion with 50 ml/kg of packed cells should be done to restore the oxygen-carrying capacity of the blood.)
- DVET may also be considered when the bilirubin-to-albumin ratio exceeds age-specific cutoffs.

A new 'escalation of care' bilirubin threshold has been recently introduced at TSB 2 mg/dl below the exchange threshold. Above this threshold, intensive phototherapy and intravenous hydration are recommended, and in case of isoimmune hemolytic disease, using 0.5–1 g/kg IVIG can also be considered. We do not use IVIG for hemolytic jaundice in our unit.[2]

The adverse effects of ET include infection, electrolyte disturbances (hypocalcemia, hypomagnesemia, hypernatremia, hyperkalemia), portal vein thrombosis, thrombocytopenia, coagulopathy, GVHD, NEC, arrhythmias, and a mortality risk of 0.5–2%.

Bilirubin-induced Neurological Damage

Unbound/free bilirubin can cross the intact blood–brain barrier (BBB) and cause damage by inducing apoptosis and causing neuronal necrosis. The key factors promoting its toxicity are the low water solubility of bilirubin and its tendency to aggregate and precipitate at physiologic pH.

Factors that increase the amount of unbound bilirubin (drugs such as ceftriaxone that displace bilirubin from albumin) or factors that increase the permeability of BBB (such as anoxia, hypercarbia, and hyperosmolality) increase the risk of BIND. Premature infants have a more permeable blood-brain barrier as well as a lower affinity of albumin for bilirubin and may develop neuronal damage at lower TSB levels.

Acute bilirubin encephalopathy (ABE) is used to describe the acute manifestations of bilirubin toxicity—enlisted in Table 20.4—seen in the first weeks after birth. Modified BIND scoring is done in our unit to objectively assess and monitor these babies.

Clinical Features of ABE

Preterm neonates may not display the classical signs of ABE. Thus, close monitoring and a high index of suspicion are essential. All neonates with suspected ABE should also be evaluated for other causes of encephalopathy, such as asphyxia, sepsis, and meningitis, that can coexist with hyperbilirubinemia.

MRI in ABE or kernicterus shows a pathognomonic image of bilateral symmetric high-intensity signal in the globus pallidus. Similar changes have been reported in subthalamic nuclei, auditory brainstem, and cerebellar nuclei. All neonates with features of BIND or high bilirubin levels in the presence of risk factors should undergo hearing evaluation with auditory brainstem response (ABR) audiometry to rule out auditory involvement.

The term kernicterus is reserved for the chronic and permanent clinical sequelae of bilirubin toxicity. It is classically described

Table 20.4: Acute manifestation of bilirubin

Early	*Subtle signs like lethargy, hypotonia, poor suckle, or high-pitched cry*	
Intermediate	Tone variable (usually hypertonia), irritability, fever, seizures	Almost all infants who survive this phase are likely to develop chronic bilirubin encephalopathy; an emergent ET may reverse CNS changes in some.
Advanced	Pronounced hypertonia (opisthotonos, retrocollis), weak or shrill cry, apnea, seizures, coma	Affected infants die from intractable seizures or respiratory failure.

as a tetrad of choreoathetoid cerebral palsy with neuromotor impairment, sensorineural hearing loss, upward gaze palsy, and dental enamel dysplasia.

PROLONGED JAUNDICE

The persistence of significant jaundice for more than 2 weeks in term and 3 weeks in preterm neonates is termed prolonged jaundice. The first step in these neonates is to rule out cholestasis. After that, other common causes, such as breastmilk jaundice, hypothyroidism, and continuing hemolysis (due to ABO/Rh incompatibility or G6PD deficiency or from extravasated blood in cephalhematomas), need to be considered.

Breast milk jaundice is a common and mostly benign cause, occurring in up to 30% of infants. It is observed in infants otherwise gaining adequate weight. A few proposed theories for its occurrence are high free fatty acid concentration in breast milk (causing bilirubin displacement from albumin), high beta-glucuronidase activity, and inhibition of UGT1A activity by breast milk contents. Interruption of breastfeeding is seldom required.

A mutation in the promotor region of UGT1A1 causes Gilbert syndrome. It is typically not detected until after puberty. The appearance of mild jaundice seen at times of stress (without concurrent evidence of hemolysis), with response to phenobarbital, would point towards the diagnosis.

Infants with Criggler–Najjar syndrome type I have almost nil UGT1A1 activity and develop severe jaundice requiring exchange transfusion in the first week of life. There is no response to phenobarbital, and these infants must be managed on home PT, usually at night in the post-neonatal period. Liver transplantation is the only curative treatment option. Criggler–Najjar syndrome type II patients have less severe jaundice that responds to phenobarbital and less commonly develop kernicterus.

REFERENCES

1. Global Burden of Disease Study 2016 (GBD 2016) Data Resources | GHDx [Internet]. [cited 2023 Apr 21]. Available from: https://ghdx.healthdata.org/gbd-2016.
2. Kemper AR, Newman TB, Slaughter JL, Maisels MJ, Watchko JF, Downs SM, et al. Clinical Practice Guideline Revision: Management of Hyperbilirubinemia in the Newborn Infant 35 or More Weeks of Gestation. Pediatrics. 2022 Aug 5;150(3):e2022058859.

3. Nagar G, Vandermeer B, Campbell S, Kumar M. Reliability of Transcutaneous Bilirubin Devices in Preterm Infants: A Systematic Review. Pediatrics. 2013 Nov 1;132(5):871–81.
4. Bhutani VK, Maisels MJ, Schutzman DL, Castillo Cuadrado ME, Aby JL, Bogen DL, et al. Identification of risk for neonatal haemolysis. Acta Paediatr. 2018 Aug;107(8):1350–6.
5. Hyperbilirubinemia S on. Management of Hyperbilirubinemia in the Newborn Infant 35 or More Weeks of Gestation. Pediatrics. 2004 Jul 1;114(1):297–316.
6. Tridente A, De Luca D. Efficacy of light-emitting diode versus other light sources for treatment of neonatal hyperbilirubinemia: a systematic review and meta-analysis. Acta Paediatr Oslo Nor 1992. 2012 May;101(5):458–65.
7. Kumar P, Chawla D, Deorari A. Light-emitting diode phototherapy for unconjugated hyperbilirubinaemia in neonates. Cochrane Database Syst Rev. 2011 Dec 7;2011(12): CD007969.
8. Van Rostenberghe H, Ho JJ, Lim CH, Abd Hamid IJ. Use of reflective materials during phototherapy for newborn infants with unconjugated hyperbilirubinaemia. Cochrane Database Syst Rev. 2020 Jul 1;7:CD012011.
9. Hammerman C, Kaplan M. Hyperbilirubinemia in the Term Infant. Clin Perinatol. 2021 Aug;48(3):533–54.
10. Anderson NB, Calkins KL. Neonatal Indirect Hyperbilirubinemia. NeoReviews. 2020 Nov 1;21(11):e749–60.

CHAPTER

21

Feeding of Low Birth Weight Infants

Globally about 20.5 million infants are born with a birth weight of <2500 g every year, with Southern Asia having the highest prevalence of low birth weight (LBW) infants (26.4%) in the world.[1] Though these LBW infants constitute only about 15% of the total live births, they account for 80% of neonatal deaths.[2] Most of these deaths can be prevented with extra attention to warmth, prevention of infections, and more importantly, optimal feeding. Nutritional management influences the immediate survival and subsequent growth and development of LBW infants. Simple interventions such as early initiation of breastfeeding and avoidance of prelacteal feeding have been shown to improve their survival in a resource-restricted settings.[3] Early nutrition could also influence long-term neurodevelopmental outcomes.

HOW IS THE FEEDING OF LBW INFANTS DIFFERENT?

Term infants with normal birth weight can feed directly from their mother's breasts. In contrast, feeding LBW infants is relatively challenging because of the following limitations:

1. Many LBW infants are born premature and have inadequate feeding skills; they might not be able to breastfeed and would require other feeding methods.
2. They are prone to have significant illnesses that often preclude enteral feeding in the first few weeks of life.
3. Because intrauterine accretion of nutrients occurs mainly in the later part of the third trimester, preterm VLBW infants have low body stores at birth requiring supplementation of nutrients after birth.
4. Because of gut immaturity, they are more likely to experience feed intolerance necessitating adequate monitoring and treatment.

DECIDING THE INITIAL METHOD OF FEEDING

It is essential to categorize LBW infants into two major groups—*sick* and *healthy*—before deciding on the initial feeding method.

Sick Infants

This group constitutes infants with significant respiratory distress requiring assisted ventilation, shock requiring inotropic support, seizures, symptomatic hypoglycemia/hypocalcemia, electrolyte abnormalities, acute kidney injury or other organ failures, surgical conditions of the gastrointestinal tract, necrotizing enterocolitis (NEC), hydrops, etc. These infants are usually started on intravenous (IV) fluids. Enteral feeds should be initiated as soon as they are hemodynamically stable. Even infants with respiratory distress on assisted ventilation can be started on enteral feeds once the acute phase is over and their saturation and perfusion have improved. Similarly, sepsis—unless associated with shock/sclerema—is not a contraindication for enteral feeding.

Healthy LBW Infants

Enteral feeding should be initiated immediately after birth in healthy LBW infants with the appropriate feeding method determined by their gestation and oral feeding skills.

Maturation of oral feeding skills: Breastfeeding requires effective sucking, swallowing, and proper coordination between sucking/swallowing and breathing. These complex skills mature with increasing gestation (Table 21.1).

How to Decide on the Initial Feeding Method

Traditionally, the initial feeding method in LBW infants was decided based on their birth weight. This is not ideal because the feeding ability depends mainly on gestation rather than birth weight.

Table 21.1: Maturation of oral feeding skills in LBW infants[4]

Gestational age	*Maturation of feeding skills*
<28 weeks	No proper sucking efforts No propulsive motility in the gut
28–31 weeks	Sucking bursts develop No coordination between suck/swallow and breathing
32–34 weeks	Slightly mature sucking pattern Coordination between breathing and swallowing begins
>34 weeks	Mature sucking pattern More coordination between breathing and swallowing

However, not all infants born at a particular gestation would have the same feeding skills. Hence the ideal method would be to evaluate if the feeding skills expected for the gestation are present and then decide accordingly (Fig. 21.1).

All stable LBW infants should be put on their mother's breasts, irrespective of their initial feeding method. The immature sucking observed in preterm infants born before 34 weeks might not meet their daily fluid and nutritional requirements but helps in the rapid maturation of their feeding skills and improves the milk secretion in their mothers (*'non-nutritive sucking'*).

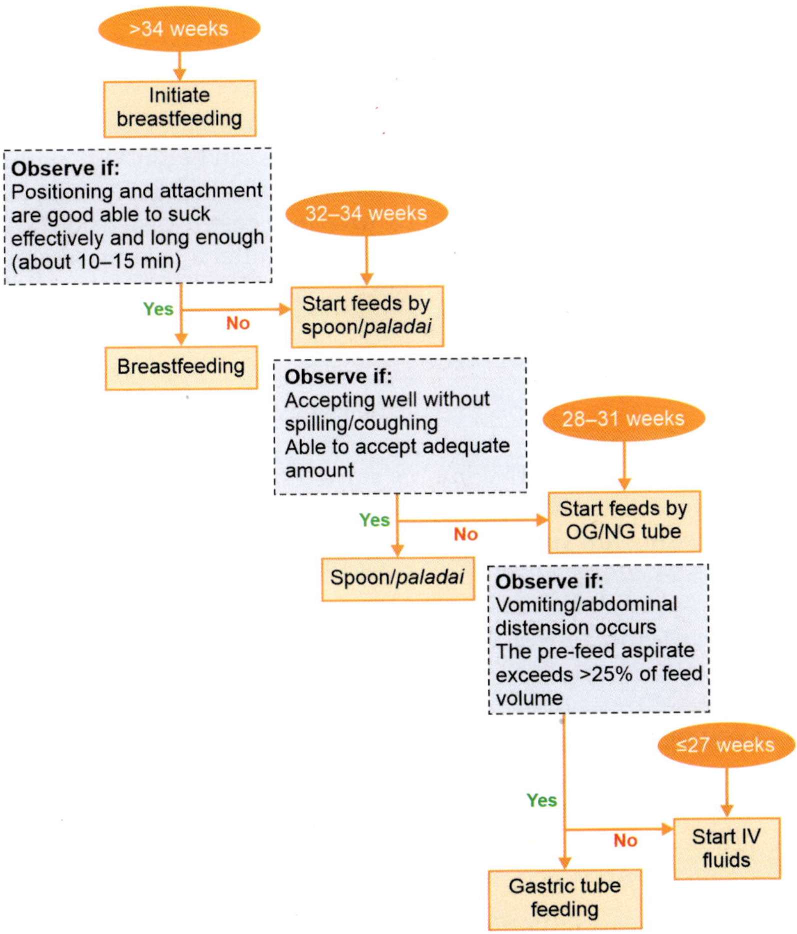

Fig. 21.1: Initial feeding method

Special Situations

Extreme preterm infants: They are usually started on parenteral nutrition from day one of life. Enteral feeds—trophic feeding or minimal enteral nutrition (MEN)—are initiated once the infant is hemodynamically stable. Further advancement is based on the infant's ability to tolerate the feeds.[5]

Antenatally detected Doppler flow abnormalities: Fetuses with abnormal Doppler flow, such as absent/reversed end diastolic flow (A/REDF) in the umbilical artery, are likely to have had mesenteric ischemia *in utero*. After birth, they have a significant risk of developing feed intolerance and NEC.[6,7] Enteral feeding in preterm neonates with A/REDF is usually delayed for 24 hours (*see* Volume 3 Chapter 10: Feeding of Neonates with Umbilical Artery Doppler Abnormalities).

Infants on CPAP/ventilation: These infants can be started on OG tube feeds once they are hemodynamically stable. It is essential to leave the tube open intermittently to reduce gastric distension. We usually keep the tube closed for 30 minutes after a feeding session and leave it open until the next feed.

PROGRESSION OF ORAL FEEDS

All LBW infants, irrespective of their gestation and birth weight, should ultimately be able to feed directly from the mother's breast. For preterm LBW infants started on IV fluids/OG tube/ *paladai* feeding, the steps of progression to direct and exclusive breastfeeding are summarized in Fig. 21.2. *Slower advancement of feeds (15–24 ml/kg/day) has not been shown to have any advantage over faster daily increments (30–40 mL/kg/day).*[8] Term LBW infants started on IV fluids (because of their sickness) should be put on the breast once they are hemodynamically stable.

Choice of Milk

All LBW infants should receive only breast milk regardless of their initial feeding method. This can be ensured even in infants fed by *paladai* or gastric tube by giving expressed breast milk (mother's own milk or human donor milk).

Expressed breast milk (EBM): All preterm infant's mothers should be counseled and supported in expressing their own milk for

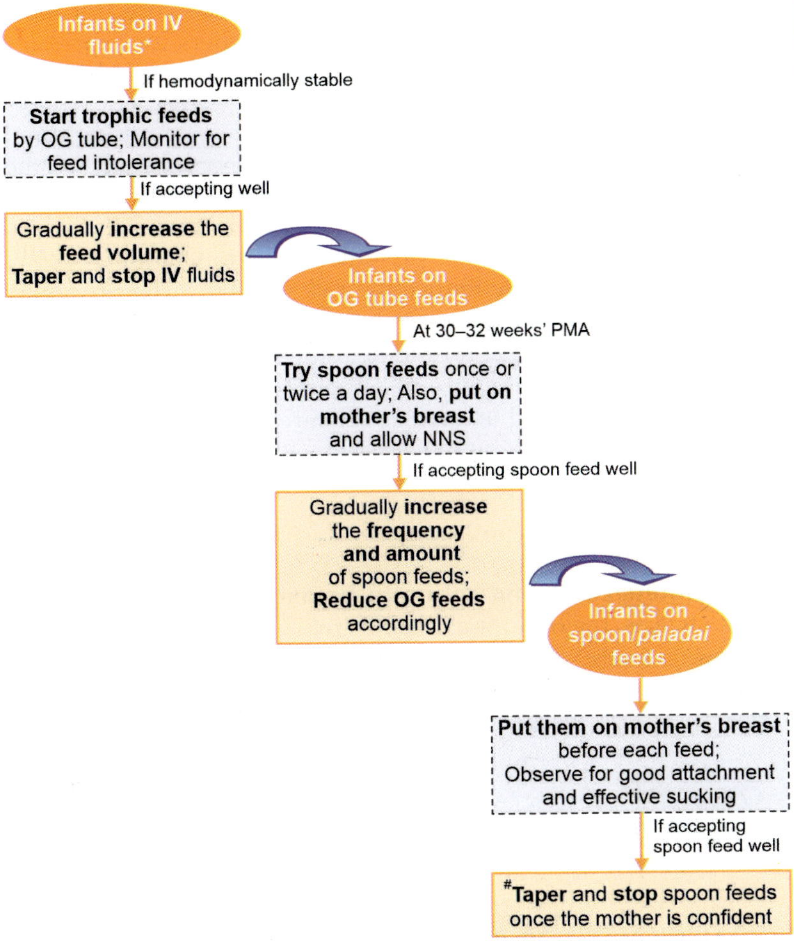

Fig. 21.2: Progression of oral feeding in preterm LBW infants

IV: Intravenous; *OG:* Oro-gastric tube; *PMA:* Postmenstrual age; *NNS:* Non-nutritive sucking

*Term and near-term sick infants started on IV fluids can be initiated on breastfeeding once they are hemodynamically stable;

#Some infants may have to be given spoon feeding for some period even after they start accepting breastfeeding

feeding their infants. Milk expression should ideally be initiated within hours of delivery for the infant to get the benefits of feeding colostrum. After that, it should be done every 2–3 hours to facilitate exclusive breastmilk feeding. This would also help in maintaining lactation in the mother. Expressed breast milk can be stored for about 6 hours at room temperature. We counsel mothers for expression of breast milk soon after delivery by demonstration and by using posters and videos (available on our website: www.newbornwhocc.org).

Donor human milk: In centers where optimal milk banking facilities are available, donor human milk can be used. Pasteurized donor human milk (PDHM) is preferable to formula milk in VLBW neonates because it may reduce the risk of NEC.[9] The process of pasteurization inactivates certain beneficial bioactive factors, and hence it is not a substitute for mother's own milk (MOM). Though there has been a recent surge in establishing human milk banks in India, there is a need to scale up, ensure quality assurance, and strengthen existing services to help bridge the demand–supply gap of PDHM.[10]

Special Situations

Sick mothers/contraindication to breastfeeding: In these rare circumstances, the options available are:

1. Formula feeds:
   a. Preterm formula—in VLBW infants and
   b. Term formula—in infants weighing >1500 g at birth
2. Animal milk, e.g. cow's milk

Once the mother's condition becomes stable (or the contraindication to breastfeeding no longer exists), these infants should be started on exclusive breastfeeding.

HOW MUCH MILK IS TO BE GIVEN?

Calculating the fluid requirements and feed volumes is essential for infants on paladai/gastric tube feeding. The daily fluid requirement is determined based on the estimated insensible water loss, other losses, and urine output. Extreme preterm infants need more fluids in the initial weeks of life because of the high insensible water loss.

We usually start fluids at 80 ml and 60 ml/kg/day for infants with <1500 g and ≥1500 g, respectively. We usually allow rapid increments of 30–40 ml/kg/day for enteral feeds, depending on the tolerance. We typically reach a maximum of 180 ml/kg/day by day 14.[11]

Nutritional Supplementation in LBW Infants

LBW infants, especially those born preterm, require supplementation of various nutrients to meet their high demands. The requirements of VLBW infants differ significantly from those with birth weights of 1500 to 2499 grams.

Supplementation in VLBW Infants

These infants, usually born before 32–34 weeks ofgestation, have inadequate body stores of most nutrients. The amount of protein, energy, calcium, phosphorus, trace elements (iron, zinc), and vitamins (D, E and K) present in expressed breast milk is often unable to meet their high daily requirements (Table 21.2). Hence, these infants require multi-nutrient supplementation till they reach term gestation (40 weeks of PMA).

Multi-nutrient supplementation can be ensured by one of the following methods:

1. Supplementation of individual nutrients, e.g. calcium, phosphorus, vitamins, etc.
2. Fortification of expressed breast milk by using either human milk fortifiers (HMF) or preterm formula.

Supplementing with individual nutrients: The following nutrients must be added to the expressed breast milk:

1. Calcium and phosphate supplements[a]
2. Vitamin A, B complex and zinc supplements[b] usually in the form of multivitamin drops
3. Vitamin D3 drops[c]
4. Folate drops[d]
5. Iron drops[e]

Since supplementation of minerals and vitamins would not meet the high protein requirements of these infants, this method is usually not preferred. If used, the supplements should be added at different times of the day to avoid an abnormal increase in osmolality.

Fortification with HMF: Fortification of expressed breast milk with HMF increases the nutrient content of the milk without compromising its other beneficial effects, such as reduction in

[a]e.g. Syr. Ostocalcium (GlaxoSmithKline Co.), Syr.Ossopan-D (TTK Healthcare)
[b]e.g. Dexvita (Tridoss Co.), Visyneral-zinc drops (Lifeon Co.)
[c]e.g. Arbivit (Raptakos, Brett & Co.), Sunsips (Endura Co.)
[d]e.g. Folium (Speciality Meditech Co.), Folvite (Wyeth Lederle Co.)
[e]e.g. Ferrochelate (Albert David Co.), Tonoferon (East India Co.)

Table 21.2: Recommended dietary allowance (RDA) of nutrients in preterm LBW infants and their estimated intake with fortified and unfortified human milk

	RDA (Units/kg/day)[9]*	*At daily intake of 180 mL/kg*							
		Only expressed breast milk (EBM)#	*EBM fortified with new Lactodex-HMF (4 g/100 ml)*	*EBM fortified with HIJAM-HMF (4 g/100 ml)*	*EBM fortified with NiQuHMoF (4 g /100 ml)*	*EBM fortified with Preterm formula (4 g/100 ml; Dexolac Special care)*	*Lactodex LBW formula*	*PreNAN LBW formula*	*Dexolac Special Care formula*
Energy (kcal)	115–140	117	141	142	141.5	152.2	144.2	144	142.5
Protein (g)	3.5–4.0€	2.5	4.4	4.3	4.66	3.68	3.96	4.7	4.8
Carbohydrates (g)	11.0–15.0	11.6	15.1	12	15.2	15.5	15.4	15.1	15.9
Fat (g)	4.8–8.1	6.8	7.1	8.6	7.1	8.4	7.8	7.2	6.7
Calcium (mg)	120–200	43	157	223	151	88.4	187.8	178.1	183.7
Phosphate (mg)	70–115	22	79	112	79.6	44.7	93.9	89.1	91.8
Vitamin A (IU)	1330–3330	680	2120	1796	4040	1192	1878	1752	2074
Vitamin D (IU)	400–700 (<1000)	3.5	960	724	1155	47	188	175	175
Vitamin E (mg)	2.2–11	1.8	7.8	6.3	5.8	2.9	4.8	3.5	4.6

(Contd.)

Table 21.2: Recommended dietary allowance (RDA) of nutrients in preterm LBW infants and their estimated intake with fortified and unfortified human milk (*Contd.*)

	RDA[*] (Units/kg/ day)[9]	*At daily intake of 180 mL/kg*							
		Only expressed breast milk (EBM)[#]	*EBM fortified with new Lactodex-HMF (4 g/100 ml)*	*EBM fortified with HIJAM-HMF (4 g/ 100 ml)*	*EBM fortified with NiQuHMoF (4 g /100 ml)*	*EBM fortified with Preterm formula (4 g/100 ml; Dexolac Special care)*	*Lactodex LBW formula*	*PreNAN LBW formula*	*Dexolac Special Care formula*
Folic acid (µg)	23–100	6	96	150	99.6	22.2	57.8	55.5	65.6
Zinc (mg)	2–3	0.6	0.88	0.89	1.58	1.1	1.1	1.87	2.1
Iron (mg)	2–3	0.2	2.4	2.8	3.08	0.92	3.5	2.6	2.9
Remarks		Deficient in protein, calcium, phosphate, vitamins B_6 and D, and zinc	Deficient in zinc	Deficient in zinc	Deficient in zinc	Deficient in calcium, phosphate, vitamins A, D, and folic acid, zinc, and iron	Deficient in vitamin D and zinc	Deficient in vitamin D and zinc	Deficient in vitamin D

[*]ESPGHAN 2022
[#]Based on the milk of mothers who have delivered preterm neonates (after 2–3 weeks of delivery)
[€]increased up to 4.5 g/kg/day if growth is slow with no other causes of suboptimal growth
(RDA, recommended dietary allowance; EBM, expressed breast milk)

NEC, infections, etc. The Cochrane review on fortification found short-term improvement in in-hospital weight gain, linear and head growth without any increase in adverse effects such as NEC. However, more evidence for benefits on long-term growth and neurodevelopment outcomes is needed.[12]

The preparations of HMF available in India include Lactodex-HMF (1 g/sachet; Raptakos, Brett and Co. Ltd; ₹28.5/- per sachet) *HIJAM* (1 g/sachet; Endocura Pharma; ₹25/- per sachet), and NiQuHMoF (0.6 g/sachet and 1g/sachet; NeoWinn Biotech; ₹46/- and ₹76/- per sachet, respectively); *Similac HMF* (0.9 g/sachet; Abbott Nutrition) is costlier and not readily available. The recommended dietary allowances (RDA) and the estimated intakes with fortified human milk are given in Table 21.2. *As the table shows, VLBW infants on fortified breast milk with HMF would require zinc supplementation.*

Fortification with the preterm formula: The other option available for fortification is adding preterm formula powder (e.g. *Dexolac Special Care* [Wockhardt Co.], *Pre-NAN* [Nestle Co.], Lactodex LBW [*Raptakos*, Brett and Co. Ltd]). The recommended concentration is 0.4 g per 10 mL of breast milk. A study from our center showed that fortification with preterm formula was non-inferior to human milk fortifier and could serve as a cost-effective alternative.[13] Though more economical, this method has two significant drawbacks:

1. It is difficult to measure such small amounts of formula powder; and
2. The RDA of calcium, phosphorus, vitamin D, folic acid, etc. are not met even after fortification.

While the former issue can be managed by using a small scoop of 1 g size for 25 ml of milk, the latter needs to be addressed by additional supplementation (Table 21.2).

The protocols for nutritional supplementation in VLBW infants until 40 weeks PMA and beyond are described in Tables 21.3 and 21.4.

We use fortification with preterm formula powder for all preterm (<32 weeks) or VLBW (<1500 g) infants. Fortification is started once the infants reach 100 mL/kg/day of enteral feeds. Since calcium, phosphorus, vitamin D, zinc, and iron intake is low even after fortification with preterm formula, we supplement these nutrients additionally (Table 21.3).

We continue fortification till the infant reaches 40 weeks PMA or attains 2 kg (whichever is earlier).

Table 21.3: Nutritional supplementation in preterm VLBW infants until 40 weeks PMA

Nutrients	*EBM fortified with Lactodex-HMF**	*EBM fortified with preterm formula*
Calcium	Not needed	Start calcium supplements to meet the RDA once the infant is on 100 mL/kg/day. (e.g. *Syr. Ostocalcium at 5–6 ml/kg/d*)
Phosphorus	Not needed	Same as above
Zinc and vitamins A, B_6, etc.	Start multivitamin supplements once the infant is on 100 ml/kg/day (e.g. *ViSyneral zinc/ Dexvita* drops at 1.0 ml/day)	Start multivitamin supplements once the infant is on 100 mL/kg/day. (e.g. *ViSyneral zinc/Dexvita drops at 1.0 ml/day*)
Vitamin D	Not needed	Start vitamin D_3 drops if the total intake is less than the RDA. (e.g. *Arbivit/Sunsips at 0.5 ml/day*)
Folic acid*	Not needed	Start supplements once the infant is on 100 ml/kg/day. (e.g. *Folvite/folium at 0.1 ml/day*)
Iron	Not needed	Start iron (2 mg/kg/d) at 4–6 weeks of life. (e.g. *Tonoferon drops at 2 drops/kg/day*)

PMA: Postmenstrual age; *EBM:* Expressed breast milk; *HMF:* Human milk fortifier

Note: The examples quoted are only indicative; Readers are encouraged to use similar products.

*Needed only if the iron drops/syrup does not have folic acid.

Table 21.4: Nutritional supplementation in preterm VLBW infants after 40 weeks PMA

Nutrients	*Method of supplementation*	*Dose*	*Till when?*
Vitamin D*	Vitamin D_3 drops	800–1000 IU/day	Till 2 years of age
Iron	Iron drops/syrup	2 mg/kg/day (maximum 15mg/day)	Till 2 years of age

Supplementation for Infants with birth Weights of 1500–2500 g

These infants who are more likely to be born at term or near-term gestation (>32 weeks) do not require multinutrient supplementation

Table 21.5: Nutritional supplements for infants with birth weights of 1500–2499 g

Nutrients	*Method of supplementation*	*Dose*	*When to start*	*Till when?*
Vitamin D	Multivitamin drops/syrup	1 ml/day (to provide 400 IU/ day of vitamin D)	2 weeks of age	Till 2 years of age
Iron	Iron drops/syrup	2 mg/kg/day (maximum 15 mg/day)	4 weeks of age	Till 2 years of age

or fortification of breast milk (cf. VLBW infants). However, vitamin D, iron, and zinc might still have to be supplemented in them.

We supplement both vitamin D and iron in infants with birth weights of 1500–2499 grams; vitamin D (400 IU) is started at 2 weeks and iron (2 mg/kg/day) at 4 weeks of life; both are continued till 2 years of age (Table 21.5).

Growth Monitoring of LBW Infants

Regular growth monitoring helps assess the nutritional status and adequacy of feeding; it also identifies those infants with inadequate weight gain. All LBW infants should be weighed daily until discharge from the hospital. Other anthropometric parameters, such as length and head circumference, should be recorded weekly. Both term and preterm LBW infants tend to lose weight (about 10% and 15%, respectively) in the first 7 days of life; they regain their birth weight by 10–14 days. After that, the weight gain should be at least 15–20 g/kg/day till a weight of 2–2.5 kg is reached. After this, a gain of 20–30 g/day is considered appropriate (refer to the protocol on 'Postnatal growth monitoring').[14]

LBW infants should be discharged after they:

- Reach 34 weeks PMA and are above 1500–1600 g and
- Show consistent weight gain for at least three consecutive days.

Feed Intolerance

The inability to tolerate enteral feedings in extremely premature infants is a significant concern in the NICU. Feed intolerance is often the predominant factor affecting the infant's hospitalization duration. There are no universally agreed-upon criteria to define feed intolerance in preterm infants.[9] Various clinical features that are usually considered to be the indicators of feed intolerance are summarized in Table 21.6.

Table 21.6: Indicators of feed intolerance[9]
Symptoms:
• Vomiting (altered milk/bile or blood-stained)*
• Systemic features: lethargy, apnea
Signs:
• Abdominal distension (with or without visible bowel loops)*
• Increased gastric residuals: >2 mL/kg or any change from previous pattern
• Abdominal tenderness
• Reduced or absent bowel sounds
• Systemic signs: cyanosis, bradycardia, etc.

**Common signs*

Of these, vomiting, abdominal distension, and increased gastric residual volume form the 'triad' for defining feed intolerance.

Vomiting: The characteristic of vomitus is essential in assessing the cause: while altered milk is usually innocuous, bile- or blood-stained vomiting should be thoroughly investigated.

Abdominal distension: Monitoring the abdominal girth in all preterm VLBW infants admitted to the ICU is essential. This helps in the early identification of feed intolerance and eliminates the need for routine gastric aspirate.

Gastric residual volume: It indicates the rapidity of gastric emptying. Since several factors (both systemic and local) influence gastric emptying, the residual volume is a poor and nonspecific indicator of fed intolerance. Measures to enhance the specificity, such as quantifying the volume or using different cut-offs for defining feed intolerance, are not much useful. Moreover, repeated gastric aspiration to look for residuals could injure the delicate mucosa aggravating the local pathology.

We monitor the abdominal girth every 2 hours in all preterm LBW infants admitted to the nursery. We do not routinely aspirate the gastric contents before giving the next feed. *Aspiration is done only if there is an increase in abdominal girth by ≥2 cm from the baseline.*

Management of Feed Intolerance

The common factors attributed to feed intolerance in preterm infants are immature intestinal motility, immaturity of digestive enzymes, underlying medical conditions such as sepsis, inappropriate feed volume, hyperosmolar medications/feedings, and, importantly,

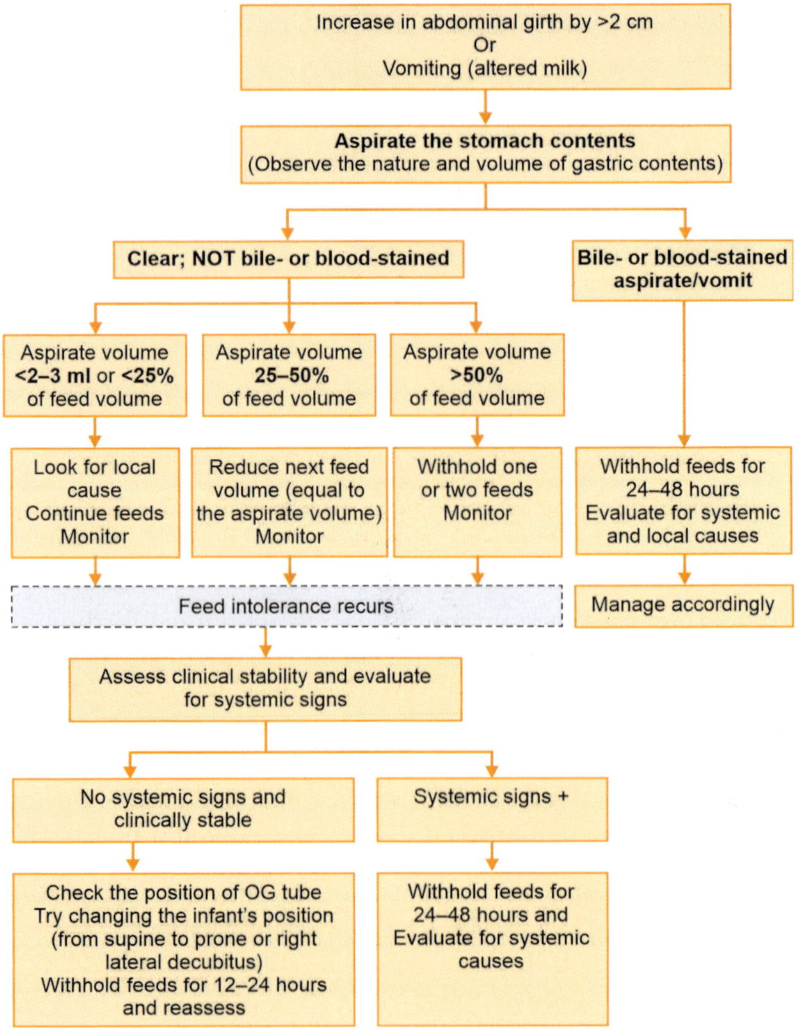

Fig. 21.3: Approach to feed intolerance in LBW infants

necrotizing enterocolitis (NEC). The steps in evaluating and managing an infant with feed intolerance are given in Fig. 21.3.

REFERENCES

1. UNICEF-WHO Low birthweight estimates: Levels and trends 2000–2015 | UNICEF [Internet]. 2019 [cited 2023 Apr 21]. Available from: https://www.unicef.org/reports/UNICEF-WHO-low-birthweight-estimates-2019.

2. Blencowe H, Krasevec J, Onis M de, Black RE, An X, Stevens GA, et al. National, regional, and worldwide estimates of low birthweight in 2015, with trends from 2000: a systematic analysis. The Lancet Global Health. 2019 Jul 1;7(7):e849–60.
3. Edmond KM, Kirkwood BR, Tawiah CA, Owusu Agyei S. Impact of early infant feeding practices on mortality in low birth weight infants from rural Ghana. J Perinatol. 2008 Jun;28(6):438–44.
4. Kara Gross Margolis, Joseph A Piccaro. Fetal and Neonatal Physiology. 5th ed. Vol. 2. 881–7 p.
5. Mishra S, Agarwal R, Jeevasankar M, Deorari AK, Paul VK. Minimal enteral nutrition. Indian J Pediatr. 2008 Mar;75(3):267–9.
6. Dorling J, Kempley S, Leaf A. Feeding growth restricted preterm infants with abnormal antenatal Doppler results. Archives of Disease in Childhood - Fetal and Neonatal Edition. 2005 Sep 1;90(5):F359–63.
7. Martini S, Annunziata M, Della Gatta AN, Aceti A, Brunetti M, Pilu G, et al. Association between Abnormal Antenatal Doppler Characteristics and Gastrointestinal Outcomes in Preterm Infants. Nutrients. 2022 Jan;14(23):5121.
8. Oddie SJ, Young L, McGuire W. Slow advancement of enteral feed volumes to prevent necrotising enterocolitis in very low birth weight infants. Cochrane Database of Systematic Reviews [Internet]. 2021 [cited 2023 Apr 21];(8). Available from: https://www.cochranelibrary.com/cdsr/doi/10.1002/14651858.CD001241.pub8/full.
9. Embleton ND, Moltu SJ, Lapillonne A, van den Akker CHP, Carnielli V, Fusch C, et al. Enteral Nutrition in Preterm Infants (2022): A Position Paper From the ESPGHAN Committee on Nutrition and Invited Experts. J Pediatr Gastroenterol Nutr. 2023 Feb 1;76(2):248–68.
10. Sachdeva RC, Mondkar J, Shanbhag S, Sinha MM, Khan A, Dasgupta R. A Landscape Analysis of Human Milk Banks in India. Indian Pediatr. 2019 Aug 15;56(8):663–8.
11. Chawla D, Agarwal R, Deorari AK, Paul VK. Fluid and electrolyte management in term and preterm neonates. Indian J Pediatr. 2008 Mar;75(3):255–9.
12. Brown JVE, Lin L, Embleton ND, Harding JE, McGuire W. Multi-nutrient fortification of human milk for preterm infants. Cochrane Database of Systematic Reviews [Internet]. 2020 [cited 2020 Sep 16];(6). Available from: https://www.cochranelibrary.com/cdsr/doi/10.1002/14651858.CD000343.pub4/full.
13. Chinnappan A, Sharma A, Agarwal R, Thukral A, Deorari A, Sankar MJ. Fortification of Breast Milk With Preterm Formula Powder vs Human Milk Fortifier in Preterm Neonates: A Randomized Noninferiority Trial. JAMA Pediatrics [Internet]. 2021 May 10 [cited 2021 Jun 22]; Available from: https://doi.org/10.1001/jamapediatrics.2021.0678.
14. Colaizy T, DeMauro SB, Mcnelis K, Poindexter BB. Enteral nutrition for the High-risk neonate. In: Avery's Disease of the Newborn. 10th ed. p. 1009–22.

CHAPTER

22 Postnatal Growth Monitoring and Extrauterine Growth Restriction

GROWTH MONITORING IN NICU

Assessment of growth in the NICU involves accurate weight, length, and head circumference measurement, as depicted in Table 22.1. The parameters must be plotted on an appropriate growth chart.

Growth Charts for Growth Monitoring

Using a growth chart is a simple and effective way to monitor growth. Serial plotting of weight and other anthropometric indicators in the growth chart allows the individual infant's growth

Table 22.1: Desired gains in anthropometric parameters

Parameter	*Frequency of measurement*	*Expected normal range*	*Remarks*
Weight Weight gain velocity	Daily Weekly	• 15–20 g/kg/day till 36 weeks PMA • 20–35 g/day from 36 weeks PMA to 2 months corrected age[1]	• Weight gain (g/kg/day) = (current weight- previous week weight)/(average of current and previous week weight × 7) • g/kg/day or g/day ignore the previous growth velocity pattern • Weight velocity calculation avoided in first 7 days (to exclude postnatal weight loss phase)
Length	Weekly	0.7–1 cm/week	Measured using infantometer
Head circumference	Weekly	0.7–1 cm/ week	Occipitofrontal circumference using a non-stretchable tape

PMA: Postmenstrual age

to be compared with expected growth and helps in the early identification of abnormal growth patterns.

Two types of growth charts are commonly used for growth monitoring in preterm infants: intrauterine and postnatal growth charts (Table 22.2).

In our unit, we use Fenton's chart for monitoring the growth of preterm VLBW neonates, followed by the WHO growth charts from 40 weeks PMA. For term LBW infants, we follow the WHO MGRS growth charts. The available options according to hypothetical scenarios are presented in Table 22.3. Certain commonly used growth charts for postnatal growth are discussed here.

a. **Fenton growth charts (2013, revised):** These charts provide sex-specific weight, HC, and length curves between 22 and 50 weeks of postmenstrual age. Derived from retrospective data from six countries involving more than 4 million preterm neonates, the data between 36 weeks and 50 weeks PMA were interpolated (smoothening) without any actual measurements to account for the disjunction between Fenton and WHO growth charts. They are used to classify 'size-at-birth' and to monitor postnatal growth till 50 weeks PMA, which can then be continued with WHO MGRS charts.

Table 22.2: Growth charts used in the NICU

Intrauterine growth charts	*Postnatal growth charts*
'Standard' or 'Prescriptive'	'Reference' or 'Descriptive'
Illustrate 'ideal' growth	Illustrate 'actual' growth
Created using cross-sectional anthropometric birth data for each gestation	Created using longitudinal data
Useful for estimating 'size at birth'	Useful for monitoring postnatal growth
Do not account for initial postnatal weight loss when used to monitor postnatal growth; prevalence of EUGR/SGA higher	Initial weight loss accounted in reference curve; more realistic representation of the true postnatal growth; prevalence of EUGR/SGA lower
Examples: Lubchenco (1963), Babson (1970), AIIMS (1991), Olsen (2010), Fenton (2013), Intergrowth-21 Newborn cross-sectional study – size standards	**Examples:** Dancis, Wright's, Ehrankranz, Intergrowth-21 PPFS – Preterm postnatal follow up study, WHO MGRS

Table 22.3: Suggested options for the use of growth charts in common scenarios		
Scenario	*Appropriate growth charts*	*Comments–merits/demerits*
30-week gestation/1.2 kg weight for postnatal growth monitoring	Ehrenkranz (1994–1995)	Older charts, no standardized nutrition intake. Not available for birth weight >1500 g
	Fenton (2013)	Does not account for initial postnatal weight loss when used to monitor postnatal growth; prevalence of EUGR/SGA higher. Smoothening of curves to match WHO MGRS (gap between 36–50 weeks is an extrapolation) Targeting the growth curve parallel to the reference curve after the initial weight loss phase can be done.
	Intergrowth (PPFS)	Though the chart provides curves from 26–37 weeks, it is primarily developed from neonates >33 weeks.
40 week/2.9 kg for postnatal growth monitoring	WHO MGRS	–

b. **Intergrowth–21 growth charts:** The Intergrowth consortium assessed fetal growth and newborn size prospectively in eight geographically defined diverse urban populations to provide various growth charts:

Newborn cross-sectional study (NCSS): Provides gender-specific centiles for weight, length, and HC; derived from 20,486 observations, they depict the standards for size at birth from 33–42 weeks.

Preterm postnatal follow-up study (PPFS): Derived from 201 neonates, this provides longitudinal postnatal curves for preterm neonates between 26 and 37 weeks of gestation. It can be used till 64 weeks PMA, after which they merge with the WHO growth charts. However, the number of observations for gestation less than 34 weeks is very small.

c. **Ehrenkranz growth charts:** Derived from 1660 observations during the 1994–1995 period limited to the United States of America, these charts provide postnatal growth curves for

VLBW infants (501–1500 g) for weight, length, HC, and mid-arm circumference from birth to 120 days. The sampling excluded major congenital anomalies; however, nutrition intake was not standardized.

Growth Pattern of Preterm VLBW Neonates

The traditional concept of targeting growth of the preterm neonate in the NICU to match that of the fetal standards is seldom achieved in practice. Fetal growth cannot be used as reference standard to monitor postnatal growth. Hence, there is no consensus on how the growth of preterm neonate must be monitored. One way to examine postnatal growth is subtracting z-score at a given time point on growth curve from that at birth. Healthy preterm neonates (nourished according to protocols) average around –0.8 z-scores after the initial postnatal weight loss.[2] After the initial weight loss phase, weight gain trajectory is parallel to the intrauterine growth chart curves[3] (Fig. 22.1). Targeting return of weight centile to birth z-score in the first week of life hence may not be appropriate.[4]

EXTRAUTERINE GROWTH RESTRICTION

Extrauterine growth restriction (EUGR) in preterm VLBW neonates is a common problem across the globe. In a large series of VLBW

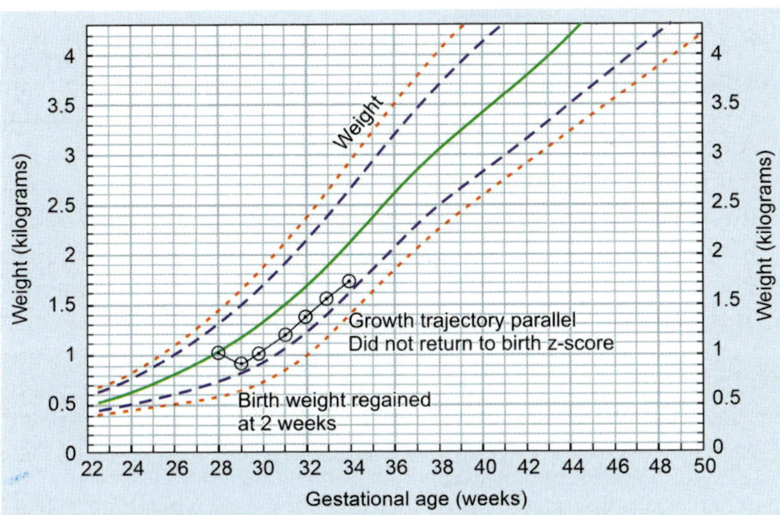

Fig. 22.1: Growth curve of a 28 week/1 kg baby, depicting initial weight loss and following parallel growth trajectory

neonates, more than 50% were growth restricted at discharge.[5] The incidence of EUGR at 40 weeks postmenstrual age (PMA) was 73% and 81% in preterm VLBW neonates receiving preterm formula fortification and HMF, respectively, in our unit.[6] The incidence varies inversely with gestational age at birth.

Definition

An ideal definition of EUGR should:

1. Correlate well with the neurodevelopmental outcome, and
2. Consider the weight, length, head circumference, genetic potential, expected postnatal weight loss, body composition, and the risk of metabolic syndrome in later life.

The definition of EUGR has been a widely debated topic with controversy largely revolving along the following issues:

- Which charts to use?
- What cutoff to be used—absolute value or change from baseline?
- When to measure—36 weeks or 40 weeks of gestation or at discharge?
- What to measure—weight or length or head circumference or a combination?

The commonly used definition of EUGR—less than 10th percentile at 36–40 weeks' PMA—is fraught with controversies which include the following:

- It is based only on weight without any consideration of other aspects of growth.
- It does not recognize the postnatal weight loss and the usual subsequent growth patterns in preterm neonates.
- It is based on an arbitrary statistical cutoff.
- It is assessed before the growth slowing of the reference fetus, which is around 36–40 weeks, thereby overestimating EUGR.
- The doubtful association with adverse neurodevelopmental outcomes.

Evidence

In a review of 355 preterm infant growth studies, 19% of the studies described rates of EUGR.

62% of these 67 studies used <10th percentile cutoff, 10% used <3rd percentile cut-off and 18% used loss of >2 z-scores. Timing for EUGR assessment also varied, 63% conducted this assessment at discharge, 21% at term age, and 20% at 36 weeks.[7]

EUGR and Neurodevelopmental Outcome

Poor in-hospital weight gain in ELBW infants was associated with a significantly higher risk of adverse neurodevelopmental outcomes at 18–22 months corrected age in a multi-cohort study of infants with birth weights from 501 to 1000 g.[8] Quantifying the degree of abnormal growth (z-score) was better than an arbitrary cutoff of <10th percentile. Head circumference and linear growth were also associated with better neurodevelopment (not weight gain alone).

Evidence

Weight <10th percentile at 36 weeks PMA had a high sensitivity (88%) but low specificity (13%) for Bayley II mental developmental and psychomotor developmental indices <70.8 A 1-point decrease in weight-for-age z-score was associated with 5.6 point decrease in MDI.[9] In contrast, an 1 SD increase in length-for-age z-score was associated with 4 point increase in cognitive scores at 24 months CA.[10] Infants with a suboptimal head size at the age of three months had a significantly lower median IQ than those with a normal head size.[11]

Postnatal trajectories deviate from intrauterine growth trajectory due to one-time irreversible contraction of extravascular space and abrupt loss of placental supply. Neonates may follow an individualized growth curve of –0.8 z-scores remerging after 42 weeks. Infants who followed the individualized growth trajectories had the lowest values of fat mass percentage for their corresponding weight at term-equivalent age.[10] Causes of EUGR are depicted in Table 22.4.

Table 22.4: Causes of EUGR[11]	
Antenatal factors	Uteroplacental insufficiency, maternal malnutrition, chorioamnionitis, lack of antenatal steroids
Postnatal factors	Extreme prematurity, requirement of ventilation, male gender, sepsis, inadequate postnatal nutrition, GER, feed intolerance
Increased energy expenditure	BPD, drug withdrawal, sepsis
Medications	Postnatal steroids, diuretics
Metabolic causes	Anaemia, hyponatremia, hypothermia, micronutrient deficiency, pain
Surgical causes	NEC, intestinal atresia, intestinal perforation, infantile hypertrophic pyloric stenosis
Malabsorption	Cow milk protein allergy, glucose-galactose malabsorption, lactose intolerance

Strategies to Prevent EUGR

- Use of breastmilk
- Early "aggressive" nutrition: TPN initiation
- Early enteral feeding
- Fortification

Breast milk is associated with better neurodevelopment despite suboptimal initial weight gain. So, the mother's own milk (MOM) is the first choice in feeding preterm infants. It provides short- and long-term benefits, including protection against NEC, ROP, BPD sepsis, and neurocognitive improvement (Table 22.5).

Fortification Strategies

Standard Fortification

A fixed amount of fortifier (as per the manufacturers' instructions) is added to a fixed volume of human milk in standard fortification. Despite this, many VLBW infants have suboptimal growth, predominantly due to protein undernutrition. Individualized milk fortification tries to address the pitfalls of standard fortification.

Table 22.5: Potential strategies to prevent EUGR

Period	*Optimal nutrition interventions in the NICU*
Acute stage	Early aggressive parenteral nutrition. First week protein and energy intakes are associated with better developmental outcomes in extremely low birth weight infants. Goal: To reduce cumulative calorie and protein deficits. To minimize postnatal weight loss and the time taken to regain birth weight
	Trophic feeding and early enteral feeding Start enteral feeding from day 1 if no contraindication to feeding
	Rapid advancement
Intermediate stage	Fortification
	Micronutrient supplementation
	Higher calories and protein for conditions like NEC, sepsis, BPD, and postoperative period
Post discharge	Fortification is to be continued up to 40 weeks PMA
Other measures	Temperature maintenance
	Prevention of infection
	Adequate respiratory support during NICU stay

Individualized Human Milk Fortification

a. **Adjustable fortification:** Protein adequacy is monitored, and extra protein is added to the fortification accordingly.

b. **Targeted fortification:** Macronutrient concentrations in human milk are analyzed, based on the results of which the milk is supplemented with extra protein and/or fat.

Evidence

In an RCT of preterm infants with birth weights of 600–1750 g and gestation of 26–34 weeks, the mean measured protein intake was higher in the 'adjusted fortification' group (3.5 g/kg/day) than the standard group (2.8 g/kg/day). The former group had better weight and head circumference gains compared to the latter group (17 vs 14 g/kg/day and 1.0 vs 0.7 cm/week, respectively).

REFERENCES

1. Fenton, T. R. et al. Accuracy of preterm infant weight gain velocity calculations vary depending on method used and infant age at time of measurement. Pediatr. Res. 85, 650–4 (2019).
2. Rochow, N. et al. Physiological adjustment to postnatal growth trajectories in healthy preterm infants. Pediatr. Res. 79, 870–9 (2016).
3. Pediatric nutrition. (American Academy of Pediatrics, 2020).
4. Fenton, T. R. et al. "Extrauterine growth restriction" and "postnatal growth failure" are misnomers for preterm infants. J. Perinatol. 40, 704–14 (2020).
5. Horbar, J. D. et al. Weight Growth Velocity and Postnatal Growth Failure in Infants 501 to 1500 Grams: 2000–2013. Pediatrics 136, e84–e92 (2015).
6. Chinnappan, A. et al. Fortification of Breast Milk With Preterm Formula Powder vs Human Milk Fortifier in Preterm Neonates: A Randomized Noninferiority Trial. JAMA Pediatr. 175, 790–6 (2021).
7. Fenton, T. R. et al. Preterm Infant Growth Velocity Calculations: A Systematic Review. Pediatrics 139, e20162045 (2017).
8. Ehrenkranz, R. A. et al. Growth in the Neonatal Intensive Care Unit Influences Neurodevelopmental and Growth Outcomes of Extremely Low Birth Weight Infants. Pediatrics 117, 1253–61 (2006).
9. Goldberg, D. L. et al. Identifying Malnutrition in Preterm and Neonatal Populations: Recommended Indicators. J. Acad. Nutr. Diet. 118, 1571–82 (2018).
10. Landau-Crangle, E. et al. Individualized Postnatal Growth Trajectories for Preterm Infants. J. Parenter. Enter. Nutr. 42, 1084–92 (2018).
11. Peila, C. et al. Extrauterine Growth Restriction: Definitions and Predictability of Outcomes in a Cohort of Very Low Birth Weight Infants or Preterm Neonates. Nutrients 12, 1224 (2020).

CHAPTER

23

Necrotizing Enterocolitis

Necrotizing enterocolitis (NEC) is one of the commonest gastrointestinal emergencies seen in the neonatal intensive care unit. The incidence of NEC varies among different centers, with endemic and epidemic occurrences. More than 85% of cases of NEC occur among preterm (<32 weeks' gestation) VLBW neonates. Studies from developed countries report an incidence of 2–7% among VLBW infants.[1] The incidence of NEC among VLBW neonates in our unit in 2021 was 5.8%.

Risk factors for NEC: Prematurity, hypoxia, sepsis, abnormal colonization of the bowel, ischemic-reperfusion injury, umbilical arterial catheterization, H_2 blockers, broad-spectrum antibiotics, and antenatally detected umbilical artery blood flow abnormalities (absent/reversed end–diastolic flow) are the common risk factors of NEC.

Exclusive breast milk feeding protects against NEC by altering gastric pH, increasing intestinal motility, decreasing epithelial permeability, and altering the composition of intestinal bacterial flora. There is no increased risk of NEC with early introduction of feeds or faster rate of enhancement of feeds.[2–3]

Type of milk and NEC: What is the evidence?

Meta-analysis of 12 RCTs comparing formula feeds versus donor human milk in preterm infants showed that preterm infants fed with formula had approximately twice the incidence of NEC: typical RR 1.87 (95% CI 1.23–2.85).[4]

PATHOGENESIS

The pathogenesis of NEC is multifactorial, with an immature host immunologic system, altered intestinal microbiome (dysbiosis), milk substrate, and mucosal injury/inflammation playing key roles. The most common site of involvement is the distal small intestine and proximal large intestine. The pathologic hallmarks are coagulation (hemorrhagic–ischemic) necrosis, inflammation, and bacterial overgrowth.

CLINICAL FEATURES

NEC commonly presents as a fulminant and rapidly progressive illness; however, it may also present as a slowly progressive illness with abdominal distension and features of sepsis and ileus (Table 23.1). In extremely preterm neonates, a high index of suspicion is required for early diagnosis.

The age of onset is inversely related to the postmenstrual age (PMA) at birth, with a mean of around 12 days and a PMA of 29–31 weeks. The typical clinical features include the following:

Table 23.1: Staging of NEC (modified Bell's staging)[5]

Stage	*Systemic signs*	*Local signs*	*Radiological signs*	*Treatment*
Stage I	Temperature instability, apnea, bradycardia	Increased pre-feed residuals, mild abdominal distension, and occult blood in stool (stage IA) or gross blood in the stool (stage IB)	Normal or mild ileus	NPO; consider antibiotics for 3 days pending culture report
Stage IIA	Same as stage I	Same as I plus absent bowel sounds, prominent abdominal distension, abdominal tenderness	Ileus, **pneumatosis intestinalis**	NPO, antibiotics for 7–10 days
Stage IIB	Same as stage I plus mild metabolic acidosis and thrombocytopenia	Same as IIA plus abdominal wall edema with palpable loops and tenderness	Same as IIA plus **portal venous gas**, with or without ascites	NPO, antibiotics for 14 days

(Contd.)

Table 23.1: Staging of NEC (modified Bell's staging)* (*Contd.*)				
Stage	*Systemic signs*	*Local signs*	*Radiological signs*	*Treatment*
Stage III A	Same as IIB plus hypotension bradycardia, mixed acidosis, DIC	Same as II with worsening abdominal wall edema, erythema, and induration (signs of generalized peritonitis), marked tenderness	Same as IIB with **definite ascites**	Same as above; may require fluids up to 200 ml/kg/day, inotropes, assisted ventilation, abdominal paracentesis
Stage III B	Same as IIIA with worsening shock, deterioration in laboratory values and vital signs	Same as IIIA	Same as IIB plus **pneumoperi-toneum**	Same as above plus surgical intervention

Systemic signs: Respiratory distress with increased episodes of apnea/bradycardia and temperature instability, lethargy or irritability with poor feeding, decreased peripheral perfusion and pallor, acidosis, hypo/hyperglycemia, oliguria, and bleeding diathesis.

Abdominal signs (usually predominate): These include increased gastric aspirates, abdominal distension or tenderness, blood in stools, peritonitis, abdominal wall erythema, vomiting (bile or blood-stained), and ascites.

INVESTIGATIONS

Laboratory findings: There may be anemia, neutropenia with a shift to the left, thrombocytopenia, metabolic acidosis, hyponatremia, and occult blood in the stool. Blood cultures are positive in up to 40% of cases. Severe refractory hyponatremia, persistent metabolic acidosis, and thrombocytopenia comprise the classic metabolic triad in NEC.

Abdominal X-ray: Both AP and left lateral decubitus (useful for detection of a small pneumoperitoneum) or cross-table lateral

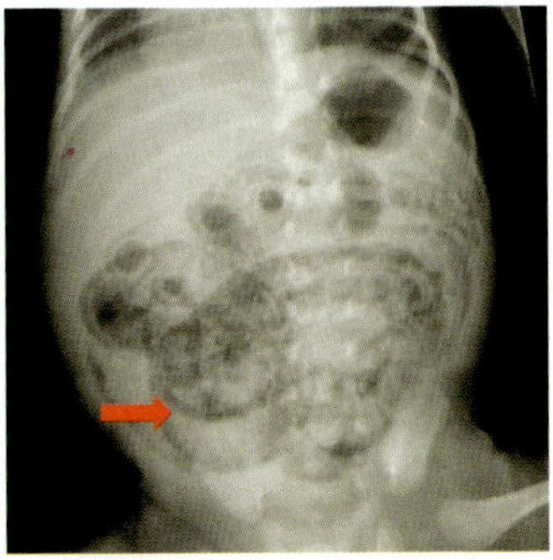

Fig. 23.1: Pneumatosis intestinalis: (Arrow indicates intramural gas in bowel wall; the radiologic hallmark)

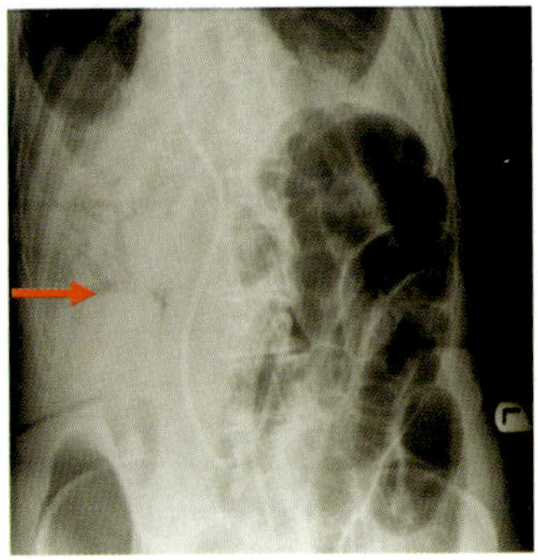

Fig. 23.2: Portal venous gas: (Arrow indicates portal venous gas)

views (avoids the need to move and position these sick neonates) may be required for diagnosis. The common features include bowel wall edema, pneumatosis intestinalis (the radiologic hallmark; Fig. 23.1), portal venous gas (Fig. 23.2), gasless abdomen indicating ascites, fixed position of bowel loop on serial X-rays (same appearance of a dilated loop of bowel on radiography over 24 hours). The frequency of repeating X-rays depends on the severity of NEC and may vary from 6 to 24 hours and at clinical deterioration.

USG abdomen: This may help detect ascites, bowel wall thickness, and bowel wall perfusion; pneumatosis intestinalis and portal vein gas can also be seen.

Practical tip: X-ray abdomen

ELBW neonates often have only abdominal distension and ileus and are more likely to have pneumoperitoneum; pneumatosis intestinalis is more common after 30 weeks PMA.[6]

Near-infrared spectroscopy (NIRS): NIRS is a clinical tool that noninvasively measures oxygen consumption of tissues in real-time and can assess potential ischemia of the bowel, which can aid in the early diagnosis of NEC. Evidence suggests that a reduction in regional splanchnic saturation (rSO_2) may be an early warning sign of NEC in vulnerable neonates. Moreover, monitoring of NIRS in preterm neonates with NEC may predict complications such as bowel necrosis, perforation, need for surgical intervention, and death in the first 48 hours after the onset of symptoms of NEC.[7,8]

Biomarkers: Recent studies have evaluated the role of biomarkers in predicting and diagnosing NEC. Among them, fecal calprotectin, intestine fatty acid binding protein, claudins, and Trefoil factor 3 appear most promising.[9]

MANAGEMENT

Prevention

- **Antenatal strategies**
  - *Antenatal steroids:* The incidence of NEC is significantly reduced with antenatal steroids given to pregnant women with preterm labor or premature rupture of membranes.[10]
- **Feeding and nutrition**
  - *Human milk feeding:* Newborns exclusively breastfed have a reduced risk of NEC.[4] In addition, human milk has a dose-dependent effect on the reduction of NEC.
  - *Oropharyngeal administration of colostrum:* Limited studies show that colostrum, rich in immunological factors, can stimulate the oropharyngeal immune system and protect against NEC in preterm neonates. However, the meta-analysis of studies has shown only a trend toward beneficial effects in the reduction of NEC.[11]
  - *Standardized enteral feeding:* Minimal enteral nutrition and standard feeding guidelines have proven benefits in decreasing the incidence of NEC.[12]
- **Pharmacological measures**
  - *Probiotics:* Meta-analysis of 56 trials has shown that probiotics may reduce the risk of NEC (relative risk 0.54; CI 0.45–0.65).[13] The ESPGHAN Working Group for Probiotics recommends *L rhamnosus* GGATCC 53103 alone at a dose of 1×10^9 CFU or a combination of *infantis* Bb-02, B lactis Bb-12, and *Str thermophilus* TH-4 at a dose of 3×10^8 CFU (of each strain) for prevention of NEC stage 2 or 3.[14]
  - *We occasionally use L rhamnosus* GGATCC 53103 at the dose mentioned above in ELGANs.
  - *Lactoferrin:* Lactoferrin has been shown to attenuate lipopolysaccharide-mediated proinflammatory cytokine release from monocytic cells, and stimulate enterocyte proliferation, which is vital in maintaining intestinal mucosa integrity. Supplementation of lactoferrin with or without probiotics has been shown to reduce the incidence of late-

onset sepsis and NEC. However, the Cochrane review of 12 RCTs showed that enteral lactoferrin supplementation decreased late-onset sepsis but showed no benefit in reducing NEC. Enteral lactoferrin, along with probiotics, have been shown to reduce late-onset sepsis and severe NEC.[15]

- *L-arginine:* Arginine is a substrate for nitric oxide production and may help prevent NEC. Moderate quality evidence from three trials showed a significant reduction in the incidence of any stage NEC (RR 0.38; 95% CI 0.23–0.64). However, given the small number of neonates enrolled, more trials are needed to make a definite recommendation.[16]
- *Restricting the use of empirical antibiotics:* Prolonged use of empirical antibiotics for more than 5 days in ELBW neonates with negative blood cultures has been associated with an increased risk of NEC or death.[17]
- *Restricting the use of histamine-2 receptor antagonists:* H_2 receptor antagonists have been associated with an increased risk of infection and NEC.[18]

Medical Management

- All neonates with suspected/established NEC should be kept nil per oral with continuous gastric aspiration; volume-by-volume replacement of aspirates should be done with N/2 saline.
- Total parenteral nutrition may be required, particularly in neonates with stage II/III NEC.
- Remove umbilical arterial or venous catheters, if any (to prevent ongoing intestinal ischemia).
- Initiate appropriate respiratory support in the form of CPAP or mechanical ventilation.
- Circulatory support: If there are any features of shock, manage with normal saline bolus and inotropes with continuous monitoring of arterial blood pressure.
- Metabolic derangements like acidosis and electrolyte imbalances should be corrected.
- Blood cultures must be sent with broad-spectrum antibiotics as per the NICU protocol (with anaerobic cover when there is evidence of peritonitis or bowel perforation).
- Pain control and minimal handling of the neonate are recommended.
- Maintain hematocrit; arrange PRBC and FFP if evidence of DIC.

- Renal function monitoring: Monitor urine output, urea, creatinine, serum electrolytes, and fluid management as indicated.
- Serial monitoring with abdominal X-rays and abdominal girth monitoring is recommended.
- Consultation with a pediatric surgeon for further management (see below).

Surgical Management

Absolute indications for surgery:

1. Pneumoperitoneum (indicating bowel perforation).
2. Presence of necrotic bowel (severe and persistent metabolic acidosis and/or thrombocytopenia, persistent fixed loop on serial X-rays with lack of response to medical management).

The surgical options include:

1. **Laparotomy:** The standard procedure is laparotomy with resection of gangrenous bowel and enterostomy formation. Resection and primary anastomosis may be tried in a few neonates.
2. **Primary peritoneal drainage (PPD):** Consider PPD in ELBW neonates who are too unstable to undergo laparotomy.

Laparotomy vs.PPD: What is the evidence?

Rao et al.[19] found no significant benefits or harms of peritoneal drainage over laparotomy. However, they included only 2 RCTs and had a small sample size of 185 neonates. The trials also did not distinguish isolated intestinal perforation from NEC. One trial found that 74% of neonates initially treated with primary peritoneal drainage required a rescue laparotomy.

PROGNOSIS

The overall mortality of NEC ranges from 20% to 40% but approaches 100% in neonates with the most severe form of the disease.1 Other complications in severe NEC requiring surgical intervention include intestinal strictures, short bowel syndrome, cholestasis, and growth failure. There is also a significant risk of neurodevelopmental sequelae on follow-up.[19]

REFERENCES

1. Battersby C, Santhalingam T, Costeloe K, Modi N. Incidence of neonatal necrotising enterocolitis in high-income countries: a systematic review. Arch Dis Child Fetal Neonatal Ed. 2018 Mar;103(2):F182–9.

2. Oddie SJ, Young L, McGuire W. Slow advancement of enteral feed volumes toprevent necrotising enterocolitis in very low birth weight infants. CochraneDatabase Syst Rev. 2021;8:CD001241.
3. Young_L, Oddie_SJ, McGuire_W.. Delayed introductionof progressive enteralfeeds to prevent necrotising enterocolitis in very low birth weight infants.Cochrane Database Syst Rev. 2022;(12):CD001970.
4. Quigley M, Embleton ND, McGuireW. Formula versus donor breast milk for feeding preterm or low birth weight infants. Cochrane Database of Systematic Reviews 2018;(4): CD002971.
5. Gordon PV, Swanson JR, Attridge JT, Clark R. Emerging trends in acquiredneonatal intestinal disease: is it time to abandon Bell's criteria? J Perinatol 2007;27:661–71.
6. Sharma R, Hudak ML, Tepas JJ 3rd, Wludyka PS, Marvin WJ, Bradshaw JA, PieperP. Impact of gestational age on the clinical presentation and surgical outcome ofnecrotizing enterocolitis. J Perinatol 2006;26:342–7.
7. Patel AK, Lazar DA, Burrin DG, et al. Abdominal near-infrared spectroscopy measurements are lower in preterm infants at risk for necrotizing enterocolitis. Pediatr Crit Care Med 2014;15(8):735–41.
8. Schat TE, Schurink M, van der Laan ME, et al. Near-infrared spectroscopy to predict the course of necrotizing enterocolitis. PLoS One 2016;11(5):e0154710.
9. Agakidou E, Agakidis C, Gika H, Sarafidis K. Emerging biomarkers for prediction and early diagnosis of necrotizing enterocolitis in the era of metabolomics and proteomics. Frontiers in Pediatrics. 2020;8:602255.
10. McGoldrick E, Stewart F, Parker R, Dalziel SR. Antenatal corticosteroids for accelerating fetal lung maturation for womenat risk of preterm birth. Cochrane Database Syst Rev.2020;(3):CD004454.
11. Tao J, Mao J, Yang J, Su Y. Effects of oropharyngeal administration of colostrum on the incidence of necrotizing enterocolitis, late-onset sepsis, and death in preterm infants: a meta-analysis of RCTs. European Journal of Clinical Nutrition. 2020;74(8):1122–31.
12. Kim JH.Necrotizing enterocolitis:the road to zero.Semin Fetal Neonatal Med2014 ;19:39–44
13. Sharif S, Meader N, Oddie SJ, Rojas-Reyes MX, McGuire W. Probiotics to prevent necrotising enterocolitis in very preterm or very low birth weight infants. Cochrane Database Syst Rev. 2020 Oct 15;10(10):CD005496.
14. van den Akker CHP, van Goudoever JB, Shamir R, Domellöf M, Embleton ND, Hojsak I, et al. Probiotics and Preterm Infants: A Position Paper by the European Society for Paediatric Gastroenterology Hepatology and Nutrition Committee on Nutrition and the European Society for Paediatric Gastroenterology Hepatology and Nutrition Working Group for Probiotics and Prebiotics. J Pediatr Gastroenterol Nutr. 2020 May;70(5):664–80.
15. Pammi M, Gautham KS. Enteral lactoferrin supplementation for prevention of sepsis and necrotizing enterocolitis in preterm infants. Cochrane Database Syst Rev.202028;(6):CD007137.
16. Shah PS, Shah VS, Kelly LE. Arginine supplementation for prevention of necrotising enterocolitis in preterm infants. Cochrane Database Syst Rev. 2017 11;(4):CD004339.

17. Cotten CM, Taylor S, Stoll B, Goldberg RN, Hansen NI, Sánchez PJ, Ambalavanan N, Benjamin DK; NICHD Neonatal Research Network. Prolonged duration of initial empirical antibiotic treatment is associated with increased rates of necrotizing enterocolitis and death for extremely low birth weight infants. Pediatrics 2009; 123: 58–66.
18. Santos VS, Freire MS, Santana RNS, Martins-Filho PRS, Cuevas LE, Gurgel RQ (2019). Association between histamine-2 receptor antagonists and adverse outcomes in neonates: Asystematic review and meta-analysis. PLoS ONE 14(4): e0214135.
19. Rao SC, Basani L, Simmer K, Samnakay N, Deshpande G. Peritoneal drainageversus laparotomy as initial surgical treatment for perforated necrotizingenterocolitis or spontaneous intestinal perforation in preterm low birth weightinfants. Cochrane Database Syst Rev. 2011;(6):CD006182.

Section

7

Infections

CHAPTER

24

Neonatal Sepsis

Sepsis is one of the most common causes of neonatal mortality globally.[1] Most infection-related neonatal deaths occur in low and middle-income countries due to poor hygiene and suboptimal infection control practices. Sepsis-related mortality is largely preventable with the prevention of sepsis itself, timely recognition, rational antimicrobial therapy, and aggressive supportive care.

EPIDEMIOLOGY: INDIAN DATA

The Delhi Neonatal Infection Study (DeNIS) collaboration reported a 6.2% and 14.3% incidence of culture-positive sepsis and total (culture-positive or culture-negative) sepsis among all NICU admis-sions.[2] Nearly two-thirds of sepsis episodes occurred at or before 72 hours of life (early-onset sepsis). Two-thirds of the isolates were gram-negative, including, *Acinetobacter* spp. (22%), *Klebsiella* spp. (17%), and *Escherichia coli* (14%), with high rates of multi-drug resistance among these isolates. The common gram-positive pathogens were coagulase-negative *Staphylococcus* (15%), *Staphylococcus aureus* (12%), and *Enterococcus* spp. (6%). The profile of organisms responsible for early-onset and late-onset sepsis (i.e. after 72 hours) was not different. Nearly a quarter of neonatal deaths were attributable to sepsis.

Neonatal sepsis is a clinical syndrome of a dysregulated host response to bloodstream infection in the first 28 days of life. It encompasses various systemic infections such as septicemia, meningitis, pneumonia, arthritis, osteomyelitis, and urinary tract infections. Superficial infections (umbilical infections, conjunctivitis, and oral thrush) are not usually included under neonatal sepsis.

CLASSIFICATION

Neonatal sepsis can be classified into two major categories depending on the onset of symptoms.

Early-onset sepsis (EOS) presents at or before 72 hours of life. In severe cases, the neonate may be symptomatic at birth. Infants with EOS usually manifest with respiratory distress and pneumonia. The source of infection has been traditionally believed to be the maternal genital tract.

Based on the literature, the following risk factors seem to be associated with EOS:[3–5]

1. Spontaneous preterm labor in absence of PROM
2. Foul-smelling liquor
3. Prelabor rupture of membranes >24 hours (PROM)
4. Confirmed or suspected intrauterine inflammation, infection, or both (*Triple I*[6])
5. Single unclean vaginal examination during labor
6. Prolonged labor (sum of 1st and 2nd stage of labor >24 hours)
7. Severe perinatal asphyxia (Apgar score <4 at 1 minute).

Late-onset sepsis (LOS): It presents after 72 hours of life. LOS can be either healthcare-associated (HAI) or community-acquired infection. The neonates usually present with septicemia, pneumonia, or meningitis. Various factors predispose to an increased risk of HAI, includingprematurity, low birth weight, admission to the intensive care unit, mechanical ventilation, presence of invasive lines, administration of parenteral fluids, and use of stock solutions. Factors that might increase the risk of community-acquired LOS include poor hygiene, poor cord care, bottle feeding, and prelacteal feeds.

CLINICAL FEATURES

Nonspecific features: The earliest signs of sepsis are often subtle and nonspecific. Indeed, a high index of suspicion is needed for early diagnosis. Neonates with sepsis may present with one or more of the following symptoms or signs:

a. Hypothermia or fever (the former being more common in preterm neonates).
b. Lethargy, poor cry or refusal to suck.
c. Poor perfusion, prolonged capillary refill time.
d. Hypotonia, absent neonatal reflexes.
e. Bradycardia/tachycardia.
f. Respiratory distress, apnea and gasping respiration.
g. Hypo/hyperglycemia.
h. Metabolic acidosis.

Clinical features specific to various systems:

- **Central nervous system:** Bulging anterior fontanelle, vacant stare, high-pitched cry, excess irritability, stupor/coma, seizures, neck retraction/retrocollis.

  The presence of these features should raise clinical suspicion of meningitis.
- **Cardiovascular:** Hypotension, cyanosis, shock.
- **Gastrointestinal:** Increased gastric residuals, vomiting, diarrhea, abdominal distension, paralytic ileus.
- **Hepatic:** Direct hyperbilirubinemia (especially with urinary tract infections).
- **Renal:** Acute renal failure.
- **Hematological:** Bleeding, petechiae, purpura.
- **Skin changes:** Multiple pustules, abscess, sclerema, mottling, umbilical redness and discharge.

INVESTIGATIONS

Treatment should be initiated in a neonate suspected to have sepsis without any delay—only minimal and rapid investigations should be undertaken.

1. **Blood culture:** It is the gold standard for the diagnosis of sepsis and must be performed in all neonates with suspected sepsis. A positive blood culture with a known sensitivity pattern of the isolated organism is the best guide to antimicrobial therapy. Therefore, following the proper procedure for collecting the blood culture is essential. One ml of blood is adequate for a blood culture bottle containing 5–10 ml of culture broth. The samples from indwelling catheters should be avoided because of the risk of the growth of contaminants.

   Blood cultures should be observed for at least 72 hours before they are reported as sterile. It is now possible to detect bacterial growth within 12–24 hours using improved bacteriological techniques such as BACTEC and BACT/ALERT culture systems. These systems are based on using carbohydrate substrates in culture media and subsequent production of CO_2 by growing microorganisms, detected through their impact on pH by either a colorimetric or a fluorescent sensor placed at the bottom of the bottle.[7]
2. **Sepsis screen:**[8,9] Neonates suspected to have sepsis should undergo a sepsis screen to corroborate the diagnosis. However,

the decision to start antibiotics need not be conditional on the sepsis screen result if there is a strong clinical suspicion of sepsis and the neonate is too sick.

The various components of the sepsis screen include total leukocyte count (TLC), absolute neutrophil count (ANC), immature to total (I/T) neutrophil ratio, microerythrocyte sedimentation rate, and C reactive protein (CRP). The ANC varies considerably in the immediate neonatal period, and the standard reference ranges are available from Manroe's charts for term neonates.[10] The lower limit of ANC begins at $1800/cm^3$ at birth, rises to $7200/cm^3$ at 12 hours of age and then declines and persists at $1800/cm^3$ after 72 hours of age. The reference ranges for VLBW infants are available from Mouzinho's charts.[11]

The I/T ratio is ≤0.16 at birth and reaches a nadir of 0.12 after 72 hours of age. While using a kit-based semiquantitative assay of CRP, always check for the cutoff (usually set at 0.6 or 0.8 mg/L), which can give a higher false positivity rate. The sepsis screen used in our unit is described in Table 24.1.

The presence of two abnormal parameters in a screen is associated with a sensitivity of 93–100%, specificity of 83%, and positive and negative predictive values of 27% and 100%, respectively, in detecting sepsis, especially after the first week of life.[9] Presence of two (or more) abnormal parameters is considered a positive screen, and the neonate may be started on antibiot-ics. If the screen is negative but clinical suspicion persists, it may be repeated within 12 hours. If the screen is still negative, sepsis can be excluded with reasonable certainty.

3. **Procalcitonin (PCT):** PCT is an acute phase protein secreted by several tissues in response to various endogenous and exogenous stimuli such as cytokines and lipopolysaccharides.

Table 24.1: Components of sepsis screen

Component	*Abnormal value*
Absolute neutrophil count	Low counts as per Manroe's chart for the term and Mouzinho's chart for VLBW infants
Immature/total neutrophil ratio	>0.2
Micro-ESR	>15 mm in 1st hour
C reactive protein (CRP)	>1 mg/L

ESR: Erythrocyte sedimentation rate

In healthy neonates, plasma PCT values increase gradually after birth, reach peak values after 24 hours of age (mean 1.5–2.5 ng/ml, range 0.1–20 ng/ml) and then decrease to typical values below 0.5 ng/ml by 48–72 hours of age.[12] Age-specific cutoffs have been devised for preterm, late preterm, and term infants within the first 5 days.[13] A recent meta-analysis found only a moderate accuracy with a sensitivity of 85% and specificity of 54% at a cut-off of 2–2.5 ng/ml.[14] We do not use PCT to diagnose sepsis in our unit.

4. **Other biomarkers:** Other biomarkers, besides CRP and PCT, have been evaluated for early diagnosis of sepsis in neonates, including serum amyloid A, hepcidin, CD64, CD11b, IL-1, IL-6, IL-8, TNF-α, soluble TNF receptor, E-selectin, ICAM, etc.[15] Among these, serum amyloid A has shown some promising results; however, none of these biomarkers are currently in routine use.
5. **Molecular assays:** Molecular pathogen detection methods are based on the hybridization or amplification of pathogen DNA. Neonatal studies have been conducted using amplification methods (e.g. polymerase chain reaction; PCR) that can be completed in less than 12 hours and may have better sensitivity than microbial cultures. A recent Cochrane review in 2017 concluded that molecular assays may perform well as 'add-on' tests.[16] However, molecular assays do not provide information on antibiotic susceptibility. These are not recommended for routine practice, given insufficient evidence, high cost, and lack of widespread availability.
6. **Lumbar puncture (LP):** The incidence of meningitis in neonatal sepsis has varied from 0.3 to 3% in various studies.[2] The clinical features of sepsis and meningitis often overlap; it is possible to have meningitis without any specific symptomatology. This justifies the extra-precaution of performing LP in neonates suspected of sepsis.

   In EOS, lumbar puncture is performed in the presence of a positive blood culture in an asymptomatic neonate with a maternal risk factor or if the neonate is symptomatic with a clinical picture consistent with sepsis. It is not indicated if antibiotics have been started solely because of risk factors in asymptomatic neonates. In late-onset sepsis, LP should be done in all neonates before antibiotics because up to 1/3rd of VLBW neonates with meningitis can have negative blood cultures. Lumbar puncture may be postponed in critically sick neonates. It should be performed as soon as the clinical condition stabilizes. The cerebrospinal fluid characteristics are unique in the newborn period, and normal values are given in Table 24.2.[17,18]

The NNF CPG guidelines[19] summarize the performance of cellular and biochemical parameters in diagnosing neonatal meningitis. The guidelines recommend using CSF WBC count and protein but not CSF glucose for diagnosis.

7. **Radiology:** Chest X-ray should be considered in the presence of respiratory distress or apnea.

   An abdominal X-ray is indicated in the presence of abdominal signs such as abdominal distension. Neuroimaging should be performed in neonates suspected to have complications secondary to meningitis (intracranial abscesses, ventriculitis, hydrocephalus, etc.).

8. **Urine culture:** Urine cultures have a low yield and are not indicated routinely. However, neonates at risk for fungal sepsis, with urogenital malformation or vesicoureteral reflex, or suspected urinary tract infection (crying during micturition) should have a urine examination to exclude UTI. Urine cultures are obtained by suprapubic puncture, bladder catheterization, or clean catch samples from midstream urine.

   UTI is defined as the growth of a single uropathogenic organism with a colony count of ≥50,000 CFU/ml or between 10,000 and 50,000 CFU/ml with associated pyuria (WBC >5/HPF) detected on a midstream clean catch urine sample or any organism in urine which is obtained by suprapubic aspiration. However, the optimal definition for UTI based on a catheterized specimen in neonates has still not been established.

Table 24.2: Normal CSF parameters in term and preterm neonates

CSF Components	*Term neonates*	*Preterm* very low birth weight neonates
Cells/mm^3	8 (0–32)	5 (0–44)
PMN (%)	60%	8% (0–66)
CSF protein (mg/dl)	90 (20–170)	148 (54–370)
CSF glucose (mg/dl)	52 (34–119)	67 (33–217)

Values expressed as median (range)

MANAGEMENT

Supportive

Adequate and proper supportive care is crucial in sick neonates with sepsis. The neonates should be nursed in a thermoneutral environment to avoid hypo/hyperthermia. Oxygen saturation should be maintained at 91–95%; mechanical ventilation may have to be initiated if needed. If the infant is hemodynamically unstable, intravenous fluids should be administered, and the infant should be monitored for hypo/hyperglycemia. Volume expansion with crystalloids and judicious use of inotropes are essential to maintain normal tissue perfusion and blood pressure. Packed red cells and fresh frozen plasma may be required in anemia or bleeding diathesis.

Antibiotic Therapy

i. **Early-onset sepsis:** In high-income countries, various approaches have been described to identify neonates at risk of EOS based on perinatal risk factors to make a timely and rational decision for antibiotic therapy.[20,21] However, due to inherent pathogen related and other differences in developing countries compared to high-income countries, these approaches may not be generalizable to our settings.

   Currently, we consider antibiotics in a neonate with any one of the following:

   a. Presence of ≥3 risk factors for early onset sepsis (*see above*).
   b. Suspected or confirmed Triple I.
   c. Presence of ≥2 risk factor(s) *and* a positive sepsis screen.
   d. A strong clinical suspicion of sepsis.

ii. **Late-onset sepsis:** The indications for starting antibiotics in LOS include:

   a. A positive sepsis screen or
   b. A strong clinical suspicion of sepsis.

iii. **Prophylactic antibiotics:** *We do not use prophylactic antibiotics in any circumstance*, including neonates receiving IV fluids/ TPN or with meconium aspiration syndrome or after exchange transfusion.

iv. **Choice of antibiotics:** Empirical antibiotic therapy should be unit-specific and determined by the prevalent spectrum of etiological agents and their antibiotic sensitivity pattern. Antibiotics, once started, should be modified according to the sensitivity pattern. A simplified stepwise approach to facilitate the choice of an empiric antibiotic regimen is outlined in Table 24.3.

The empirical choice of antibiotics is dependent upon the probable source of infection. A combination of ampicillin or penicillin with gentamicin may be good first-line therapy for infections that are likely to be community-acquired where resistant strains are unlikely.[22] Cloxacillin should be considered if there is evidence of staphylococcal infection.

A combination of beta-lactam antibiotics with an aminoglycoside may be instituted for infections acquired during the hospital stay. However, except in cases of multi-drug resistance, monotherapy with beta-lactam is usually adequate for infections due to common organisms; the addition of an aminoglycoside is proven to be unnecessarily broad with no added survival advantage but an increased risk of toxic effects.[23] Third-generation cephalosporins were considered a good choice for managing nosocomial infections and meningitis. However, recent reports suggest that at least 60–70% of gram-negative organisms are now resistant to them.[24]

A combination of piperacillin-tazobactam with amikacin should be considered if *Pseudomonas* sepsis is suspected. Penicillin-resistant *Staphylococcus aureus* should be treated with cloxacillin, nafcillin, or methicillin. Methicillin-resistant *Staphylococcus aureus* (MRSA) should be treated with vancomycin or oxacillin with an aminoglycoside.

Table 24.3: A stepwise approach for framing empiric antibiotic therapy for a unit

1. Collate the frequency table of isolates and their antibiogram of the last 6–12 months.
2. First-line antibiotics: Combination of common antibiotics that together cover 60–70% of iso-lates.
3. Second-line antibiotics: Other antibiotic combinations cover 80–90% of isolates.

Note:

- The antibiotic regimen needs to be reviewed every 6–12 months.
- Cephalosporins are generally avoided as the first-line antibiotics since they are known to induce ESBL (extended-spectrum beta-lactamases)/cephalosporinases rapidly and are associated with high predilection for fungal colonization.
- Reserve drugs like colistin, meropenem, vancomycin, or linezolid should not be used empirically.

Ciprofloxacin has excellent activity against gram-negative and gram-positive organisms; however, it does not have good CSF penetration. It may be used to treat resistant gram-negative bacteremia after excluding meningitis. For *Enterococcus* sepsis, a combination of ampicillin and gentamicin is a good choice for initial therapy. *Enterococcus* is inherently resistant to cephalosporins. Vancomycin should be used to treat *Enterococcus* resistant to first-line antibiotics.

v. **Rationalization of antibiotic usage:** Once initiated, it is essential to regularly review the need for antibiotics to minimize the development of antibiotic resistance. A few salient principles of antibiotic stewardship are highlighted below:

1. Downgrade to a narrower spectrum or lower-cost antibiotic to which the organism is sensitive, irrespective of clinical response to antibiotics already being used.
2. A single sensitive antibiotic should suffice for almost all pathogens except *Pseudomonas*.
3. In the case of pan-resistant organisms with intermediate sensitivity to one or the other antibiotics, consider a higher dose of that antibiotic, preferably in combination.
4. Antibiotic usage can further be rationalized using risk scores or prediction modeling techniques to detect sepsis using maternal and neonatal characteristics. The web-based EOS calculator[25] has been shown to reduce antibiotic usage by 50% in high-income countries.[26] The generalisability of the calculator is, however, limited due to striking differences between high-income countries (where it is developed) and low-income countries. Further, it incorporates maternal group B *Streptococcus* colonization as a risk factor which is extremely rare in our population. Also, it only applies to neonates more than 35 weeks of gestation, limiting its usage in our NICUs.

vi. **Reserve antibiotics:** Newer antibiotics like aztreonam, meropenem, and imipenem are classified as 'reserve' antibiotics based on the AWaRe classification by WHO. Aztreonam has excellent activity against gram-negative organisms, while meropenem is effective against most bacterial pathogens except MRSA and *Enterococcus*. Imipenem is generally avoided in neo-nates because of a reported increase in seizures following its use. Empiric use of these

Table 24.4: Duration of antibiotic therapy in neonatal sepsis

Diagnosis	*Duration*
Meningitis (with or without positive blood/CSF culture)	21 days
Blood culture positive but no meningitis	14 days
Culture-negative sepsis (clinical course consistent with sepsis)	5–7 days

antibiotics should be avoided; they should be reserved only for situations where the sensitivity of the isolated organism warrants its use.

vii. **Duration of antibiotic therapy:** The antibiotic therapy duration depends upon clinical course, culture positivity and presence of absence of meningitis (Table 24.4).

Adjunctive Therapy

i. **Exchange transfusion (ET):** ET removes inflammatory cytokines and bacterial products, offering an immunological advantage. One study demonstrated a 50% reduction in sepsis-related mortality following double-volume exchange transfusion in septic neonates with sclerema.[27] In another study, ET conferred cardiovascular and hematological benefits without reducing mortality.[28] A recent narrative review discussed the pros and cons of ET and cautioned against using it as a last resort in cases of sclerema and multi-organ failure.[29]

ii. **Immunotherapy:** A recent network meta-analysis evaluated therapy with immunoglobulins (IgG, IgM enriched IgG, and colony-stimulating factors [G-CSF or GM-CSF]).[30] None of them were superior to placebo in reducing all-cause mortality. A Cochrane review of the use of immunoglobulin conclusively declared no benefit of the same for suspected or proven sepsis.[31]

iii. **Lactoferrin:** A Cochrane review evaluating the use of lactoferrin in preterm infants reported a significant decrease in the incidence of sepsis and necrotizing enterocolitis by 18%.[32]

Another updated meta-analysis revealed a limited but significant reduction in sepsis in very low birth weight neonates. However, the data were considered insufficient to guide clinical practice.[33] We do not use lactoferrin to prevent sepsis.

REFERENCES

1. Liu L, Oza S, Hogan D, Perin J, Rudan I, Lawn JE, et al. Global, regional, and national causes of child mortality in 2000-13, with projections to inform post-2015 priorities: an updated systematic analy-sis. Lancet Lond Engl. 2015 Jan 31;385(9966):430–40.
2. Investigators of the Delhi Neonatal Infection Study (DeNIS) collaboration. Characterisation and antimicrobial resistance of sepsis pathogens in neonates born in tertiary care centres in Delhi, India: A cohort study. Lancet Glob Health. 2016 Oct;4(10):e752–60.
3. Beck C, Gallagher K, Taylor LA, Goldstein JA, Mithal LB, Gernand AD. Chorioamnionitis and Risk for Maternal and Neonatal Sepsis: A Systematic Review and Meta-analysis. Obstet Gynecol. 2021 Jun 1;137(6):1007–22.
4. Takkar VP, Bhakoo ON, Narang A. Scoring system for the prediction of early neonatal infections. Indian Pediatr. 1974 Sep;11(9):597–600.
5. Baltimore RS. Neonatal nosocomial infections. Semin Perinatol. 1998 Feb;22(1):25–32.
6. Peng CC, Chang JH, Lin HY, Cheng PJ, Su BH. Intrauterine inflammation, infection, or both (Triple I): A new concept for chorioamnionitis. Pediatr Neonatol. 2018 Jun 1;59(3):231–7.
7. Kirn TJ, Weinstein MP. Update on blood cultures: how to obtain, process, report, and interpret. Clin Microbiol Infect Off Publ Eur Soc Clin Microbiol Infect Dis. 2013 Jun;19(6):513–20.
8. Philip AG. Detection of neonatal sepsis of late onset. JAMA. 1982 Jan 22;247(4):489–92.
9. Gerdes JS, Polin RA. Sepsis screen in neonates with evaluation of plasma fibronectin. Pediatr Infect Dis J. 1987 May;6(5):443–6.
10. Manroe BL, Weinberg AG, Rosenfeld CR, Browne R. The neonatal blood count in health and disease. I. Reference values for neutrophilic cells. J Pediatr. 1979 Jul;95(1):89–98.
11. Mouzinho A, Rosenfeld CR, Sánchez PJ, Risser R. Revised reference ranges for circulating neutrophils in very-low-birth-weight neonates. Pediatrics. 1994 Jul;94(1):76–82.
12. Pontrelli G, De Crescenzo F, Buzzetti R, Jenkner A, Balduzzi S, Calò Carducci F, et al. Accuracy of serum procalcitonin for the diagnosis of sepsis in neonates and children with systemic inflammatory syndrome: a meta-analysis. BMC Infect Dis. 2017 Apr 24;17:302.
13. Eschborn S, Weitkamp JH. Procalcitonin versus C-reactive protein: review of kinetics and performance for diagnosis of neonatal sepsis. J Perinatol Off J Calif Perinat Assoc. 2019 Jul;39(7):893–903.
14. Fukuzumi N, Osawa K, Sato I, Iwatani S, Ishino R, Hayashi N, et al. Age-specific percentile-based reference curve of serum procalcitonin concentrations in Japanese preterm infants. Sci Rep. 2016 Apr 1;6:23871.
15. Hedegaard SS, Wisborg K, Hvas AM. Diagnostic utility of biomarkers for neonatal sepsis—a systematic review. Infect Dis Lond Engl. 2015 Mar;47(3):117–24.

16. Pammi M, Flores A, Versalovic J, Leeflang MM. Molecular assays for the diagnosis of sepsis in neonates. Cochrane Database Syst Rev. 2017 Feb 25;2017(2):CD011926.
17. Sarff LD, Platt LH, McCracken GH. Cerebrospinal fluid evaluation in neonates: Comparison of high-risk infants with and without meningitis. J Pediatr. 1976 Mar;88(3):473–7.
18. Rodriguez AF, Kaplan SL, Mason EO. Cerebrospinal fluid values in the very low birth weight infant. J Pediatr. 1990 Jun;116(6):971–4.
19. nnf_guidelines-2011.pdf [Internet]. [cited 2022 Jul 11]. Available from: http://babathakranwala.in/iapneochap/uploads/acd-corner/nnf_guidelines-2011.pdf.
20. Puopolo KM, Benitz WE, Zaoutis TE, Committee on Fetus and Newborn, Committee on Infectious Diseases, Cummings J, et al. Management of Neonates Born at ≥35 0/7 Weeks' Gestation With Suspected or Proven Early-Onset Bacterial Sepsis. Pediatrics. 2018 Dec 1;142(6):e20182894.
21. Puopolo KM, Benitz WE, Zaoutis TE, Committee on Fetus and Newborn, Committee on Infectious Diseases, Cummings J, et al. Management of Neonates Born at ≤34 6/7 Weeks' Gestation With Suspected or Proven Early-Onset Bacterial Sepsis. Pediatrics. 2018 Dec 1;142(6):e20182896.
22. Fuchs A, Bielicki J, Mathur S, Sharland M, Van Den Anker JN. Reviewing the WHO guidelines for antibiotic use for sepsis in neonates and children. Paediatr Int Child Health. 2018 May 23;38(Suppl 1):S3–15.
23. Cantey JB, Lopez-Medina E, Nguyen S, Doern C, Garcia C. Empiric Antibiotics for Serious Bacterial Infection in Young Infants: Opportunities for Stewardship. Pediatr Emerg Care. 2015 Aug;31(8):568–71.
24. Deorari AK. Changing Pattern of Bacteriologic Profile in Neonatal Sepsis Among Intramural Babies. J Neonatol. 2006 Mar 1;20(1):8–15.
25. Puopolo KM, Draper D, Wi S, Newman TB, Zupancic J, Lieberman E, et al. Estimating the probability of neonatal early-onset infection on the basis of maternal risk factors. Pediatrics. 2011 Nov;128(5):e1155–63.
26. Kuzniewicz MW, Walsh EM, Li S, Fischer A, Escobar GJ. Development and Implementation of an Early-Onset Sepsis Calculator to Guide Antibiotic Management in Late Preterm and Term Neonates. Jt Comm J Qual Patient Saf. 2016 May;42(5):232–9.
27. Sadana S, Mathur NB, Thakur A. Exchange transfusion in septic neonates with sclerema: effect on immunoglobulin and complement levels. Indian Pediatr. 1997 Jan;34(1):20–5.
28. Somasekhara Aradhya A, Sundaram V, Kumar P, Ganapathy S, Jain A, Rawat A. Double Volume Exchange Transfusion in Severe Neonatal Sepsis. Indian J Pediatr. 2015 Jul 28;83.
29. Iijima S. Exchange Transfusion in Neonatal Sepsis: A Narrative Literature Review of Pros and Cons. J Clin Med. 2022 Jan;11(5):1240.
30. Li Y, Yang S, Wang G, Liu M, Zhang Z, Liu H, et al. Effects of immunotherapy on mortality in neonates with suspected or proven sepsis: a systematic review and network meta-analysis. BMC Pediatr. 2019 Aug 5;19(1):270.
31. Alsaleem M. Intravenous Immune Globulin Uses in the Fetus and Neonate: A Review. Antibodies Basel Switz. 2020 Nov 4;9(4):E60.

32. Pammi M, Suresh G. Enteral lactoferrin supplementation for prevention of sepsis and necrotizing enterocolitis in preterm infants. Cochrane Database Syst Rev. 2020 Mar 31;3:CD007137.
33. Gao Y, Hou L, Lu C, Wang Q, Pan B, Wang Q, et al. Enteral Lactoferrin Supplementation for Preventing Sepsis and Necrotizing Enterocolitis in Preterm Infants: A Meta-analysis with Trial Sequential Analysis of Randomized Controlled Trials. Front Pharmacol. 2020 Aug 7;11:1186.

CHAPTER

25

Perinatal HIV

An estimated 160,000 children under-five years of age were newly infected with HIV in 2020, with most of the transmission occurring during the perinatal period. Most children living with HIV acquire the infection through mother-to-child transmission (MTCT). HIV infection can be transmitted from an infected mother to her baby during pregnancy, delivery, or breastfeeding. Though HIV can be transmitted as early as the first trimester of pregnancy, transmission from mother to the fetus occurs most commonly in the perinatal period.

RISK FACTORS FOR PERINATAL HIV TRANSMISSION[1]

Viral factors: High viral load, nonsyncytium inducing phenotype, HIV-1 infection.

Maternal factors: Advanced disease (low CD4 count, symptoms of AIDS), primary infection during pregnancy, rupture of membranes more than 4 hours, maternal bleeding, mother not on antiretroviral therapy, vaginal delivery, other sexually transmitted diseases.

Fetoplacental factors: Chorioamnionitis, placenta previa, first of twins, prematurity.

Postnatal factors: Breastfeeding, higher breast milk virus load, mastitis or maternal nipple lesions, maternal seroconversion during breastfeeding, infant having thrush at less than 6 months of age (if on exclusive breastfeeding).

PREVENTION OF PERINATAL HIV

Breastfeeding

Breastfeeding is an important mode of transmission of HIV infection in developing countries. The risk of HIV infection via breastfeeding is highest in the initial months of breastfeeding. With effective ART in the antenatal period,persistent maternal viral suppression to <1000 RNA copies/ml at delivery and continuing ART therapy in the mother during breast feeding, the overall risk of mother-to-child transmission is low (0.25–2%).

The WHO 2016 guidelines recommend that mothers living with HIV should breastfeed for at least 12 months and may continue for up to 24 months or beyond while being fully supported for ART adherence. Exclusive replacement feeds may be started if the mother has died, has a terminal illness, or decides not to breastfeed despite adequate counselling. In such a case, commercial infant formula milk is given as a replacement feed when AFASS (Affordable, Feasible, Acceptable, Sustainable, and Safe) criteria are met. Replacement feeding should be provided by a *katori* spoon; bottle feeds should be avoided. Mixed feeding, breastmilk plus replacement feeds, is better than no breastfeeding at all and can be given if needed. After 6 months, WHO recommends that complementary feeds can be initiated along with direct breast feeds till 24 months of age.

MODE OF DELIVERY

The national guidelines for preventing MTCT (mother-to-child transmission) recommends that cesarean section (CS) in HIV-positive pregnant women be performed only for obstetric indications.[2] The WHO guidelines (2016) also do not recommend elective CS in resource-limited settings unless there is any obstetric or medical indication.

MTCT is increased by a prolonged duration of rupture of membranes, multiple vaginal examinations, episiotomy, instrumental delivery (vacuum or forceps), and invasive fetal monitoring procedures (scalp/fetal blood monitoring). Hence, the membranes should not be artificially ruptured unless there is fetal distress or delay in the progress of labor, repeated vaginal examinations should be minimized, any invasive procedure on the fetus are to be avoided, and instrumental delivery should be avoided unless there is fetal distress or significant maternal fatigue. Routine episiotomy is avoided as far as possible. In women on ART with HIV RNA $\leq$1000 copies/ml, the duration of ruptured membranes is not associated with an increased risk of perinatal transmission.

ARV REGIMENS

For Treating Pregnant Women[2]

The 2021 National AIDS Control Organization (NACO) guidelines recommend an optimized, fixed-dose combination ART regimen of Tenofovir 300 mg (TDF), lamivudine 300 mg (3TC), and dolutegravir 50 mg (DTG) to be given once daily for all pregnant and breastfeeding women with HIV infection. Lifelong ART is initiated as soon as possible, including the entire duration of breastfeeding. ART initiation should not be delayed while awaiting CD4 test results. Alternate regimens include TDF +3TC+Efavirenz (EFV); Zidovudine (AZT)+3TC+EFV; AZT+3TC+Nevirapine (NVP); or TDF+3TC+NVP. Pregnant women already on ART should continue to receive whatever regimen they are on if they respond adequately.

For Infants for Prevention of MTCT

- If the woman received ART adequately and regularly in the antenatal period with suppressed viral load <1000 RNA copies/ml from 32 weeks till delivery:
  - **Infant exclusively breastfeeding:** Daily nevirapine (NVP) prophylaxis at birth and continued for 6 weeks.
  - **Infant on exclusive replacement feeding:** Daily NVP prophylaxis or twice-daily AZT at birth and continued for 4–6 weeks.[3]
- Following infants are at a **higher risk** of acquiring infection:[2]
  - Mother is not on ART or received <4 weeks of ART at the time of delivery.
  - Mother has unknown or high viral load—defined as RNA more than 1000 copies/ml—from 32 weeks of pregnancy to delivery.
  - Mother newly identified during the current pregnancy or within 6 weeks of delivery.

  The high-risk infants should receive the following regimen:
  - **Two drugs:** AZT (given twice daily) and NVP (once daily) for the first 12 weeks in case of exclusive breastfeeding and for the first 6 weeks of life in case of exclusive replacement feeding. The mothers should be started on or continue to receive ART.[2] For those requiring ART beyond 6 weeks, NVP alone can also be used (in place of NVP+AZT) for the next 6 weeks (Table 25.1).

POSTNATAL DIAGNOSIS OF HIV INFECTION[2,4,5]

In children younger than 18 months, diagnosis of HIV infection is based on a positive virological test at 6 weeks for HIV or its components—usually by HIV-DNA PCR—by dry blood spot (DBS). In case of a positive DBS result, the diagnosis should be confirmed by a second test on a separate whole blood sample repeated at the earliest (Fig. 25.1).[6]

The revised WHO Guidelines (2021) recommend considering additional nucleic acid testing (NAT) at birth to identify *in utero*

Table 25.1: Drugs used for the prevention of mother-to-child transmission[10,13]

Infant age	*Birth weight*	*Nevirapine (NVP) dosing*	*Zidovudine (AZT) dosing*
Birth to 6 weeks	<2000 g	2 mg/kg/dose OD (0.2 ml/kg once daily)	5 mg per dose BD (0.5 ml of syrup twice daily)
	2000–2449 g	10 mg OD (1 ml of syrup once daily)	10 mg per dose BD (1 ml of syrup twice daily)
	≥2500 g	15 mg OD (1.5 ml of syrup once daily)	15 mg per dose BD (1.5 ml of syrup twice daily)
>6 weeks to 12 weeks	–	20 mg OD (2.0 ml of syrup once daily)	Dose not established for prophylaxis; Use a treatment dose of 60 mg BD (6 ml syrup twice daily)

NB: Preterm neonates less than 35 weeks of gestation should be dosed using expert guidance. Administer the first dose of NVP within 6–12 hours of delivery
(Composition: Nevirapine syrup 1 mL = 10 mg; zidovudine syrup 1 mL = 10 mg).

transmission of infection.[4] Infants with positive NAT at birth are likely to have been infected *in utero*. These infants will have a faster disease progression and will likely experience high mortality in the first few months of life if not treated. ART must be started in such infants immediately after obtaining a blood sample for the second test to confirm the infection. A third NAT should be done if the second test is negative before stopping ART.

Positive antibody testing is not recommended for confirmatory diagnosis of HIV infection in children until 18 months of age. Confirmation of HIV infection must be done at or after 18 months using three rapid tests.[2] If breastfeeding is continued beyond 18 months, antibody testing should be undertaken at least 3 months after cessation of breastfeeding to allow for the development of HIV antibodies.

Cotrimoxazole Prophylaxis

Cotrimoxazole prophylaxis is recommended for all HIV-exposed infants under 18 months of age. It must be started at 4–6 weeks of age and continued until HIV infection can be excluded.[7] In children <6 months, the dose is 2.5 ml once a day (trimethoprim 40 mg and sulphamethoxazole 200 mg/5 ml).

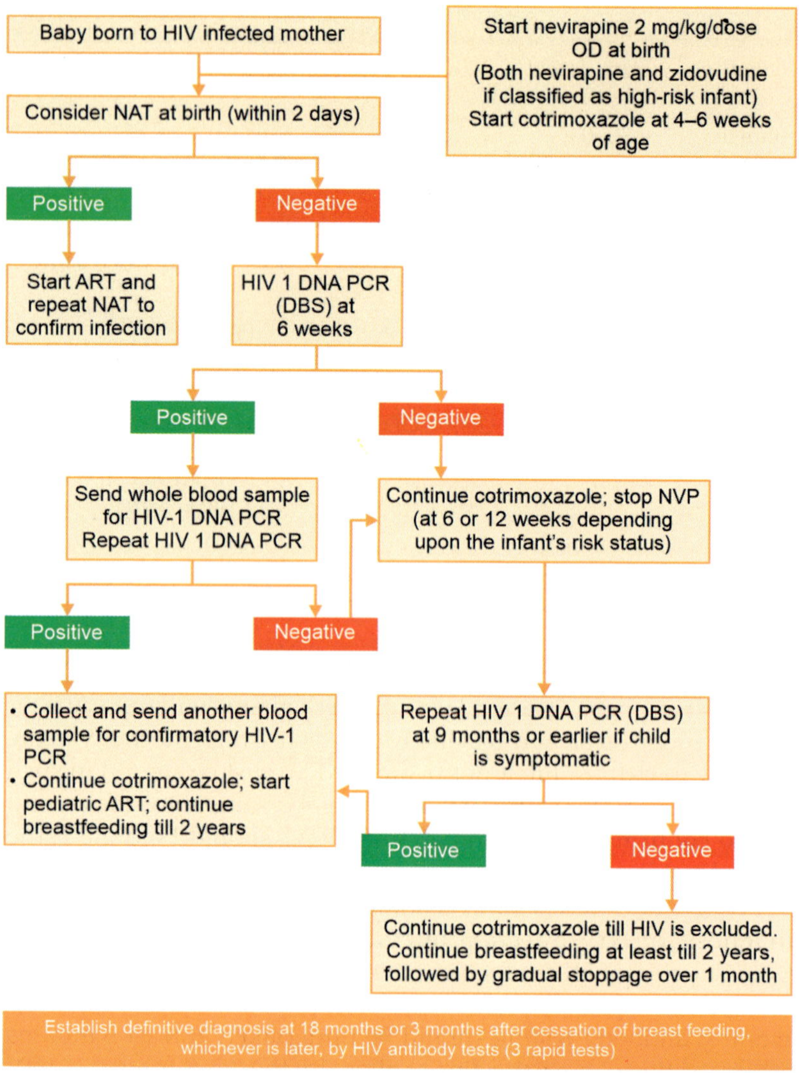

Fig. 25.1: Diagnostic algorithm for HIV-exposed infants less than 6 months (WHO 2021 and NACO 2021)

TREATMENT OF HIV-INFECTED NEONATE

If treatment is not initiated, more than 50% of infected neonates will die within two years. However, the US FDA has approved only five drugs for use in term newborns—zidovudine, lamivudine, emtricitabine, NVP, and raltegravir. Of these, only zidovudine has been studied adequately in preterm neonates.

Two NRTIs and one of the following classes of medications—an integrase strand transfer inhibitor, non-NRTI, or a protease inhibitor—are recommended immediately or within a few days of diagnosis. The WHO 2021 guidelines recommend zidovudine (ZDV) + lamivudine (3TC) + raltegravir (RAL) or NVP till two weeks of age, followed by ZDV + 3TC + ritonavir booster (LPV/r) after two weeks.[4]

Immunization

HIV-exposed or infected but asymptomatic children should receive all standard vaccines as per the national schedule.[8] HIV infected children with immune suppression or symptoms should receive all standard vaccines except BCG, OPV, and varicella. Measles-containing vaccines (MR or MMR) are allowed in infants with HIV (except in the terminal phase). Consider HiB and pneumococcal vaccines in all HIV-exposed children (irrespective of symptoms or CD4 count).

REFERENCES

1. Havens P, Waters D. Management of the infant born to a mother with HIV infection. Pediatr Clin North Am 2004;51:909–37.
2. National Guidelines for HIV Care and Treatment 2021 [online]. Available at: http://naco.gov.in/sites/default/files/National_Guidelines_for_HIV_Care_and_Treatment_2021.pdf [Accessed September 2023].
3. Coovadia HM, Brown ER, Fowler MG, Chipato T, Moodley D, Manji K, et al. Efficacy and safety of an extended nevirapine regime in infant children of breastfeeding mothers with HIV-l infection for prevention of postnatal HIV-l transmission (HPTN 046): a randomized, double blind, placebo-controlled trial. Lancet. 2012;379:221–8.
4. World Health Organization. (2021). Updated recommendations on HIV prevention, infant diagnosis, antiretroviral initiation and monitoring [online]. Available at: https://www.who.int/publications/i/item/9789240022232.
5. Chantry CJ, Cooper ER, Pelton SI, Zorilla C, Hillyer GV, Diaz C. Seroreversion in human immunodeficiency virus-exposed but uninfected infants. Pediatr Infect Dis J 1995;1–1:382–7.
6. Consolidated guidelines on the use of antiretroviral drugs for treating and preventing HIV infection – What's new. November 2015 Policy Brief [online]. Available at: http://apps.who.int/iris/bitstream/handle/10665/198064/9789241509893_eng.pdf;sequence=1 [Accessed September 2023].
7. Guidelines on co-trimoxazole prophylaxis for HIV-related infections among children, adolescents and adults. [online] Available at: http://www.who.int/hiv/pub/guidelines/ctx/en/ [Accessed 11 Apr. 2018].
8. Immunization in special circumstances. In: Shah RC, Shah NK, Kukreja (Eds). IAP Guidebook on Immunization, Mumbai: IAP Committee on Immunization 2005–2006;52–4.

CHAPTER

26 Management Algorithms of Infants Born to Mother with Various Infections

a. Neonates Born to Mothers with Tuberculosis (TB)

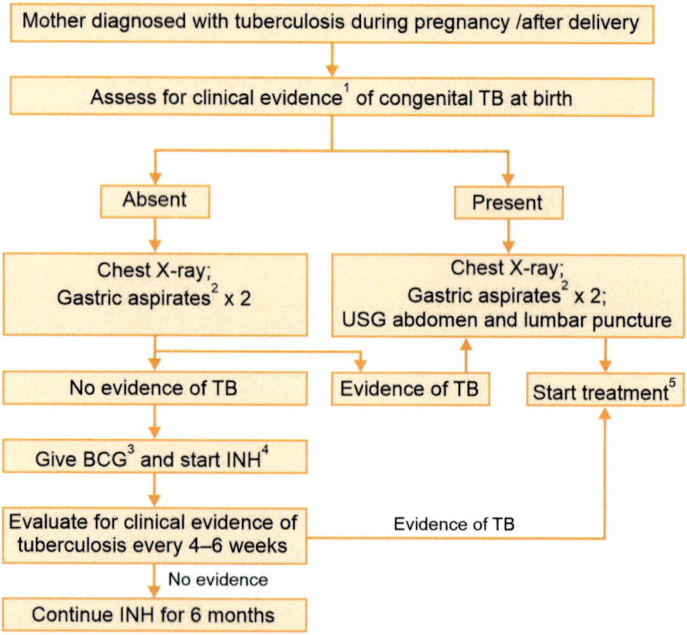

[1]Clinical features of congenital TB: respiratory distress, hepatosplenomegaly, lymphadenopathy, fever, poor feeding, and poor weight gain.

[2]Gastric aspirates are required only in the presence of respiratory findings or radiological evidence. They should be preferably sent for TB Gene Xpert; however, if the latter is not available, they may be sent for AFB staining.

[3]Give BCG at birth as INH does not interfere with BCG uptake.

[4]Dose of INH: 10 mg/kg/day. Adjust the dose at each postnatal visit according to weight. It is advisable to co-administer pyridoxine at 5–10 mg/day. No prophylaxis is recommended for drug-resistant TB due to toxicity and non-established efficacy of 2nd line drugs.

[5]Recommended treatment: 2 HRZE + 4 HR(E). Daily doses for isoniazid 7–15 mg/kg, rifampicin 10–20 mg/kg, ethambutol 15–25 mg/kg, pyrazinamide 30–40 mg/kg. If ethambutol is given in a dose of 20 mg/kg/day or lesser and for 2 months, the risk of optic neuritis is negligible.

Reassure the mother that it is safe to breastfeed her baby with proper cough hygiene (mask use, cough etiquette). Separation of mother and neonate is necessary only if mother is sick/non-adherent to treatment/sputum positive/has drug-resistant TB.

b. Neonates Born to Mothers with Hepatitis B Virus (HBV) Infection

Neonate born to mother with HBV infection
(*Prenatal testing of all pregnant women for HBsAg is recommended*)

↓

At birth: Give hepatitis B vaccine along with HBIG (100 IU/0.5 ml intramuscular) in different thighs (*preferably within* 12 *hours but not later than* 48–72 *hours of birth*)

↓

Follow up: Complete HBV immunization as per schedule
(*Four-dose schedule under the Universal Immunization Program*)

↓

Follow-up testing: Perform anti-HBs antibodies and HBsAg testing at **9–12 months** of age for

↓

- Anti-HBs titre ≥10 mIU/ml and HBsAg negative: immune; no further action required
- Anti-HBs <10 mIU/ml and HBsAg negative: No HBV infection but failed to respond to immunization; repeat vaccination (3 doses) and test anti-HBs after 1–2 months of last dose
- Anti-HBs negative and HBsAg positive: HBV infection; follow up with pediatric gastroenterologist

---

- Risk of vertical transmission:
  - When mother is HBsAg +ve but HBeAg –ve: 5–20%
  - When mother is HBsAg +ve and HBeAg +ve: 70–90%
- 90% of infected neonates become chronic carriers.
- HBV infection is not a contraindication to breastfeeding.
- Hepatitis B vaccine gives 70–90% of active immunity; Hepatitis B immune globulin gives additional 10–30% immunity. Higher dose (200 IU) of HBIG offers no advantage over standard dose (100 IU) in terms of efficacy. If HBIG is unaffordable or unavailable, administer only the vaccine.
- For mothers with unknown HBsAg status at birth (antenatal testing not done):
  - Perform urgent maternal testing for HBsAg.
  - Give hepatitis B vaccine to the neonate within 12 hours of birth.
  - If mother is positive for HBsAg or the maternal results are delayed: give HBIG within 12 hours to neonates with birth weight <2 kg and within 7 days of life to neonates with birth weight ≥2 kg.

c. Neonate Born to Mother with Hepatitis C Virus (HCV) Infection[1]

Pregnant woman with HCV infection: Prenatal and intrapartum care appropriate for obstetric risk factors
(No currently known intervention to reduce MTCT[2])

↓

Neonate born to mother with HCV infection
(Mode of delivery has no effect on perinatal infection risk[3])

↓

Exclusive breastfeeding
(Breastfeeding is not contraindicated, except when the mother has cracked, damaged, or bleeding nipples, when she can express and discard breastmilk and resume breastfeeding once nipples have healed)

↓

Follow up testing:[4] Should be done **at or after 18 months** of age for anti-HCV antibodies

↓

- Negative: HCV infection ruled out; no action required
- Positive: HCV infection; HCV-RNA assay after age 3 year to confirm chronic HCV infection[5]
  - ↓ Consultation with a pediatric gastroenterologist, treatment with direct-acting antiviral (DAA) regimens if approved for child's age irrespective of disease severity

[1]Based on recommendations from the Infectious Diseases Society of America, the American Association for the Study of Liver Diseases, and the International Antiviral Society–USA (www.hcvguidelines.org)

[2]Risk of mother-to-child transmission (MTCT):

- Mother HCV RNA +ve: 5–6%
- Mother co-infected with (untreated) HIV infection: 10–20%

[3]However, invasive fetal monitoring, vaginal lacerations, and prolonged rupture of membranes (>6 hours) increase the risk of transmission.

[4]Testing with an HCV-RNA assay can be considered in the first year of life, but the optimal timing of such a test is unknown.

[5]About 25–50% of infected infants recover spontaneously (loss of previously detectable HCV RNA) by 3 years of age.

d. Neonates Born to Mothers with Syphilis*

Routine serological testing for syphilis (STS) must be undertaken in all women at the first prenatal visit.
In high-risk cases, it should be repeated at 28 weeks and delivery.
(Routine STS in neonates for screening purposes is not helpful because of high false-negative rates)

Mother with syphilis (reactive VDRL/RPR and confirmed by reactive TPHA/FTA-ABS)

↓

Evaluate the neonate:
- Assess adequacy of maternal treatment.
- Pathologic examination of the placenta or umbilical cord.
- Dark field microscopy of suspicious lesions or body fluids.
- Clinical examination of infant for evidence of syphilis (non-immune hydrops, anemia, jaundice, hepatosplenomegaly, rhinitis, skin rash, pseudo paralysis).
- Quantitative VDRL/RPR in serum (NOT cord blood). No need for TPHA/FTA-ABS.

↓

S. No.	*Scenario*	*Additional evaluation*	*Treatment*
1.	**Proven/highly probable disease** **Presence of any one of the three:** 1. Physical abnormalities suggestive of congenital syphilis 2. VDRL/RPR: 4X higher titer than the mother's titer 3. Positive darkfield test of body fluid(s)	1. CSF (VDRL, cell, protein) 2. CBC with differential and platelet count 3. Long-bone radiographs 4. Other tests as clinically indicated (chest X-ray, LFTs, neuroimaging, ophthalmologic examination, and BERA)	Aqueous crystalline penicillin G (1–1.5 lakh units/kg/day) IV for 10 days (50,000 units/kg/dose q 12 h during first 7 days of life and q 8 h thereafter; **preferred**) **OR** Procaine penicillin G 50,000 units/kg/dose IM in a single daily dose for 10 days
2.	**Possible congenital syphilis:** **Presence of all three:** 1. Normal physical examination 2. VDRL/RPR ≤4X of maternal titer 3. Mother: Not treated / inadequately treated/ treated with non-penicillin regimen/treated <4 wk before delivery.	As above (scenario 1)	As above (scenario 1) if complete evaluation not done or follow up uncertain. **OR** Benzathine penicillin G 50,000 units/kg/ dose IM in a single dose **only** if complete evaluation normal and follow up certain.

(Contd.)

(*Contd.*)

S. No.	*Scenario*	*Additional evaluation*	*Treatment*
3.	**Congenital syphilis less likely** **Presence of all three:** 1. Normal physical examination. 2. VDRL/RPR ≤4X of maternal titer. 3. Mother: adequately treated during pregnancy and ≥4 weeks before delivery and does not have any reinfection or relapse.	No evaluation required	Benzathine penicillin G 50,000 units/kg as a single IM injection (**preferred**) **OR** Strict follow-up with no treatment for neonate whose mother's VDRL/RPR titers decreased 4X after appropriate therapy for early syphilis or remained stable at low titer.
4.	**Congenital syphilis unlikely** **Presence of all three:** 1. Normal physical examination 2. VDRL/RPR titer ≤4X of maternal titer 3. Mother: adequately treated before pregnancy and her VDRL/RPR titer remained low and stable before and during pregnancy and at delivery.	No evaluation required	No treatment required **OR** Benzathine penicillin G 50,000 units/kg as a single IM injection if follow-up uncertain and VDRL/RPR in the neonate is reactive.

**Based on CDC 2021 guidelines (https://www.cdc.gov/std/treatment-guidelines/congenital-syphilis.htm)*

e. Neonates Born to Mothers with Toxoplasmosis*

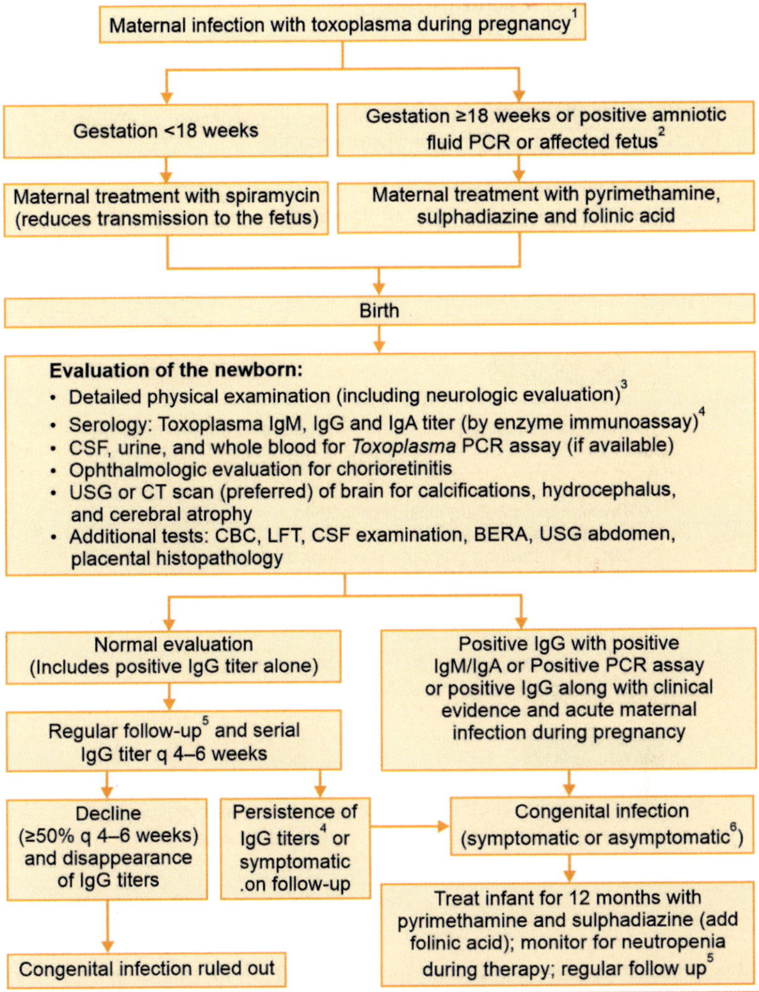

*For details, see Maldonado YA, Read JS, AAP Committee on Infectious Diseases. Diagnosis, treatment, and prevention of congenital toxoplasmosis in the United States. Pediatrics. 2017;139(2):e20163860.

[1]For details on management of maternal infection during pregnancy: Montoya JG, Remington JS. Management of *Toxoplasma gondii* infection in pregnancy. Clin Infect Dis 2008;47:554–66.

[2]Fetal abnormalities in USG include hydrocephalus, brain, splenic and hepatic calcifications, hepatosplenomegaly, and ascites.

[3]Majority of the infants are asymptomatic at birth. Clinical evidence include: hepatosplenomegaly, hydrocephalus, pneumonia, thrombocytopenia, lymphadenopathy, chorioretinitis, intracranial calcifications, myocarditis.

[4]Positive serum IgM (after 5 days of life) and/or IgA (after 10 days of life) in the neonate, along with a positive IgG, is considered diagnostic of congenital toxoplasmosis. Persistence of positive *Toxoplasma* IgG antibodies beyond 12 months of age is considered the gold standard for diagnosis of congenital toxoplasmosis.

[5]Includes neurologic and ophthalmologic examinations at three-monthly interval for first 2 years, six-monthly intervals in the 3rd year and annually thereafter until adolescence.

[6]High incidence of long-term sequelae (e.g. chorioretinitis) in untreated infants even if asymptomatic at birth.

f. Approach to neonates with suspected congenital cytomegalovirus (CMV) infection

Consider congenital CMV infection in neonates with one or more of the following:
- Symptomatic disease: a constellation of signs like IUGR, jaundice, purpura, hepatosplenomegaly, microcephaly and retinitis
- Abnormal imaging consistent with CMV infection: periventricular calcifications, PVL, ventriculomegaly, vasculitis and polymicrogyria
- Abnormal fetal ultrasound: echogenic bowel, IUGR, microcephaly or abnormal fetal brain imaging, hepatic calcifications, fetal hydrops or ascites
- Born to mother with CMV infection during pregnancy[1]

↓

Perform urine/saliva PCR within first 3 weeks

- **Positive** → Congenital infection
- **Negative** → Congenital infection ruled out

Congenital infection ↓

Perform:
- Physical examination including detailed neurological evaluation
- CBC, LFT, hearing and ophthalmological evaluation
- USG cranium, CT/MRI (if neurological symptoms/signs or microcephaly)

↓

Neonate with no or mild symptoms or isolated sensorineural hearing loss[2]

- **Yes** → Follow up till 2 years[3]
- **No** → Moderate-to-severe symptomatic congenital infection[4] → Treat with oral valganciclovir (preferred) or IV ganciclovir for 6 months[5]

[1]Suspected or confirmed maternal infection includes seroconversion during pregnancy, positive CMV IgG and IgM, or mononucleosis-like illness during pregnancy.

[2]Rawlinson WD, Boppana SB, Fowler KB, et al. Congenital cytomegalovirus infection in pregnancy and the neonate: consensus recommendations for prevention, diagnosis, and therapy. Lancet Infect Dis. 2017 Jun;17(6):e177-e188.

[3]Most infected infants (90%) are asymptomatic at birth. However, 15% of them will develop long term sequelae (e.g. SNHL) within first 2 years of life mandating regular follow-up with hearing evaluation.

[4]Defined as multiple findings attributable to CMV infection (petechiae, thrombocytopenia, hepatomegaly, splenomegaly, hepatitis, IUGR, etc.); or central nervous system involvement (microcephaly, radiological findings, abnormal CSF, chorioretinitis, sensorineural hearing loss, or the detection of cytomegalovirus DNA in CSF, etc.).

[5]Treatment is indicated for moderate to severe symptomatic congenital infection diagnosed within 1 month of life (efficacy of initiating treatment in infants >1 month is not known). Dose of valganciclovir is 16 mg/kg/dose q 12 hourly orally and that of ganciclovir is 6 mg/kg/dose IV q 12 hourly (in case of unreliable GI absorption). Absolute neutrophil count and aminotransferases need to be monitored during treatment for neutropenia and transaminitis.

g. Neonates Born to Mothers with Varicella Infection

Birth

Onset of maternal rash with respect to birth of baby (days)															
Day of life	←	−7	−6	−5	−4	−3	−2	−1	1	2	3	4	5	6	→
Likelihood of neonatal infection	Neonate has protective antibodies **AND** the likelihood of severe disease is low			Neonate does not have protective antibodies **AND** the likelihood of severe neonatal disease is high							Neonate does not have protective antibodies **BUT** the likelihood of severe neonatal disease is low				
Isolation[1]	Do not separate the neonate from the mother; continue breastfeeding. Isolate dyad from other mothers and neonates.			Separate the mother and the neonate until maternal lesions have dried up and crusted.[2] If the neonate develops rash, he stays with the mother. Mother/baby with active vesicles to be isolated from others.							Separate the mother and the neonate until maternal lesions have dried up and crusted.[2] If the neonate develops rash, he stays with the mother. Mother/baby with active vesicles to be isolated from others.				
Treatment	No VZIG IV Acyclovir,[4] if the neonate develops severe disseminated varicella.			VZIG or IVIG within 72 hours of exposure[3] (Not required if the mother has zoster) IV Acyclovir,[4] if the neonate develops varicella of any severity.							No VZIG IV acyclovir,[4] if the neonate develops severe disseminated Varicella.				

[1]Incubation period of varicella is 10–21 days, and up to 28 days for those who have received VZIG or IVIG. Therefore, the period of isolation for a person exposed but without rash continues from day 8 of exposure (period of infectivity) till day 21 (or day 28 if received VZIG or IVIG), and for a person with rash continues until all lesions have dried up and crusted. Isolation is not required if the mother has zoster.

[2]Give expressed breast milk even if mother–baby dyad is separated unless there are lesions on the breast. Breastfeeding is allowed once mother becomes noninfectious.

[3]Dose of VZIG: 62.5 IU IM for infants ≤2 kg and 125 IU IM for infants weighing >2 kg. If VZIG unavailable, IVIG can be given at a dose of 400 mg/kg. VZIG or IVIG can be administered within 10 days of exposure.

[4]Dose of Acyclovir: 30 mg/kg per day in 3 divided doses for 10 days. Severe disease includes pneumonia, encephalitis, thrombocytopenia, and severe hepatitis.

Exposure of a hospitalized neonate to health care provider with varicella

- All exposed susceptible patients should be discharged as soon as possible.
- All exposed susceptible patients who cannot be discharged should be placed in isolation from day 8–21 (or day 28 if they received VZIG or IVIG).
- Ascertain gestation of infant and take the maternal history of varicella:
  - Infant <28 weeks: Give VZIG or IVIG regardless of the maternal history of varicella.
  - Infant 28–36 weeks and no maternal history of varicella: Give VZIG or IVIG.
  - For healthy term infants (37 weeks or more): No need for VZIG (regardless of the maternal history).

h. Neonates Born to Mothers with Active Herpes Genital Lesions

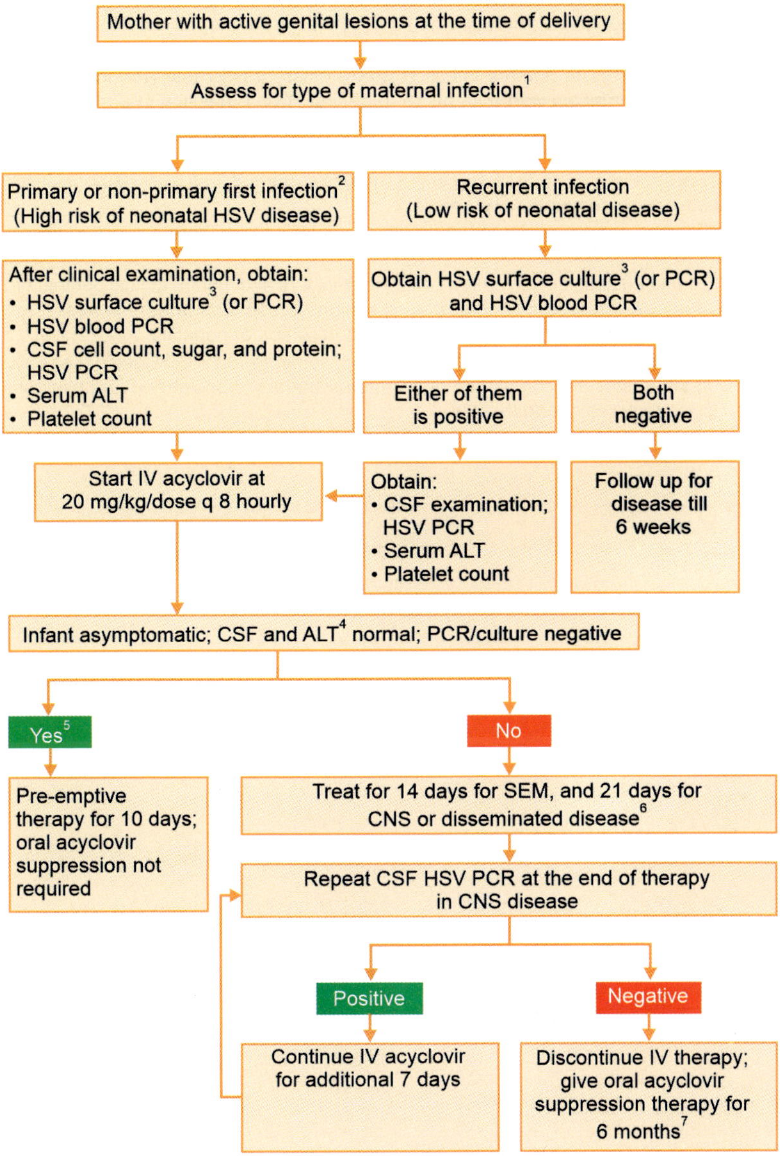

[1]For details on diagnosis of maternal infection: Kimberlin DW, Baley J; Committee on Infectious Diseases, Committee on Fetus and Newborn. Guidance on management of asymptomatic neonates born to women with active genital herpes lesions. Pediatrics 2013;131(2):383-6

[2]Non-primary refers to primary infection with a different HSV serotype in a person who is already infected with a serotype (e.g., first HSV-1 infection in a mother with HSV-2 infection).

[3]Take samples from all the sites: conjunctivae, mouth, nasopharynx, and rectum.

[4]Serum ALT values more than two times the upper normal limit may be considered suggestive of disseminated HSV disease.

[5]Breastfeeding can be continued in stable neonates unless there are active breast lesions.

[6]SEM disease- disease involvement limited to skin, eye and mouth; topical ophthalmic drugs may be required in ocular disease; signs of disseminated disease- CNS abnormalities, fever, rash, shock, DIC, pneumonitis and/or hepatitis.

[7]Acyclovir suppression given at 300 mg/m^2/dose, administered in 3 divided doses daily for 6 months after the completion of parenteral therapy; absolute neutrophil count monitoring required during therapy.

Index

W

Z

Volume 2

AIIMS Protocols in Neonatology

Core Protocols

Third Edition

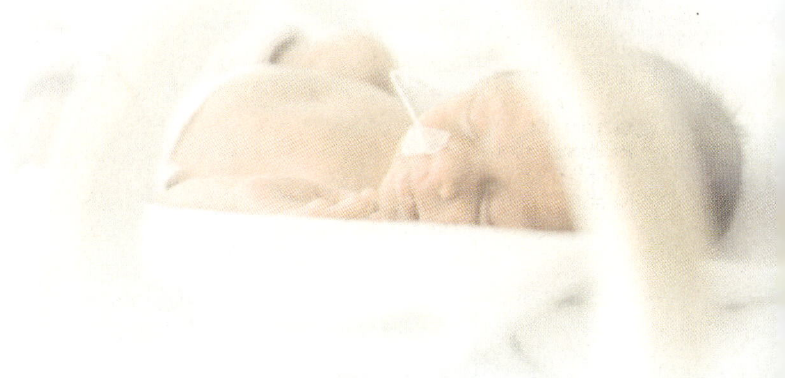

The volumes in the set

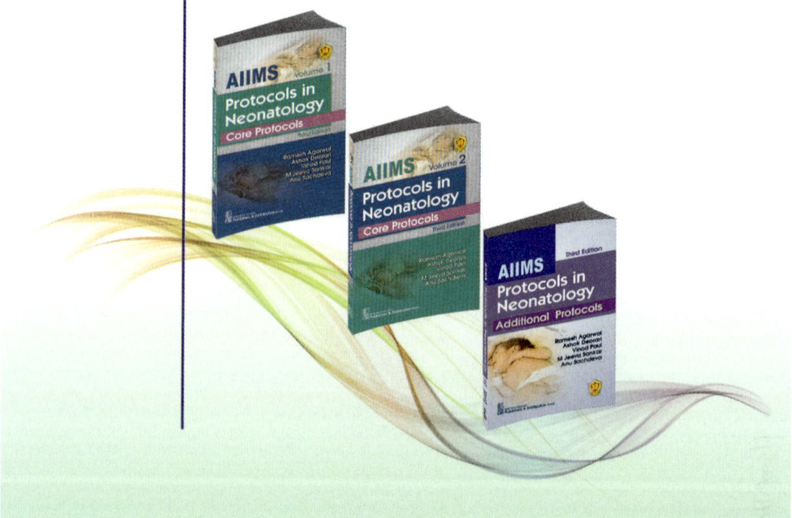

Volume 2

AIIMS Protocols in Neonatology

Core Protocols

Third Edition

Ramesh Agarwal
MD DM (Neonatology)
Professor*

Ashok Deorari
MD FAMS
Principal and Dean, Himalayan Institute of Medical Sciences
Swami Rama Himalayan University, Dehradun
Former Professor and Head*

Vinod K Paul
MD PhD DNB FAMS FIAP FNNF
Member, NITI Aayog, Government of India
Former Professor and Head*

M Jeeva Sankar
MD DM
Additional Professor*

Anu Sachdeva
MD DM
Additional Professor*

***Department of Pediatrics**
WHO Collaborating Centre for Education and Research in Newborn Care
All India Institute of Medical Sciences, New Delhi, India
www.newbornwhocc.org

[PDFs of the protocols are available online: www.newbornwhocc.org]

CBSPD

CBS Publishers & Distributors Pvt Ltd

New Delhi • Bengaluru • Chennai • Kochi • Kolkata • Lucknow • Mumbai
Gujarat • Hyderabad • Jharkhand • Nagpur • Patna • Pune • Uttarakhand

Disclaimer

Science and technology are constantly changing fields. New research and experience broaden the scope of information and knowledge. The authors have tried their best in giving information available to them while preparing the material for this book. Although all efforts have been made to ensure optimum accuracy of the material, yet it is quite possible some errors might have been left uncorrected. The publisher, the printer and the authors will not be held responsible for any inadvertent errors, omissions or inaccuracies.

The protocols are context-specific, and readers are advised to modify and adapt the protocols for their settings.

AIIMS Volume 2

Protocols in Neonatology

Core Protocols

Third Edition

ISBN: 978-93-5466-921-7

Third Edition: 2024

Reprint: 2025, 2026, **2027**

First Edition 2015

Second Edition 2019

Published by Satish Kumar Jain and produced by Varun Jain for

CBS Publishers & Distributors Pvt Ltd

4819/XI Prahlad Street, 24 Ansari Road, Daryaganj, New Delhi 110 002, India
Ph: 011-23289259, 23266838 Website: www.cbspd.com e-mail: delhi@cbspd.com

Corporate Office: 204 FIE, Industrial Area, Patparganj, Delhi 110 092, India
Ph: 011-4934 4934 Fax: 011-4934 4935 e-mail: publishing@cbspd.com; publicity@cbspd.com

Branches

- **Bengaluru:** Seema House 2975, 17th Cross, KR Road, Banasankari 2nd Stage, Bengaluru 560 070, Karnataka, India
  Ph: +91-80-26771678/79 Fax: +91-80-26771680 e-mail: bangalore@cbspd.com
- **Chennai:** 18/8B, Subbaraya Street, Shenoy Nagar, Chennai 600 030, Tamil Nadu, India
  Ph: +91-44-42032115, 45022115 e-mail: chennai@cbspd.com
- **Kochi:** 42/1325, 1326, Power House Road, Opposite KSEB, Ernakulum Kochi 682 018, Kerala, India
  Ph: +91-484-4059061-65 Fax: +91-484-4059065 e-mail: kochi@cbspd.com
- **Kolkata:** 147, Hind Ceramics Compound, 1st Floor, Nilgunj Road, Belghoria, Kolkata 700 056, West Bengal, India
  Ph: +91-33-25633055/56 e-mail: kolkata@cbspd.com
- **Lucknow:** Basement, Khushnuma Complex, 7 Meerabai Marg (behind Jawahar Bhawan), Lucknow 226 001, UP, India
  Ph: +91-522-4000032 e-mail: tiwari.lucknow@cbspd.com
- **Mumbai:** PWD Shed, Gala no 25/26, Ramchandra Bhatt Marg, Next to JJ Hospital Gate no. 2, Opp. Union Bank of India, Noorbaug, Mumbai 400 009, Maharashtra, India
  Ph: +91-22-66661880/89 e-mail: mumbai@cbspd.com

Representatives

- **Gujarat** • **Hyderabad** • **Jharkhand** • **Nagpur** • **Patna** • **Pune** • **Uttarakhand**

For trade terms please contact customercare@cbspd.com
For general enquiries please contact info@cbspd.com

Printed at: HT Media Ltd, Greater Noida, UP, India

to
Newborn Infants

Contributors

Aathira Ravindranath DM
Consultant Pediatric
Gastroenterologist
Apollo BGS Hospital, Mysuru
aathira.r@gmail.com

Abin Sheref Mohammed MBBS
Junior Resident
Department of Pediatrics
All India Institute of Medical Sciences
New Delhi
Abinsheref.1997@gmail.com

Aditi Sinha PhD
Additional Professor
Department of Pediatrics
All India Institute of Medical Sciences
New Delhi
aditisinhaaiims@gmail.com

Akash Sharma
Consultant Neonatologist and
Pediatrician
In-charge NICU, Surya Hospitals
Jaipur, drakash.jpr@gmail.com

Akash Singhal MD
Senior Resident
Department of Neonatology
All India Institute of Medical Sciences
New Delhi

Alec Reginald Errol Correa DM
Medical Geneticist
Lifecell International
Pune
aleccorrea88@hotmail.com

Alisha Gupta MCh
Ex-Senior Resident
Department of Pediatric Surgery
All India Institute of Medical Sciences
New Delhi
doc.alishagupta@gmail.com

Amanpreet Sethi DM
Assistant Professor
Department of Pediatrics
Guru Gobind Singh Medical College
Faridkot, Punjab
sethi.amanpreet702@gmail.com

Amit Upadhyay DM
Consultant Neonatologist
Nutema Hospital, Meerut
au.llrm@gmail.com

Anapti Anil MD
Senior Resident
Department of Obstetrics and
Gynaecology
All India Institute of Medical Sciences
New Delhi, anapti.garg9@gmail.com

Anjan Kumar Dhua MCh
Additional Professor
Department of Pediatric Surgery
All India Institute of Medical Sciences
anjandhua@hotmail.com

Ankit Meena DM
Senior Resident
Department of Pediatrics
All India Institute of Medical Sciences
New Delhi
ankit.aiims.meena@gmail.com

Ankita MBBS
Junior Resident
Department of Pediatrics
All India Institute of Medical Sciences
New Delhi
ankiagar23@gmail.com

Ankit Verma MD
Assistant Professor
Department of Pediatrics
All India Institute of Medical Sciences
New Delhi
ankitverma0486@gmail.com

Ankitha Ravishankar MBBS
Junior Resident
Department of Pediatrics
All India Institute of Medical Sciences
New Delhi
ankitha.ravishankar@gmail.com

Anubhuti Rana MD
Assistant Professor
Department of Obstetrics and Gynaecology
All India Institute of Medical Sciences
New Delhi, anubhuti_rana@yahoo.com

Aparna Chandrasekaran DM
Chief Neonatologist
Krishna Institute of Medical Sciences (KIMS), Cuddles
Kondapur, Hyderabad
appubanu@gmail.com

Aparna K Sharma MD
Professor
Department of Obstetrics and Gynaecology
All India Institute of Medical Sciences
New Delhi
kaparnasharma@gmail.com

Arunambika Chinnappan MD
Senior Resident
Department of Neonatology
All India Institute of Medical Sciences
Bhubaneswar
arunambika.chinnappan@gmail.com

Arun Sasi DM
Consultant Neonatologist
Royal Children's Hospital, Melbourne
Mercy Hospital for Women, Melbourne
Adjunct Clinical Lecturer
Department of Obstetrics and Gynecology
University of Melbourne
Melbourne, Australia

Arvind Bagga MD
Director and Sr Consultant
Department of Pediatric Nephrology
Indraprastha Apollo Hospitals
New Delhi, arvindbagga@hotmail.com

Ashish Jain DM
Associate Professor and Head
Department of Neonatology
Maulana Azad Medical College
New Delhi
neoashish2008@gmail.com

Ashutosh Kapoor DM
Consultant Neonatologist and Pediatrician
In-charge NICU
Chandan Hospital, Lucknow
ashukap22@gmail.com

Biswaroop Chakrabarty DM
Additional Professor
Department of Pediatrics
All India Institute of Medical Sciences
New Delhi
biswaroopchakrabarty@gmail.com

Chandrakumar Natarajan DM
Senior Consultant and Head
Department of Neonatology
KKCTH Hospital
Nungambakkam, Chennai
drchandrakumar@gmail.com

Deena Thomas DM
Consultant Neonatologist
Muthoot Hospital
Kozhencherry, Kerala
deenathomas87@gmail.com

Deepak Chawla DM
Professor
Government Medical College and Hospital, Chandigarh
drdeepakchawla@gmail.com

Deepika Kainth DM
Assistant Professor
All India Institute of Medical Sciences
New Delhi
aiims.deepika@gmail.com

Delona Treesa Joseph MBBS
Senior Resident
Department of Pediatric Surgery
All India Institute of Medical Sciences
New Delhi
delonatreeza@gmail.com

Deula Candida D'Cruz MD
Senior Resident
Department of Pediatrics
All India Institute of Medical Sciences
New Delhi
deulacandidadcruz@gmail.com

Devi S Saranya MD
Senior Resident
Division of Genetics
Department of Pediatrics
All India Institute of Medical Sciences
New Delhi
devisaranyas92@gmail.com

Dhinakaran Raman DM
Consultant Neonatologist
Prashanth Hospital
Velachery, Chennai
dhina.mmc@gmail.com

Dilip Kumar MBBS
Junior Resident
Department of Pediatrics
All India Institute of Medical Sciences
New Delhi

Girish Gururaj DM
Apollo Hospital, Mysuru

Gitanjali Jain MD
Senior Resident
Department of Neonatology
All India Institute of Medical Sciences
New Delhi
gitanjali_jain@yahoo.co.in

Haleemath Afrah MBBS
Junior Resident
Department of Pediatrics
All India Institute of Medical Sciences
New Delhi
helloafrah@gmail.com

Harshita Nori MD
Senior Resident
Department of Neonatology
All India Institute of Medical Sciences
New Delhi
harshita.nori@gmail.com

Jagjit Singh Dalal DM
Senior Professor and Head
Department of Neonatology
Pandit BD Sharma PGIMS
Rohtak
jagjit.dr@gmail.com

Kamal Arora DM
Professor
Division of Neonatology
Department of Pediatrics
Dayanand Medical College and
Hospital, Ludhiana
dockamalpaeds@yahoo.com

Kapil Sikka MS
Professor
Department of Otorhinolaryngology
and Head–Neck Surgery
All India Institute of Medical Sciences
New Delhi
kapil_sikka@yahoo.com

Krishna Mohan Gulla MD, FNB (PICU) DM
Resident
Division of Pediatric Pulmonology
and Intensive Care
All India Institute of Medical Sciences
New Delhi
mohangulla35@gmail.com

Lalit Takia DM
Assistant Professor
Department of Pediatrics
All India Institute of Medical Sciences
New Delhi, lalitpgims@gmail.com

Likhita P MBBS
Junior Resident
Department of Pediatrics
All India Institute of Medical Sciences, New Delhi
likhu13@gmail.com

Lumchio Levis Murry MSc (Nursing)
Associate Professor
All India Institute of Medical Sciences
New Delhi, levis.murry@gmail.com

Madhulika Kabra MD
Professor
All India Institute of Medical Sciences
New Delhi
madhulikakabra@hotmail.com

Madhumati Bose
Certified Neonatal Oro-Motor Assessment Scale
Consultant on Autism for State Initiative on Disabilities (SID), Kerala; Honorary Consultant
All India Institute of Medical Sciences
Holy Family Hospital, New Delhi
madhumatibose@gmail.com

Mahesh V DM (Pediatric Nephrology)
Assistant Professor
Department of Pediatrics
All India Institute of Medical Sciences
Mangalagiri, Andhra Pradesh
vmaahi46@gmail.com

Manas Upadhyay DM
Consultant Neonatologist
Cuttack, Odisha
manl013456@gmail.com

Manisha Jana MD, FRCR
Professor
All India Institute of Medical Sciences
New Delhi
manishajana@gmail.com

Manju Saksena PhD
Physician Scientist
All India Institute of Medical Sciences
New Delhi
manjusaksena@gmail.com

Mayank Priyadarshi DM
Assistant Professor
Department of Neonatology
All India Institute of Medical Sciences
Rishikesh, Uttarakhand
priyadarshi.aiims@gmail.com

Mehak Sehgal MCh (Pediatric Surgery)
Ex-Senior Resident
All India Institute of Medical Sciences
New Delhi
mehak.sehgal91@gmail.com

Mohammad Tousifullah DM
Consultant Neonatologist
Jaswant Rai Speciality Hospital
Meerut, drmdtousif@gmail.com

Mudit Agarwal MBBS
Junior Resident
Department of Pediatrics
All India Institute of Medical Sciences
New Delhi
mudit.agarwal07@gmail.com

Mukul Kumar Mangla DM
Senior Medical Officer
Safadarjung Hospital and VMMC
New Delhi
drmanglamukul@yahoo.com

Narendra Kumar Bagri MD
Additional Professor
Division of Pediatric Rheumatology and Clinical Immunology
Department of Pediatrics
All India Institute of Medical Sciences
New Delhi
drnarendrabagri@gmail.com

Neerja Gupta DM
Additional Professor
Division of Genetics
Department of Pediatrics
All India Institute of Medical Sciences
New Delhi, neerja17aiims@gmail.com

Nidhi Garg MD
Senior Resident
Department of Neonatology
All India Institute of Medical Sciences
New Delhi
ng5620@gmail.com

Parminder Singh Rooprai MD
Senior Resident
Department of Neonatology
All India Institute of Medical Sciences
New Delhi
param_rules@yahoo.co.in

Pavneet Kaur MD
Junior Resident
Department of Pediatrics
All India Institute of Medical Sciences
New Delhi
dr.pavneetkaurthind@gmail.com

Poonam Coshic MBBS, MBA (Healthcare Administration)
Chief Medical Officer
Blood Bank (H)
All India Institute of Medical Sciences
New Delhi
poonamcoshic@gmail.com

Pradeep Kumar Sharma DM
Senior Consultant
Deep Hospital, Ludhiana
psaiims@yahoo.co.in

Prashant Jauhari DM
Additional Professor
Department of Pediatrics
All India Institute of Medical Sciences
New Delhi
pjauhari0@gmail.com

Pratima Anand DM
Neonatologist
Department of Neonatology
Lady Hardinge Medical College and Associated Hospitals
New Delhi
anandpratima@gmail.com

Pragya Tyagi MASLP
Audiologist
Department of Otorhinolaryngology and Head–Neck Surgery
All India Institute of Medical Sciences
New Delhi
pragyatyagi@hotmail.com

Praveen George Paul MD, DM
Senior Resident
Department of Pediatric Endocrinology
All India Institute of Medical Sciences
New Delhi
praveenpaul388@gmail.com

Priyanka Gupta MD, DM
Senior Resident
Department of Pediatric Endocrinology
All India Institute of Medical Sciences
New Delhi
prigupta552@gmail.com

Priyanka Khandelwal DM (Pediatric Nephrology), International Pediatric Nephrology Fellow
Department of Pediatrics
Great Ormond Street Hospital for Children
London,
drpriyanka8588@gmail.com

Priyanka Singh MD
Senior Resident
Department of Neonatology
All India Institute of Medical Sciences
New Delhi
priyanka09singh@gmail.com

Puneet Kumar Choudhary DM
Senior Resident
Department of Pediatrics
All India Institute of Medical Sciences
New Delhi
shinepuneet@gmail.com

Purna Chandra Guggilum DM
Senior Resident
Department of Pediatrics
All India Institute of Medical Sciences
New Delhi
chandra.puri12@gmail.com

Rahul Kumar MBBS
Junior Resident
Department of Pediatrics
All India Institute of Medical Sciences
New Delhi
mailtorahulkumarsuman@gmail.com

Raja Ashok Koganti DM (Neonatology)
Consultant Neonatologist
Ankura Hospital for Women and Children, Vijayawada
drrajaashok@gmail.com

Rajiv Aggarwal Fellowship in Neonatology
Director and Senior Consultant
Department of Pediatrics and Neonatology
Narayana Health City, Bengaluru
drrajivaggarwal@hotmail.com

Rajni Sharma MD
Additional Professor
All India Institute of Medical Sciences
New Delhi
email:drrajnisharma@yahoo.com

Rakesh Lodha MD
Professor
Department of Pediatrics
All India Institute of Medical Sciences
New Delhi
rlodha1661@gmail.com

Ranjith Kumar Manokaran DM
Associate Professor
Sri Ramachandra Institute of Higher Education and Research
Porur, Chennai
doct.ranjith@gmail.com

Ravneet Kaur DM
Associate Consultant
Division of Medical Genetics
Fortis Hospital
Mohali, Punjab
docravneet@gmail.com

Richie Dalai DM
Assistant Professor
Department of Neonatology
All India Institute of Medical Sciences
Patna
richie.aiims@gmail.com

Rinchen Zangmo MD
Ex-Assistant Professor
Department of Obstetrics and Gynaecology
All India Institute of Medical Sciences
New Delhi
rinchhen.zn@gmail.com

Rishika Potharaju MBBS
Junior Resident
Department of Pediatrics
All India Institute of Medical Sciences
New Delhi

Rohan Malik DM
Additional Professor
All India Institute of Medical Sciences
New Delhi
dr.rohanmalik@gmail.com

Sachit Anand MCh
Assistant Professor
Department of Pediatric Surgery
All India Institute of Medical Sciences
New Delhi
kanu.sachit@gmail.com

Sai Srinivas Gurram MD
Senior Resident
Department of Neonatology
All India Institute of Medical Sciences
New Delhi
srinivassai982@gmail.com

Satish Mishra DM
Consultant Neonatologist and Pediatrician
NEO Center for Advanced Neonatology and Child Health
Sagar, Madhya Pradesh
drmishrasatish@gmail.com

Satya Prakash MD, DM
Senior Resident
Department of Neonatology
All India Institute of Medical Sciences
New Delhi
satyaprakash1994@gmail.com

Saurabh Kumar Gupta
MD (Pediatrics), DM (Cardiology)
Professor
Department of Cardiology
All India Institute of Medical Sciences
New Delhi
drsaurabhmd@gmail.com

Seema Singhal MD
Additional Professor
Department of Obstetrics and Gynaecology
All India Institute of Medical Sciences
New Delhi
drseemasinghal@gmail.com

Shamnad Madathil MD, DM
Consultant Neonatologist
Baby Memorial Hospital
Kozhikode
shamnadmadathil@gmail.com

Shashank S Koundinya MBBS
Junior Resident
Department of Pediatrics
All India Institute of Medical Sciences
New Delhi
shashankskoundinya007@gmail.com

Shridhar Gopalakrishnan
DM (Neonatology)
Professor
Department of Pediatrics
Armed Forces Medical College, Pune
shri27cat@gmail.com

Sindhu Sivanandan DM
Consultant Neonatologist and Clincal Lead
Kauvery Hospital, Chennai
drsindhusivanandan@gmail.com

Srikanth Kulkarni DM (Neonatology)
Consultant Neonatologist
Rainbow Children's Hospital
Marathahalli
Bengaluru
sskulkarni151@gmail.com

Srinivasavaradan S Govindarajan MD, DM
Senior Resident
Department of Pediatric Nephrology
All India Institute of Medical Sciences
New Delhi
kavisrini.1993@gmail.com

Subhash Chandra Shaw DM
Professor
Department of Pediatrics
Army Hospital Research and Referral
Delhi
drscshaw@rediffmail.com

Subramanian Sreeram DM
Consultant
Paramitha Children Hospital and NEO BBC Children Hospital
Hyderabad
drsreeraman@yahoo.co.in

Suman Chaurasia MD, PhD
Assistant Professor
All India Institute of Medical Sciences
Rishikesh, Uttarakhand
sumanyss@gmail.com

Suma S DM
Consultant Neonatologist
Bai Jerbai Wadia Hospital for Children
Mumbai, suma.sund@gmail.com

Sunil Kushwah MD, DM
Senior Resident
Department of Pediatric Nephrology
Post Graduate Institute of
Medical Education and Research
(PGIMER), Chandigarh
drsunilkushwah04@gmail.com

Sunil Saharan MD
Assistant Professor
Division of Congenital Interventional
Cardiology, New York University
Langone Medical Center, New York
sunilsaharan@gmail.com

Surjeet Kumar Bhardwaj MD, DM (Neonatology)
Assistant Professor
Department of Pediatrics
DrYSPGMC, Nahan, HP
drsurjeet99@gmail.com

Suvasini Sharma DM
Associate Professor
Lady Hardinge Medical College,
New Delhi
sharma.suvasini@gmail.com

Tanushree Sahoo MD, DM
Assistant Professor
Department of Neonatology
All India Institute of Medical Sciences
Bhubaneswar
tanushree_sony206@yahoo.co.in

Tejo Pratap Oleti DM
Senior Consultant and Head
Department of Neonatology
Fernandez Hospital, Hyderabad
tejopratap@gmail.com

Umang Bhardwaj MD
Senior Resident
Department of Neonatology
All India Institute of Medical Sciences
New Delhi
umangbhardwaj51@gmail.com

Vandana Jain MD
Professor
All India Institute of Medical Sciences
New Delhi
drvandanajain@aiims.edu

Vasudha Kohli MD
Senior Resident
Department of Pediatrics
All India Institute of Medical Sciences
New Delhi
kohli.vasudha@gmail.com

Venkatesan Sampath Kumar MS
Associate Professor
Department of Orthopaedics
All India Institute of Medical Sciences
New Delhi
venkatortho4@gmail.com

Venkatnarayan Kannan DM
Officer on Special Duty
NITI Aayog, Government of India
New Delhi
venkatnarayan_kannan@yahoo.co.in

Vishesh Jain MCh
Assistant Professor
Department of Pediatric Surgery
All India Institute of Medical Sciences
New Delhi
dr.vishesh79@gmail.com

Vivek Kumar MD
Consultant (Research)
Department of Pediatrics
All India Institute of Medical Sciences
New Delhi
vivekneoaiims@gmail.com

Vivek Tiwari MS
Senior Orthopaedic Consultant
Apollo Sage Hospital, Bhopal
vivek_tiwari50@yahoo.com

V Prakash MD
All India Institute of Medical Sciences
New Delhi

Preface to the Third Edition

We take immense pleasure in presenting the third edition of *AIIMS Protocols in Neonatology*. In this updated edition, we have introduced 39 new protocols and deleted nine protocols from the second edition, expanding the compendium to encompass 106 protocols. Our primary aim is to provide valuable resources that enhance our readers' education and patient care.

These protocols are thoughtfully categorized into two distinct packages: Core Protocols, spanning two volumes, cater to the management of common neonatal conditions, while Additional Protocols are dedicated to practitioners handling critically ill neonates and to DM and DNB fellows. This categorization empowers readers to delve into all protocols or focus exclusively on the Core ones.

Our unwavering commitment throughout the development of this edition has been to ensure that these protocols are firmly rooted in evidence-based practices. Our team has diligently reviewed the extensive body of literature, including guidelines from reputed bodies such as the World Health Organization (WHO), American Academy of Pediatrics (AAP), American College of Obstetrics and Gynecology (ACOG), National Institute of Clinical Excellence (NICE), Government of India, and National Neonatology Forum (NNF), meticulously contextualized the information, and presented it in a user-friendly format.

We emphasize that the protocols primarily apply to our own or similar institutions and *may have to be adapted to the users' context.* We highly recommend appropriate diligence in this regard.

Creating this edition has demanded a monumental collaborative effort. Faculty members, fellows, residents from our division, colleagues from other divisions within our department and various departments across our institution, and colleagues from other institutions have invested their time and expertise into its development. We extend our heartfelt gratitude to all those who have contributed to this endeavor.

We are grateful to the readers of the second edition who provided us with their valuable feedback. Your insights have been instrumental in refining this edition. We have diligently incorporated relevant changes and rectified any errors to make this version more comprehensive and reliable.

We extend our heartfelt gratitude to Mr YN Arjuna and the dedicated team at CBS, our new publisher, for their exceptional commitment and hands-on involvement in supervising the entire publication process of this third edition.

We acknowledge the possibility of mistakes in this edition. We value your feedback, as it has been invaluable in the past. Please send any observations or suggestions to us via email at ra.aiims@gmail.com, jeevasankar@gmail.com, or dranuthukral@gmail.com.

Ramesh Agarwal
Ashok Deorari
Vinod K Paul
M Jeeva Sankar
Anu Sachdeva

Preface to the First Edition

Protocols are instrumental for adoption of evidence-based practices and elimination of unnecessary or potentially harmful practices. Protocol based approach makes sure that there is a uniform clinical practice irrespective of disparate players and their views. Unit protocols also facilitate learning of the trainee doctors and nurses.

Protocols have been an integral part of NICU life at AIIMS right since its inception. As part of its philosophy of unrestricted sharing of the knowledge and resources, the neonatology faculty at AllMS decided way back to publish the protocols in Indian Journal of Pediatrics. There was an overwhelming response from the neonatal fraternity to the extent that AIIMS protocols practically became part of majority of the neonatal units in India as well as other countries in South East Asia. For postgraduate students, it served as first hand resource for learning neonatology. The AIIMS protocols have been cited for over 400 times across the globe including in many major publications of recent times.

Initially, we published the protocols in Indian Journal of Pediatrics, which were periodically updated. Subsequently, the journal published them in form of a manual that enhanced their usability and outreach. The full texts of the protocols were made available on our website (wwwnewbornwhocc.org), which was one of the reasons of its popularity receiving nearly 200,000 hits over the last few years.

This publication is a manifestation of our desire to bring out a physician manual that contains relevant protocols based on context specific and updated evidence as well as other necessary resources and tools for day-to-day neonatology practice in level 2 and 3 neonatal units in South East Asia. The current manual has 33 protocols. These are focused on the operational aspects of a condition rather than discussing the theory. There are summaries of relevant evidence and management algorithms at appropriate places. There is a substantial amount of additional resource material such as resuscitation algorithm, hand hygiene poster, BP charts, drugs to be avoided in G6PD deficiency, online resources for self-learning and drugs use in pregnancy and lactation. There is a section that deals with main findings on chest X-ray of common conditions. A section on drug dosages has also been included.

India produces over 1200 postgraduate theses in pediatrics every year; however, the quality of research is too low to teach research methods to the students and generate a good piece of evidence. We have included a section that provides a number of research questions and optimum design to be used and relevant outcomes to be studied.

AIIMS protocols have been an outcome of intense efforts of the faculty, scientists and many past and present residents and fellows over a long time. All of them have shown an extraordinary commitment for this cause. We wish to acknowledge the immense contribution of Drs M Jeeva Sankar, Anu Thukral, Deepak Chawla, Kamal Arora and Aparna Chandrasekaran who not only contributed substantially in terms of contents but also in process of editing. We wish to thank Mr YN Arjuna of CBS Publishers who patiently accommodated our changing philosophy and style.

No book is flawless and we are unlikely to be exception. We would really appreciate your constructive criticism (ra.aiims@gmail.com).

Ramesh Agarwal
Ashok Deorari
Vinod K Paul

Contents

Section 12: Therapeutic Modalities

Annexures

Section

8

Metabolic, Hematological, Immunological, Genetics and Endocrine Disorders

CHAPTER

27

Hypocalcemia

Hypocalcemia is a common clinical and laboratory abnormality in neonates. Ionized calcium is essential for many biological processes, including coagulation, neuromuscular functioning, integrity of cell membrane, and many cellular enzymatic reactions.

CALCIUM HOMEOSTASIS DURING THE FETAL AND NEONATAL PERIOD

Calcium (Ca) is actively transferred from mother to fetus during the last trimester, as demonstrated by a significantly higher level of total Ca concentration in cord blood compared to maternal serum.[1] Serum Ca (SCa) in the fetus is 10 –11 mg/dl at term that maintains a gradient of maternal-to-fetal calcium of 1:1.4. Parathyroid hormone (PTH) and calcitonin (CT) do not cross the placental barrier. PTH-related peptide (PTHrP) is the primary regulator of the positive Ca balance across the placenta. Though vitamin D is critical for mineral ion homeostasis and bone development during adult life, fetal mineral ion homeostasis is mostly independent of it.

After birth, the SCa levels in neonates depend on PTH secretion, dietary calcium intake, renal calcium reabsorption, and skeletal calcium and vitamin D status. Hence, after delivery, SCa levels start decreasing—the rate and extent of decrease are inversely proportional to the gestation—and reach a nadir of 7.5–8.5 mg/dl in healthy term neonates by day 2 of life. This postnatal drop in SCa may be related to decreased PTH level, end-organ unresponsiveness to PTH,[2] abnormalities of vitamin D metabolism, hyperphosphatemia, hypomagnesemia, and hypercalcitonemia, which occur by 12–24 hours of age.[3] PTH levels increase gradually in the first 48 hours of life, and normal levels of SCa are achieved by the 3rd to 4th day of life.[4] Efficacy of the intestinal absorption and the renal handling of Ca mature by 2–4 weeks. This transition phase is responsible for the increased risk of early-onset hypocalcemia in high-risk neonates.

DISTRIBUTION OF CALCIUM IN THE BODY

Body Ca exists in two major compartments: skeleton (99%) and extracellular fluid (1%). Ca in the extracellular fluid is present in three forms[5]—bound to albumin (40%), bound to anions like phosphorus, citrate, sulfate, and lactate (10%), and as free ionized form (50%). Ionized serum calcium (iSCa) is crucial for many biochemical processes, including blood coagulation, neuromuscular excitability, cell membrane integrity and function, and cellular enzymatic and secretory activity.

Measurement of the total serum Ca (tSCa) concentration alone can be misleading because the relationship between tSCa and iSCa is not always linear. The correlation between the two is poor when the serum albumin concentration is low and, to a lesser degree, with disturbances in acid-base status, which occur frequently in premature or sick infants. With hypoalbuminemia, tSCa is low, while iSCa is normal. Falsely low iSCa may be recorded in alkalosis and with heparin contamination of blood samples. The tSCa falls by about 0.8 mg/dl (0.2 mmol/L) for every 1.0 g/dl fall in the plasma albumin concentration.

Therefore, the estimation of tSCa is a poor substitute for measuring the iSCa.

DEFINITION

Hypocalcemia is defined by different tSCa and iSCa cutoffs in preterm and term infants (Table 27.1).[6]

Hypocalcemia is usually classified into two categories based on the age of onset. Early-onset hypocalcemia presents within the first 72–96 hours and usually requires short-term calcium supplementation. In contrast, late-onset hypocalcemia usually presents after 96 hours and requires long-term therapy.

Table 27.1: Definition of hypocalcemia

Gestation	*Total serum calcium*	*Ionic serum calcium*
Preterm	<7 mg/dl (1.75 mmol/L)	<4 mg/dl (1 mmol/L)
Term	<8 mg/dl (2 mmol/L)	<4.8 mg/dl (1.2 mmol/L)

SCa is usually reported in different units viz. mg/dl, mEq/l, and mmol/l. The relationship among these units is related to the following equations:

mmol/L = [mg/dl × 10] ÷ molecular wt; mEq/L = mmol/L × valency

Since the molecular weight of Ca is 40, and the valence is +2, 1 mg/dl is equivalent to 0.25 mmol/L and 0.5 mEq/L. Thus, values in mg/dl may be converted to molar units (mmol/L) by dividing it by 4.

EARLY-ONSET NEONATAL HYPOCALCEMIA (ENH)

This condition is relatively common and seen within the first 3–4 days of life in the following clinical settings (Table 27.2).

There is no universal recommendation regarding routine screening of at-risk infants for ENH. However, it may be considered in the following categories of infants:

a. Preterm infants born before 32 weeks of gestation.
b. Infants of diabetic mothers.
c. Infants born after severe perinatal asphyxia (defined as an Apgar score <4 at 1 minute of age)

Schedule for screening: at 24 and 48 hours of age.

Clinical Presentation

Asymptomatic: ENH is usually asymptomatic (unlike the late onset hypocalcemia) and is incidentally detected.

Symptomatic: The symptoms may be neuromuscular irritability – myoclonic jerks, jitteriness, exaggerated startle, and seizures. They may represent cardiac involvement like tachycardia, heart failure, prolonged QT interval, and decreased contractibility. More often, they are nonspecific and unrelated to the severity of hypocalcemia. Apnea, cyanosis, tachypnea, vomiting, and laryngospasm are other symptoms.

Diagnosis

Laboratory: by measuring total or ionized serum calcium. Ionized calcium is the preferred mode for the diagnosis of hypocalcemia.

ECG: QoTc >0.22 seconds or QTc >0.45 seconds

$$QTc = \frac{\text{QT interval in seconds}}{\sqrt{\text{R - R interval in seconds}}}$$

Table 27.2: Causes of early-onset hypocalcemia
Prematurity
Preeclampsia
Infants of diabetic mother
Perinatal stress/asphyxia
Maternal intake of anticonvulsants (phenobarbitone, phenytoin sodium)
Maternal hyperparathyroidism
Iatrogenic (alkalosis, use of blood products, diuretics, phototherapy, lipid infusions, etc.)

$$\text{QoTc} = \frac{\text{QT interval in seconds}}{\sqrt{\text{R - R interval in seconds}}}$$

(QT interval is measured from the origin of the q wave to the end of the T wave on ECG; QoT is measured from the origin of the q wave to the origin of the T wave).

A diagnosis of hypocalcemia based only on ECG criteria is likely to yield a high false-positive rate. Although these parameters have a reasonable correlation with hypocalcemia in LBW infants (sensitivity of 77% and specificity of 94.4%), [7] neonates suspected to have hypocalcemia by ECG criteria should have the diagnosis confirmed by measurement of serum calcium levels.

Treatment

Asymptomatic hypocalcemia: Infants detected to have hypocalcemia on screening but are otherwise asymptomatic should receive 80 mg/kg/day of elemental calcium (8 ml/kg/day of 10% calcium gluconate; 1 ml = 9.4 mg of elemental calcium) for 48 hours. This may be tapered to a 50% dose for another 24 hours and then discontinued. Neonates tolerating oral feeds may be treated with oral calcium (IV preparation may be used orally).

Symptomatic hypocalcemia: These infants should receive a bolus dose of 2 ml/kg/dose diluted 1:1 with 5% dextrose over 10 minutes under cardiac monitoring. When there is severe hypocalcemia with poor cardiac function, calcium chloride 20 mg/kg may be given through a central line over 10–30 minutes (because calcium chloride, unlike gluconate salt, does not require metabolism by the liver for the release of free calcium). This should be followed by continuous IV infusion of 80 mg/kg/day elemental calcium for 48 hours. Continuous infusion is preferred to IV bolus doses (1 ml/kg/dose q 6 hourly). Calcium infusion should be dropped to 50% of the original dose for the next 24 hours and then discontinued. Normal calcium values should be documented at 48 hours (i.e. before weaning the infusion). The infusion may be replaced with oral calcium therapy on the last day.

Precautions and Side Effects

Bradycardia and arrhythmia are known side effects of bolus IV calcium administration. Hence, bolus doses of calcium should be diluted 1:1 with 5% dextrose and given slowly over 10–30 minutes under cardiac monitoring. Continuous infusion is preferred to IV bolus. An umbilical venous catheter (UVC) may be used to administer calcium after ensuring that the tip is positioned in the inferior vena cava. Hepatic necrosis may occur if the tip of the UVC lies in a branch of the portal vein. The umbilical artery catheter (UAC) should never be used for giving calcium injections. Accidental injection into the umbilical artery may result in arterial spasms and intestinal necrosis.

Skin and subcutaneous tissue necrosis may occur due to extravasation. Hence, IV sites where calcium is infused should be checked at least two hourly to monitor for extravasation.

Prolonged or Resistant Hypocalcemia

This condition should be considered in the following situations:

- Symptomatic hypocalcemia unresponsive to adequate doses of calcium therapy.
- Infants needing calcium supplements beyond 72 hours of age.
- Hypocalcemia presenting at the end of the first week.

These infants should be investigated for causes of LNH (see below).

LATE ONSET NEONATAL HYPOCALCEMIA (LNH)

It usually presents at the end of the first week of life. It is usually symptomatic in the form of neonatal tetany or seizures and is generally caused by high phosphate intake (iatrogenic). The common causes are listed in Table 27.3.

Examination

Neonates with LNH should have an examination with particular emphasis on cataracts, hearing, and any evidence of basal ganglia involvement (movement disorder) in the follow-up.

Investigations

Investigations listed in Table 27.4 should be considered in LNH or if the hypocalcemia does not respond to adequate doses of calcium. The workup is vital to determine the etiology.

Hypoparathyroidism should be strongly suspected if hypocalcemia is present with hyperphosphatemia and a normal renal function (*See* Table 27.5 for interpretation of diagnostic investigation).

Table 27.3: Causes of late-onset hypocalcemia
1. Increased phosphate load: cow milk, renal insufficiency
2. Hypomagnesemia
3. Vitamin D deficiency
4. Maternal vitamin D deficiency
5. Malabsorption
6. Hepatobiliary disease
7. PTH resistance
8. Transient neonatal pseudo-hypoparathyroidism
9. Hypoparathyroidism a. *Primary:* hypoplasia/aplasia (DiGeorge's syndrome, CATCH 22 syndrome), activating mutations of the calcium sensing receptor (CSR) b. *Secondary:* maternal hyperparathyroidism, metabolic syndromes (Kenny–Caffey syndrome, long-chain fatty acyl CoA dehydrogenase deficiency, Kearns–Sayre syndrome.
10. Autosomal dominant hypocalcemic hypercalciuria
11. Iatrogenic: Citrated blood products, lipid infusion, bicarbonate therapy, loop diuretics, glucocorticoids, phosphate therapy, aminoglycosides (mainly gentamicin), viral gastroenteritis, phototherapy

Table 27.4: Investigations required in infants with persistent/late-onset hypocalcemia

First line	*Second line*
Serum phosphate Serum alkaline phosphatase (SAP) Liver function tests Renal function tests (RFT) X-ray chest/ wrist Arterial pH	Serum magnesium (Mg) Serum parathormone levels (PTH) 25-hydroxyvitamin D levels (25-OH D) Urine calcium creatinine ratio Maternal calcium, phosphate, and alkaline phosphatase

Table 27.5: Interpretation of investigations

Disorder causing hypocalcemia	*Findings*
Hypoparathyroidism	High: phosphate Low: SAP, PTH, 25-OH D
Pseudohypoparathyroidism	High: SAP, PTH, Phosphate Low: 25-OH D
Chronic renal failure	High: phosphate, SAP, PTH, deranged RFT Low: 25-OH D, pH (acidotic)

(Contd.)

Table 27.5: Interpretation of investigations (*Contd.*)	
Disorder causing hypocalcemia	*Findings*
Hypomagnesemia	High: PTH Low: phosphate, Mg, 25-OH D
VDDR I	High: SAP, PTH Low: Phosphate, 25-OH D
VDDR II	High: SAP, 25-OH D, PTH Low: Phosphate

VDDR: Vitamin D dependent rickets

Treatment

The initial treatment of LNH is the same as that of ENH. This should be followed by specific management according to the etiology and may, in certain conditions, be life-long.

1. **Hypomagnesemia:** Symptomatic hypocalcemia unresponsive to adequate doses of IV calcium therapy is usually due to hypomagnesemia. It may present either as ENH or later as LNH. The neonate should receive two doses of 0.2 ml/kg of 50% $MgSO_4$ injection 12 hours apart, deep IM, followed by a maintenance dose of 0.2 ml/kg/day of 50% $MgSO_4$ PO for 3 days.
2. **High phosphate load:** These infants have hyperphosphatemia with near-normal calcium levels. This results from feeding animal milk with a high phosphate load (e.g. cow's milk). Exclusive breastfeeding should be encouraged, and animal milk should be discontinued. Phosphate-binding gels must be avoided.
3. **Hypoparathyroidism:** High phosphate levels in the absence of high phosphate intake (cow's milk) and normal renal functions suggest hypoparathyroidism.[8]

   Supplementing calcium may lead to calcium deposition and tissue damage if the phosphate level is high. Thus, reduction of the phosphate load must be attempted to keep the calcium and the phosphate product less than 55.[9] These neonates should be supplemented with calcium (50 mg/kg/day in 3 divided doses) and 1,25$(OH)_2$ vitamin D_3 (0.5–1 µg/day). Therapy may be stopped in hypocalcemia secondary to maternal hyperparathyroidism after 6 weeks.
4. **Vitamin D deficiency states:** These infants have hypocalcemia associated with hypophosphatemia due to an intact parathormone response in the kidneys. They benefit from 1,25$(OH)_2$ vitamin D_3 supplementation in a dose of 30–60 ng/kg/day.

After starting treatment, neonates with LNH must be monitored for SCa, phosphate, 24-hour urinary calcium, and calcium creatinine ratio. Try to keep the calcium in the lower range, as defective distal tubular absorption leads to hypercalciuria and nephrocalcinosis.[10]

PROGNOSIS AND OUTCOME

Most cases of ENH resolve within 48–72 hours without any significant sequelae. LNH caused by exogenous phosphate load and magnesium deficiency also responds well to phosphate restriction and magnesium repletion, respectively. When caused by hypoparathyroidism, hypocalcemia requires continued therapy with vitamin D and calcium. The treatment period depends on the nature of the hypoparathyroidism, which can be transient, last several weeks to months, or be permanent.

REFERENCES

1. Schauberger CW, Pitkin RM, Maternal-perinatal calcium relationships. ObstetGynecol 1979;53:74–6.
2. Linarelli LG, Bobik J, Bobik C. Newborn urinary cyclic AMP and developmental responsiveness to parathyroid harmone. Pediatrics 1972;50:14–23.
3. Hillman,Rajanasathit S, slatopolsky E, haddad JG. Serial measurements of serum calcium, magnesium, parathyroid hormone, calcitonin, and 25-hydroxy-vitamin D in premature and term infants during the first week of life. Pediatr Res 1977;11:789–44.
4. Salle BL, Delvin EE, Lapillonne A, Bishop NJ, Glorieux FH. Perinatal metabolism of vitamin D. Am J Clin Nutr 2000;71(5 suppl):1317S–24S.
5. Singh J, Moghal N, Pearce SH, Cheetham T. The investigation of hypocalcaemia and rickets. Arch Dis Child. May 2003;88(5): 403–7.
6. Oden J, Bourgeois M. Neonatal endocrinology. Indian J Pediatr 2000;67:217–23.
7. Nekvasil R, Stejskal J, Tuma A. Detection of early onset neonatal hypocalcemia in low birth weight infants by Q-Tc and Q-oTc interval measurement. Acta Paediatr Acad Sci Hung. 1980;21(4):203–10.
8. Marx SJ. Hyperparathyroid and hypoparathyroid disorders. N Engl J Med 2000;343:1863–75.
9. Sharma J, Bajpai A, Kabra M et al. Hypocalcemia – Clinical, biochemical, radiological Profile and follow-up in a Tertiary hospital in India. Indian Pediatrics 2002;39:276–82.
10. Rigo J, Curtis MD. Disorders of Calcium, Phosphorus and Magnesium Metabolism in Richard J Martin, Avory A Fanaroff, Michele C Walsh(eds) . Neonatal-Perinatal Medicine- Diseases of the fetus and infant. 8th edition; Elsevier, Philadelphia, 2006: p1508–14.

CHAPTER

28

Hypoglycemia

There is no universal definition for hypoglycemia. The "normal" range of blood glucose is variable. It depends upon factors like birth weight, gestational age, body stores, feeding status, availability of alternative energy sources (such as ketones, lactate, and free fatty acids), as well as the presence or absence of conditions that affect energy demand, such as sepsis and birth asphyxia.

DEFINITION

There is no concrete evidence to show the causation of adverse long-term outcomes by a particular level or duration of hypoglycemia. While studies have shown that persistent hyperinsulinism has a definite association with adverse neurological outcomes, there are no concrete data on the long-term adverse effects of asymptomatic hypoglycemia in at-risk neonates.[1] Hence, an "operational threshold" has been defined by consensus. It is defined as a *plasma or whole blood glucose concentration at which clinicians should consider intervention*. A blood glucose level (BGL) of less than 40 mg/dl (plasma glucose <45 mg/dl) has been taken as the operation threshold for intervention. The WHO defines hypoglycemia as a BGL of less than 45 mg/dl (2.2 mmol/L).

Blood glucose levels as low as 30 mg/dl within 1–2 hours of birth are common in normal newborns. The term "transitional neonatal hypoglycemia" (TNH) has been used to describe this transient phenomenon.[2] TNH occurs in up to 10% of normal newborns and represents a normal physiological adaptation to postnatal life.[3] The American Academy of Pediatrics (AAP) has provided guidelines for screening at-risk newborns and an algorithmic approach to management if the plasma glucose is lower than 40 mg/dl in the first 24 hours.[4]

We define hypoglycemia as a blood glucose level (BGL) of less than 40 mg/dl (plasma glucose <45 mg/dl) irrespective of age of the infant.

SCREENING FOR HYPOGLYCEMIA

Screening for hypoglycemia is recommended in following high-risk infants (Table 28.1).

In newborns considered to be at high risk of persistent hypoglycemia disorders (e.g. genetic/syndromic disorders or congenital hyperinsulinism), it is advisable to screen for hypoglycemia and also for the ability to maintain PG >70 mg/dl if one feed is missed (i.e. ability to tolerate fasting for 6–8 hours) before discharge.[6]

Schedule for Screening

There is a paucity of literature on the optimal timing and intervals of glucose monitoring. The lowest blood sugar values are seen at 2 hours of life. IDMs frequently experience asymptomatic hypoglycemia very early, viz. 1–2 hours, and rarely beyond 12 hours (range 0.8–8.5 hours), supporting the need for early screening for this population. However, preterm and SGA may be at high risk for up to 36 hours of life.

Some SGA and preterm infants may develop hypoglycemia when feeding is not established. Based on these assumptions and current

Table 28.1: Indication of routine blood glucose screening[5]
1. Birth weight <2000 g
2. Gestational age ≤35 weeks
3. Small for gestational age infants (SGA)
4. Infant of diabetic mothers (IDM)
5. Large for gestational age (LGA) infants
6. Neonates with Rh-hemolytic disease
7. Neonates born to mothers receiving therapy with terbutaline/propranolol/labetalol/oral hypoglycemic agents
8. Neonates with morphological features of growth restriction like three or more loose folds of skin around buttocks and thighs, loss of subcutaneous fat, a difference between head and chest circumference of >3 cm
9. Any sick neonate, e.g. those with perinatal asphyxia, polycythemia, sepsis, shock, etc. during the acute phase of illness
10. Family history of a genetic form of hypoglycemia
11. Congenital syndromes (e.g. Beckwith–Wiedemann), abnormal physical features (e.g. midline facial malformations, microphallus)
12. Neonates on total parenteral nutrition

Table 28.2: Schedule of blood glucose monitoring	
Category of infants	*Time schedule*
1. At-risk neonates (Table 28.1)	*2, 6, 12, 24, 48, and 72 hours of life* (72 hours for S No 3,7, and 8 in Table 28.1)
2. Sick neonates (sepsis, asphyxia, polycythemia, shock during acute phase of illness)	Every 6–8 hours (individualize as needed)
3. Neonates on parenteral nutrition	Initial 72 hours: every 6–8 hours After 72 hours: once a day

Infants exhibiting signs compatible with hypoglycemia at any time also need to be investigated

knowledge, Table 28.2 elaborates on the schedule and frequency of monitoring in different situations.

Parents should be informed that their infant is at-risk for hypoglycemia and therefore requires blood tests at regular intervals. This will ensure appropriate parental participation in monitoring and allay fears if further interventions are needed.

Infants in Whom Screening is Not Required

Screening for hypoglycemia is not recommended in healthy, breastfed, term appropriate-for-gestational age (AGA) infants. However, term infants with poor feeding, cold stress, or born to mothers with inadequate lactation may be considered for screening.

Method of Blood Glucose Level Estimation

Point-of-care (POC) reagent strips (glucose oxidase method): Though widely used, glucose estimation by this method is unreliable, especially at levels in which therapeutic intervention is required, such as BGL <40–50 mg/dl. They are useful for screening purposes, but low values must be confirmed by laboratory testing. However, treatment of hypoglycemia may be initiated based on the results of the reagent strips.

It is crucial to consider the variations between capillary and venous, blood and plasma, and immediate and stored samples (whole blood sugar value is about 15% less than that of plasma value, and the BGL can fall by 14–18 mg/dl per hour in samples that await analysis).[7] Arterial samples have slightly higher values than venous or capillary samples.

The newer generation glucose reagent strips generate a current when glucose reacts with enzymes such as glucose oxidase or glucose dehydrogenase. The amount of current is proportional to the amount of glucose in plasma. These second-generation glucose readers are more accurate than the previous version but still unreliable in infants with low BGL. A novel approach to measuring dermal glucose concentration using highly sensitive sensors based on glucose binding protein (GBP) technology has also been developed.[8]

Recently **continuous glucose monitoring sensors** (CGMS) have been used in glucose monitoring in newborns.[9] Monitoring by CGMS helps detect hypoglycemia that may be missed on routine screening. However, many of these episodes may be clinically insignificant and thus may lead to overtreatment. Also, there are practical issues in the use of CGMS in NICU because the use of CGMS requires inserting a probe into the subcutaneous tissue, which might increase the risk of infection. Future studies are needed to determine the safety and efficacy of CGMS in the neonatal population.

Laboratory diagnosis: This is the gold standard for measuring blood glucose. Glucose can be measured by either the glucose oxidase (calorimetric) method or the glucose electrodes (used in blood gas machines). Blood samples should be analyzed quickly to avoid erroneously low glucose levels. Therefore, samples must be transported in tubes containing glycolytic inhibitors such as fluoride.

SYMPTOMS OF HYPOGLYCEMIA

It is well known that low BGL may not manifest clinically and be asymptomatic.[10] There is considerable controversy regarding the need to treat infants with low BGLs but without any symptoms.[11]

A smaller proportion of infants with hypoglycemia can be symptomatic. Symptoms of hypoglycemia include neurogenic (autonomic) and neuroglycopenic symptoms. Neurogenic symptoms occur due to sympathetic nervous discharge triggered by hypoglycemia and include both adrenergic and cholinergic responses. Neuroglycopenic symptoms result from a deficient supply of primary fuel (glucose) to the brain. Clinical signs of hypoglycemia are variable and may include stupor, jitteriness, tremors, apathy, episodes of cyanosis, convulsions, intermittent apneic spells or tachypnea, weak and high-pitched cry, lethargy, and difficulty in feeding. Episodes of sweating, sudden pallor, hypothermia, and cardiac arrest have also been reported in neonates.

DIAGNOSIS

- **Asymptomatic hypoglycemia** is said to be present when BGL is less than 40 mg/dl (to be confirmed by laboratory estimation), but the infant does not manifest any clinical features.
- **Symptomatic hypoglycemia** should be diagnosed if hypoglycemia (BGL is <40 mg/dl) coexists with clinical symptoms. Neonates generally manifest nonspecific signs that result from a variety of illnesses. Therefore, careful evaluation should be done to look for all possible causes, especially those attributed to hypoglycemia.

If clinical signs attributable to hypoglycemia persist despite intravenous glucose, then other causes of persistent/resistant hypoglycemia should be explored.

MANAGEMENT

Asymptomatic Hypoglycemia

Figure 28.1 summarizes the management of an infant with asymptomatic hypoglycemia.

Direct breastfeeding is the best option for a trial of oral feeding. If the infant cannot suck, expressed breast milk may be given. Breast milk promotes ketogenesis (ketones are important alternative sources for the brain, along with other sources such as pyruvate, free fatty acids, glycerol, and amino acids). If breast milk is not available, then formula feeds may be given.

Recently buccal dextrose gel has been used to prevent and treat asymptomatic hypoglycemia. Commercially available dextrose gel (200 mg/kg) is applied to the dried buccal mucosa, and the infant is encouraged to feed. Blood glucose is rechecked 30 minutes after gel administration. It has been found to reduce the number of episodes of hypoglycemia, recurrence rates, and need for admission to NICU and to improve exclusive breastfeeding rates at discharge in at-risk late preterm and term neonates.[12]

A few randomized clinical trials in SGA[13] and large-for-gestational age[14] infants found that the sugar or sucrose-fortified milk (5 g sugar per 100 ml milk) raises blood glucose and prevents hypoglycemia. Such supplementation may be tried in asymptomatic neonates with blood sugar levels between 20 and 40 mg/dl. However, this practice can compromise breastfeeding rates, so one should be prudent in exercising this option.

Symptomatic Hypoglycemia

All symptomatic infants should be treated with IV fluids. A 2 ml/kg bolus of 10% dextrose (200 mg/kg) should be given for symptomatic hypoglycemia (including seizures). The bolus should be followed by continuous glucose infusion at 6–8 mg/kg/min. BGL should be checked after 30 min and then every 6 hours until blood sugar is >50 mg/dl (Fig. 28.1). If BGL stays below 50 mg/dl despite bolus and glucose infusion, glucose infusion rate (GIR) should be increased in steps of 2 mg/kg/min every 15–30 min until a maximum of 12 mg/kg/min.

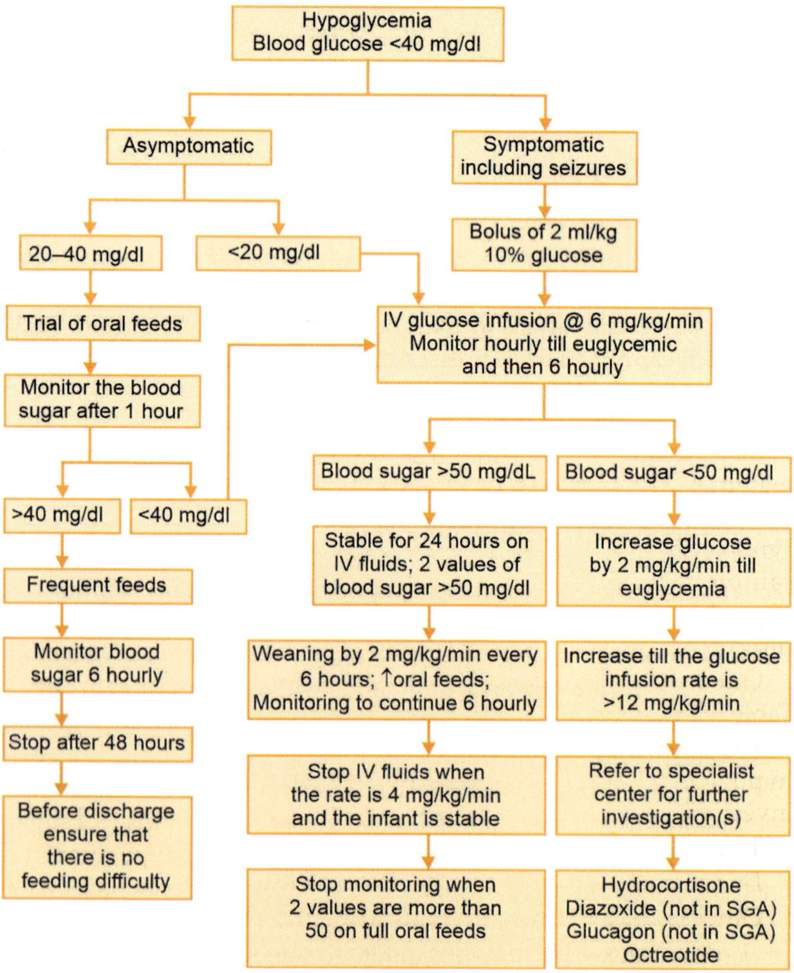

Fig. 28.1: Algorithm for management of neonatal hypoglycemia

After 24 hours of IV glucose therapy, once two or more consecutive BGLs are >50 mg/dl, the infusion can be tapered off at 2 mg/kg/min every 6 hours with BGL monitoring. A concomitant increase in oral feeds must accompany tapering. Once a rate of 4 mg/kg/min of glucose infusion and adequate oral intake is achieved, and the BGLs are consistently above 50 mg/dl, the infusion can be stopped.

It is vital to ensure continuous glucose infusion, preferably using an infusion pump without interruption. Do not stop glucose infusion abruptly, as severe rebound hypoglycemia may occur. Avoid using more than 12.5% dextrose infusion through a peripheral vein due to the risk of thrombophlebitis.

Practical tip

If there is persistent hypoglycemia, check the intravenous line for patency. Also, recheck the intravenous fluid preparation and infusion rate.

Recurrent/resistant Hypoglycemia

This condition should be considered when the infant fails to maintain normal BGL despite a GIR of 12 mg/kg/min or when stabilization is not achieved by 7 days of therapy. High levels of glucose infusion may be needed in these infants to achieve euglycemia. Hyperinsulinism must be excluded because it is the most common cause of persistent hypoglycemia. Hyperinsulinemic hypoglycemia can be congenital (due to mutations affecting the regulation of insulin secretion from the pancreas) or acquired (neonates with maternal diabetes, birth asphyxia, polycythemia, Rh incompatibility, and severe intrauterine growth restriction, Beckwith–Wiedemann syndrome, etc.). Diagnosis of hyperinsulinism is based on critical sample assay, and the criteria are given below in Table 28.3. Typical critical sample assay should include (i) glucose, (ii) insulin, (iii) cortisol, and (iv) beta-hydroxybutyrate and free fatty acids.

Other important causes of resistant hypoglycemia are listed in Table 28.4.

Besides increasing GIR, a few drugs may also be tried for resistant hypoglycemia. Before administration of drugs, take the samples to investigate the cause (Table 28.5).

The drugs that are used are listed in Table 28.6.

Do not use diazoxide or glucagon in small-for-gestational age infants.

Other management options in resistant hypoglycemia are:

1. **Mammalian target of rapamycin (mTOR) inhibitors like sirolimus, everolimus:**[16] Usually given orally in

Table 28.3: Criteria for diagnosis of hyperinsulinism
Critical sample must be drawn at time of hypoglycemia (blood glucose <40 mg/dl)
1. Detectable insulin (>2 mIU/L); usual levels with hyperinsulinism are >5–10 mIU/L.
2. Low free fatty acids (<1.5 mmol/L).
3. Low ketones (plasma β hydroxybutyrate <2.0 mmol/L).
4. Inappropriate glycemic response to 0.1 mg/kg intravenous glucagon at the time of hypoglycemia (normally glucose rise >30 mg/dl in 20 minutes).

Table 28.4: Important causes of resistant hypoglycemia[15]
A. Hyperinsulinemic hypoglycemia: K_{ATP} channel defects Glutamate dehydrogenase (GLUD1) activating mutation Glucokinase activating mutation Short-chain 3-hydroxy acyl coA dehydrogenase (SCHAD) mutation Beckwith–Wiedemann syndrome (BWS)
B. Normoinsulinemic hypoglycemia: Counterregulatory hormone deficiency Cortisol deficiency (central or adrenal, e.g. hypopituitarism, congenital adrenal hyperplasia) Growth hormone deficiency (congenital hypopituitarism) Inborn errors of metabolism Glycogen storage disease (I, III, VI) Disorders of gluconeogenesis Defects in fatty acid catabolism and ketogenesis Organic acidurias Galactosemia Hereditary fructose intolerance

doses of 0.5 mg/m^2/day divided into 1–2 doses targeting a 5–15 ng/ml drug level. They act by inhibiting insulin production. Further trials are needed before incorporating them into routine use.

2. **Glucagon-like peptide 1 (GLP1) receptor antagonist:** Role in congenital hyperinsulinism. Further trials on safety and efficacy are required.
3. **Surgical treatment (near-total pancreatectomy):** In infants unresponsive to medical treatment. Consider 18F-fluro-L-DOPA PET before this to detect focal lesions in the pancreas.[17]

Table 28.5: Investigations to be done in resistant hypoglycemia*	
Blood	*Urine*
• Serum insulin levels, C-peptide, IGFBP3, thyroid hormones • Serum cortisol levels • Growth hormone levels Serum ammonia • Serum lactate levels, free fatty acids, blood BOHB Galactose 1 phosphate uridyl transferase levels • Tandem Mass spectroscopy (TMS) Genetic testing for mutations like SUR1 and KiR6.2	• Urine ketones • Urine reducing substances • Urine GCMS

**Samples should be taken at the time of hypoglycemia*

Table 28.6: Treatment options in resistant hypoglycemia				
Drug	*Dose*	*Route*	*Mode of action*	*Side effects*
Hydrocortisone	10 mg/kg/ day BD	PO /IV	Reduces peripheral glucose utilization Increases gluconeogenesis Increases glucagon effect	Hyperglycemia, hypertension
*Diazoxide**	5–15 mg/ kg/day TDS	PO	K channel agonist	Fluid retention, *hypertrichosis, cardiac failure*
Octreotide	5–35 mcg/ kg/day TDS/QID	S/C	Somatostatin analogue inhibits insulin secretion	Cholelithiasis, transient growth impairment, tachyphylaxis
*Glucagon**	0.2 mg/kg	S/C or IM	Glycogenolysis, increased gluconeogenesis	Nausea, vomiting, skin rash, rebound hypoglycemia

**Do not use diazoxide or glucagon in small-for-gestational age infants.*

Some of the practically helpful formulae in the management of hypoglycemia are given in Table 28.7. The concentration of 10%

Table 28.7: Useful formulae
1. $GIR(mg/kg/min) = \frac{\% \text{ of dextrose being infused} \times \text{rate (ml/hour)}}{\text{body weight (in kg)} \times 6} - \frac{(D \times \text{rate})}{(6 \times \text{weight})}$
2. $\text{Infusion rate (mg/kg/min)} = \frac{\text{IV rate (mL/kg/day)} \times \% \text{ of dextrose}}{144}$
3. Infusion rate (mg/kg/min) = Fluid rate (ml/kg/day) × 0.007 × % of dextrose infused

Table 28.8: Achieving appropriate glucose infusion rate at different daily fluid intakes

Daily fluid volume (ml/kg/day)	*Glucose infusion rate (GIR)*					
	6 mg/kg/min		*8 mg/kg/min*		*10 mg/kg/min*	
	D10	*D25*	*D10*	*D25*	*D10*	*D25*
60	42	18	24	36	5	55
75	68	7	49	26	30	45
90	90	–	74	16	55	35
105	85*	–	99	6	80	25
120	100*	–	120	–	97	18

**Add 20 ml/kg of normal saline to provide 3 mEq/kg of sodium.*

dextrose and 25% dextrose to achieve appropriate glucose infusion rate (GIR) at different daily fluid intakes are given in Table 28.8.

FOLLOW-UP AND OUTCOME

The outcome of neonatal hypoglycemia is determined by factors like duration, degree of hypoglycemia, rates of cerebral blood flow and cerebral utilization of glucose, and comorbidities. Particular attention should be paid to the neurodevelopmental outcome, overall IQ, reading ability, arithmetic proficiency, and motor performance. The infants must be assessed at one month corrected age for vision. At 3, 6, 9, 12, and 18 months of corrected age, they need to be followed up for growth, neurodevelopment, vision, and hearing loss. Vision can be assessed with the Teller acuity cards, while hearing is assessed by brainstem-evoked auditory responses. Neurodevelopment must be evaluated by the clinical psychologist using DASII/similar scales. MRI at 4–6 weeks provides a good estimate of hypoglycemic injury and should be considered in the follow-up of such infants.[18]

Hypoglycemia and neurodevelopment outcome—what is the evidence?

- A systemic review involving 18 studies concluded that there is no good correlation between hypoglycemia and neurodevelopment outcome, and further well-designed, high-quality studies are needed.[19]
- Patterns of cerebral injury and neurodevelopmental outcomes were studied in 35 neonates with symptomatic hypoglycemia without evidence of HIE, and it was seen that 94% had white matter abnormalities; on follow-up at 18 months of age, 65% had impairment in development.[20]
- The recently published 'Children with Hypoglycemia and their Later Development (CHYLD)' study that prospectively evaluated the long-term effects of neonatal hypoglycemia in 477 at-risk late preterm and term neonates reported that hypoglycemia was not associated with increased risk of combined neurosensory impairment at 4.5 years but was associated with a dose-dependent increased risk of poor executive function and visual motor function; severe, recurrent and undetected episodes of hypoglycemia increased this risk.[21]

REFERENCES

1. Adamkin DH, Polin R. Neonatal hypoglycemia: is 60 the new 40? The questions remain the same. J Perinatol. 2016;36:10–2.
2. Adamkin DH. Neonatal hypoglycemia. Semin Fetal Neonatal Med. 2017;22:36–41.
3. Stanley CA, Rozance PJ, Thornton PS, De Leon DD, Harris D, Haymond MW, et al. Re-Evaluating "Transitional Neonatal Hypoglycemia": Mechanism and Implications for Management. J Pediatr. 2015;166:1520–5.e1.
4. Committee on Fetus and Newborn. Postnatal Glucose Homeostasis in Late-Preterm and Term Infants. PEDIATRICS. 2011;127:575–9.
5. Kalhan S, Parimi P. Gluconeogenesis in the fetus and neonate. Semin Perinatol. 2000;24:94–106.
6. Thornton PS, Stanley CA, De Leon DD, Harris D, Haymond MW, Hussain K, et al. Recommendations from the Pediatric Endocrine Society for Evaluation and Management of Persistent Hypoglycemia in Neonates, Infants, and Children. J Pediatr. 2015;167:238–45.
7. Cowett RM, Damico LB. Capillary (heel stick) versus venous blood sampling for determination of glucose concentration in neonate. Biol Neonate. 1992. 62–6.
8. Woo HC, Tolosa L, El-Metwally D, Viscardi RM. Glucose monitoring in neonates: need for accurate and non-invasive methods. Arch Dis Child Fetal Neonatal Ed. 2014;99:F153–7.
9. Rozance PJ, Hay WW Jr. New approaches to management of neonatal hypoglycemia. Matern Health Neonatol Perinatol. 2016 May 10;2:3.
10. Lucas A, Morley R. Outcome of neonatal hypoglycemia. Br Med J. 1999;318:194.

11. Filan PM, Inder TE, Cameron FJ, et at. Neonatal hypoglycemia and occipital cerebral injury. J Pediatr. 2006;552–5.
12. Edwards T, Liu G, Battin M, Harris DL, Hegarty JE, Weston PJ, Harding JE. Oral dextrose gel for the treatment of hypoglycaemia in newborn infants. Cochrane Database Syst Rev. 2022 Mar 18;3:CD011027.
13. Singhal PK, Singh M, Paul VK. Prevention of hypoglycemia: A controlled evaluation of sugar fortified milk feeding in small- for- date infants. Indian Pediatr. 1992;29(11):1365–9.
14. Singhal PK, Singh M, Paul VK. A controlled study of sugar fortified milk feeding in prevention of neonatal hypoglycemia. Indian J Med Res. 1991;94:342–5.
15. Thompson-Branch A, Havranek T. Neonatal Hypoglycemia. Pediatr Rev. 2017 Apr;38(4):147–57.
16. Güemes M, Hussain K. Hyperinsulinemic Hypoglycemia. Pediatr Clin North Am. 2015;62:1017–36.
17. Eichenwald EC, Hansen AR, Martin C, Stark AR, editors. Cloherty and Stark's manual of neonatal care. Eighth edition. Philadelphia: Wolters Kluwer; 2017.
18. Duvanel CB, Fawer CL, Cotting J. Long term effects of neonatal hypoglycemia on brain growth and psychomotor development in small-for-gestational age preterm infants. J Pediatr. 1999;134(4):492–8.
19. Boluyt N, Kempen A van, Offringa M. Neurodevelopment After Neonatal Hypoglycemia: A Systematic Review and Design of an Optimal Future Study. Pediatrics. 2006 Jun 1;117(6):2231–43.
20. Burns CM, Rutherford MA, Boardman JP, Cowan FM. Patterns of cerebral injury and neurodevelopmental outcomes after symptomatic neonatal hypoglycemia. Pediatrics. 2008;122:65–74.
21. McKinlay CJD, Alsweiler JM, Anstice NS, Burakevych N, Chakraborty A, Chase JG, et al. Association of Neonatal Glycemia With Neurodevelopmental Outcomes at 4.5 Years. JAMA Pediatrics. 2017;171:972.

CHAPTER

29

Polycythemia

Polycythemia—increased hematocrit—is associated with hyperviscosity of blood. As the blood viscosity increases, there is an impairment of tissue oxygenation and perfusion and a tendency to form microthrombi. Significant damage may occur if these events occur in the cerebral cortex, kidneys, and adrenal glands. Hence, polycythemia requires urgent diagnosis and prompt management.

The viscosity of blood is directly proportional to hematocrit and plasma viscosity and inversely proportional to the deformability of red blood cells. Symptoms of hypoperfusion correlate better with viscosity as compared to hematocrit. Viscosity is, however, difficult to measure at the bedside. Hyperviscosity is therefore suspected in the presence of an abnormally high hematocrit with or without suggestive symptoms.

The relationship between viscosity and hematocrit is almost linear, up to a hematocrit of 65% and exponential thereafter.[1,2] The polycythemia–hyperviscosity syndrome is thus usually confined to infants with hematocrits of more than 65%; it is very rare with hematocrits of <60%.

DEFINITION

Polycythemia is diagnosed in the presence of a venous hematocrit of more than 65% or a venous hemoglobin concentration of more than 22 g/dl. Hyperviscosity is defined as a viscosity greater than 14.6 centipoise at a shear rate of 11.5 per second.[3]

INCIDENCE

The incidence of polycythemia varies from 1.5 to 4% of all live births.[4,5] The incidence was 0.7% of live births in the last 7 years in our unit. Incidence is higher in small-for-gestational age (SGA) and large-for-gestational age (LGA) infants. About 15% of term

SGA infants develop polycythemia compared to 2% of term AGA infants.[6]

Neonates born at high altitudes also have a higher incidence of polycythemia.[1] Maternal smoking is an important risk factor for polycythemia.[7] Term neonates born to mothers engaged in smoking during pregnancy are 2.5 times more likely to require a partial exchange transfusion for polycythemia than the counterparts of non-smoker mothers.[7] Infants born by cesarean section have lower hematocrit values than those delivered vaginally.[8] Infants subjected to delayed cord clamping also carry a higher risk of asymptomatic polycythemia.[9]

PHYSIOLOGICAL CHANGES IN POSTNATAL LIFE

Significant changes occur in the hematocrit from birth through the first 24–48 hours of life. The hematocrit peaks at around 2 hours of age, and values up to 71% may be normal at this age.[10–11] It gradually declines to 68% by 6 hours and usually stabilizes by 12–24 hours. The initial rise in hematocrit is related to a transudation of fluid out of the intravascular space.

ETIOLOGY OF POLYCYTHEMIA (TABLE 29.1)[12]

Table 29.1: Risk factors of polycythemia

Increased erythropoiesis	*Secondary to transfusions*
1. Intrauterine hypoxia a. Placental insufficiency b. Small-for-gestational-age infant c. Post-maturity d. Gestational hypertension e. Drugs (e.g. propranolol) f. Severe maternal heart disease g. Maternal smoking 2. Maternal diabetes 3. Neonatal hyperthyroidism or hypothyroidism 4. Congenital adrenal hyperplasia 5. Chromosome abnormalities a. Trisomy 13 b. Trisomy 18 c. Trisomy 21 (Down syndrome) 6. Beckwith–Wiedemann syndrome	1. Delayed cord clamping • Intentional • Unassisted delivery 2. Maternal-to-fetal transfusion 3. Twin-twin transfusion

CLINICAL FEATURES

Polycythemia can result in a wide range of symptoms involving several organ systems (Table 29.2). About 50% of neonates with polycythemia develop one or more symptoms. However, most of these symptoms are nonspecific, and may be related to the underlying conditions rather than due to polycythemia *per se*.

SCREENING FOR POLYCYTHEMIA

Screening for polycythemia should be done in certain high-risk groups (Table 29.3).

Table 29.2: Clinical features ascribed to polycythemia and hyperviscosity
Central nervous system
Early: Hypotonia and sleepiness, irritability, jitteriness, seizures and infarcts.
Late: motor deficits, lower achievement and IQ scores.
Metabolism
Hypoglycemia
Jaundice
Hypocalcemia
Heart and lungs
Tachycardia, tachypnea, respiratory distress
Cyanosis, plethora
Chest X-ray: cardiomegaly, pulmonary plethora
Echocardiography: increased pulmonary resistance, decreased cardiac output
Gastrointestinal tract
Poor suck, vomiting
Feed intolerance—abdominal distension
Necrotizing enterocolitis
Kidneys
Oliguria
Transient hypertension
Renal vein thrombosis
Hematology
Mild thrombocytopenia
Thrombosis (rare)
Miscellaneous
Peripheral gangrene
Priapism
Testicular infarction

Table 29.3: Screening for polycythemia

Table 29.3: Screening for polycythemia
Eligible candidates a. Small-for-gestational age (SGA) b. Infants of diabetic mothers (IDM) c. Large-for-gestational age (LGA) d. Mono-chorionic twins, especially the larger twin. e. Infants with morphological features of intrauterine growth restriction such as three or more loose folds of skin around the buttock and thighs, loss of subcutaneous fat, a difference of head circumference and chest circumference of >3 cm.
Schedule 2 hours of life; if high, repeat at 6, 12, 24, and 48 hours
Method Centrifuge venous blood in heparinized capillaries for 3–5 min @ 10000 to 15000 rpm.

Any infant with clinical features suggestive of polycythemia should be investigated for the same.

Blood samples for hematocrit can be obtained by either heel-prick (capillary hematocrit) or venipuncture (venous hematocrit). Capillary hematocrit measurements are, however, unreliable and highly subject to variations in blood flow. They are significantly higher than venous hematocrits. This difference is even more apparent in infants receiving a large placental transfusion.[13]

Practice tip

Capillary samples may be used for screening, but all high values should be confirmed by a venous sample for the diagnosis of polycythemia.

METHODS OF HEMATOCRIT DETERMINATION

Two methods are available:

1. **Automated hematology analyzer:** This calculates the hematocrit from a direct measurement of mean cell volume and hemoglobin.
2. **Microcentrifuge:** Blood is collected in heparinized micro-capillaries (110 mm length and 1–2 mm internal diameter) and centrifuged at 10,000–15,000 rotations per minute (rpm) for 3–5 minutes. Plasma separates and the packed cell volume is measured to give the hematocrit.

An automated analyzer gives lower values as compared to hematocrits measured by the centrifugation method.[14] Most of the reported data on polycythemia is on centrifuged hematocrits.

MANAGEMENT

Before the diagnosis of polycythemia is considered, it is mandatory to exclude dehydration. If the birth weight is known, reweighing the baby and looking for excessive weight loss (>10–15%) would help diagnose dehydration. Dehydration, if present, should be corrected by increasing fluid/feed intake. The hematocrit should be measured again after the correction of dehydration. Once a diagnosis of polycythemia is made, associated metabolic problems, including hypoglycemia, should be excluded.

Management of polycythemia is dependent upon two factors (Fig. 29.1):

1. Presence of symptoms suggestive of polycythemia and
2. Absolute value of hematocrit.

a. Symptomatic Polycythemia

The definitive treatment for polycythemia is to perform a partial exchange transfusion (PET). PET involves removing some of the blood volume and replacing it with normal saline to decrease the hematocrit to a target hematocrit of 55%. Following PET, symptoms like jitteriness may persist for 1–2 days despite lowering the hematocrit to physiological ranges.

The volume of blood to be exchanged is given by the formula in Table 29.4.

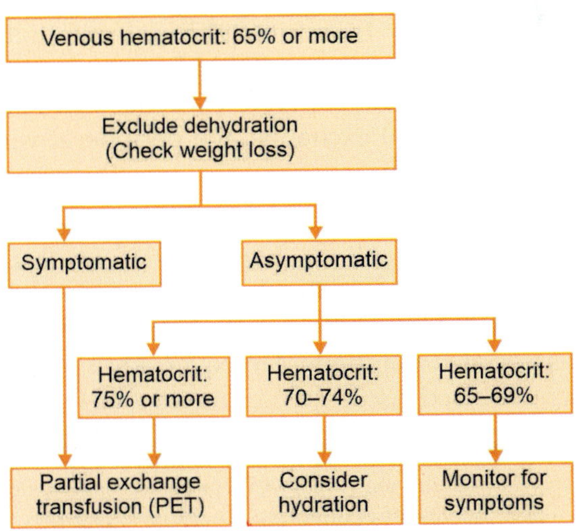

Fig. 29.1: Management algorithm of polycythemia

Table 29.4: Volume to be exchanged in PET

Volume to be exchanged

$$= \frac{\text{Blood volume}^{*} \times (\text{observed hematocrit} - \text{desired hematocrit})}{\text{Observed hematocrit}}$$

For example, for a 35 weeks gestation newborn weighing 2 kg (assumed blood volume 90 ml/kg) and observed hematocrit of 75% and desired hematocrit of 55%, the amount of blood to be exchanged would be:

$$= 2 \times 90 \times \frac{75-55}{75}$$

= 48 ml of blood to be exchanged with normal saline to bring hematocrit from 75–55%

Rule of thumb: Volume of blood to be exchanged is usually 20 ml/kg

**Refer Rawlings chart[15] for estimating the blood volume; as a rough guide, it is 80–90 ml/kg in term babies and 90–100 ml/kg in preterm babies.*

PET: peripheral vs. umbilical route: PET may be carried out via the peripheral or the central route. In the former, blood is withdrawn from the peripheral arterial line and replaced with saline simultaneously via a peripheral venous line. In the central route, blood is withdrawn from the umbilical venous catheter, while saline is replaced by a peripheral vein. Alternatively, the umbilical venous catheter may be used in the central route to withdraw blood and replace saline (pull-and-push technique similar to double volume exchange transfusion for severe jaundice), or the blood is withdrawn from the umbilical arterial line and saline replaced from the umbilical venous line.

One prospective study found increased infection rates without increased risk of NEC following partial exchange using the umbilical vein.[16] Though there is no concrete evidence against using the umbilical vein for partial exchange, the peripheral venous route seems to be a safer option.

PET: choice of exchange fluid: Crystalloids such as normal saline (NS) are preferred over colloids because they are less expensive and are easily available. Crystalloids produce a nearly comparable reduction in hematocrit as colloids[17,18] and do not have the risk of transfusion-associated infections. Moreover, adult plasma has been shown to increase blood viscosity when mixed with fetal erythrocytes.

Evidence: Choice of exchange fluid for PET

A systematic review determined efficacy of crystalloid versus colloid solutions to identify the best fluid for PET:[17]

(Contd.)

(Contd.)

Evidence: Choice of exchange fluid for PET
• Clinically unimportant difference in hematocrit favoring colloids than crystalloids: – at 2–6 hours: 2.3% (95% CI 1.3–3.3%) – at 24 hours: 1.7% (95% CI 0.8–2.7%) • This difference was more significant when NS was compared to plasma but absent when compared with 5% albumin. • No side effects of using colloids were found.

We use only normal saline for partial exchange transfusion.

b. Asymptomatic Polycythemia

The line of management in infants with asymptomatic polycythemia depends upon their hematocrit values.

i. **Hematocrit 75% or more:** These infants are usually managed with PET.

ii. **Hematocrit between 70 and 74%:** Conservative management with hydration is tried in these infants. An extra fluid/feeds of 20 ml/kg may be added to the daily fluid requirements. The additional fluid may be ensured by either enteral (supervised feeding) or parenteral route (IV fluids). Rationale for this therapy is that additional fluids result in hemodilution thereby reducing the blood viscosity.

iii. **Hematocrit between 65 and 69%:** These infants only need monitoring for symptoms of polycythemia and reestimation of hematocrit. Further management depends upon the repeat hematocrit values. The RCT on fluid supplementation (20–25 ml/kg over 6–8 hours) vs. no fluid supplementation in 55 late preterm and term neonates with asymptomatic polycythemia (hematocrit: 65–70%) found no significant difference in the need for partial exchange transfusion between the two groups.[19]

Evidence for Management of Polycythemia

Evidence: Partial exchange transfusion for polycythemia
A Cochrane review (2010)[20] on this issue showed: • No effect on neonatal mortality (one study; RR 5.23; 95% CI 0.66–41.3). • No difference in developmental delay (4 low quality studies; RR 1.45, 95% CI 0.83–2.54). • Increased risk of NEC in infants receiving PET (2 studies; RR 11.18, 95% CI 1.49, 83.64). • No differences in short-term complications including hypoglycemia (two studies) and thrombocytopenia (one study).

PET reverses the physiological abnormalities associated with polycythemia–hyperviscocity syndrome. It improves capillary perfusion, cerebral blood flow, and cardiac function. However, there is little data to suggest that PET improves long-term outcomes in patients with polycythemia. The Cochrane review (2010) concluded that there are no proven clinically significant short or long-term benefits of PET in polycythemic infants who are clinically well or who have minor symptoms related to hyperviscosity. Also, PET may increase the risk of NEC.[20]

However, the studies included in the review were of low quality; also, most surviving infants were not assessed for developmental outcomes, and therefore, the true risks and benefits of PET are unclear. The study by Iris et al. showed that restrictive management of polycythemia does not increase short-term complications.[21]

Given the uncertainty regarding the long-term outcomes, it is preferable to restrict PET in symptomatic infants with a hematocrit of >65% and in asymptomatic neonates with a hematocrit of >75%.

REFERENCES

1. Mackintosh TF, Walkar CH. Blood viscosity in the newborn. Arch Dis Child 1973;48:547–53.
2. Phibbs RH. Neonatal Polycythemia. In: Rudolph AB(ed): Pediatrics, 16th ed. New York: Appleton Century Crofts, 1997, pp 179.
3. Ramamurthy RS, Brans WY. Neonatal Polycythemia I. Criteria for diagnosis and treatment. Pediatrics 1981;68:168–74.
4. Wirth FH, Goldberg KE, Lubchenco LO: Neonatal hyperviscocity I. Incidence. Pediatrics 1979;63:833–6.
5. Stevens K, Wirth FH. Incidence of neonatal hyperviscosity at sea level. Pediatrics 1980;97:118.
6. Bada HS, Korones SB, Pourcyrous M, et al. Asymptomatic syndrome of polycythemic hyperviscocity: effect of partial exchange transfusion. J Pediatr 1992;120:579–85.
7. Awonusonu FO, Pauly TH, Hutchison AA. Maternal smoking and partial exchange transfusion for neonatal polycythemia. Am J Perinatol 2002;19: 349–54.
8. Lubetzky R, Ben-Shachar S, Mimouni FB, et al. Mode of delivery and neonatal hematocrit. Am J Perinatol 2000;17:163–5.
9. Hutton EK, Hassan ES. Late vs early clamping of the umbilical cord in full-term neonates: systematic review and meta-analysis of controlled trials. JAMA 2007;297:1241–52.
10. Shohat M, Merlob P, Reisner SH: Neonatal Polycythemia. I. Early diagnosis and incidence relating to time of sampling. Pediatrics 1984;73:7–10.

11. Shohat M, Reisner SH, Mimouni F, et al. Neonatal polycythemia II. Definition related to time of sampling. Pediatrics 1984;73:11–3.
12. Oski FA, Naiman JL: Hematologic problems in the newborn, ed 3, Philadelphia, 1982, WB Saunders.
13. Oh W. Neonatal polycythemia and hyperviscosity. Pediatr Clin North Am 1986;33:523–32.
14. Goldberg K, Wirth FH, Hathaway WE, et al. Neonatal hyperviscocity II. Effect of partial exchange transfusion. Pediatrics 1982;69:419–25.
15. Rawlings JS, Pettett G, Wiswell TE, et al. Estimated blood volumes in polycythemic neonates as a function of birth weight. J Pediatr 1982;101: 594–9.
16. Rodriguez-Balderrama I, Rodriguez-Juarez DA, Cisneros-Garcia N, et al. Comparison of 2 methods of partial exchange transfusion in newborns with polycythemia: peripheral-peripheral and central-peripheral]. Bol Med Hosp Infant Mex 1993;50:633–8.
17. de Waal KA, Baerts W, Offringa M. Systematic review of the optimal fluid for dilutional exchange transfusion in neonatal polycythaemia. Arch Dis Child Fetal Neonatal Ed 2006;91:F7–10.
18. Deorari AK, Paul VK, Shreshta L, Singh M. Symptomatic neonatal polycythemia: Comparison of partial exchange transfusion with saline versus plasma. Indian Pediatr 1995; 32:1167–71.
19. Sundaram M1, Dutta S, Narang A. Fluid Supplementation versus No Fluid Supplementation in Late Preterm and Term Neonates with Asymptomatic Polycythemia.Indian Pediatr. 2016 Nov 15;53(11):983–6.
20. Ozek E, Soll R, Schimmel MS. Partial exchange transfusion to prevent neurodevelopmental disability in infants with polycythemia. Cochrane Database Syst Rev 2010 Jan 20;(1):CD005089.
21. Morag I, Strauss T, Lubin D, Schushan-Eisen I, Kenet G, Kuint J. Restrictive management of neonatal Polycythemia. Am J Perinatol 2011;28:677–82.

CHAPTER

30

Approach to Bleeding Neonate

Compared to older children and adults, neonates have quantitative and qualitative differences in components of the hemostatic system: the platelets tend to be hyporeactive, levels of coagulation factors (vitamin K dependent factors II, VII, IX, X) are decreased, and contact factors (XI, XII) are reduced to about 50% of typical adult values, translating to prolonged prothrombin time (PT) and activated partial thromboplastin time (aPTT). However, the increased bleeding risk is counteracted by factors that promote hemostasis (high levels of vWF, elevated hematocrit, and reduced levels of natural anticoagulants). The overall hemostatic system in healthy neonates is thus well-balanced; however, systemic diseases can tilt this balance and result in bleeding.[1]

ETIOLOGY OF BLEEDING

Bleeding can be due to a defect in any of the steps in the hemostatic pathway (Fig. 30.1).[2,3]

CLINICAL FEATURES

Neonate with bleeding diathesis can present with significant bleeding (intraventricular hemorrhage, pulmonary hemorrhage, lower gastrointestinal hemorrhage) or minor bleeding events (petechiae, mucosal bleeds, cephalhematoma, blood-tinged endotracheal tube secretions in mechanically ventilated infants, and oozing from the umbilical stump or sites of blood draws, etc.)

Platelet disorders usually present with petechiae, small mucosal bleeds, and ecchymosis. Immune thrombocytopenia, particularly NAIT, can have a varied presentation ranging from mild to moderate bleeding resolving within a week to severe intracranial hemorrhage (ICH) leading to death or neurodevelopmental sequelae. Untreated cases can present with ICH in 10–20% of patients and sequelae in 20% of survivors.

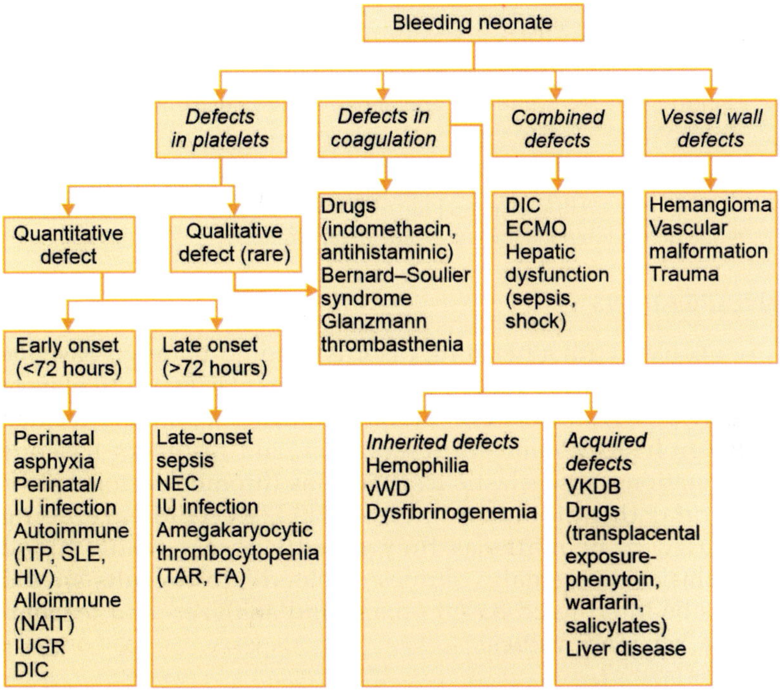

Fig. 30.1: Algorithmic approach to etiology of bleeding

DIC: Disseminated intravascular coagulation; *NAIT:* Neonatal alloimmune thrombocytopenia; *NEC:* Necrotizing enterocolitis; *ITP:* Immune thrombocytopenia; *SLE:* Systemic lupus erythematosus; *VKDB:* Vitamin K deficiency bleeding; *ECMO:* Extracorporeal membrane oxygenation; *SDH:* Subdural hemorrhage; *TAR:* Thrombocytopenia absent radii; *IU:* Intrauterine; *IUGR:* Intrauterine growth retardation; *HIV:* Human immunodeficiency virus; *FA:* Fanconi anemia; *vWD:* von Willebrand disease

Coagulation disorders are often acquired, though inherited coagulation disorders like hemophilia A, B, and vWD can manifest in the neonatal period. Hemophilia in the neonatal period presents with iatrogenic bleeding (oozing/hematoma following venipuncture, IM injections) or spontaneous hemorrhage (intracranial/extracranial hemorrhage). Rarely, severe deficiencies of fibrinogen and factors VII, X, and XIII present in the neonatal period with soft tissue bleeds and umbilical stump bleeding (80% cases of factor XIII deficiency).

Fresh bleeding from the GI tract in an otherwise well neonate may be fetal or maternal in origin. The alkali denaturation test, commonly known as the Apt–Downey test or Apt test, may be done to differentiate fetal from maternal blood (Table 30.1).

Table 30.1: Steps of APT test
1. Mix one part of the bloody stool or vomitus with five parts of sterile water.
2. Centrifuge it for 2 minutes and separate the clear pink supernatant (hemolysate).
3. Add 1 ml of 0.25 N (1%) sodium hydroxide to 4 ml of hemolysate.
4. Hemoglobin A (HbA) changes from pink to yellow-brown (maternal blood), while hemoglobin F (HbF) stays pink (fetal blood).

INVESTIGATIONS

Any neonate with a bleeding disorder should undergo baseline investigations, including complete blood count (CBC) with platelet count (PC), PT, and aPTT (Table 30.2). Further workup is decided based on history, clinical presentation, and results of baseline investigations. Viscoelastic tests such as thromboelastography/ rotational thromboelastometry (TEG/ROTEM) are being evaluated in neonates as they rapidly assess whole blood hemostasis using small volumes of blood.[4] Test results should always be interpreted based on age and analyzer- and reagent-specific reference values.

Table 30.2: Investigations in a neonate with suspected bleeding disorder[5]	
Level 1	Blood count Prothrombin time (PT) Activated partial thromboplastin time (aPTT) Fibrinogen/D-dimer (in sick neonates)
Level 2	Peripheral smear (differential diagnosis of thrombocytopenia) Human platelet antigen analysis (suspect NAIT) Single clotting factor assay depending on PT/aPTT constellation Mixing study (useful in presence of factor inhibitors)
Level 3	Platelet function analysis (Platelet aggregometry)

Practical tips

- Use venous blood samples for diagnosing coagulation disorders: avoid capillary samples.
- Use 3.2% trisodium citrate (light blue capped tubes) as the anticoagulation agent for taking samples; avoid the heparinized source.
- Underfilling (<90%) and overfilling (>110%) of collection tube result in prolongation/ shortening of clotting time, respectively.
- The sample should be capped and transported at room temperature within 1 hour; avoid refrigeration or transportation in ice.

- **Platelet count:** Platelet count <150 × 10^9/L denotes thrombocytopenia. The mean platelet count is ≥200 × 10^9/L in most preterm infants, but the 5th centile may be as low as 104 × 10^9/L for those ≤32 weeks gestation and 123 ≤10^9/L for late preterm and term neonates. Nevertheless, a platelet count of <100 × 10^9/L warrants evaluation.

When to suspect NAIT in neonatal thrombocytopenia?

Diagnosis: All criteria necessary

- Fetal or neonatal thrombocytopenia.
- Identification of a paternal, fetal, or neonatal platelet antigen that the mother lacks.
- Identification of maternal antibodies to that antigen.

Human platelet antigen (HPA) analysis* is useful in suspected NAIT wherein the presence of antiplatelet antibodies directed against HPA [most commonly HPA 1a (80%), HPA 5b (10–15%)] is tested. If negative for common antigens, cross-react the mother's sera with the father's platelets for rare HPA antigens.

*Human platelet antigen genotyping done at the National Institute of Immunohematology, Mumbai.

- **Peripheral smear:** Useful in the differential diagnosis of thrombocytopenia. 1 platelet/oil immersion field in a peripheral smear corresponds to a count of 10000–15000/mm^3. Look for platelet size (giant platelets indicate hyper utilization) or fragmented RBCs (>10% of schistocytes suggest DIC) in the peripheral smear.
- **Coagulation pathway:** Tests assessing the coagulation pathway should begin with PT and aPTT (Table 30.3). Subsequent tests are ordered based on clinical presentation. Vitamin K deficiency bleeding (VKDB) is characterized by prolonged PT and aPTT (the latter may be normal in early vitamin K deficiency). Mild vitamin K deficiency is characterized by elevated 'Proteins induced by vitamin K absence' (PIVKA) levels. Factor XII deficiency is a distinct entity that causes isolated aPTT prolongation with no clinical bleeding. Reference ranges for coagulation tests are available for term and preterm neonates (Table 30.4).
- **Fibrinogen levels:** Decreased in sepsis, hypoxia, liver disease, and consumptive states.
- **D-dimer assay:** Increased in sepsis, DIC, liver disease, and thromboembolism.

An algorithmic approach to a bleeding neonate is given in Fig. 30.2.

Table 30.3: Interpretation of coagulation tests		
Prolonged PT (Assesses factors V, VII, X, and fibrinogen)	*Prolonged aPTT (Assesses factors VIII, IX, XI, V, and X)*	*Prolonged PT and aPTT*
Factor VII deficiency Vitamin K deficiency (mild) Warfarin therapy	Factor deficiency (VIII, IX, XI) Severe vWD Dysfibrinogenemia Heparin contamination	Disseminated intravascular coagulation (DIC) Liver disease Vitamin K deficiency (severe) Afibrinogenemia Dysfibrinogenemia

Table 30.4: Neonatal reference ranges for common coagulation tests measured on day of life 1[5]

	PT (s)	*aPTT (s)*	*Fibrinogen (mg/dl)*
<27 weeks*	14.4–36.7	40.5–158.5	70–480
28–34 weeks**	13.9–20.6	30–57	87–470
30–36 weeks*	10.6–16.2	27.5–79.4	150–373
Full Term#	10.1–15.9	31.3–54.5	167–399

*Reference ranges reflect 2.5th–97.5th percentiles.

**Reference ranges reflect 5th–95th percentiles.

#Reference ranges calculated from mean ±SD (2SD below and above the mean)

MANAGEMENT

I. If Definite Etiology is Not Known

Consider giving the following:

1. **Vitamin K:** 1 mg IV/IM, if not received at birth or status unknown. Infants on prolonged antibiotic therapy (>2 weeks) may be given vitamin K IM/IV 0.5 mg weekly.
2. **Fresh frozen plasma (FFP):** 15–20 ml/kg for significant or active bleeding; repeat q 8–12 hours, if needed. However, specific factor deficiencies must be treated with factor concentrates whenever available (*refer to* the Chapter 51: Blood Component Therapy).
3. **Platelets:** Neonates, particularly high-risk neonates, have a favorable outcome when a lower platelet count threshold is used for transfusion (Table 30.5).
4. **Whole blood/packed red blood cell (PRBC):** Usually given in severe blood loss. Ensure to take pretransfusion samples for diagnostic testing before transfusion; if not done, wait for 2 weeks

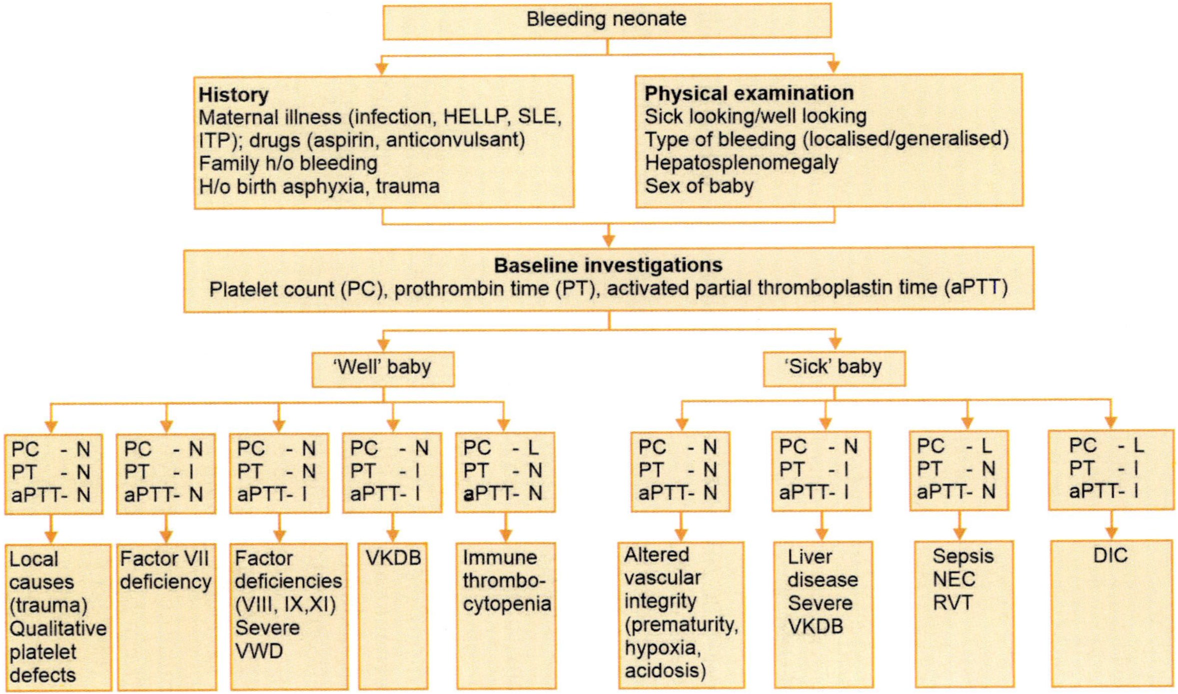

Fig. 30.2: Algorithmic approach to a bleeding neonate. *N:* Normal; *I:* Increased; *L:* Low; *PC:* Platelet count; *DIC:* Disseminated intravascular coagulation; *SLE:* Systemic lupus erythematosus; *ITP:* Immune thrombocytopenic purpura; *HELLP:* Hemolysis, elevated liver enzymes, low platelet; *VKDB:* Vitamin K deficiency bleeding; *NEC:* Necrotizing enterocolitis; *CBC:* Complete blood count; *RVT:* Renal vein thrombosis

Table 30.5: Suggested thresholds of platelet count for neonatal platelet transfusion[6]

Platelet count	*Condition*
<25,000 /mm^3	Neonates with no bleeding (including neonates with NAIT if no bleeding and no family history of ICH)
<50,000 /mm^3	• Neonates with bleeding • Current coagulopathy • Before surgery • NAIT if previously affected sibling with ICH
<1,00,000 /mm^3	Major bleeding, e.g. significant IVH Major surgery NAIT with ICH

NAIT: Neonatal alloimmune thrombocytopenia; *ICH:* Intracranial hemorrhage; *IVH:* Intraventricular hemorrhage

in case of PRBC/platelet transfusion and 4 weeks in case of whole blood transfusion.

5. **Clotting factor concentrates:** Concentrates are available for factors VIII, IX, VII, and XIII.

II. If a Specific Etiology is Known

A. Immune thrombocytopenia[7,8]

1. **NAIT**
   a. Antenatal management: IVIG (1–2 g/kg/week) with or without steroids (prednisolone 0.5–1.0 mg/kg/day) in pregnant women with a history of serologically confirmed fetal or alloimmune thrombocytopenia and previous fetus or newborn with intracranial hemorrhage.[11]
   b. Postnatal management (Table 30.6)
      i. Do cord platelet count
      ii. Do USG Cranium to rule out ICH

2. **Autoimmune thrombocytopenia**
   a. Perform platelet count (PC) on day one or from cord blood:
      i. If PC is normal, repeat on day three; if normal, no further evaluation.
      ii. If PC is between 100 and 150 × 10^9/L, repeat between days 3 and 5 of life.
      iii. If PC <100 × 10^9/L, repeat PC daily; more frequently if clinical bleeding or PC <50 × 10^9/L.

Table 30.6: Postnatal management of NAIT		
Platelet count	*Treatment*	*Dose*
<25,000 /mm^3 in asymptomatic neonates with no family history of ICH <50,000 /mm^3 in preterm neonates or neonates with a family history of intracranial bleed <1,00,000 /mm^3 in neonates with ICH	Random donor platelets* (RDP)	10 ml/kg
<50,000 /mm^3 in asymptomatic neonates immediately following platelet therapy	Intravenous immunoglobulin (IVIG)	1 g/kg/d for 2 days OR 400 mg/kg/day for 5 days
Thrombocytopenia refractory to both platelets and IVIG	Methylprednisolone	1 mg/kg BD for 3–5 days

**Antigen negative platelets (preferred, if available). Blood banks should be immediately notified in cases of suspected NAIT*

b. Perform cranial ultrasound to rule out intracranial bleeding in neonates with PC <50 × 10^9/L.

c. Management
   i. PC <30 × 10^9/L: RDP + IVIG (1 g/kg/day × 2 days)
   ii. PC of 30–50 × 10^9/L: IVIG alone

Unlike NAIT, donor-pooled platelets are usually destroyed by the ubiquitous circulating antibodies in autoimmune etiology, making platelet transfusion less efficacious. RDPs serve as a temporary measure, while IVIG remains the treatment of choice and rapidly raises platelet count.

B. Vitamin K deficiency bleed (VKDB)

The different types of VKDB, possible causes, their clinical presentation, and management are given below in Table 30.7.

C. Hemophilia

Factor replacement therapy is the treatment of choice for hemophilias A and B. Replacement therapy should be monitored because neonates require higher doses.[9] One of the most severe complications associated with factor replacement therapy is the formation of neutralizing antibodies (inhibitors). Both plasma-derived and recombinant factor concentrates carry this risk, although the risk may be lower with 3rd generation plasma-derived factor concentrates. Also, cranial ultrasound should

Table 30.7: Vitamin K deficiency syndromes				
Type	*Time of onset*	*Cause*	*Site of bleed*	*Treatment*
Early	First 24 hours after birth	Maternal medications (anticonvulsants, antibiotics, antitubercular drugs)	Cephalhematoma, umbilical stump, intracranial	Consider FFP for clinical bleed Vitamin K usually not effective
Classic	1–7 days after birth	Lack of prophylactic vitamin K; Poor feeding (breastfed)	Gastrointestinal, mucocutaneous, post-circumcision, umbilical stump; rarely intracranial	Parenteral vitamin K Consider FFP for clinical bleed
Late	1–8 weeks after birth	Fat malabsorption (biliary atresia, alpha-1-antitrypsin deficiency), poor feeding, liver and gastrointestinal disorders	Gastrointestinal, mucocutaneous, intracranial	Parenteral vitamin K Consider FFP for clinical bleed Recombinant factor VIIa (for mild cases)

be undertaken before discharge in all neonates with severe or moderate hemophilia.

Consider one of the following:

a. **FFP/cryoprecipitate:** In case of severe bleeds.
b. **Factor VIII concentrate in Hemophilia A:** 1 IU/kg raises factor levels by 2%.
c. **Factor IX concentrate in Hemophilia B:** 1 IU/kg raises factor levels by 1%.

REFERENCES

1. Revel-Vilk S. The conundrum of neonatal coagulopathy. Hematol Am Soc Hematol Educ Program 2012;2012:450–4.
2. Roberts I, Murray NA. Neonatal thrombocytopenia: causes and management. Arch Dis Child-Fetal Neonatal Ed 2003;88:F359–64.
3. Aronis-Vournas S. The bleeding neonate. In: Hematology Meeting Reports (formerly Haematologica Reports) [Internet]. 2009 [cited 2017 May 5]. Available from: http://www.pagepress.org/journals/index.php/hmr/article/view/454.

4. Eberl W. Diagnostic Challenges in Newborns and Infants with Coagulation Disorders. Hamostaseologie. 2020;40:84–7.
5. Davenport P, Sola-Visner M. Hemostatic Challenges in Neonates. Front Pediatr. 2021 Mar 2;9:627715.
6. New HV, Berryman J, Bolton-Maggs PHB, Cantwell C, Chalmers EA, Davies T, et al. Guidelines on transfusion for fetuses, neonates and older children. Br J Haematol 2016;175:784–828.
7. Batton E, Leibel SL. Immune-Mediated Neonatal Thrombocytopenia. Neoreviews. 2022 Jul 1;23:e462–71.
8. Eichenwald EC, Hansen AR, Martin C, Stark AR, editors. Cloherty and Stark's manual of neonatal care. Eighth edition. Philadelphia: Wolters Kluwer; 2017.
9. Chalmers E, Williams M, Brennand J, Liesner R, Collins P, Richards M, et al. Guideline on the management of haemophilia in the fetus and neonate. Br J Haematol 2011;154:208–15.

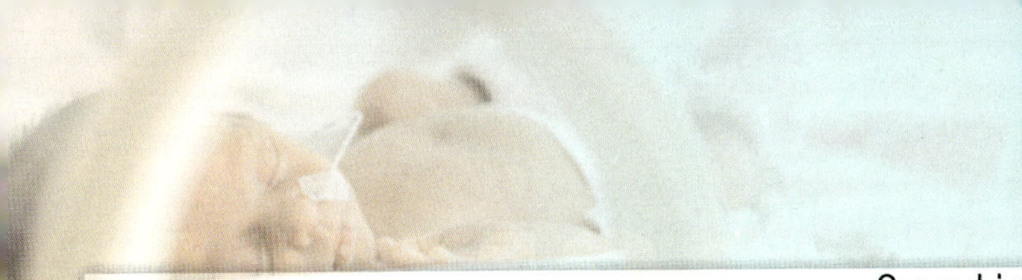

Section

9

Genitourinary Tract

CHAPTER

31

Acute Kidney Injury

Acute kidney injury (AKI), common morbidity among sick neonates, is an independent risk factor for mortality.[1] The old term acute renal failure has now been replaced with 'acute kidney injury (AKI) to emphasize the importance of early recognition and intervention at the time of injury rather than waiting until complete organ failure. AKI is defined as an abrupt (within 7 days) reduction in kidney function: an increase of serum creatinine either more than or equal to 0.3 mg/dl (26.4 µmol/L) or more than equal to 50% (1.5-fold) from the baseline, or oliguria of <1 ml/kg per hour over 24 hours.[2]

INCIDENCE

A large multicentre study (AWAKEN) reported an AKI incidence in 29.9% of neonates. The incidence of AKI varies from 1 to 56%, depending on the study population.[3] Among the neonates with AKI, more than 65% are within seven days of life.[4]

At-risk Population

- Sick and small neonates, especially extremely low birth weight neonates.
- Perinatal asphyxia.
- Neonates with other concurrent morbidities (malformations, intraventricular hemorrhage, and necrotizing enterocolitis).
- PDA (hemodynamically significant).
- Congenital cardiac defects (post-surgery).
- Bronchopulmonary dysplasia.
- Nephrotoxic medications (aminoglycosides, ACE inhibitors).

Staging

In 2013, the Working Group on the Kidney Diseases: Improving Global Outcomes (KDIGO) clinical practice guidelines published a classification for AKI that applied to the pediatric population.

Table 31.1: Classification of Neonatal AKI[2]

Stage	*Change in serum creatinine (S Cr)*	*Urine output over 24 hours*
0	No change or rise <0.3 mg/dl within 48 hours	>1 ml/kg/hour
1	Rise in serum creatinine by 0.3 mg/dl within 48 hours or ≥1.5–1.9 times rise in serum creatinine from the lowest previous value within seven days	≤1 ml/kg/hour
2	≥2–2.9 times increase in serum creatinine from the lowest previous value	≤0.5 ml/kg/hour
3	≥3 times rise in serum creatinine from the lowest previous value or ≥2.5 mg/dl or the initiation of dialysis	≤0.3 ml/kg/hour

Fulfilling either serum creatinine-based or urine output-based criteria classifies the neonate in that particular stage. The lowest previous value of serum creatinine should be considered as the baseline, preferably on day 3 of life or later.

Later, the KDIGO definition was modified for defining neonatal AKI (Table 31.1).[2]

Practical tip

- Even an increase in serum creatinine by 0.3 mg/dl is sufficient to suspect AKI.
- SCr of 2.5 mg/dl represents glomerular filtration rate of less than 10 ml/min/1.73 m^2.

HISTORY

a. **Prenatal history:**
   - Maternal drug intake like ACE inhibitors (enalapril) or NSAIDs (indomethacin).
   - Maternal uncontrolled diabetes (associated with genitourinary malformations).
   - Oligohydramnios (fetal oliguria due to bilateral congenital renal disease, bilateral/lower urinary tract obstruction, or maternal drugs).

b. **Family history** of polycystic kidney disease, renal tubular disorders, and congenital nephrotic syndrome.

c. **Birth and postnatal history:** Perinatal asphyxia, respiratory distress, sepsis, and shock may predispose the kidneys to anoxic injury culminating in acute tubular necrosis or oliguria in asphyxia.

d. **Micturition history:** About 7% of neonates do not void in the first 24 hours; hence no passage of urine beyond 24 hours has to be evaluated. The most common cause of delayed micturition is inadequate perfusion of the kidneys. However, intrinsic renal disorders and urinary tract obstruction must be ruled out.

Examination

Assess for:

a. Hydration status (edema/dehydration).
b. **Signs of dehydration:** Tachycardia, sunken fontanel, sunken eyes, or dry mucous membrane.
c. **Signs of hypervolemia:** Edema over dependent areas like labia, scrotum, and posterior scalp.
d. **Hemodynamic stability:** Heart rate, blood pressure, and respiratory rate.
e. Dysmorphism (abnormal ears, preauricular pits, ambiguous genitalia, hypospadias, abdominal wall defects, aniridia, or Potter facies).
f. Urine stream and/or dribbling.
g. **Any abdominal mass:** Suprapubic mass could indicate a palpable bladder, post void residual bladder suggests a posterior urethral valve (PUV), or assess for palpable kidneys.
h. Input and output of fluids and electrolytes.
   Fluid overload percentage is calculated in critically ill infants

$$\text{Fluid overload (\%)} = \frac{\text{Input (L)} - \text{Output (L)} \times 100}{\text{Premorbid weight (kg)}}$$

Markers of AKI: At present, serum creatinine and urine output remain the best available markers of AKI. Newer biomarkers like serum cystatin C and urine neutrophil gelatinase-associated lipocalin are still under evaluation.

Serum creatinine: The limitations of serum creatinine in identifying AKI in neonates are:[2]

- Serum creatinine levels during the first 48 hours of life reflect maternal creatinine levels.
- It declines at varying rates depending on the gestational age. In preterm infants, it can initially be higher than maternal levels peaking at roughly four days due to reabsorption in the renal tubules and decreased total body fluid, followed by a gradual decline to normal levels by 3–4 weeks.

- It rises late and may remain normal during the first 24–48 hours after renal injury and until about 25–50% of renal function is lost
- It does not indicate the nature and timing of the renal injury

Urine output: Oliguria is defined as a urine output of less than 1 ml/kg/hour after the first day of life in term and preterm neonates. However, urine output has the following limitations:

- Not all AKI is associated with oliguria. AKI in neonates can be oligo-anuric (40%) or nonoliguric (60%). Asphyxiated neonates can have nonoliguric AKI.[3]
- Some term neonates may void for the first time at around 24 hours of life.
- Oliguria can also occur in the syndrome of inappropriate ADH (SIADH) secretion without AKI.
- VLBW infants without AKI may have an oliguric phase that resolves spontaneously in the first few days of life.

Practical tip

Neonatal AKI may be nonoliguric and can be missed if serum creatinine is not monitored in patients at high-risk of AKI.

Newer Techniques

Near-infrared spectroscopy: Near-infrared spectroscopy (NIRS) is a non-invasive tool to identify inadequate renal tissue oxygenation. Previous literature has shown a correlation between low renal tissue oxygenation ($RrSO_2$) in the first 24 hours of age and the later development of AKI. $RrSO_2$ persistently below 50 for 8–12 hours had a sensitivity of 64% and specificity of 71% with AUC-0.98.[5]

Novel biomarkers: Urinay NGAL and cystatin C have been evaluated in preterm neonates and found to have a sensitivity of 90% and 80%, respectively; however, higher cost and limited evidence preclude their use in routine practice.

ETIOLOGY

Based on the site of origin of insult, it can be three types: [6]

1. Prerenal (75–80%)
2. Intrinsic renal (10–15%)
3. Post-renal (5%)

Although prerenal or post-renal causes can be reversible during the early phase, persistent insult can progress to intrinsic AKI. Although widely used, this classification is imprecise due to overlapping pathophysiological mechanisms.[7] This distinction has blurred with the increasing recognition of AKI as a continuum of volume responsiveness through unresponsiveness. Practically, response to fluid resuscitation has a definite role in reversing renal damage in the former.[7]

EVALUATION

Laboratory investigations: The affected neonates require evaluation for the cause and the complications of AKI. Besides serum creatinine and blood urea, serum electrolytes, arterial blood gas, urine sodium, and creatinine are generally required.

Role of indices: While differentiation of prerenal and intrinsic renal failure may be based on urinary indices (Table 31.2), their clinical utility is limited. The urine sample for measuring indices must be obtained *before the fluid and diuretic challenge*. Preterm neonates lose more sodium in the urine due to tubular immaturity. A FENa of more than 2.5–3.0% is associated with intrinsic AKI. Hence a FENa of more than 6% can be used to define intrinsic AKI in neonates born between 29–32 weeks.[8] As the values overlap in newborns with and without AKI, FENa has limited usefulness in neonates. Likewise, a renal failure index (RFI) of more than 4 in term and more than 8 in preterm neonates <32 weeks suggests intrinsic AKI.

Urine complete and microscopy: The presence of granular and hyaline casts, RBC, protein, and tubular cells suggests an intrinsic cause. In asphyxia, there is an increase in epithelial cells and transient microscopic hematuria with leucocytes.

Table 31.2: Renal indices to differentiate prerenal from intrinsic renal failure[1]

Parameters	*Prerenal*	*Intrinsic renal*
Urinary Na	≤20 mEq/L	>50 mEq/L
Renal failure index*	Low <1	High >4
Fractional excretion of sodium (FENA)%$	≤1	>3

*Renal failure index (RFI): $\frac{\text{Urinary Na} \times \text{Serum creatinine}}{\text{Urine creatinine}}$

$Fractional excretion of sodium (FENa)%: $\frac{\text{Urinary Na} \times \text{serum creatinine} \times 100}{\text{Serum sodium} \times \text{urine creatinine}}$

Genitourinary Tract

Urinary biomarkers: The excretion of low molecular weight proteins like beta$_2$-glycoprotein is a sensitive indicator of tubular damage, as in asphyxia. The role of urine and serum biomarkers in predicting AKI in neonates is evolving. Promising biomarkers of AKI include serum and urine neutrophil gelatinase-associated lipocalin (NGAL), urine interleukin-18 (IL-18) and kidney injury molecule-1 (KIM-1), β-2-microglobulin and serum cystatin C.[9]

Ultrasonography and Doppler: Renal ultrasonography helps diagnose congenital anomalies like polycystic kidneys, renal dysplasia, and obstructive uropathy. Renal Doppler studies are performed when renal vascular lesions are suspected.

Glomerular Filtration Rate (GFR)

GFR is calculated using the Schwartz formula as follows:[10]
Estimated GFR (eGFR in mL/min/1.73 m^2)

$$= \frac{K \times \text{Length (cm)}}{\text{Serum creatinine (mg / ml)}}$$

K = 0.33 in preterm infants aged <1 year and 0.45 in term infants aged <1 year

MANAGEMENT

There are no specific drugs to prevent or treat AKI. Treatment relies on supportive care, correction of fluid and electrolyte abnormalities, acid–base homeostasis, treatment of complications, avoidance of nephrotoxins, and renal replacement therapy whenever required. A detailed description of drug dose modification in AKI is provided[5] (*see* Annexure 3).

Initial Management: When a baby has not passed urine for 12 hours, examine the baby for the distended bladder by palpating the abdomen or ultrasound (if available at bedside). *Avoid bladder catheterization to prevent infection*, but it may be necessary for sick neonates. If required, it has to be done with a 5 Fr lubricated feeding tube under strict asepsis. *Compression of the bladder (suprapubic pressure) should be avoided, especially in preterm infants, for fear of vesicoureteric reflex and rarely bladder rupture.*[6]

The common causes of prerenal azotemia are hypovolemia, systemic hypotension, and hypoxia (in nearly 80% of cases). After confirming the absence of urine in the bladder, a fluid challenge can be given.[6] In the absence of obvious signs of fluid overload, a normal

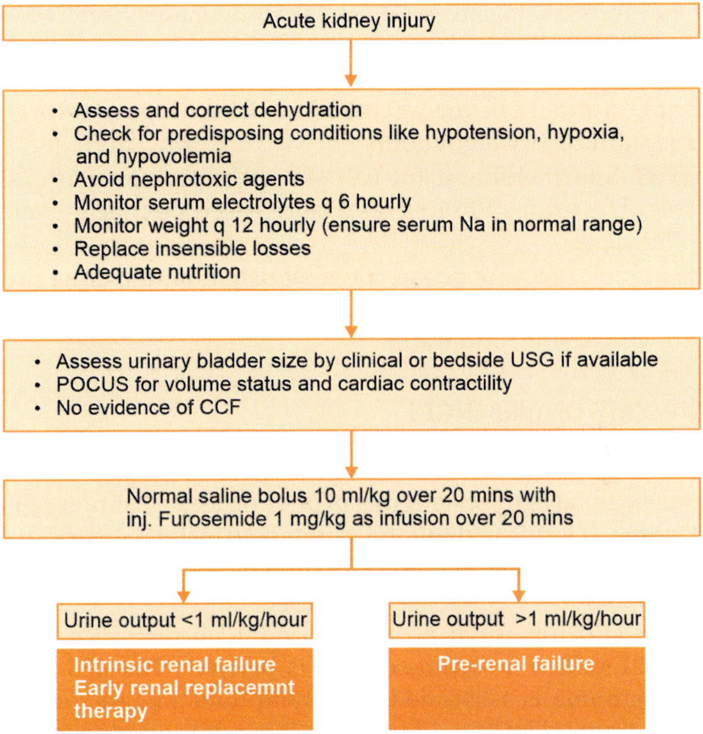

Fig. 31.1: Management algorithm for neonatal AKI
UOP: Urine output; *CCF:* Congestive cardiac failure

saline bolus of 10–20 ml/kg can be given over 60 min.[3] Despite the fluid challenge, if urine output fails to ensue, furosemide in a single dose of 1 mg/kg can be given (in a non-dehydrated patient) (Fig. 31.1).

The only use of diuretics in patients with incipient or established fluid overload with AKI does not improve the outcomes as diuretics by itself cause acute tubular injury and may not be effective when intrinsic AKI had already set in. Neonates who do not pass urine after furosemide are unlikely to improve urine output. Due to the high incidence of progressive AKI in such patients, renal replacement therapy should be considered.

Fluid Management

Fluids must be restricted to insensible water loss (IWL) plus urinary (and other) losses. The urinary loss must be replaced volume for volume. The IWL in a term neonate is approximately 20 ml/kg/day

(400 ml/body surface area). In preterm neonates, this can vary between about 40 and 80 ml/kg/day depending on gestation, postnatal age, use of radiant warmers, phototherapy, etc.[11] Fluids prescription should be revised based on urine output, weight, and volume status every eight hours.

In oligo-anuric children, the IWL should be replaced with 5–10% dextrose. The urine output should be replaced volume by volume with *N/5 saline*.[7]

During the polyuric phase, meticulously monitor urine output serum electrolytes and replace them with appropriate amounts of sodium, potassium, and water.[3]

ELECTROLYTE DISTURBANCES

Hyponatremia

Neonates can have hyponatremia in oliguric as well as non-oliguric renal failure. It is due to dilution secondary to water retention; hence, it must be corrected with fluid restriction. In most cases, there is no sodium deficit.

Serum sodium must be monitored 12 hourly. Restricting fluids will suffice if serum sodium is between 120–135 mEq/L. If hyponatremia is associated with symptoms like seizures, or if serum sodium is less than 120 mEq/L, it requires prompt correction with 3% hypertonic saline over 2 hours, using the formula.

$$\text{Na required (mEq)} = [\text{Na desired} - \text{Na actual}] \times \text{body weight (kg)} \times 0.8$$

Hyponatremia unresponsive to the above therapy is an indication of dialysis. Neonates with nonoliguric AKI may have urinary sodium losses of up to 10 mEq/kg/day, which must be replaced. Care should be taken not to increase the serum sodium by more than 0.5 mEq/L/hour.

Hyperkalemia

Hyperkalemia (K^+ >6.5 mEq/L[1]) is one of the most dangerous complications of AKI. It results from reduced glomerular filtration rate, urinary potassium secretion, acidosis, immature tubular response to aldosterone, and cellular breakdown.

Practical tip

If hyperkalemia is associated with hypoglycemia, hyponatremia and hypotension, consider adrenal insufficiency.

The first step in managing hyperkalemia is to stop potassium-containing fluids and the drugs which can accentuate hyperkalemia (indomethacin, ACE inhibitors, and potassium-sparing diuretics). ECG will help in diagnosing the cardiac effects of hyperkalemia. If ECG changes are evident, IV calcium gluconate 10% is given. This will decrease the myocardial excitability but will not lower the potassium levels.

This should immediately be followed by methods to decrease potassium levels. Hyperkalemia in AKI is an indication for starting peritoneal dialysis; all three medical measures should be instituted while awaiting initiation of dialysis (Table 31.3).

Practical tips

- Saturate the plastic tubing with insulin solution before infusing to the baby.
- Oral or rectal administration of resins is avoided because it is associated with the risk of concretions, hypernatremia and fluid overload, especially in VLBW infants and those with poor peristalsis; adding resins to milk feed and using decanted supernatant is useful in managing patients with chronic hyperkalemia.
- Salbutamol aerosol may not be very effective in neonates.

Table 31.3: Management of Hyperkalemia[3]

Medication	*Dose*	*Mechanism/ Degree of effect*	*Onset of action*
Calcium gluconate (10%)	0.5–1 ml/kg over 5–10 min	Modifies myocardial excitability, with no decrease in K levels	5–10 min
Glucose and insulin	0.5 g/kg/h of glucose and 0.1 U/kg/hour infusion of insulin	Intracellular uptake of potassium	30 min
Salbutamol IV infusion	4 μg/kg over 20 min	Intracellular uptake of potassium	30–40 min
Peritoneal dialysis	Use a dialysate with no K^+ concentration	Dialysis	Minutes
Cation exchange resin (Na/Ca polystyrene sulfonate)	1 g/kg intrarectally q 6 h*; alternatively, add to milk feed at 0.5–1 g per mEq K^+, decant supernatant, and discard residue**	Exchange of K for Na or Ca. 1g/kg reduces K levels by 1 mEq/kg	1–2 hours, may take up to 6 hours

*Carries risk of intestinal perforation and hypernatremia.

**Often used in chronic than acute hyperkalemia.

Hypocalcemia

Hypocalcemia occurs due to hyperphosphatemia and resistance to parathyroid hormone. Symptomatic hypocalcemia should be corrected by infusing 10% calcium gluconate at a dose of 0.5–1 ml/kg over 5–10 min under cardiac monitoring, followed by maintenance calcium at 8 ml/kg/day added intravenously. Also, during the oliguric phase, no intake of phosphorous/magnesium is to be provided. Calcium carbonate preparations are preferred if the baby is fit for enteral feeds.

Role of dopamine: The Cochrane meta-analysis of three studies concluded that dopamine has no role in the management of acute renal failure due to indomethacin.[12]

Dopamine acts via DA_1 and DA_2 receptors at doses less than 5 µg per kg per min to increase renal blood flow. Preterm infants are hypersensitive to alpha receptors; hence, low amounts of dopamine can cause vasoconstriction and raise renal vascular resistance.[13] This may explain the difficulty in using dopamine to improve renal function. While dopamine, combined with frusemide, causes natriuresis and diuresis in preterm infants with RDS and oliguria, current guidelines do not recommend its use in managing patients with AKI.[14]

Theophylline: KDIGO guidelines recommend a single dose of theophylline (5–8 mg/kg) in neonates with severe perinatal asphyxia for prevention. We do not routinely use theophylline in neonates with severe asphyxia.

Fenoldopam

It is a selective dopamine-1 receptor agonist causing renal vasodilatation resulting in increased blood flow and GFR. Therapy with fenoldopam for preventing or treating neonatal AKI is not recommended.

Nutrition

The goal is to provide 100 kcal/kg/day as neonates with AKI are catabolic. Proteins or amino acids can be provided in a dose of 1–2 g/kg/day. If enteral feeding is possible, breast milk should be used as its content of phosphorous and potassium are low, failing which, low phosphate formula can be given. Caloric density can be increased by adding medium-chain triglycerides. A central venous catheter may be needed to infuse hypertonic glucose to prevent hypoglycemia if the baby is on parenteral nutrition.

Acidosis

Mild metabolic acidosis is common in neonates with AKI. If pH is <7.2 and bicarbonate <18 mEq/L, sodium bicarbonate is given in a dose of 1–2 mEq/kg over 3–4 hours while monitoring for fluid overload, hypernatremia, intracranial hemorrhage, and hypocalcemia. Neonates with severe or persistent acidosis in the presence of AKI require dialysis.

Hypertension

Fluid overload in neonatal AKI can result in hypertension, which can be controlled with fluid restriction and antihypertensive agents. The development of severe hypertension should raise suspicion for renal artery or venous thrombosis. Neonates with severe hypertension are managed with continuous IV infusion of nitroprusside, labetalol, or nicardipine. Commonly used antihypertensives in newborns are oral amlodipine (0.1–0.3 mg/kg/dose q 12–24 hourly) and enalapril (0.1–0.4 mg/kg/day q 6–12 hourly). Other drugs that may be administered include beta blockers and hydralazine. Cautious use of ACE inhibitors is required, particularly in premature neonates; lower doses may lead to renal hypoperfusion and progression of renal injury.[1]

Renal Replacement Therapy

The indications of renal replacement therapy (RRT) are:

- Hyperkalemia
- Hyponatremia with volume overload (pulmonary edema, severe hypertension)
- Metabolic acidosis (pH<7.20 despite medical management)
- Hypocalcemia
- Hyperphosphatemia refractory to therapy
- Inability to provide adequate nutrition due to fluid restriction.

While anuria, along with the above, is an absolute indication for initiating renal replacement therapy (RRT), dialysis should begin early to prevent catastrophic metabolic complications and the risk of mortality associated with more than 15–20% fluid overload.

The two purposes of RRT are ultrafiltration (removal of water) and dialysis (removal of solutes), and it can be provided by acute peritoneal dialysis (PD), intermittent hemodialysis, or continuous renal replacement (CRRT).

OUTCOME AND FOLLOW-UP

Non-oliguric AKI has a better prognosis when compared to oliguric renal failure. Mortality ranges from 25 to 78% in oligo anuric AKI.[15] Newborns who have had AKI are predisposed to developing chronic renal failure in the future. While most studies are retrospective, prospective studies have also shown decreased GFR (5–23%), proteinuria (12–17%), hyperfiltration (11–13%), and hypertension (3–19%) during follow-up. Neonates with AKI (RIFLE groups injury and failure) had a 4-times higher risk of developing hypertension or CKD than those without AKI.[16] Therefore, all neonates who develop AKI need follow-up, especially since prematurity and low birth weight are independent predictors for the development of CKD.[16] Adequacy of growth and nutrition, blood pressure, proteinuria, and renal function status has to be monitored at least three months after the resolution of AKI and long-term after that.

REFERENCES

1. Askenazi DJ, Griffin R, McGwin G, et al. Acute kidney injury is independently associated with mortality in very low birth weight infants: a matched case-control analysis.Pediatr Nephrol 2009;24:991–7.
2. Zappitelli M, Ambalavanan N, Askenazi DJ, et al. Developing a neonatal acute kidney injury research definition: a report from the NIDDK neonatal AKI workshop. Pediatr Res. 2017;82(4):569–73.
3. Nada A, Bonachea EM, Askenazi DJ. Acute kidney injury in the fetus and neonate.SeminFetal Neonatal Med. 2017;22(2):90–7.
4. Jetton JG, Boohaker LJ, Sethi SK, et al. incidence and outcomes of neonatal acute kidney injury (AWAKEN): a multicentre, multinational, observational cohort study. *Lancet Child Adolesc Health*.2017;1(3):184–94.
5. Harer MW, Adegboro CO, Richard LJ, McAdams RM. Non-invasive continuous renal tissue oxygenation monitoring to identify preterm neonates at risk for acute kidney injury.Pediatr Nephrol.2021 Jun;36(6):1617–25.
6. Hentschel R, Lodige B, Bulla M. Renal insufficiency in the neonatal period. Clin Nephrol 1996: 46:54–8.
7. Bagga A, Sinha A, Gulati A. Protocols in Pediatric Nephrology, 1st e, CBS publishers and Distributors Pvt Ltd.
8. Ishizaki Y, etal, evaluation of diagnostic criteria of acute renal failure in premature infants.ActaPaediatrJpn 1983,35:311–5.

9. Marin T, DeRossett B, Bhatia J. Urinary Biomarkers to Predict Neonatal Acute Kidney Injury: A Review of the Science.J Perinat Neonatal Nurs. 2018 Jul/Sep;32(3):266–74.
10. Basalely, A., Liu, D. &Kaskel, F.J. Big equation for small kidneys: a newly proposed model to estimate neonatal GFR.Pediatr Nephrol 35, 543–6 (2020).
11. Chawla D, Agarwal R, Deorari AK, Paul VK.Fluid and electrolyte management in term and preterm neonates.AIIMS-NICU protocols 2008.
12. Friedrich JO, Adhikari N, Herridge MS. Meta-analysis: Low dose dopamine increases urine output but does not prevent renal dysfunction or death.Ann Intern Med 2005;142:510–24.
13. Seri I. Effects of low dose dopamine infusion on cardiovascular and renal functions cerebral blood flow and plasma cathecolamines levels in sick preterm neonates.Pediatric Res 1993, 34:742–9.
14. Tulassy T, Seri I, Acute oliguria in preterm infants with hyaline membrane disease; interaction of dopamine and frusemide. Acta PediatrScand 1986,75:420–4.
15. Chevalier R. Prognostic factors in neonatal acute renal failure.Pediatrics 1984; 74:165–272.
16. Chaturvedi S, Ng KH, Mammen C. The path to chronic kidney disease following acute kidney injury: a neonatal perspective.Pediatr Nephrol.2017; 32(2):227–41.

CHAPTER

32

Management of Antenatally Diagnosed Hydronephrosis

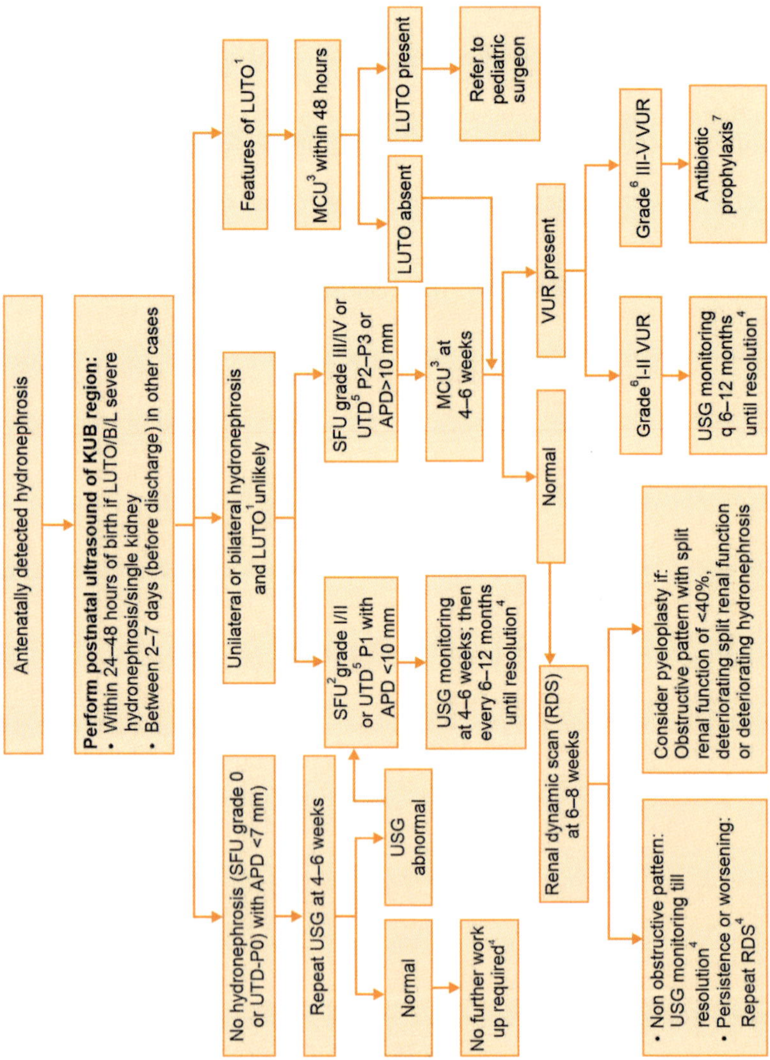

Fig. 32.1: Management of antenatally diagnosed hydronephrosis

APD: Anteroposterior diameter of renal pelvis; *LUTO:* Lower urinary tract obstruction; *MCU:* Micturating cystourethrogram; *USG:* Ultrasound; *VUR:* Vesicoureteric reflux

[1]Lower urinary tract obstruction (LUTO) is suggested by bilateral hydroureteronephrosis associated with oligohydramnios, bladder wall thickening and/ or dilatation

[2]Society of Fetal Urology (SFU) grading for hydronephrosis

- Grade 0: No Splitting of renal pelvis
- Grade I: Urine in pelvis barely splits pelvis
- Grade II: Urine fills intra-renal pelvis ± extra-renal pelvis and one or few major calyces dilated
- Grade III: SFU grade II and minor calyces uniformly dilated and normal parenchymal thickness
- Grade IV: SFU grade III and thin parenchyma

[3]Give antibiotic prophylaxis on the day of procedure (amoxicillin 40 mg/kg one hour prior to, and 20 mg/kg after 6 hours of the procedure).

[4]Counsel parents regarding increased risk of urinary tract infections due to VUR; perform urinalysis and urine culture for any fever without focus and consult pediatrician.

[5]Urinary Tract Dilatation (UTD) classification for hydronephrosis: Postnatal (P) staging beyond 48 hr of life, as follows:

UTD-P0: Normal pelvi-calyceal system and APD <10 mm

UTD-P1: Pelvis and central calyces dilated and APD 10 mm to <15 mm

UTD-P2: Central and peripheral calyces dilated; *abnormal ureter* and APD ≥15 mm

UTD-P3: Central and peripheral calyces dilated; abnormal ureter or bladder; abnormal renal parenchymal thickness or appearance and APD ≥15 mm

[6]Grades of VUR (International reflux study committee)

Grade I: Reflux that involves only the ureter

Grade II: Reflux that involves the ureter, pelvis and the calyces with no dilatation of the and normal calyceal fornices

Grade III: Reflux that involves moderate dilatation and/or tortuosity of the ureter, moderate dilatation of the pelvis and no or slight blunting of the fornices

Grade IV: Reflux that involves moderate dilatation of the pelvis and the blunting of the fornices

Grade V: Reflux that involves gross dilatation of the and tortuosity of the ureter, pelvis and the calyces

[7]Antibiotic prophylaxis: Cephalexin at a dose of 10 mg/kg single daily dose

CHAPTER

33

Posterior Urethral Valve

Posterior urethral valves (PUV) are the most common cause of lower urinary tract obstruction (LUTO). The incidence ranges from 1 in 4000–8000 live births.

CLASSIFICATION

PUV has three categories:

a. **Type 1 (90–95%)** is composed of a ridge, which is continuous from the verumontanum, that divides into two fork-like leaflets and gets attached to the anterior urethra.
b. **Type 2 is** no longer considered a form of PUV but a dissection artifact, which was reported to extend from the verumontanum to the internal sphincter and the bladder neck
c. **Type 3 (5–10%)** is found at various levels of the posterior urethra that forms a diaphragm with a small opening in the center.

CLINICAL PRESENTATION[1,2]

a. **Antenatal:** Severe obstruction can lead to oligohydramnios. The increased urinary bladder pressure may rupture the renal calyx resulting in urinary ascites or perinephric urinoma.
b. **Postnatal:** Neonates with severe PUV can present with respiratory distress secondary to lung hypoplasia. There can be signs of severe systemic illness, such as lethargy and poor feeding. Lung hypoplasia occurs due to oligohydramnios during the canalicular phase of lung development (16–28 weeks of gestation).The abdomen may be distended because of urinary ascites, hydronephrosis, or distended bladder. Vesicoureteric reflux (VUR) is present in approximately one-third of the patients.

DIAGNOSIS

a. **Antenatal:** Prenatal ultrasonography can identify a third of cases. The findings include bilateral hydroureteronephrosis, dilated and thickened bladder (normal bladder thickness up to 3 mm), and the posterior urethra (keyhole sign). Severe cases would have large bladder diverticula or patent urachus. A thickened bladder is a better predictor of PUV than the keyhole sign.

b. **Postnatal:** Ultrasonography shows variable degrees of hydroureteronephrosis, thick bladder wall, and dilated posterior urethra. Voiding cystourethrogram (VCUG) shows the hallmark findings of an enlarged and elongated posterior urethra and bladder neck hypertrophy. Following VCUG, a cystoscopy is done to confirm the results, followed by ablation.[3]

Management[4,5]

a. **Antenatal:** Vesico-amniotic shunt can reverse the oligohydramnios but does not change the overall outcome. Fetal cystoscopy and ablation of the valves have been tried, but it has high complication rates (Fig. 33.1).

b. **Postnatal**
   1. **Drainage of the bladder:** Insert a small catheter (without balloon) or feeding tube to drain the bladder. If it is impossible to catheterize, place a suprapubic catheter, do a VCUG and leave the catheter until the neonate is stable enough for valve ablation.
   2. **Valve ablation:** Once the neonate is stable enough with stable creatinine levels, PUV can be ablated. A check cystoscopy or a VCUG is performed to confirm the procedure's effectiveness. If the urethra is too small to pass a fetal cystoscope, consider suprapubic diversion until valve ablation can be performed safely.
   3. **High urinary diversion:** Despite adequate bladder drainage, if there is still progressive dilatation of the upper tract, no improvement in renal function, or recurrent urinary tract infections, consider high urinary diversion.
   4. **Vesicostomy:** Cutaneous vesicostomy is an alternative to the suprapubic catherization. Vesicostomy is a temporary procedure that stabilizes the urinary tract and allows somatic growth until ablation of the valves can be carried out. However, it could decrease the bladder's capacity.
   5. **Vesicoureteric reflux:** Give antibiotic prophylaxis in high-grade VUR in the initial months. High grade reflux is usually associated with a poorly functioning kidney.
   6. A poorly functioning bladder may respond to early initiation of oxybutynin. High post-void residue might require clean intermittent catheterization (CIC).

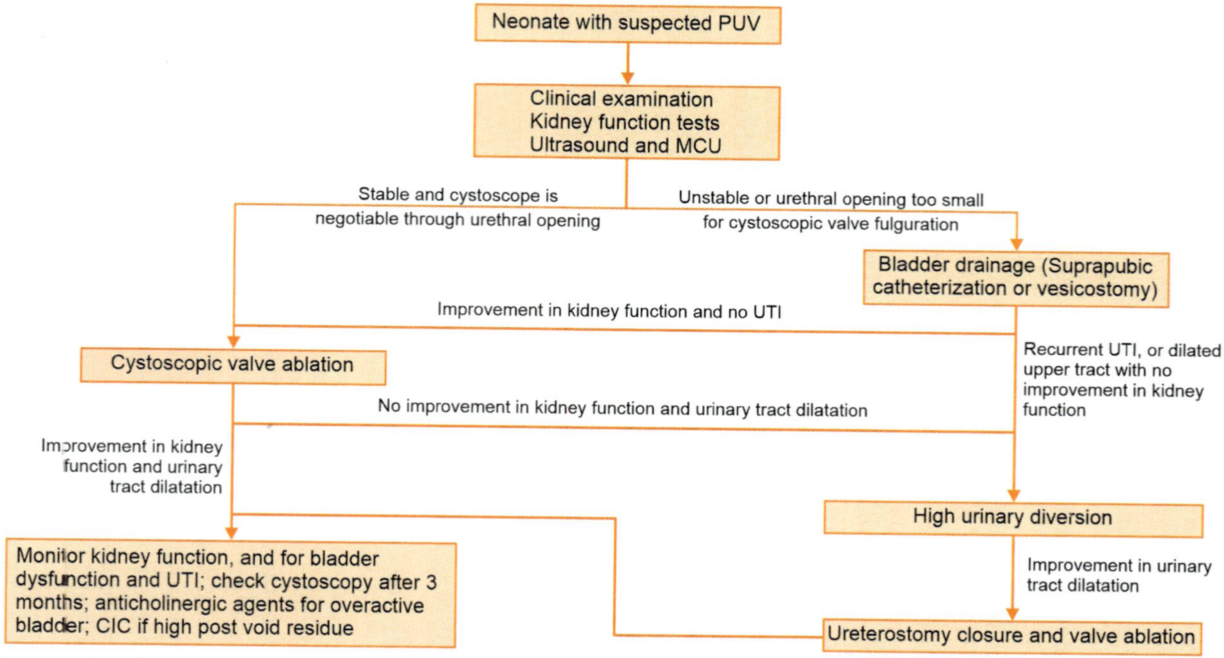

Fig. 33.1. An algorithmic approach for managing a neonate with suspected posterior urethral valves (PUV). A neonate with suspected PUV is considered 'unstable' in the presence of impaired kidney function, dyselectrolytemia, or urosepsis with or without hemodynamic instability.

CIC: Clean intermittent catheterization; *MCU:* Micturating cystourethrography; *UTI:* Urinary tract infections

OUTCOMES[6]

Ten-year survival is more than 90% for those diagnosed with PUV in the first year of life. The primary determinant of mortality in the neonatal period is pulmonary hypoplasia. The risk of chronic kidney disease is nearly 20%, and end-stage kidney disease is 11%. Infants with PUV post-ablation need lifelong monitoring as bladder dysfunction and day/night incontinence are significant concerns. High baseline creatinine in the first year, associated renal dysplasia, and severe bladder dysfunction are risk factors for end-stage kidney disease progression.In the first six months of age, male infants with lower renal parenchymal area in the renal ultrasound are at higher risk for progression to CKD/ESRD.

REFERENCES

1. Ansari MS, Gulia A, Srivastava A, Kapoor R. Risk factors for progression to end-stage renal disease in children with posterior urethral valves. J Pediatr Urol. 2010;6:261–4.
2. Bilgutay AN, Roth DR, Gonzales ET Jr, Janzen N, Zhang W, Koh CJ, et al. Posterior urethral valves: Risk factors for progression to renal failure. J Pediatr Urol. 2016;12:179.e1–7.
3. Oktar T, Acar O, Sancaktutar A, Sanlı O, Tefik T, Ziylan O. Endoscopic treatment of vesicoureteral reflux in children with posterior urethral valves. Int Urol Nephrol 2012;44:1305–9.
4. Morris RK, Malin GL, Quinlan-Jones E, Middleton LJ, Hemming K, Burke D, et al. Percutaneous vesicoamniotic shunting versus conservative management for fetal lower urinary tract obstruction (PLUTO): a randomised trial. Lancet Lond Engl 2013;382:1496–506.
5. Nassr AA, Shazly S a. M, Abdelmagied AM, Araujo Júnior E, Tonni G, Kilby MD, et al. Effectiveness of vesicoamniotic shunt in fetuses with congenital lower urinary tract obstruction: an updated systematic review and meta-analysis. Ultrasound Obstet Gynecol Off J Int Soc Ultrasound Obstet Gynecol. 2017;49:696–703.
6. Pulido JE, Furth SL, Zderic SA, Canning DA, Tasian GE. Renal parenchymal area and risk of ESRD in boys with posterior urethral valves. Clin J Am Soc Nephrol. 2014;9(3):499–505.

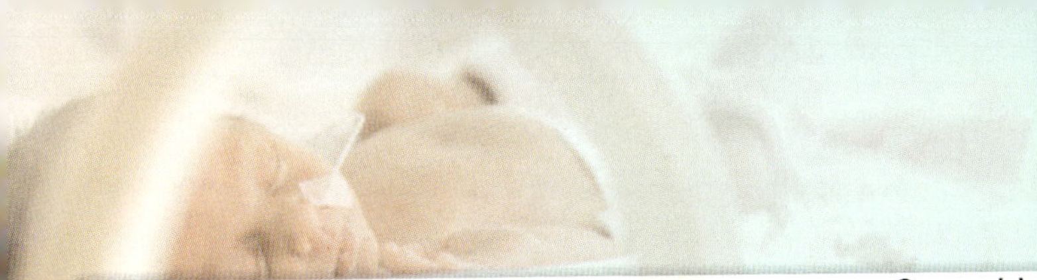

Section

10

Miscellaneous

CHAPTER

34

Follow-up of High-risk Neonates

Improving perinatal-neonatal care has led to increased survival of newborns[1] at high risk of post-discharge morbidities, including growth failure, ongoing medical illnesses, neurosensory impairment, and developmental deficits.

What is the evidence?

A recent systematic review[2] has reported a high prevalence of long term neurodevelopmental sequelae after different intrauterine and neonatal insults,: sepsis 40.0%, meningitis 42.0%, HIE 31.0%, preterm birth 31.0%, jaundice 18.0%, tetanus 26.0%, CMV infection 41.0%.

Most common sequelae: Learning difficulties, cognition or developmental delay; cerebral palsy; hearing impairment and visual impairment.[3,4]

An appropriate and comprehensive follow-up program for high-risk infants will help detect and manage any morbidity associated with perinatal events early. It shall ensure intact survival, optimum growth, and optimal quality of life for these infants.

SETTING-UP–FOLLOW-UP CARE SERVICES

High-risk Clinic: Follow-up of high-risk infants should be done in a dedicated high-risk clinic (HRC). A detailed description is provided under "Procedure for follow-up."

High-risk Follow-up Team: High-risk infant follow-up requires a multidisciplinary approach and an experienced and dedicated team, including personnel from various specialties. Ideally, the team should comprise a neonatologist/pediatrician, a clinical psychologist and an early interventionist, a physiotherapist, an occupational therapist, a neurophysiologist and speech therapist, a nutritionist, and a medical social worker. An ophthalmologist and pediatric neurologist should also be a part of the team, available for ready referral.

The neonatologist/pediatrician is the nodal person of the team who provides and coordinates for holistic management of the high-risk infant and counsels the family. The responsibilities include assessing the child on each visit, including growth and nutrition, managing ongoing morbidities, neurodevelopmental screening, and coordinating care with different specialists involved in managing the infant. Clinical psychologist performs formal developmental evaluation and manages behavioral and other domain-specific problems, while early interventionists work to enhance and facilitate the development of milestones in all domains of action; the physiotherapist is primarily responsible for the assessment and grading of muscle tone and power and plan appropriate training for an infant with tone abnormalities, prescription of appliances/casts and rehabilitation of infants with impairment/disability and the occupational therapist works to promote neuro-motor coordination and perceptual skills, fine motor functions, oro-motor coordination and training in activities of daily living like feeding, bathing, and dressing of children with special needs. Nutritionist can provide detailed complementary feeding advice and serves to manage infants with failure to thrive and those with special conditions (e.g. inborn errors of metabolism). The medical social worker is an essential interface between the follow-up care team and family, who helps to address parental expectations and social and socio-economic issues and coordinates for rehabilitation and integration of infants with impairment/disability. An ophthalmologist is required for treatment and follow-up of ROP and visual assessment and management of refractory errors, strabismus, etc. Neurologist aids in drug therapy and long-term management of neurological illnesses such as refractory seizures. Other specialists from pediatric genetics, pediatric surgery, pediatric cardiology, pediatric gastroenterology, hematology, etc. may be consulted as and when required.

As outlined above, all setups may not have a complete team of specialists. It is, therefore, essential that simple tools be available and the nodal person of the team have working knowledge of all the domains. Ideally, all the services should be provided under one roof as far as possible, and appropriate referrals should be sought as required. The days and timings of the different clinics and the appointment schedule should be marked on the patient's records, and multiple visits should be avoided.

WHO NEEDS FOLLOW-UP CARE?

A rigorous follow-up of all the neonates discharged from a particular health facility would neither be practical nor feasible. Therefore, selecting a cohort of neonates at a higher risk of developing adverse outcomes is essential—'at-risk' or 'high-risk' infants are critical. Selection of high-risk infants should be based on the gestational age, birth weight, occurrence and severity of perinatal/neonatal illnesses, interventions received in the neonatal intensive care unit (NICU), presence of malformations, etc.

There are no standardized criteria for defining high-risk infants, even in tertiary care centers. Commonly used criteria have been outlined here (Table 34.1). These may be modified depending on the level of neonatal care provided by the unit and the mix of the neonatal population the unit caters to.

PREREQUISITES FOR FOLLOW-UP

Discharge planning. Discharge planning should ideally begin many days before discharge. This gives adequate time to the caretakers to ask questions and practice skills. The following criteria should be fulfilled before discharging a high-risk infant:

- Hemodynamically stable; able to maintain body temperature in an open crib.
- On full enteral feeds (either direct breastfeeding or by paladai/spoon).

Table 34.1: High-risk neonates who need follow-up care in a tertiarly care setting
1. Birth weight <1500 grams.
2. Gestation <32 weeks.
3. Infants with BW of 1500 g or more OR gestation 32 week or more AND a. Intrauterine growth <3rd centile. b. Meningitis. c. Received mechanical ventilation for 48 hours or more. d. Hypoxic ischemic encephalopathy stage 2 or higher. e. Major malformations. f. Inborn error of metabolism/chromosomal or genetic disorders/intrauterine infections. g. Symptomatic hypoglycemia. h. Symptomatic polycythemia. i. Retrovirus positive mother. j. Hyperbilirubinemia requiring exchange transfusion OR Rh isoimmunization/cholestasis. k. Abnormal neurological examination at discharge/seizures. l. Major morbidities such as chronic lung disease, IVH grade III or more (Papile's classification), and periventricular leucomalacia.

- Parents are confident enough to take care of the infant at home.
- Has crossed birth weight and showing a stable weight gain for at least three consecutive days; in case of very low birth weight infants, weight should be at least 1600 g before considering discharge.
- Not on any medications (except for vitamins and iron supplementation). Ideally, preterm infants on theophylline/ caffeine therapy for apnea of prematurity should be off treatment for at least 5 days to ensure no recurrence.
- Received vaccination as per schedule (based on postnatal age).

These criteria can be individualized to meet the infant and family's needs.

Counseling before discharge: Counseling is essential in caring for these high-risk infants at home; regular counseling sessions should be done before discharge. Parents should be advised regarding the following:

- Temperature regulation—proper clothing, cap, socks, kangaroo mother care, etc.
- Feeding—The focus should be on exclusive breastfeeding. If required, other types and amounts of milk, method of administration, and nutritional supplementation, if any, should be advised as per the child's need.
- Prevention of infections—handwashing, avoidance of visitors, etc.
- Follow-up visits—where and when (refer to Table 34.2).
- Danger signs—recognition and where to report if symptoms are present.
- Vaccination—schedule, next visit, etc.
- Special needs—e.g. subsequent visits for ROP screening, USG/ MRI brain, etc.

If possible, the family should be provided with the telephone number of the nursery/health care provider, e.g. the on-duty doctor, in case the family needs to consult for the infant's illness in an emergency or otherwise.

PROCEDURE FOR FOLLOW-UP

The family must be provided with a structured discharge summary, including the details of important events during the hospital stay, investigations and treatment received, and the schedule of follow-up visits. The venue and follow-up dates should be indicated on the discharge summary.

High-risk Clinic: A specified site should be earmarked for follow-up services. The venue, days, and timings of the clinic should be fixed. Prior appointments should be given, and ad-hoc visits should be discouraged. Registration procedures at the clinic should be simplified to avoid any undue delays.

Venue: Dedicated room(s) in the OPD premises should be designated for high-risk follow-up.

Days and Timing: One or more fixed days and times of the week should be allocated for the clinic.

Registration: The high-risk infant should be registered at the clinic on the first visit following hospital discharge. An OPD card for the same should be made.

Record Maintenance: A separate file for each high-risk infant should be made on the day of infant registration in the HRC. The HRC case file should have a uniform format and include the following information for each infant:

- Demographic and contact details of infants' family.
- Detailed diagnosis at discharge.
- Details of any intermittent morbidities/any critical investigations, e.g. cranial USG/MRI brain.
- Reports of hearing and vision (ROP) screening, as applicable.
- Nutritional details.
- Anthropometry (weight, head circumference, and length).
- Developmental screening chart.
- Neurological assessment proforma.
- Immunization details.
- Doctor's evaluation and note.

A copy of the discharge summary should be maintained in all these files for a ready referral. Essential details and advice should also be noted in the OPD card.

WHEN TO FOLLOW-UP

The follow-up schedule should be explained to the parents at discharge and should also be mentioned in the discharge summary (*see* below).

For follow-up visits, at-risk infants can be grouped under two major categories:

Table 34.2: Follow-up schedule for at-risk infants
Very preterm infants (<32 weeks or <1500 g) • After 3–7 days of discharge to check if the infant has adjusted well in the home environment. • Every 2 weeks until a body weight of 3 kg (6, 10 and 14 week immunization visits to be covered during these visits). • At 3, 6, 9,12, 15 and 18 months of corrected age and then every 6 months until 8 years of age. • More visits if required.
Infants with other conditions • Two weeks after discharge • At 6, 10, 14 weeks of age • At 6, 9, 12, 15 and 18 months of corrected/postnatal age, as applicable and then every 6 months until 8 years of age • More visits if required.

- Very preterm or very low birth weight (VLBW; <1500 g) infants and
- Infants with other conditions

The follow-up schedule for both these categories has been summarized in Table 34.2. This schedule represents a minimum number of visits for high-risk neonates. More frequent visits are recommended if the infant has ongoing issues or illness. Note that first contact of the infant with the health providers after discharge is essential and helps identify adjustment problems at home. Ideally, this contact should be achieved by the home visit, preferably within the first week of discharge.

Very low birth weight infants or those born at less than 32 weeks gestation (or bigger and sick infants) should be followed up for an eye check-up for retinopathy of prematurity till the postnatal age of 44 weeks (*see* chapter 35: ROP protocol).

Some neurological abnormalities identified in the first year of life are transient or improve, whereas findings in other children may worsen over time.[5] Standard follow-up for many multicenter networks is currently at 18–24 months corrected age. By 12 months, corrected age, the cognitive and language assessment can be done. By 18–24 months of corrected age, there is an improved prediction of early school-age performance.[6–8] Long-term follow-up is essential because minor neurological disabilities may not be detected early and become apparent only with increasing age.

Practice tip!

Corrected age: Age of the child since the expected date of delivery. The correction for gestational immaturity at birth should be done until 24 months age. All anthropometric parameters and developmental milestones are assessed according to corrected age to compensate for the prematurity. The initiation of complementary feeds is also according to corrected age.

Postnatal age: Age of the child since birth. Immunization is done according to postnatal age.

WHAT SHOULD BE DONE AT FOLLOW-UP?

Table 34.3 summarizes the follow-up plan.

1. **Assessment of feeding and dietary counseling:** Parents should be asked about the infants' diet and offered dietary counseling at each visit. Breastfeeding frequency and adequacy should be assessed. The amount, dilution, and feeding mode should be noted if supplemental feeding is given. It is a good idea to enquire about the source of milk as milk supplied by local vendors is often diluted (dilution has the same impact on the infant whether done by the family or the vendor!). It is also essential to record the duration of exclusive breastfeeding. If an infant is not gaining adequate weight on exclusive breastfeeding, take care of any illness or maternal problems which may interfere with feeding and milk output. Supplementation may be considered if poor weight gain persists despite all measures to improve breast milk output.

   We start complementary feeding at six months of corrected age. Initially, semisolids should be advised as per the local cultural practices. Spend adequate time explaining what and how to give. Giving too little or dilute complementary food, such as rice-water, dal-water, too much juice, etc. should be discouraged (Table 34.4).[9]

   Complementary foods (CF) should include a variety and adequate quantities of food groups (meat, poultry, fish, or eggs, as well as vitamin A-rich fruits and vegetables) daily. If not possible, use fortified foods and vitamin-mineral supplements to ensure adequate nutrient intake. As infants age, complementary foods should change from semisolid to solid, and the variety of foods should also increase. By eight months, infants should eat 'finger foods.' By 12 months of age, most children eat family food.

   Micronutrient supplementation: The LBW Feeding protocol may be referred to for the same.

Table 34.3: Follow-up plan for high-risk infants

Assessment	*Age in months*								
	1	2	3	6	9	12	15	18	24........8 years
Assessment of feeding and dietary counseling	All visits								
Growth monitoring	All visits								
Immunization	As per schedule (based on postnatal age)								
Ongoing morbidities	All visits and as and when required								
Neurological examination			*	*	*	*	–	*	*
Developmental screening	All visits								
Formal developmental assessment			*	¶	¶	*	–	*	*
Hearing (BERA)			*	¶	¶	¶	–	¶	¶
Ophthalmic evaluation	ROP screening				*	¶	–	¶	¶
USG/MRI brain	As indicated								

¶ *If the previous test abnormal*

Table 34.4: Amount and frequency of complementary foods

Age	*Foods*	*Frequency*
6–8 months	Thick, soft porridge (khichri/dalia); add sugar and oil mixed with either milk or pounded ground nuts. Mixtures of mashed foods made of potatoes or millet or rice; mix with fish or beans or pounded groundnuts; add green vegetables	Breastfeeding plus 2–3 meals per day
9–11 months	–Do– Give nutritious snacks between meals, like eggs, bananas, or bread	Breastfeeding plus 3–4 meals/day plus one snack between meals
12–24 months	–Do– Family foods, chopped or mashed if necessary	3–4 meals/day plus two snacks between meals

2. **Growth monitoring:** Growth (including weight, head circumference, and length) should be monitored and plotted on an appropriate growth chart at each visit. The infant's growth pattern (slope of the curve) is compared with the standard curve; any deviation should be noted and appropriate remedial action taken. We use Fenton's charts (till 50 weeks postmenstrual age; PMA)[10] and WHO growth charts after that for growth monitoring of preterm neonates.[11]

   Anthropometry should be taken during follow-up visits. Weight and head circumference should be monitored at each visit and length three monthly. These should be marked on the gender-specific WHO-MGRS growth charts. The **Corrected age** of the child should be used while using these charts for preterm infants.

3. **Immunization:** Parents should be offered the option of additional vaccines such as hepatitis B, *Hemophilus influenza* B, and MMR (where not in the routine immunization schedule) if they can afford them. Immunization should be ensured according to chronological age.

4. **Ongoing morbidity surveillance and management:** Ongoing morbidity and its management is one of the essential services a follow-up clinic is meant to provide. These may relate to prolonged jaundice, recurrent exacerbations of respiratory distress in a child with chronic lung disease, gastroesophageal reflux or other feeding difficulties or inadequate weight gain in

a preterm infant, anemia in an infant with Rh immunization, cardiac failure in an infant with congenital heart disease, diagnostic evaluation and intermittent illnesses in an infant born to HIV positive mother, etc. The details of any such intermittent morbidity/hospitalization should be systematically recorded in the high-risk file as well as the OPD card of the infant.

5. **Developmental follow-up:**[12] Early identification of infants who are at risk of developmental disability allows for appropriate parent counseling and for planning for the child's future. This counseling and planning should consider the uncertainty of standardized developmental screening tests that should be performed at 3, 6, 9, 18, and 24 months of corrected age. Regular screening is more helpful than a single screening to identify problems, especially in later-developing skills such as language. Screening does not help in making a diagnosis or designing a treatment plan but helps identify areas where a child's development differs from same-age norms.

   Early identification of developmental problems should lead to further developmental and medical evaluation, diagnosis, and treatment, including early developmental intervention. A pediatrician/neonatologist must be well-versed in the normal developmental milestones and be able to use the available screening tools effectively so that a formal developmental evaluation is required only for the most deserving cases.

   We currently use Trivandrum Developmental Screening Chart (TDSC) in our clinic. DDST-II is also used in some places, though it requires some training before it may be used. Table 34.5 lists the commonly available and used screening tests in India.

Practice tip!

Waiting until a child misses a major milestone such as walking or talking may delay the recognition of a problem that deprives the child benefits of early intervention.

Additional tools like VSMS, CBCL, and M-CHAT may be used beyond infancy (beginning at 18 months of age) for social, emotional, behavioral, and autism evaluation, respectively (Table 34.6).

A formal developmental assessment is done using DASII, which is the Indian adaptation of BSID-II and is considered to be the gold standard to date in Indian settings. It measures motor and mental domains using 230 items in children between 0–30 months

Table 34.5: Developmental screening tests commonly available in India

Test	*Domains assessed*	*Age range*	*No. of items*	*Psychometric properties*
Trivandrum Development Screening Test (TDSC)[13]	Gross motor, Fine motor, Vision/hearing, and personal/ social/language	0–2 years	17	Sensitivity 66.7%; Specificity 78.8%; validated against DDST
Denver Developmental Screening Test-II (DDST-II) or/ Denver-II	Gross motor, Language, Fine motor—adaptive, and personal-social. Also, a behavior rating scale	0–6 years	123	Sensitivity 83%; Specificity 43%[14]
Baroda Development Screening Test (BDST)[15]	Motor and mental	0–30 months	54	Sensitivity and specificity of 65–95%

Table 34.6: Other tools relevant to developmental evaluation early in life

Test	*Brief description*	*Age*
Screening tools		
Modified checklist of autism for toddlers (M-CHAT)	To identify children who may benefit from a more thorough developmental and autism evaluation	16–30 months
Vineland social maturity scale (VSMS)	Indian adaptation by Malins is available Assesses personal and social skills in the following areas: Self- help general, self-help eating, self-help dressing, self-direction, occupation, communication, locomotion, and socialization	0–15 years
Vineland adaptive behavior scale-II	It is a revision of the Vineland social maturity scale (VSMS) Assesses personal and social adaptive behavior skills in five domains-communication, daily living skills, socialization, motor skills, and maladaptive behavior (optional)	Birth–90 years

(Contd.)

Table 34.6: Other tools relevant to developmental evaluation early in life (*Contd.*)

Test	*Brief description*	*Age*
Screening tools		
Child Behavior Checklist-Language development survey (CBCL-LDS $1^1/_2$)	Assesses different domains of behavior like emotionally reactive, anxious depressed, somatic complaints, withdrawn, sleep problems, attention problems, and aggressive behavior, along with language	1.6–5 years

of age. However, such tools are considered ideal to be periodically revalidated to account for secular trends. Also, since the arrival of BSID-III, which helps assess neurodevelopment in different domains (Cognitive, Language-receptive and expressive, fine and gross motor, socio-emotional, and adaptive behavior) till 42 months of age, it should be adapted and validated for use in India. Additional diagnostic tools for autism, intelligence, and specific learning disabilities may also be required as the child grows up (Table 34.7).

Table 34.7: Few diagnostic tools relevant to high-risk infants

Test	*Brief description*	*Age*
Development Assessment Scale for Indian Infants (DASII)	• An Indian adaptation of Bayley-II, standardized on the Indian population. • Assesses two domains—Motor and mental. • Gives the developmental age of a child expressed as the percentile of normal. • Provides developmental quotients comparing the developmental and corrected age of the child.	Birth–30 months
Childhood Autism Rating Scale (CARS)	• Behavior rating scale. • Assessment on fifteen items—relationship to people, imitation, emotional response, use of body and object, adapt to change, visual and listening response, response to taste-smell-touch, presence of fear and nervousness, verbal and non-verbal communication, activity level, intellectual response, and general impression.	3–22 years

(*Contd.*)

Table 34.7: Few diagnostic tools relevant to high-risk infants (*Contd.*)

Test	*Brief description*	*Age*
Wechsler Preschool and Primary Scale of Intelligence-Third Edition (WPPSI-III)	• Test of Intelligence for younger children. • Provides verbal IQ, performance IQ, and full-scale IQ. • Comprises 14 subsets of three types: core, supplemental, or optional, which are - receptive vocabulary, block design, information, object assembly, picture naming, similarities, symbol search, vocabulary, word reasoning, coding, comprehension, picture completion, matrix reasoning, and picture concepts. • Children in the two years 6 months – 3 years 11 months age band are administered only the initial five subtests.	Divided into two age bands: 2 years 6 months to 3 years 11 months and 4–7 years 3 months
Malins Intelligence Scale for Indian Children (MISIC)	• An Indian adaptation of Wechsler's Intelligence Scale for Children. • Gives verbal and performance IQ. • Assess the following items: – *Verbal IQ*-Information, comprehension, arithmetic, similarities, vocabulary, digit span. – *Performance IQ*-Picture completion, picture arrangement, block design, object assembly, coding, and mazes. • Based on test scores, the intelligence grades are provided as extremely Low, borderline, low average, average, high average, superior and very superior.	6–15 years 11 months
NIMHANS Battery for specific learning disabilities	• The battery of tests for evaluating children suspected of having learning disabilities (dyslexia, dysgraphia, dyscalculia). • Consists of 2 levels for assessment of pre-academic skills for 5–7 years (includes evaluation of attention, auditory and visual discrimination, visual and auditory memory, speech and language, visual-motor, and writing and number skills) and academic skills at level 2 for age 8–12 years (which include attention, reading, spelling, perceptual-motor, visual-motor integration, memory, and arithmetic skills).	Two age bands: 5–7 years and 8–12 years

Also, if feasible, an objective assessment of the home environment shall be a good adjunct to any developmental evaluation of such children.

6. **Neurologic examination:** The main focus of neurological assessment during the high-risk follow-up visits is usually the evaluation of muscle tone besides vision and hearing. However, a complete neurological examination should be performed if indicated in a particular child. Amiel Tison's neurological assessment is currently the most widely used neurological examination tool during early follow-up of infants.

   Evaluation of muscle tone is an integral part of the neurological examination. A waxing and waning pattern of neuromotor development from 28 weeks of gestation to the end of the first year of life was reported by Amiel-Tison. From 28 to 40 weeks gestation, muscle tone and motor function acquisition spread from the lower extremities towards the head (caudo-cephalic progression). After full term, the process is reversed so that relaxation and motor control proceed downwards for the next 12–18 months (cephalocaudal). So, the upper limbs begin to relax and acquire skills before the lower limbs. The axial tone follows a similar pattern. Head control appears first, followed by the ability to sit, stand and walk. Hypertonia or hypotonia should be examined by measuring the following angles: adductor angle, popliteal angle, ankle dorsiflexion, and scarf sign; any asymmetry between the extremities should also be recorded. Any history of seizures or involuntary movements should also be recorded.

   The following angles should be measured to assess tone, as shown in Table 34.8:

   The Hammersmith Neonatal Neurological Examination (HNNE) is a practical and easy-to-perform neonatal neurological examination that has 34 items assessing tone, motor patterns, observation of spontaneous movements, reflexes, visual and auditory attention, and behavior.[16] Each of the 34 items is

Table 34.8: Muscle tone norms (Amiel-Tison)

Age (mo)	*Adductor angle*	*Popliteal angle*	*Dorsiflexion angle*	*Scarf sign*
0–3	40–80°	80–100°	60–70°	The elbow does not cross the midline
4–6	70–110°	90–120°	60–70°	Elbow crosses midline
7–9	110–140°	110–160°	60–70°	The elbow goes beyond the axillary line
10–12	140–160°	150–170°	60–70°	–

assigned a score ("raw score"). Each row for a particular item is scored as 1,2,3,4,5 and if an item falls between two columns, it is given ½ score, e.g. 3.5. Individual optimality score is assigned for each item based on the raw score and the total optimality score is calculated by adding individual optimality score. The maximum possible score is 34. The presence of a suboptimal score does not mean that a neonate is abnormal. It just means that the neonate needs to be reassessed. The number of items falling outside the 90th centile is a better predictor of the severity of the outcome than global optimality. Preterm infants at term are more hyperexcitable and have less flexor tone in the limbs and less extensor tone in the neck in the sitting posture. They have a wider range in individual optimality scores than term. They generally have a wide range and lower scores and it may be difficult to define an optimality cutoff.

Cerebral palsy usually presents with definitely abnormal neurological examination with upper motor neuron signs with motor developmental delay. Hypertonia in lower limbs is defined as when either adductor angle is restricted to less than the age-specific norms as per Amiel–Tison or if there is scissoring or tight tendo-Achilles or restriction of ankle dorsiflexion on extension of knee. Hypertonia in upper limbs is defined as when the scarf sign does not cross the midline at one year corrected age. Hypertonia of the neck extensors can be inferred by an increased gap between the nape of the neck and examination table with the infant lying in the supine position. Truncal extensor hypertonia is present when the body tends to go into hyperextension or opisthotonus. Any tone abnormality requires a detailed evaluation and management by a trained physiotherapist.

The level of function in cerebral palsy should be categorized according to the Gross Motor Functional Classification System (GMFCS). Notably, even in children without cerebral palsy, the prevalence of motor impairment is 19% for moderate impairment and 40% for mild-moderate impairment.[17] With advances in neonatal intensive care, a new era of this no-CP "high-risk neonates" may be emerging. To identify these issues the first formal assessment is done at 3 months corrected age. As a single assessment is not sufficient, longitudinal follow-up is required up to at least two years.

During follow-up, at the end of 12 months, three major patterns can be identified:

a. Normal at all examinations,
b. Tone abnormalities and developmental delay suggests a definite brain injury, or
c. Abnormal development at 3, 6 months age and improving at 9 months and normal at 12 months age.

This third pattern of transient tone abnormalities has been described in preterm infants as neurological abnormalities which present early and disappear by 1 year of age. These infants have similar IQ compared to normal children but have significantly poor scores in cognitive function and are more likely to present as learning difficulties as they grow older.

7. **Hearing evaluation:** High-risk infants have a higher incidence of moderate to profound hearing loss (2.5–5% vs. 1% in normal infants). Since clinical screening is often unreliable, brainstem auditory evoked responses (BAER/BERA) should be performed on these infants before three months of postnatal age.

We do a screening BERA (*A*utomated *A*uditory *B*rainstem *R*esponse-AABR) initially in all cases before discharge.[18] Those who fail on the first screen are re-screened before discharge to minimize the false positivity rates.[19] Those failing on the second screen are referred for a diagnostic BERA in the Department of ENT.

- OAEs may be used at both steps in infants without risk factors, but for infants with risk factors, it is imperative to use an AABR for the initial screen so that neural hearing loss will not be missed.
- For premature infants (born at <34 weeks of gestation), hearing screening should ideally be done after they reach 34 weeks postmenstrual age as it has been shown to decrease false positive results.
- For readmissions in the first month of life for all infants at high risk (e.g. hyperbilirubinemia requiring exchange transfusion or meningitis), a repeat hearing screening is recommended before discharge.
- Any infant missing the initial screen should be instructed to return for a screen after six weeks, which may coincide with the immunization visit (to minimize fallouts).

However, even after a two-stage screening with an OAE pass followed by an AABR pass, permanent hearing loss has been significant.[20] Therefore, it is essential to continue hearing follow-ups.[21]

8. **Vision assessment:** Besides the check-up for retinopathy of prematurity which should start in the NICU and continue till 40–44 weeks postconceptional age or till the retinal vessels have matured (*refer to* Chapter 35: Retinopathy of Prematurity), the children should have an assessment for eye problems in the newborn period and then at all subsequent routine health supervision visits. The eye evaluation during follow-up should include the following:[22]

   Ocular history: Parents' observations are valuable and should be sought. Ask questions such as:
   a. Is the child able to see well?
   b. If the child holds objects close to her eyes while focusing?
   c. Do they find the child's eyes straight?
   d. Do the eyes seem to cross or seem hazy?
   e. Do eyes appear unusual?

   Vision assessment: The vision is evaluated by assessing the capability to fix and follow among children younger than three years or those not verbal yet. One should determine if an eye can fix and maintain it on an object and then be able to follow the object in different positions. If a child fails to do so, it indicates a significant visual impairment. The assessment should be performed with both eyes together and each eye separately. If there is a poor fixation and following binocularly after the age of 3 months, one should suspect a significant bilateral eye or brain abnormality. In such cases, a formal assessment is required. These examinations should only be done if the child is awake and alert, as disinterest or lack of cooperation may mimic a poor vision response.

   In addition, an external evaluation of the different eye structures, including lids, conjunctiva, sclera, cornea, and iris, should be performed, and ocular alignment should be checked. Strabismus can occur at any age, indicating serious orbital, intraocular, or intracranial disease. Examine pupils and red reflex to detect opacities in the visual axis, such as cataracts, corneal abnormality, or abnormalities in the posterior side of the eye, including retinal detachment. Examination of both eyes together permits the detection of potentially amblyopic conditions like asymmetric refractive errors or strabismus.

   Visual acuity should be formally assessed at nine months of age using the Cardiff or the Teller acuity cards. Rehabilitation for visual impairment should be early so that the child gets appropriate stimulation. The child should be provided with glasses or corrective surgery as appropriate.

9. **Role of neuroimaging:**[23]

   For very preterm neonates: Routine screening cranial ultrasound (CUS) is recommended for preterm neonates below 32 weeks gestation at the postnatal age of 7–14 days and between 36 and 40 weeks PMA. MRI brain detects more abnormalities than CUS; however, the current evidence does not support its routine use for neurodevelopmental prognosis.

   Term infants with asphyxia: The conventional (T1, T2) and diffusion weighted (DWI) MRI scans can help in diagnosis (global hypoxia-ischemia, focal infarction), time of insult, and the outcome. The conventional MRI performed during the neonatal period carries a pooled sensitivity of 91% and specificity of 51% to detect abnormal neurological outcomes at ≥1 year.

   Timing of scan: The prognostic utility of MRI has been shown from days 3–14. Late MRI (days 8–30) has higher sensitivity than early MRI (days 1 and 7) for prediction of outcome at age one year.

   Term neonates with bilirubin encephalopathy: An MRI should be considered for infants with bilirubin encephalopathy. It should be done in the newborn period once the infant is clinically stable.

Early Enrichment

The evidence concerning the usefulness of early stimulation and intervention for high-risk neonates is limited to preterm and low birth-weight infants, mostly from developed countries.[24]

What is the evidence

The Newborn Individualized Developmental Care and Assessment Program (NIDCAP) developed to stimulate preterm infants at levels adapted to the child's degree of neurological maturity shows promising findings, primarily on cognitive and motor development, though the scientific evidence on the effects is limited.[25]

Early intervention programs (beginning in NICU and post hospital discharge) suggest positive influence on cognitive and motor development.[24, 25]

Early intervention programs from birth to nine years for children with physical disabilities result in positive outcomes for both children and families.[26]

A few measures that may help have been outlined below. These include tactile, kinesthetic, auditory, and visual components:

Birth–2 months	Place your infant's head and neck on the crook of your elbow and forearm while lifting or carrying her.
2–4 months	Help your infant to roll by placing her on either side and calling her name or making a sound with the rattle from behind encouraging her to turn.
4–6 months	Play different types of music for her to listen. Make her sit in front of the mirror and imitate the sounds that she makes. Roll a medium size ball gently in front of her for her to follow. Give her small light rattles to hold in each hand. Encourage her to sit by herself leaning on her arms and taking their support. Start an activity that she enjoys and then stop to see if she moves her body in the same manner to indicate her desire to continue the play.
6–8 months	Give her a spoon to bang on a steel plate, a small drum to bang her hand on, a rattle to shake, and paper to crumble and tear (please be there when she is playing with paper). Cover your face with a plain cloth, slowly remove it and say jha or thuki, and hug her. Repeat the activities a couple of times on yourself and then take her hand to pull off the cloth. Once she is familiar with the game cover her face and you pull off the cloth, clap, and show excitement. Call the child by one name only and encourage her to respond by smiling at her if she looks. Make her sit independently for 5–10 mins by putting her brightly colored and musical toys in front of her. If she loses balance, after some time help her to sit again by holding her by the hips lightly. Encourage crawling when she is on her tummy by placing her favorite toy in front of her just a little out of her reach so that she has to stretch her hands and push herself forward. Repeat the sounds of da da, ma ma, ga ga, ba ba that she makes. Pretend you understand them and answer back in your mother tongue with different intonations. Keep talking to her and naming all the family members who come to her, hold or play with her.

(Contd.)

(Contd.)

8–10 months	Put two blocks in each hand and encourage her to bang them together while looking at them. Encourage her to clap her hands. Hold her hand and help her to take out toys one by one from a tub filled with toys. Once she has learned to take out the toys, hold her hand and encourage her to drop the toys back into the tub one by one. When a family member leaves, ask her to wave bye bye. Take her in your lap and show her picture books with single, large, colorful pictures of everyday objects and animals. You name and point at the pictures.
10–12 months	Show her the functions of objects used in daily life, like glass for drinking, mobile for talking, comb for the hair. Encourage her to hold furniture and take some steps around it.
12–15 months	Take her hand and help her to point to a toy or any food item she wants. You say the name of the toy and encourage her to take out a sound resembling the name. Hold her lightly from the back and give her the confidence to take a few steps on her own.

HOW TO ENSURE A GOOD FOLLOW-UP RATE

A good follow-up rate may be ensured through the following:

The importance of follow-up should be routinely emphasized to the parents during the hospital stay. Elder members of the family, especially grandmothers should be involved in the process.

The permanent and present addresses of the families should be maintained, along with phone numbers. It shall be ideal if a person of follow-up team like the medical social worker can make an early visit to the infant's home, either at discharge or within 48–72 hours of discharge.

1. It is highly desirable that a permanent 24 × 7 helpline no. be provided to the family at discharge to contact in case of any problem. Regular contact with the parents with inquiry about the status of the child during follow-up shall be helpful.
2. An easily accessible, less time consuming, and hassle-free organizational flow of follow-up services, including the provision of comprehensive assessments under one roof shall encourage parents to come for regular follow-ups.

3. A person who serves as care coordinator and handles all appointments and services shall add to the quality of care experience of the families coming for follow-up.

Practice tip!

The most important determinant of if the family would come for follow-up is the availability of comprehensive and reliable clinical services that family can access easily in a dignified manner.

REFERENCES

1. National neonatology forum of India, National neonatal perinatal database-2002–2003.
2. Mwaniki MK, Atieno M, Lawn JE, Newton CR. Long term neurodevelopmental outcomes after intrauterine and neonatal insults: a systematic review. Lancet 2012 Feb 4;379(9814):445–52. Epub 2012 Jan 13.
3. MKC Nair, Chacko DS, Paul MK, Nair L, George B, Kumar GS. Low birth weight infants- outcome at 13 years. Indian Pediatrics, vol 46 supplement, jan 2009 S71-S74.
4. Chaudhari S, Otiv M, Chitale A, Pandit A, Hoge m. Pune low birth weight study-cognitive abilities and ediucational performance at twelve years. Indian Pediatr 2004 Feb;41:121–8.
5. Drillien C. Abnormal neurological signs in the first year of life in low birth weight infants: possible prognostic significance. Dev Med Child Neurol 1997;14:575–84.
6. Weisglas-Kuperus N, Baerts W, Smrkovsky M, Sauer PJ. Effects of biological and social factors on the cognitive development of very low birth weight children. *Pediatrics.*1993; 92:658–65.
7. Dezoete JA, MacArthur BA, Tuck B. Prediction of Bayley and Stanford-Binet scores with a group of very low birthweight children. *Child Care Health Dev.*2003; 29:367–72.
8. Lee H, Barratt MS. Cognitive development of preterm low birth weight children at 5 to 8 years old. *J Dev* Behav Pediatr.1993; 14:242–9.
9. Guiding principles for complementary feeding of the breastfed child. Freely downloadable from WHO website (http://whqlibdoc.who.int/paho/2003/a85622.pdf).
10. Fenton TR, Nasser R, Eliasziw M, Kim JH, Bilan D, Sauve R. Validating the weight gain of preterm infants between the reference growth curve of the fetus and the term infant. BMC Pediatr. 2013 Jun 11;13:92.
11. De Onis M, Onyago AW, J, Chumlea WC, Martorell R. Measurement and standardization protocols for anthropometry used in the construction of a new international growth reference. Food Nutr Bull 2004 Mar;25(1 suppl):s27–36.
12. Council on Children with Disabilities, Section on Developmental Behavioral Pediatrics, Bright Futures Steering Committee and Medical Home Initiatives

for Children with Special Needs Project Advisory Committee. Identifying infants and young children with developmental disorders in the medical home: an algorithm for developmental surveillance and screening. Pediatrics 2006;118:405–20.

13. Nair MK, George B, Philip E, Lekshmi MA, Haran JC, Sathy N. Trivandrum Developmental Screening Chart. Indian Pediatr 1991 Aug;28(8):869–72.
14. Glascoe FP, Byrne KE, Ashford LG, Johnson KL, Chang B, Strickland B. Accuracy of the Denver-II in developmental screening. Pediatrics 1992 Jun;89 (6 Pt 2):1221–5.
15. Phatak AT, Khurana B. Baroda development screening test for infants. Indian Pediatr 1991 Jan;28(1):31–7.
16. Dubowitz L, Mercuri E, Dubowitz V. An optimality score for the neurologic examination of the term newborn. J Pediatr. 1998 Sep;133(3):406–16.
17. Williams J, Lee KJ, Anderson PJ. Prevalence of motor-skill impairment in preterm children who do not develop cerebral palsy: a systematic review. Dev Med Child Neurol. 2010 Mar;52(3):232–7.
18. Clemens CJ, Davis SA.Minimizing false-positives in universal newborn hearing screening: a simple solution. Pediatrics 2001;107:E29.
19. Coenraad S, Toll MS, Hoeve HL, Goedegebure A. Auditory brainstem response morphology and analysis in very preterm neonatal intensive care unit infants. Laryngoscope 2011 ;121:2245-9. doi: 10.1002/lary.22140. Epub 2011 Sep 6.
20. Lin HC, Shu MT, Lee KS, Ho GM, Fu TY, Bruna S, Lin G. Comparison of hearing screening programs between one step with transient evoked otoacoustic emissions (TEOAE) and two steps with TEOAE and automated auditory brainstem response. Laryngoscope 2005 Nov;115:1957–62.
21. Committee on Practice and Ambulatory Medicine, Section on Ophthalmology. American Association of Certified Orthoptists; American Association for Pediatric Ophthalmology and Strabismus; American Academy of Ophthalmology.Eye examination in infants, children, and young adults by pediatricians. Pediatrics 2003 Apr;111:902–7.
22. Ment LR, Bada HS, Barnes P, Grant PE, Hirtz D, Papile LA, Pinto-Martin J, Rivkin M, Slovis TL. Practice parameter: neuroimaging of the neonate: report of the Quality Standards Subcommittee of the American Academy of Neurology and the Practice Committee of the Child Neurology Society. Neurology 2002 Jun 25;58:1726–38.
23. Thayyil S, Chandrasekaran M, Taylor A, Bainbridge A, Cady EB, Chong WK, Murad S, Omar RZ, Robertson NJ. Cerebral magnetic resonance biomarkers in neonatal encephalopathy: a meta-analysis. Pediatrics 2010;125(2): e382–95.
24. McCormick MC, Brooks-Gunn J, Buka SL, Goldman J, Yu J, Salganik M, Scott DT, Bennett FC, Kay LL, Bernbaum JC, Bauer CR, Martin C, Woods ER, Martin A, Casey PH. Early intervention in low birth weight premature infants: results at 18 years of age for the Infant Health and Development Program. Pediatrics 2006 Mar;117:771–80.

25. Wallin L, Eriksson M. Newborn Individual Development Care and Assessment Program (NIDCAP): a systematic review of the literature. Worldviews Evid Based Nurs 2009;6:54–69.
26. Spittle AJ, Orton J, Doyle LW, Boyd R. Early developmental intervention programs post hospital discharge to prevent motor and cognitive impairments in preterm infants. Cochrane Database Syst Rev 2007 Apr 18;(2):CD005495.

CHAPTER

35

Retinopathy of Prematurity

Retinopathy of prematurity (ROP) is a vasoproliferative disorder of the retina in preterm infants. Neonates born at less than 32 weeks of gestation are at risk of developing ROP. However, preterm infants born at 32 weeks or later can also develop severe ROP if they have had a turbulent clinical course or needed prolonged oxygen therapy. Nearly one-fourth of neonates undergoing screening may show some degree of ROP, which regresses on its own in the majority. In a few infants, ROP, if untreated it can progress to the stage of retinal detachment and blindness. Timely screening and treatment of ROP can prevent blindness and minimize visual handicaps.

What is the evidence?

Studies from India have reported ROP (any stage) in 20–52% of the screened neonates.[1–10] More recent studies have reported a lower incidence of ROP (20–32.3%) and severe ROP (17.7%).[1–3]

ROP CLASSIFICATION

International Classification of ROP (ICROP) 3rd edition is used for classifying ROP.[11] ICROP-3 describes vascularization of the retina and characterizes ROP by its position (zone), severity (stage), and extent (clock hours) (Fig. 35.1 and Table 35.1).

Aggressive ROP (A-ROP): This is a type of ROP with rapidly developing pathological neovascularization along with a severe plus disease. The typical feature of A-ROP is the risk of rapid progression to retinal detachment without sequential progression through the typical stages of ROP. A-ROP may also show abnormal retinal vessels posterior to the previous edge of vascularization. If not detected and managed, A-ROP can progress rapidly to retinal detachment. Although, typically described to develop in zone I or posterior zone II (hence, previously called aggressive-posterior ROP) and in extremely preterm neonates, this form of ROP has also

Name:[ ]CR no:[ ] GA at birth:[ ] Date of screening:[/ /]

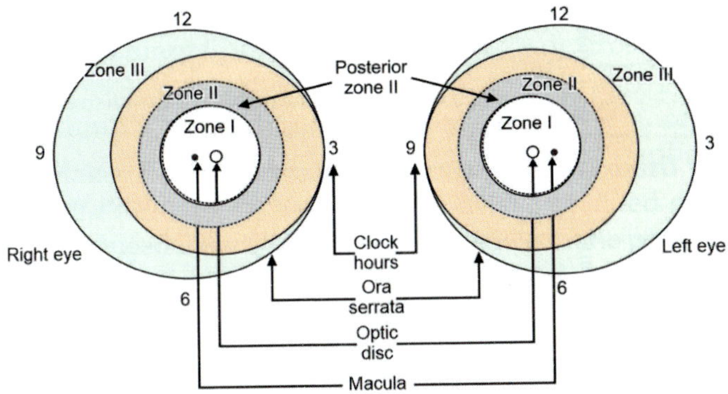

	Zone[a]	Mature retina	Iimmature No RoP	Stage 1		Stage 2		Stage 3		Stage 4	Stage 5
Right eye	I										
	II[b]										
	III										
Left eye	I										
	II[b]										
	III										

[a]If posterior-most affected zone is due to presence of a 'notch' of involvement add '(N)' to nothing, stage 2 in zone 1 (N)

[b]If posterior zone II is involved add '(P)' to the noting e.g., zone II (P)

	Type 1 ROP: Needs laser ablation
	Type 2 ROP: Re-screen after 1–2 weeks
	Needs surgical intervention
	Follow-up required after 2 weeks
	Further ROP screening not required

Next screening on ____________

Fig. 35.1: Classification of retinopathy of prematurity

Table 35.1: International Classification of Retinopathy of Prematurity		
Location	Zone I	Circle with an optic nerve at its center and a radius twice the distance from the optic nerve to the macula.
	Zone II	The concentric ring-like area from the edge of zone I to the nasal ora serrata and similar distance superiorly, inferiorly, and temporally. Within zone II, 'posterior' zone II is defined as an area of the size equal to the distance of two-disc diameters from the margin of zone I.

(Contd.)

Table 35.1: International Classification of Retinopathy of Prematurity *(Contd.)*		
	Zone III	Remaining crescent-shaped area of retina peripheral to zone II.
Severity	Stage 1	Presence of thin white demarcation line separating vascular from avascular retina
	Stage 2	Addition of height and width to the demarcation line of stage 1, so as the line becomes ridge
	Stage 3	Presence of extraretinal fibrovascular proliferation with abnormal vessels and fibrous tissue extending from ridge to vitreous
	Stage 4	Partial retinal detachment not involving macula (4A) and involving macula (4B)
	Stage 5	Complete retinal detachment: Stage 5A: Optic disc is visible by ophthalmoscopy (open-funnel detachment) Stage 5B: Optic disc is not visible because of retrolental fibrovascular tissue (maybe closed-funnel detachment) Stage 5C: Stage 5B plus anterior segment changes like, marked anterior chamber shallowing, iridocorneo-lenticular adhesions, corneal opacification (maybe closed-funnel detachment)
Plus disease		Presence of dilatation and tortuosity of retinal vessels at posterior pole of eye within zone I. Also associated with pupillary rigidity and vitreous haze.
Pre-plus disease		Presence of abnormal dilatation and tortuosity of retinal vessels insufficient for plus disease, but more than normal
Extent		Extent of ROP described in 30° clock hours (a total of twelve clock hours of 30° each)
Notch		An incursion by the ROP lesion of 1–2 clock hours into a more posterior zone. If a notch is observed on screening, the zone of the stage is defined by the posterior-most edge with a noting indicating the presence of the notch.

been reported in more anterior zones of the retina and in bigger neonates, especially in developing countries.[11]

Regression: Acute stage ROP can regress in two ways—natural spontaneous regression and treatment-induced regression. Regression of the ROP identified by thinning and whitening of neovascular tissue can be detected within 1–3 days after anti-VEGF therapy and 7–14 days after laser photocoagulation. Regression can be accompanied by continuing normal vascularization of the remaining retina or arrested vascularization, the latter being called persistent avascular retina (PAR). PAR occurs with greater frequency and may involve a larger retinal area after anti-VEGF treatment. When documenting a retinal screening examination, PAR should be described by its location and extent.[11]

Reactivation: With laser ablation, the peripheral avascular retina, the source of VEGF in pathogenesis of ROP is obliterated and can no longer produce VEGF. However, when monotherapy with anti-VEGF agents is used, the peripheral avascular retina remains viable and can continue producing VEGF. As a result, the acute stage ROP can become reactivated after a phase of regression. Reactivation of ROP can be seen at any site including original site of ROP at the junction between vascular and avascular retina, at a new edge of intraretinal vascular growth, elsewhere in the vascularized retina, or at multiple sites. Reactivation is observed most between 37–60 weeks postmenstrual age. Incidence and time of reactivation is affected by choice of different anti-VEGF agents used and their doses.[11] Reactivation should be documented specifying presence and location of new ROP features with zone and stage using the modifier 'reactivated.'[11]

SCREENING

The aim of the screening program is to detect ROP early, follow it up closely during its evolution, and treat if it assumes potentially serious severity level.

Which Infants should be Screened?

Gestational age and/or birth weight are two important parameters taken into consideration while deciding which babies to screen for ROP.

The Rastriya Bal Suraksha Karyakaram (RBSK) recommends the following criteria for screening:

a. Born at less than 34 weeks of gestation, OR
b. If gestation at birth is not known conclusively, birth weight below 2000 g, OR
c. Born at 34–36 weeks of gestation AND having ANY of the following risk factors:need of respiratory support, oxygen therapy for more than 6 hours, sepsis, episodes of apnea and need

of blood transfusion, exchange transfusion or unstable clinical course as determined by pediatrician.In absence of reliable records, admission in neonatal intensive care unit (NICU) or special care newborn unit (SCNU) can be taken as a surrogate risk factor.

> In addition to prematurity, the aforementioned risk factors for developing ROP represent level of sickness. Sickness is therefore an important underlying factor that makes higher gestation preterm neonates at risk of developing ROP.[4]

AIIMS, New Delhi instituted its ROP screening program in early 1990s. We observed a change in the epidemiology of ROP by early 2000s. Though milder ROP could be seen in infants of 32 weeks or more of gestation, ROP requiring treatment occurred only in infants of less than 32 weeks gestation or sick infants of 32–35 weeks gestation. Overall, there was a significant reduction in ROP requiring treatment. Also, AROP has occurred very rarely in our NICU. Accordingly, we changed our screening criteria to reduce the unnecessary painful ROP screening and to optimize resource utilization. We believe that happened due to high quality of care provided at AIIMS NICU. Also, a screening program being in place helps in early ROP detection.

Our current criteria of ROP screening are as follows:

a. Born at less than 32 weeks of gestation, OR
b. If gestation at birth is not known conclusively, birth weight below 1500 g, OR
c. Born at 32–35 weeks of gestation AND having ANY of the following risk factors:need of respiratory support, oxygen therapy for more than 6 hours, sepsis, episodes of apnea and need of blood transfusion, exchange transfusion or unstable clinical course as determined by pediatrician.

When and How often to Screen

First screening examination should be carried out at 32 weeks of post menstrual age (PMA) or 4 weeks of postnatal age (PNA), whichever is later.[12]

In neonates less than 28 weeks of gestation or with birth weight less than 1200 g if gestation at birth is not confirmed conclusively, the first examination for ROP should be performed at 2–3 weeks postnatal age (PNA).

Practice tip
A good rule to remember is to perform first screening at 4 weeks of PNA.

What is the evidence?

Progression of ROP follows a distinct timeline as per PMA rather than postnatal age (PNA) of the infant. ROP may not be detected before 30 weeks of PMA or before 2–3 weeks of PNA.

The median age at detection of stage 1 ROP is 34 weeks. The vascularization is complete by 40–44 weeks of gestation. The critical phase during screening is 32–38 weeks when the infant is likely to reach a severe stage of disease that may require treatment for prevention of blindness.

Follow-up examinations are normally required every 1–2 weeks depending upon ROP staging and should be recommended by the examining ophthalmologist.

ROP screening can be terminated once there is complete vascularization of retina without any ROP, or if the ROP has shown regression. This normally happens at around 40–44 weeks of PMA. However, if anti-VEGF agents are used for treatment, screening examinations need to continue to detect reactivation after regression.

Where to Examine the Baby?

Neonates are best examined in the neonatal unit itself under supervision of attending pediatrician/neonatologist. It is not wise to transport small babies to ophthalmic outpatient or ward for examination.

How to Dilate the Pupils?

Pupils are dilated with a combination of phenylephrine 2.5% and tropicamide 0.5% eye drops. The combination can be instilled 2 times at 10 min intervals half hour before screening. Alternatively, one drop of tropicamide is instilled every 10 minutes up to 2 times starting half hour before the scheduled time for examination. This is followed by phenylephrine, just one drop instilled few minutes before examination. Phenylephrine is available in 10% concentration; it should be diluted 4 times before use in neonates. Repeated instillation of phenylephrine is avoided for the fear of hypertension.

Practice tip

If pupils are not dilating despite administration of adequate mydriatic drops, AROP should be suspected. These infants should be screened on priority and appropriate and timely action taken.

What does the Examination Entail?

Screening of ROP involves indirect ophthalmoscopy (IO) using 28/30 D lens by an experienced ophthalmologist. After instilling a topical anesthetic drop like proparacaine, a wire speculum is inserted to keep the eyelids apart. First the anterior segment of the eye is examined to look for tunica vasculosa lentis, pupillary dilation, and lens/media clarity followed by the posterior pole to look for plus disease followed by sequential examination of all clock hours of the peripheral retina. A scleral depressor is often used to indent the eye externally to examine areas of interest, rotate and stabilize the eye. Use of scleral depressor increases the pain during screening examination and can be avoided if the examiner is skilled to complete the screening without it.

How to Record Findings during Screening?

Ophthalmological notes should be made after each ROP examination, detailing zone, stage and extent in terms of clock hours of any ROP and the presence of any pre-plus or plus disease. These notes should include a recommendation for the timing of the next examination (if any) and be kept with the baby's medical record.

What Precautions are Taken during Examination?

ROP screening examination can have short-term effects on blood pressure, heart rate and respiratory function in the premature baby.[14] The examination should be kept as brief as possible and precaution is taken to ensure that emergency situations can be dealt with promptly and effectively. ROP screening is a painful procedure if not done properly. It should be minimized by administrating a combination of topical anesthetic eye drops (0.5% proparacaine) 30 seconds prior to examination. Some prefer oral 24% sucrose or 25% dextrose in the dose of 0.5 ml/kg for sucking on gauze just before the insertion of eye speculum. Baby should not be fed one hour before examination to avoid vomiting and aspiration. Hand hygiene should be practiced to maintain asepsis.

What is the evidence?

A systematic review and meta-analysis comprising four studies has reported that oral sucrose reduces pain during eye examination.[13,14] Of two studies reporting the role of topical proparacaine drops has observed significant pain reduction.[15]

Use of Wide-field Digital Camera for Screening: Wide-field digital cameras capable of retinal imaging have been evaluated as an alternative to IO for screening in preterm infants. Retinal images taken by camera can be stored, transmitted to expert, reviewed, analyzed and sequentially compared over time and are useful for tele-screening purposes in community programs. However, due to high cost and variable sensitivity, wide-field digital cameras have not been used widely as replacement for IO.[16] Various lower cost alternatives have now become available. However, efficacy of these cameras is dependent not only on technical capabilities but also on the expertise and supervision of healthcare worker obtaining the retinal image, mechanism in place for timely review of images and ability to provide treatment when severe ROP is detected. A program with all these components needs to be validated before new generation wide-angle cameras are put into use.

What is the evidence?

Studies comparing wide-field retinal imaging with indirect ophthalmoscopy (IO) have reported variable sensitivity but good specificity.[16]

TREATMENT

The treatment involves ablation of peripheral normal avascular retina and thereby abolishing hypoxic drive of retina (mediated by over-expression of vascular endothelial growth factor; VEGF).This results in regression of established ROP.

Indication for Peripheral Retinal Ablation: Treatment of ROP is based on differentiation of following two types of ROP:

Type 1 ROP (needs treatment):

- Zone I, any stage ROP with plus disease
- Zone I, stage 3 ROP without plus disease
- Zone II, stage 2 or 3 ROP with plus disease

(A-ROP in any zone is also an indication of treatment)

Type 2 ROP (needs close follow up):

- Zone I, stage 1 or 2 ROP without plus disease
- Zone II, stage 3 ROP without plus disease

Peripheral retinal ablation should be conducted for all cases with type 1 ROP and continued serial examinations are advised for type 2 ROP.

What is the evidence?

Classification of ROP into type 1 and 2 is based on results of Early Treatment for Retinopathy of Prematurity Randomized Trial (ETROP).[17] Before ETROP study laser ablation was performed in neonates with threshold ROP, a classification based on location and stage of ROP.

ETROP study demonstrated improved visual outcome if laser ablation is performed in eyes with 'high-risk' pre-threshold ROP.Type 1 ROP includes threshold ROP and subset of pre-threshold ROP likely to benefit from early treatment.

Treatment modalities: ROP may be treated by laser treatment of avascular retina, intravitreal Anti-VEGF drugs or vitreoretinal surgery in advanced cases.

A. Laser Treatment

Peripheral retinal ablation is conducted by diode/double-frequency YAG laser.Ideally, laser therapy should be carried out in the NICU under the supervision of the neonatology team.

What is the evidence?

In a Cochrane systematic review peripheral retinal ablation as compared to no treatment was associated with improved structural and functional outcome in treated eyes.[18] Due to ablation of peripheral avascular retina, visual fields were reduced in treated eyes.

Preanesthetic preparation: Oral feeds should be discontinued 3 hours prior to the procedure. Baby should be started on intravenous fluids and put on cardio-respiratory monitor. Dilatation of pupil is to be ensured (as described earlier).

Anesthesia/sedation: Topical anesthesia alone provides insufficient analgesia for ROP treatment and should not be solely relied upon. Ideally, neonates should be treated under general anesthesia or analgesia plus sedation in an operation theatre.However, in absence of such options in resource limited settings, use of intravenous fentanyl (bolus of 2 µg/kg followed by infusion of 2 µg/kg/hour titrated to a maximum of 5 µg/kg/hour to reduce pain) can be considered for providing analgesia during the procedure. Use of fentanyl is associated with important but transient side effects and therefore requires continued observation of the infant for at least 24 hours after the procedure.[19]

What is the evidence?

In an open label randomized control trial (NOPAIN-ROP) with two intervention arms, regimens of intravenous fentanyl and intravenous ketamine provided adequate analgesia in only a minority of infants (16.3% and 4.5%). Even the revised higher dose regimens of fentanyl and ketamine did not improve these proportions (23.1% and 7.1%). Though, in general, the drugs were well tolerated but a minority did experience significant side effects that required prolonged monitoring (>24 hours).[19]

Procedure: Both the eyes can be treated in the same sitting unless contraindicated by instability of the baby. If baby is not able to tolerate the procedure, consider abandoning the procedure for the time being.Vital signs and oxygen saturation should be monitored very closely.

Monitoring after laser therapy: After laser therapy first examination should take place 5–7 days after treatment and should be continued at least weekly for signs of decreasing activity and regression. Treatment of any skip areas should be performed if there has been a failure of the ROP to regress.

Postoperative care:

- The baby should be closely monitored.If condition permits, oral feeds can be started shortly after the procedure.
- Premature babies, especially those with BPD may have increase or re-appearance of apneic episodes or an increase in oxygen requirement.Therefore, they should be carefully monitored for 48–72 hours after the procedure.
- Antibiotic drops (such as chloramphenicol) should be instilled 6–8 hourly for 2–3 days.

B. Intravitreal Anti-VEGF Drugs

Anti-VEGF drugslike bevacizumab or ranibizumab when injected directly into the vitreous chamber, cause regression of abnormal vessels without destroying the peripheral retina. As VEGF is an important mediator of lung growth and brain development, and there is significant systemic absorption of anti VEGF medication after intravitreal injection, there are concerns regarding toxicity of such therapy.

Intravitreal anti-VEGF drugs may be used for treatment of type 1 ROP involving zone I and zone II posterior ROP. Proper aseptic injection techniques are important to prevent iatrogenic complications like cataract and endophthalmitis. Currently there is insufficient evidence for use of anti-VEGF drugs other than bevacizumab and ranibizumab.

What is the evidence?

A systematic review suggests that there is no significant difference in incidence of complete or partial retinal detachment (RR: 1.04; 95%CI: 0.21–5.13) between bevacizumab and laser therapy.There was increased risk of recurrence of ROP with bevacizumab therapy (RR: 5.36, 95% CI: 1.22–23.50). On subgroup analysis, the risk of recurrence of ROP needing retreatment was increased in patients with zone 2 ROP while decreased in zone 1 ROP.[20]

(Contd.)

(Contd.)

In a three-arm, parallel group, superiority trial (RAINBOW study), bilateral intravitreal dose of ranibizumab 0·2 mg, ranibizumab 0·1 mg, and laser therapy were compared. The primary outcome of treatment success (defined by survival without active ROP, unfavorable structural outcome, or need for treatment switch up to 24 weeks after starting investigational treatment) occurred in 80%, 75% and 66% infants, respectively.Data on long-term effect including neurodevelopmental outcome is lacking.[21]

Long-term follow-up retinal examinations including the retinal periphery are needed till at least 60–65 weeks postmenstrual age (PMA) after the use of anti-VEGF drugs as there is a definite risk of reactivation needing a second injection or laser ablation. Other complications include retinal detachment, persistent avascular retina, macular anomalies, retinal vascular changes, vitreous hemorrhage and glaucoma. Due to lack of evidence about long-term effects including neurological outcomes, parents must be informed about the benefit and risks, and a written informed consent must be obtained for use of anti-VEGF drugs, including off-label use.

C. Vitreoretinal Surgery

Vitreoretinal surgery is done for advanced cases of ROP with retinal detachment in Stage 4–5. The outcomes of early surgery in stage 4 ROP are good, but prognosis in end stage 5 ROP is poor.

PREVENTION

Antenatal

Antenatal steroids: Use of antenatal steroids is a well-known approach to prevent respiratory distress and intraventricular hemorrhage, two important risk factors of ROP. Though antenatal steroids have not reduced occurrence of ROP, perhaps because it saves smaller babies who are at higher risk of developing ROP, but, as it reduces sickness level in preterm infants, it is likely to reduce severe ROP.

Postnatal: Most important risk factor for ROP is prematurity. It is difficult to prevent prematurity but there are other modifiable risk factors which require high quality neonatal care.

Delivery Room Interventions

- **Delayed cord clamping:** Reduces need of blood transfusion and hence reduces a potential risk factor for ROP.

- **Temperature regulation:** Maintaining normothermia reduces the risk of severe ROP.
- **Gentle respiratory management:** Avoiding injury to lungs and maintaining preductal saturation in target range for preterm infants reduces the risk of ROP.

Interventions in neonatal unit: Summarized as POINTS[22] of care:

Pain control

Oxygen management

Infection control

Nutrition

Temperature control

Supportive care

Pain control: Unnecessary painful procedures should be avoided as pain makes babies unstable and can increase oxygen requirement as well as increase the respiratory distress. Use of swaddling and oral sucrose solution or breastmilk during painful procedures helps to reduce pain.

Judicious oxygen therapy: Oxygen is a drug, and it should be used judiciously. Each neonatal unit should have a written policy regarding when and how to use oxygen and target saturations.

If a preterm neonate <32 weeks' gestation needs resuscitation at birth, inhaled oxygen concentration (FiO_2) should be titrated to prevent hyperoxia and achieve gradual increase in oxygen saturation (70% at 3 minutes and 80% at 5 minutes after birth).[23] During acute care of a sick preterm neonate, ROP is more likely to develop if partial pressure of oxygen in arterial blood is more than 80 mm Hg.

> Oxygen levels in blood should be continuously monitored using pulse oximetry keeping a saturation target of 91–95%. It is important that a work culture is inculcated wherein physicians and nurses respond to monitor alarms.
>
> **What is the evidence?**
>
> A large scale RCT (SUPPORT trial) indicated that maintaining low saturations (85% to 89%) compared to high saturations (91–95%) death preterm infants <28 week did not reduce composite outcome of in or severe ROP but it resulted in lower severe ROP and higher death rates.[24]

Therefore it is recommended that saturations in preterm neonates be maintained between 91 and 95%. Saturations should be monitored in preterm infants receiving oxygen therapy to prevent hyperoxia or hypoxia.

Infection control: Infection control bundles like hand washing, steps of hand hygiene, maintaining sterility during invasive procedures, measures to maintain skin integrity and antibiotic stewardship are often beneficial.

Nutrition: Good nutrition including early and exclusive breastmilk feeding to premature infants has proven short term as well as long term benefits, including lowering the rates of ROP. Poor postnatal weight gain is an important risk factor for significant ROP.

Other: Judicious use of blood transfusions: Transfusion of packed RBCs is another risk factor of ROP. Adult RBCs are rich in 2,3 DPG and adult Hb binds less firmly to oxygen, thus releasing more oxygen to the retinal tissue. Refer to the Chapter 51: Blood Component Therapy.

Other interventions: Supplementation of high doses of Vitamin E or reduced ambient light exposure is not associated with reduced incidence of ROP. In neonates with initial stages of ROP, administration of supplementation oxygen to achieve oxygen saturation in supraphysiological range and to reduce retinal hypoxia is not associated with halt in progression of ROP.

Quality Improvement

Protocolized Approach

- All units caring for babies at risk of ROP should have a written protocol for screening and treatment of ROP. The neonatologists have the responsibility of followingup the babies discharged from the unit till ROP screening is complete.
- If babies are transferred either before ROP screening is initiated or when it has been started but not completed, it is the responsibility of the consultant neonatologist to ensure that the neonatal team in the receiving unit is aware of the need to start or continue ROP screening.
- Whenever possible, ROP screening should be completed prior to discharge.There should be a record of all babies who require review and the arrangements for their follow-up.
- For babies discharged home before screening is complete, the first follow-up out-patient appointment must be made before hospital discharge and the importance of attendance explained to the parents.

Auditing

Following outcomes should be regularly audited in units with ROP screening and treatment program.

- Completeness of screening program: Percentage of eligible babies who receive at least one ROP eye examination.
- Timing of first screen: Percentage of eligible babies receiving first ROP screening exam by 4 weeks of postnatal age.
- Timing of treatment: Percentage of babies needing ROP treatment who are treated within 48 hours of the decision to treat being made.

REFERENCES

1. Tekchandani U, Katoch D, Dogra MR. Five-year demographic profile of retinopathy of prematurity at a tertiary care institute in North India. Indian J Ophthalmol 2021;69:2127–31.
2. Kumar P, Sankar MJ, Deorari A, Azad R, Chandra P, Agarwal R, et al. Risk factors for severe retinopathy of prematurity in preterm low birth weight neonates.Indian J. Pediatr.2011;78:812–6.
3. Sivanandan S, Chandra P, Deorari AK, Agarwal R. Retinopathy of Prematurity: AIIMS, New Delhi Experience.Indian Pediatr.2016;53 Suppl 2:S123–8.
4. Maheshwari R, Kumar H, Paul VK, Singh M, Deorari AK, Tiwari HK.Incidence and risk factors of retinopathy of prematurity in a tertiary care newborn unit in New Delhi.Natl. Med J India.1996;9:211–4.
5. Narayan S, Aggarwal R, Upadhyay A, Deorari AK, Singh M, Paul VK.Survival and morbidity in extremely low birth weight (ELBW) infants.Indian Pediatr.2003;40:130–5.
6. Charan R, Dogra MR, Gupta A, Narang A. The incidence of retinopathy of prematurity in a neonatal care unit.Indian J. Ophthalmol.1995;43:123–6.
7. Dutta S, Narang S, Narang A, Dogra M, Gupta A. Risk factors of threshold retinopathy of prematurity.Indian Pediatr.2004;41:665–71.
8. Vinekar A, Dogra MR, Sangtam T, Narang A, Gupta A. Retinopathy of prematurity in Asian Indian babies weighing greater than 1250 grams at birth: ten year data from a tertiary care center in a developing country.Indian J. Ophthalmol.2007;55:331–6.
9. Rekha S, Battu RR. Retinopathy of prematurity: incidence and risk factors. Indian Pediatr.1996;33:999–1003.
10. Gopal L, Sharma T, Ramachandran S, Shanmugasundaram R, Asha V. Retinopathy of prematurity: a study.Indian J. Ophthalmol.1995;43:59–61.
11. Chiang MF, Quinn GE, Fielder AR, Ostmo SR, Chan RP, Berrocal A, et al. International classification of retinopathy ofprematurity. Ophthalmology.2021;128(10):51–68.
12. Fierson WM, American Academy of Pediatrics Section on Ophthalmology, American Academy of Ophthalmology, American Association for Pediatric Ophthalmology and Strabismus, American Association of Certified

Orthoptists. Screening Examination of Premature Infants for Retinopathy of Prematurity.Pediatrics.2018 ;142(6):20183061.

13. Sun X, Lemyre B, Barrowman N, O'Connor M. Pain management during eye examinations for retinopathy of prematurity in preterm infants: a systematic review.Acta Paediatr.Oslo Nor. 1992. 2010;99:329–34.
14. Stevens B, Yamada J, Ohlsson A, Haliburton S, Shorkey A. Sucrose for analgesia in newborn infants undergoing painful procedures.Cochrane Database Syst. Rev. 2016;7:CD001069.
15. Dempsey E, McCreery K. Local anaesthetic eye drops for prevention of pain in preterm infants undergoing screening for retinopathy of prematurity. Cochrane Database Syst. Rev. 2011;CD007645.
16. Athikarisamy SE, Patole S, Lam GC, Dunstan C, Rao S. Screening for retinopathy of prematurity (ROP) using wide-angle digital retinal photography by non-ophthalmologists: a systematic review.Br. J. Ophthalmol. 2015;99:281–8.
17. Good WV, Early Treatment for Retinopathy of Prematurity Cooperative Group. Final results of the Early Treatment for Retinopathy of Prematurity (ETROP) randomized trial.Trans. Am.Ophthalmol.Soc. 2004;102:233–248;discussion 248–500.
18. Andersen CC, Phelps DL.Peripheral retinal ablation for threshold retinopathy of prematurity in preterm infants.Cochrane Database Syst. Rev. 2000;CD001693.
19. Madathil S, Thomas D, Chandra P, et al. 'NOPAIN-ROP' trial: Intravenous fentanyl and intravenous ketamine for pain relief during laser photocoagulation for retinopathy of prematurity (ROP) in preterm infants: A randomised trial. BMJ Open 2021;11:e046235.
20. Sankar MJ, Sankar J, Chandra P. Anti-vascular endothelial growth factor (VEGF) drugs for treatment of retinopathy of prematurity.Cochrane Database Syst Rev. 2018 08;1:CD009734.
21. Stahl A, Lepore D, Fielder A, Fleck B, Reynolds JD, Chiang MF, et al. Ranibizumab versus laser therapy for the treatment of very low birthweight infants with retinopathy of prematurity (RAINBOW): an open label randomised controlled trial.The Lancet.2019 ;S0140673619313443.
22. Deorari A, Darlow BA. Preventing sight-threatening ROP: a neonatologist's perspective. Community Eye Health.2017;30(99):50-52.
23. York JR, Landers S, Kirby RS, Arbogast PG, Penn JS. Arterial oxygen fluctuation and retinopathy of prematurity in very-low-birth-weight infants.J. Perinatol. Off.J. Calif. Perinat. Assoc. 2004;24:82–7.
24. SUPPORT Study Group of the Eunice Kennedy Shriver NICHD Neonatal Research Network, Carlo WA, Finer NN, Walsh MC, Rich W, Gantz MG, et al. Target ranges of oxygen saturation in extremely preterm infants.N. Engl. J. Med. 2010;362:1959–69.

CHAPTER

36

Hearing Screening

The hearing threshold of more than 25 decibels (dB) at the frequencies (500, 1000, 2000 and 4000 Hertz) which are important for speech recognition can result in significant auditory deficits. Hearing loss can be slight, moderate, severe or profound hearing loss based on the average threshold (Table 36.1).

Hearing loss may be conductive, sensorineural or mixed based on the site of lesion.

1. Conductive hearing loss presents in the outer or middle ear restricting the sound waves to propagate to the inner ear. It can be due to deformity in outer/middle ear such as micotia/anotia, atresia, ossicular deformity etc or due to transient obstruction of middle ear with fluid.
2. Sensorineural hearing loss ceases the conduction and processing of acoustic signals in the inner ear secondary to damage to cochlea, auditory nerve or central auditory pathway itself. It can be further subdivided into sensory loss wherein the hair cells in the cochlea are damaged and neural loss in which the auditory nerve and the neural pathway are affected.
3. Auditory neuropathy occurs when the auditory signal is either absent or processed abnormally in the auditory nerve, brainstem, or cerebral cortex.

Table 36.1: Grade of hearing impairment

Grade of Impairment	*Corresponding audiometric value in decibels (dB)*
0. No impairment	25 or better
1. Slight impairment	26–40
2. Moderate impairment	41–60
3. Severe impairment	61–80
4. Profound impairment including deafness	81 or greater

4. Mixed hearing loss is the condition when conductive component is present along with the sensorineural component.

HEARING SCREENING[1–3]

Implementation of hearing screening programme ensures early diagnosis of hearing impairment. The average age of identification of bilateral profound hearing loss has been estimated to be 24 months and impairment of lesser degree has been noted to be 48 months. This can be significantly reduced to 12 months or lesser with execution of neonatal hearing screening. It can be either "universal" or "high risk". However, high risk focused screening programmes have shown to miss out almost 50% of the congenital hearing loss cases. Therefore, several authorities have proposed to implement universal hearing screening protocol.

Two techniques are used for screening:[4]

1. **Otoacoustic emissions:** Otoacoustic emissions (OAE) are an objective, efficient and noninvasive tool to assess cochlear function. They are the reflected acoustic vibrations from the cochlea in response to the stimulus given through the testing probe. They are obtained as a result of cochlear sensory cells, primarily outer hair cell movement, and are obtained at frequencies essential for speech acquisition.

   The OAE screener consists of a probe that is placed inside the ear. The probe houses a small microphone along with the speakers. The click stimuli in case of transient evoked otoacoustic emissions (TEOAEs) or tones in case of distortion product otoacoustic emissions (DPOAE) are given through speakers and the microphone receives the reflected sound from the cochlea for SNR (Signal to noise ratio). It gives the result as 'PASS' or 'REFER'.
2. **Automated auditory brainstem response:** Automated auditory brainstem response (AABR) is a screening tool to record electrophysiological response against the auditory stimulus given at the threshold level. The AABR method produces a simple 'PASS' or 'REFER' result without requiring interpretation. It is important to note that both AABR and auditory brainstem response (ABR) are different. ABR being a diagnostic test gives the detailed information such as type and degree of hearing loss. However, AABR is a screening test that measures the response and gives the result as 'PASS' or 'REFER'. In high risk infants, OAEs alone

can assess the sound conduction through middle ear and cochlear function but will miss the condition such as Auditory Neuropathy (AN). Therefore, it is recommended to perform AABR along with OAE in such cases.

AABR screening device measures the surface signals by placing electrodes on the forehead, mastoid, and the nape of the neck. For all the high-risk infants, AABR is essentially to be used as part of screening.

Execution of screening programme can give targeted results if it follows the 1-3-6 principle (Fig. 36.1). States who meet the 1-3-6 benchmark (screening completed by 1 month, audiologic diagnosis by 3 months, enrollment in early intervention by 6 months) should strive to meet a 1-2-3 month timeline.[5,6]

- The hearing screening should be performed by one month of age either before or after discharge for all the newborns.
- The babies who fail initial and follow-up screening should undergo diagnostic audiological evaluation to confirm the degree and type of hearing loss by the age of three months.
- After the diagnosis of hearing loss, the children identified with congenital hearing loss should be intervened with appropriate medical management or amplification devices such as hearing aids or cochlear implants by the age of 6 months.

SCREENING PROTOCOL[5,7]

A two-step screening programme is the most effective and widely accepted arrangement to ensure high sensitivity of the testing protocol (Fig. 36.2). In this the babies are screened initially within 24–48 hours of birth and in case they get REFER result, they are re-screened preferably before discharge or on subsequent visit to the hospital. This reduces the number of false-positive cases due to presence of fluid in the ear during initial hours of birth.

In high-risk babies, initial screening should be carried out with both OAE and AABR. Considering the greater incidences of hearing impairment in children falling under the high-risk category, it is imperative to perform OAE as well as AABR to ensure neural hearing loss is not missed in these children. Also, to decrease false-positive results it is advisable that hearing screening is done after 34

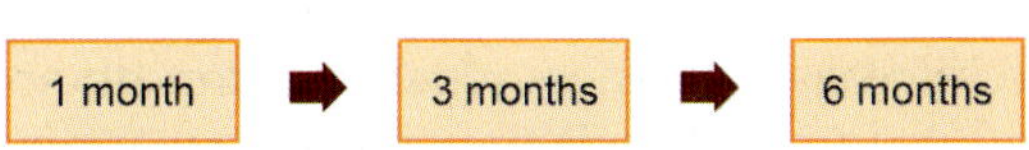

Fig. 36.1: 1-3-6 Principle for hearing screening

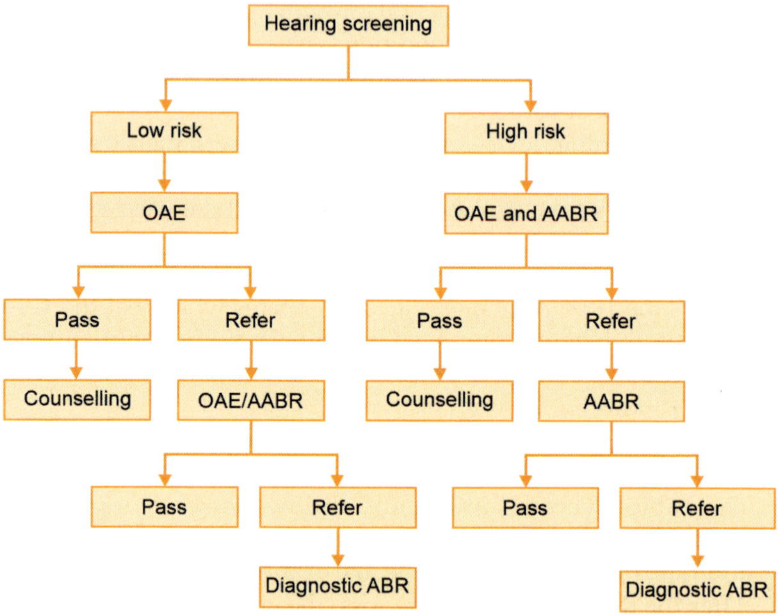

Fig. 36.2: Screening protocol for low-risk and high-risk babies

ABP: Auditory brainstem response; *AABR:* Automated ABR; *OAE:* Otoacoustic emission

weeks postmenstrual age for premature infants born at <34 weeks of gestation age (Fig. 36.2).

Evidence of two-step screening protocol and AABR for high-risk infants[4]

A retrospective study has advocated the use of two step screening protocol including Automated ABR (auditory brainstem response)/OAE (otoacoustic emissions) for well babies and inclusion of AABR along with OAE for high-risk babies.

IMPLEMENTATION[6]

The hearing screening programme needs resources such as appropriate instrumentation, isolated and less-noisy area for testing and manpower for successful implementation. Also, the execution of UNHS is majorly dependent on attitude and belief of physicians at the medical facilities involved in neonatal care. They should ensure hearing screening of all the neonates along with the appropriate test battery for well babies and high-risk infants. Counselling of parent/ caregivers to increase awareness regarding importance of hearing screening and its implication is imperative to warrant the success of screening programme.

FOLLOW-UP

All the children failing two-stage hearing screening should undergo diagnostic evaluation by 3 months of age. The test battery includes:

1. Medical evaluation: To examine the outer and middle ear and check for the presence of impacted wax or fluid.
2. Tympanometry to assess the middle ear function.
3. Otoacoustic emissions to differentially diagnose sensorineural hearing loss and auditory neuropathy.
4. Auditory brainstem responses (ABR): It is the gold standard test for threshold estimation and site of lesion analysis and also to help to determine the management option suitable.

Along with ear examination and audiological evaluation, bilateral congenital hearing loss should also prompt for genetic work-up. The genetic testing may give the opportunity to predict the possible course of impairment. It can help to establish the connection of auditory impairment with other congenital anomalies and differentiate between underlying syndrome or an isolated hearing loss.

LIMITATIONS

One of the major limitations of UNHS that poses a great challenge for the medical professionals is delayed-onset hearing loss. The late-onset progressive hearing loss, mostly associated with the known risk factors such as congenital cytomegalovirus (CMV) infection, hyperbilirubinemia, etc. can be identified with parental awareness and follow-up. However, the impairment with delayed onset and without associated risk factor can fail the purpose of screening as they cannot be captured with UNHS. The pass UNHS results may give false reassurance to parents resulting in missed or delayed identification.

How to Manage[8]

In accordance with the recommendation of WHO the rehabilitation for hearing impairment should be initiated by six months of age. It should be a multidisciplinary approach including otorhinolaryngologists, audiologists and parents. Based on the type and degree of loss, appropriate management options should be communicated to parents or caregiver. The habilitation process may include speech and language therapy along with the following options (Fig. 36.3):

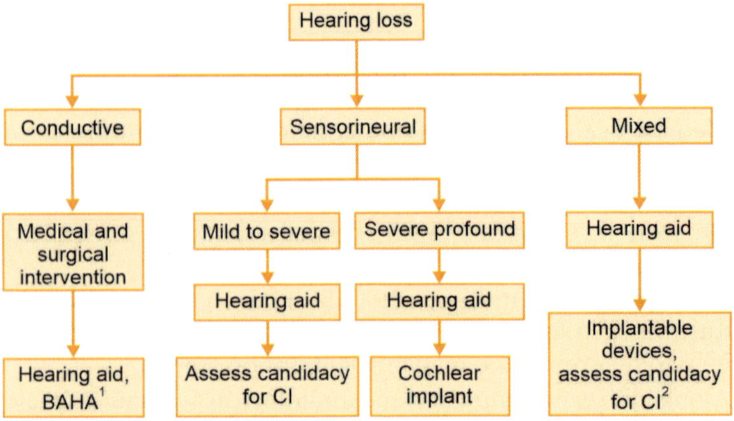

Fig. 36.3: Management of hearing loss post-diagnostic evaluation
BAHA: Bone-anchored hearing aid; *CI:* Cochlear implant

1. **Medical and surgical intervention:** Effective medical treatments are available for variety of conditions causing conductive hearing loss like middle ear effusion, chronic otitis media and acute otitis media. Some conditions like chronic tympanic membrane perforation, ear atresia and congenital ossicle abnormalities can be effectively managed by surgical correction. Immediate attention to these conditions and intervention can help to avoid delay in speech development.
2. **Hearing aids:** They can be suggested in cases of hearing loss with sensorineural component. Aids can be prescribed for hearing impairment ranging from mild to severe degree with the adequate amplification and appropriate programme. A strong follow-up and re-evaluation are critical to ensure the benefit.
3. **Bone-anchored hearing aid (BAHA):** In cases of permanent conductive hearing loss, BAHA can be suggested. It is most suitable in cases of congenital malformations of middle and external ears or chronically discharging ear. Surgical implantation should be planned considering the age of the child.
4. **Cochlear implant (CI):** In cases of severe to profound hearing loss cases, cochlear implants are the most suitable intervention option. Children with no or inadequate benefits with amplification devices can be surgically implanted with cochlear implants. The surgery performed by twelve months of age or during the critical period results in significant improvement and near normal development of speech and language skills.

Evidence of benefits from universal neonatal hearing screening

A prospective study of large cohort of children indicated towards significant benefit from early detection and intervention of hearing impairment followed by improved language outcomes.

OUTCOMES[6]

Hearing impairment when diagnosed and treated in early years of development can minimize its effects on communication skills of the child. The timely medical intervention and use of appropriate amplification device will assist children with hearing loss in achieving speech and language skills at par with their normal hearing counterparts. It will also be helpful in attaining normal cognitive development and social integration.

REFERENCES

1. Holster IL, Hoeve LJ, Wieringa MH, Willis-Lorrier RM, de Gier HH. Evaluation of hearing loss after failed neonatal hearing screening. J Pediatr. 2009;155:646–50.
2. Thompson DC, McPhillips H, Davis RL, Lieu TL, Homer CJ, Helfand M. Universal newborn hearing screening: summary of evidence. JAMA. 2001;286(16):2000–10.
3. Wrightson AS. Universal newborn hearing screening. American family phys. 2007;75:1349–52.
4. Lin HC, Shu MT, Lee KS, Ho GM, Fu TY, Bruna S, Lin G. Comparison of hearing screening programs between one step with transient evoked otoacoustic emissions (TEOAE) and two steps with TEOAE and automated auditory brainstem response. Laryngoscope. 2005;115:1957–62.
5. Bachmann KR, Arvedson JC. Early identification and intervention for children who are hearing impaired. Pediatrics in Review. 1998;19:155–65.
6. Joint Committee on Infant Hearing. Year 2019 Position Statement: Principles and Guidelines for Early Hearing Detection and Intervention Programs . The Journal of Early Hearing Detection and Intervention 2019;4(2):1–44.
7. Unlu I, Guclu E, Yaman H. When should automatic auditory brainstem response test be used for newborn hearing screening?. Auris Nasus Larynx. 2015;42:199–202.
8. World Health Organization. Hearing screening: Considerations for implementation.Geneva: World Health Organization; 2021.

CHAPTER

37

Umbilical Cord Blood Banking

Blood from the umbilical cord is a rich source of hematopoietic stem cells. These cells from the umbilical cord blood (UCB) can be used to treat certain malignancies and metabolic and immunological conditions. The process by which the umbilical cord and placental blood are salvaged at birth and stored by cryopreservation for future use is known as UCB banking. The umbilical cord blood transplantation (UCBT) may be autologous when the patient's own UCB is used or allogeneic when the donated UCB—either from relatives or unrelated donations—is used for UCBT. In either case, the UCB is obtained from a UCB bank, where it has been preserved and stored.

Cord blood banks can be classified as private, public, or hybrid. Banks that store a child's UCB for future use for herself or one of the family members are known as private cord blood banks. The banks accepting UCB donations and making them available for anyone needing a transplant are public banks. The newly emerging model is the hybrid model, where a bank offers public donations after the family makes an informed decision.

COLLECTION OF UMBILICAL CORD BLOOD

The collection of cord blood should not interfere with the baby's delivery while maintaining sterility and maximizing the yield of hematopoietic stem cells. Cord blood can be collected *in utero* (before delivery of the placenta in the delivery room) or *ex utero* (after delivery of the placenta).

The umbilical vein is cannulated via a sterile IV catheter and tubing, and the UCB flows by gravity into a sterile collection bag containing anticoagulant solution till the flow stops, which usually takes 2–5 min.[1] A total volume of at least 40 ml of blood must be collected to ensure sufficient stem cells.

Following this, the bag is transported to the cord blood bank, where it undergoes testing followed by cryopreservation, i.e. stored in liquid or vapor phase nitrogen. UCB can be cryopreserved and stored for over 15 years, transported to the transplant center, and thawed before use.

CLINICAL BENEFITS

1. UCB is helpful for all those who need allogeneic hematopoietic stem cell transplantation (HSCT) with the advantage of ease of procurement, rapid availability, expanded donor pool, no harm to the neonate, low immunogenicity, decreased chronic graft-vs-host disease (GVHD) compared to conventional HSCT from peripheral blood and bone marrow, and low relapse rate in minimal residual disease (MRD).[2]
2. UCB can be used for the allogeneic transplantation of an awaiting family member (biological parents or sibling only) who is confirmed to be suffering from an illness that allogeneic HSCT can cure. Thalassemia is an example where UCB from an unaffected matched sibling donor can be used for transplant.

LIMITATIONS OF UCB USE

1. When the disease exists in the donor's own cells, e.g. hemoglobinopathies, storage disorders, hemophagocytic lymphohistiocytosis, and primary immunodeficiencies, using one's own UCB stem cells is contraindicated.
2. In low-risk families, the risk of having a disease curable by autologous transplant is low—0.04–0.0005%. Even when there is a remote chance of having a condition where autologous stem cells are curative, e.g. in certain high-risk solid tumors, stem cells can be readily taken from the patient's marrow or peripheral blood, which provides similar results to that of using UCB.
3. Increased risk of infection following UCBT:[3] Delayed neutropenia, particularly following myeloablative regimens, increases significant vulnerability to bacterial and fungal infections. Delayed acquired immune reconstitution raises concerns about viral complications.
4. In certain hematological malignancies, the graft-versus-leukemia reaction is harnessed as a therapeutic benefit to kill the leukemia cells. UCB may have a limited role in these conditions, and allogenic stem cells from peripheral blood or bone marrow may be preferred.

5. UCB is costly, and its cost comprises testing, processing, and storage.
6. The role of UCB in diseases like BPD and HIE, where the regenerative property of the stem cells is utilized, is still under research. The use of UCB for such purposes should be limited to clinical trials.
7. A single UCB unit may not contain enough stem cells to be helpful in adults because the cell dose per kg body weight may be insufficient. A double unit umbilical cord blood transplantation has been attempted with limited benefit to mitigate this.[4] To expand functional UCB cells in vitro, using nicotinamide as part of the *ex vivo* expansion of UCB cells has been shown to achieve faster engraftment, reduced infections, and shortened hospital stays compared with an unmanipulated UCB product.[5]

RECOMMENDATIONS

The American Academy of Paediatrics, 2017, ACOG 2016; American Medical Association, 2007; American Society for Blood and Marrow Transplantation (ASBMT) 2008; and most recently, the Indian Academy of Paediatrics (IAP) consensus statement 2018 recommend the following:

1. The general public should be provided accurate information about the clinical limitations and benefits of UCB banking and transplantation (allogeneic versus autologous) as per the currently available evidence.
2. The parents of the neonate should be informed clearly that, currently, there is no scientific data to prove that autologous cord blood is of any value for regenerative medical purposes (e.g. in conditions like HIE and BPD).
3. To ensure that UCB is stored in sufficient numbers and made available for patients needing HSCT, public banking of UCB is encouraged where possible.
4. Because of the limitations of autologous UCB, storing cord blood for personal use is not recommended.
5. UCB can be stored for personal use if siblings or biological parents suffer from a disease curable by allogeneic HSCT.

At AIIMS, we do not encourage routine UCB banking; we undertake it only in specific instances, as mentioned.

REFERENCES

1. Cord blood banking for potential future transplantation: subject review. American Academy of Pediatrics. Work Group on Cord Blood Banking. Pediatrics 1999;104:116–8.
2. Milano F, Gooley T, Wood B, et al. Cord-blood transplantation in patients with minimal residual disease. N Engl J Med 2016;375:944–53.
3. Delaney C, Gutman JA, Appelbaum FR. Cord blood transplantation for haematological malignancies: conditioning regimens, double cord transplant and infectious complications. Br J Haematol 2009;147:207–16.
4. Wang L, Gu ZY, Liu SF, Ma DX, Zhang C, Liu CJ, Gao R, Guan LX, Zhu CY, Wang FY, Gao CJ, Wei HP. Single- Versus Double-Unit Umbilical Cord Blood Transplantation for Hematologic Diseases: A Systematic Review. Transfus Med Rev. 2019;33:51–60.
5. Horwitz ME, Stiff PJ, Cutler C, Brunstein C, Hanna R, et al. Omidubicel vs. standard myeloablative umbilical cord blood transplantation: results of a phase 3 randomized study. Blood 2021;138:1429–40.

Section

11

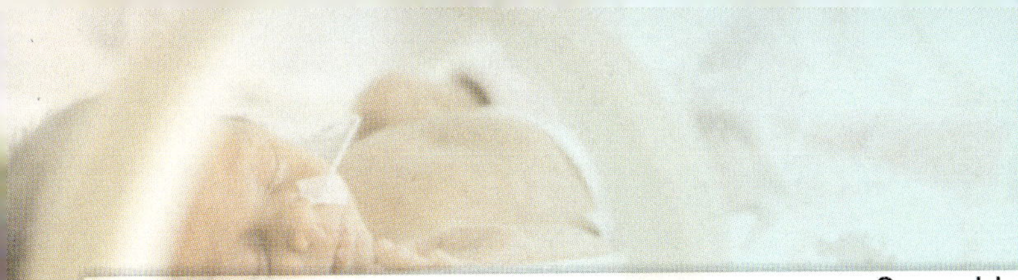

Diagnostic Modalities and Procedures

CHAPTER

38

Neonatal Chest X-ray

The chest X-ray is the most frequently ordered radiological investigation in neonatal intensive care units. It is indispensable for diagnosing pulmonary disorders in preterm and term neonates. It should ideally be performed in the neonatal ICU using portable X-ray equipment. In most cases, an anteroposterior view of the chest would provide sufficient diagnostic information. Lateral views of the chest and abdomen should only be included with a clinical indication.[1,2]

INDICATIONS[1]

1. For evaluating the initial cause of respiratory distress (such as pneumonia, pulmonary hemorrhage, collapse, airway or lung malformations).
2. For suspected cardiac or pericardial disease.
3. To check the position of the endotracheal tube, umbilical venous or arterial lines, peripherally inserted central catheters or chest tubes.
4. For evaluating the cause of worsening respiratory distress in a ventilated neonate after ruling out mechanical problems (tube block/secretions/dislodgement) or ventilator dysfunction.

Some conditions where X-rays are not indicated include:

1. Routine/daily X-rays in ventilated neonates.
2. Routine pre- or post-extubation X-rays.
3. After re-intubation in a neonate where the optimal "tip-to-lip" distance is known based on the initial X-ray.
4. Evaluation of an isolated episode of desaturation/apnea.

INTERPRETATION

All X-rays should be interpreted considering the clinical scenario. While describing an X-ray, the following vital observations need to be made:

- Projection (AP vs. PA film)
- Exposure (hard vs. soft films)
- Rotation
- Soft tissue/bone
- Lungs:
  - Expansion
  - The appearance of lung parenchyma
  - Cardiac and diaphragmatic margins
- Cardiac:
  - Cardiothoracic ratio/cardiac size
  - Pulmonary vascular markings
  - Specific chamber enlargement

Projection

The following features distinguish AP from a PA film:

- In PA films, the scapulae lie posterolaterally and are away from the lung fields, whereas they tend to overlap the lungs in AP films.
- Due to its anterior placement, the heart appears larger in AP than in PA film.
- The cervicothoracic vertebral end plates are tangential to the AP projection beam, making them prominent in the AP view, while the lamina appears more prominent in the PA view.
- The ribs appear more horizontally placed in AP than in PA view.

Practical Tip: Most neonatal chest X-rays are AP films unless the baby is made to lie in a prone position.

Exposure

- Lucency of soft tissue shadow—the darker the soft tissue, the more exposure.
- Ease of visibility of retrocardiac vertebrae—if the retrocardiac vertebrae are easily seen, the film is overexposed.
- Relative lucency of lung fields.

Rotation

The chest X-ray is said to be rotated if

- The distance between the posterior ends of the ribs from the midline of the spine is unequal on either side. The film is rotated to that side on which the distance appears greater.

- The medial end of the clavicles is not equidistant from the midline.

Usually, the side to which the chest is rotated appears more hyperlucent than the other; hence, it should be interpreted cautiously.

Soft Tissue and Bones

Carefully examining the bones cannot be overemphasized, especially for picking up changes in osteopenia and fractures. This is not discussed in detail here.

Thymus: Normal and Abnormal

The thymus may create some challenges in the interpretation of neonatal chest X-rays. Typically, the thymus appears as a bilateral, smoothly outlined superior mediastinal fullness blending with the cardiac silhouette. Some normal variants of the thymus are:

- **Notch sign:** Uniform thymus enlargement on both sides with a prominent notch on the inferior left border (corresponding to the junction of the inferior aspect of the normal thymus gland and cardiac silhouette).
- **Sail sign:** Characteristic sail-like border of the normal thymus, commonly seen on the right side.
- **Wavy thymus sign:** Undulating waviness of the lateral border of the thymus due to indentation of the ribs.

Interpretation of Lung Fields

Lung Expansion

Normal lung expansion: Up to six ribs anteriorly and eight ribs posteriorly. This follows the normal position of the diaphragm between the 5th and 7th anterior ribs. The radiological features of hyper-expansion are the presence of more than six anterior and eight posterior ribs, flattening of the diaphragm, increased lucency of lung fields (blackness), air under the heart, herniation of lung to the opposite side, and ribs more horizontal.

However, the evaluation of lung expansion by counting the number of ribs (or intercostal spaces) above the diaphragm can be tricky in newborns due to two reasons:

1. This technique represents the expansion in two dimensions only. But newborns, unlike older infants and children, have a highly compliant thoracic cage, which can quickly expand in the anteroposterior dimension.

2. Lesser diaphragmatic excursions occur during inspiration in neonates as compared to older children.

Common Disease Conditions[1,2]

Respiratory Distress Syndrome

The condition is caused by the deficiency of surfactant production by type II alveolar cells, which results in alveolar collapsibility with overinflation of larger alveoli and resultant transudation of proteinaceous fluid into alveoli, creating the classical hyaline membranes. The radiological features of the condition are:

- Under-aerated lungs
- Diffuse granularity
- Reticulogranularity (presence of air in the distended terminal bronchioles and alveolar ducts against a background of alveolar atelectasis).
- Air bronchograms (As the disease progresses, distal airways collapse, leaving the proximal bronchi, which stand out as air bronchograms. Note that the air bronchograms may be absent in an expiratory film).
- In severe cases or expiratory films, white-out lungs may replace these findings due to diffuse alveolar atelectasis.

The severity of RDS has been classified based on radiological findings as follows:

Mild: Normal/decreased aeration, reticulo-granularity

Moderate: Decreased aeration, air bronchograms, and indistinct diaphragm and heart borders

Severe: Confluent opacification of lungs with loss of mediastinal and diaphragmatic borders

RDS mimickers: A few congenital heart disorders, such as total anomalous pulmonary venous return, pulmonary vein atresia, and hypoplastic left heart syndrome, can mimic the granular pattern seen in RDS due to interstitial pulmonary edema.

Transient Tachypnoea of the Newborn (Retained Fluid Syndrome)

This results from the delayed clearance of fetal lung fluid, overloading the interstitium, lymphatics, and cardiovascular system. X-ray picture is characterized by:

- Prominent hilum with perivascular streaky shadows

- Prominent interlobar fissure
- Small pleural effusion
- There may be mild cardiomegaly
- Normal to increased lung volume

Radiographic findings usually resolve in 12–24 hours.

Pulmonary Interstitial Emphysema (PIE)

It is caused by the dissection of air from alveoli into the parenchyma and interstitium of lungs and perivascular sheaths of vessels tracking towards the hilum. X-ray appearance is characterized by:

- Radiolucent streaks- linear or irregular, branching/ cystic spaces (honeycomb-like) or pneumatoceles; seen radiating from the hilum toward the periphery of the lung.
- PIE may present with linear or cystic changes. Linear lucencies of PIE may be differentiated from air bronchograms as the latter are generally smooth and branching in contrast to interstitial air, which is coarse and nonbranching.

Pneumothorax

This results from the dissection of extra-alveolar air to the hilum, followed by rupture into pleural space. Increased radiolucency of the ipsilateral lung and sharpness of the mediastinal border are the earliest signs of pneumothorax.

The characteristic X-ray findings are:

- Clear border of a collapsed lung.
- Absent lung markings beyond the collapsed lung border (This differentiates pneumothorax from vertical skin folds).
- It may or may not be accompanied by a mediastinal shift.
- Herniation of the pneumothorax bounded by parietal pleura into the contralateral side.
- The thymus is compressed by pneumothorax, whereas it is elevated by pneumomediastinum.

Pneumomediastinum

The presence of air adjacent to the heart outlines the thymus and elevates it.

Meconium Aspiration Syndrome (MAS)

The radiological appearance may range from hyper-expansion to collapse

- Gross hyper expansion of lungs.
- Bilateral coarse patchy nodular opacities (This represents areas of focal alveolar atelectasis with focal alveolar over-distension).
- Sometimes, a large piece of meconium can obstruct the bronchus leading to emphysema of one lung/lobe and compression of the other.

Pneumonia

The radiological picture is variable and may range from reticulo-granularity to lobar or segmental consolidation

- Asymmetry of reticulogranular pattern with air bronchograms may be seen.
- Coarse granular patchy infiltrates with irregular areas of hyperinflation.

Pleural Effusion

- It was detected by the blunting of the posterior followed by lateral costophrenic angle (only in the erect film).
- In supine radiographs, the lung has decreased translucency with preserved pulmonary vascular markings.
- If enough fluid is present, it is seen as a peripheral band separating the lung and lateral chest wall.

Bronchopulmonary Dysplasia (BPD)

The radiological appearance is variable and depends on the postnatal age. (Northway et al.)[3]

- **Stage I (2–3 days):** Air bronchograms, reticulo-granularity (similar to RDS).
- **Stage II (4–10 days):** Opacification; coarse irregular densities.
- **Stage III (10–20 days):** Small generalized radiolucent cysts.
- **Stage IV (1 month):** Dense fibrotic strands, generalized cystic areas, hyper-inflated lungs.

Three Types of Bubbles in Chest X-ray

- Type I bubbles are seen in RDS. They are small, uniform, rounded, and nearly 1-2 mm in diameter. They are more prominent in lung bases. They occur due to overdistension of the terminal airways and become less pronounced on expiration.
- Type II bubbles are seen in pulmonary interstitial emphysema (PIE), are nodular and tortuous in shape, and are nearly 2–3 mm

in diameter. They are peribronchial and perivascular in location and do not empty on expiration.
- Type III bubbles are seen in focal hyper-aeration syndrome, e.g. bronchopulmonary dysplasia, and are larger than the first two types of bubbles. They are irregularly shaped and become less pronounced, like type I bubbles, on expiration.

Congenital Diaphragmatic Hernia

Bochdalek defects present with a well-defined dome-shaped soft tissue opacity usually on the left chest. They are dynamic and may "come and go" in serial films. Importantly, intestinal loops may be gasless in the first few hours of life. The herniated abdominal contents appear opaque with ipsilateral lung hypoplasia and contralateral mediastinal shift. The classical appearance of gas-filled loops in the chest may appear only a few hours after birth.

Morgagni hernias are seen as opacities adjacent to the right costophrenic angle.

Tracheoesophageal Fistula

A soft rubber tube is better than an infant feeding tube for the radiological diagnosis of TOF. The X-ray shows the coiling of the tube in the upper esophagus. If one desires to delineate the extent of the gap between the upper and lower pouch, a lateral X-ray is preferable. Absent stomach gas suggests associated esophageal atresia.

Interpretation of the Cardiac Shadow on Chest X-ray[4]

The most important features to be noted are:
1. Cardiac size
2. Pulmonary vasculature
3. Shape and size of different chambers/cardiac situs

Cardiac Size

This may be assessed simply by measuring the cardiothoracic (CT) ratio. CT ratio is the heart's largest transverse diameter divided by the chest's maximum internal diameter. A CT ratio of more than 0.6 suggests cardiomegaly in newborns.

Pulmonary Vasculature

Appreciating pulmonary vascular markings in the lateral third of the lung fields and the lung apices is usually challenging. Increased

Table 38.1: Causes of decreased and increased pulmonary blood flow in neonates

Causes of decreased PBF	*Causes of increased PBF*
Tricuspid valve • Tricuspid atresia • Ebsteinid atresia **Right ventricle** • Pulmonary stenosis (PS) • Tetralogy of Fallot **Arterial** • Peripheral pulmonary stenosis • Pulmonary atresia • Persistent truncus (type IV) • Eisenmenger syndrome	**Acyanotic defects** • Ventricular septal defect • Patent ductus arteriosus • Ostium primum/secundum ASD **Cyanotic defects** • Admixture lesions without PS • Transposition of great arteries • Total anomalous pulmonary venous drainage • Persistent truncus • Single ventricle

pulmonary vascularity is visible as pulmonary vessels are seen in the lateral third of the film or the lung apices, or if the right pulmonary artery (visible in the right hilus) appears wider than the trachea.

Decreased pulmonary blood flow (PBF; oligemia) is diagnosed by the relative blackness of lung fields with small lung hilum (Table 38.1).

Specific Chamber Enlargement

Prominent pulmonary vascular markings left atrial and ventricular enlargement may be seen in the ventricular septal defect. In an AP view, the right heart border is formed (from above downwards) by the superior vena cava (SVC), ascending aorta (AA), right atrial appendage (RAA), and right atrium (RA). The left heart border is formed by the aortic arch (AoA), main pulmonary artery (PA), left atrial appendage (LAA), and left ventricle (LV). This forms the basis for diagnosing various chamber enlargements. Note that the right ventricle (RV) does not contribute to either of the borders and usually presents with an upturned apex when enlarged, left atrial enlargement results in splaying of the carina and a double left heart border appearance. Prominent main pulmonary artery left atrial and ventricular enlargement may be seen in patent ductus arteriosus. Reverse three sign along the upper left heart border- hypoplastic aortic knob and left ventricular prominence; inferior rib border notching usually seen in co-arctation in pediatric age group and not in neonates. Other congenital heart conditions are listed in Table 38.2.

Table 38.2: Specific X-ray picture of congenital heart lesions	
Heart lesion	*X-ray picture*
Tetralogy of Fallot	"Coeur en sabot"* (boot-shaped) heart—caused by a small pedicle (atretic PA) with an upturned apex due to RV hypertrophy; Pulmonary oligemia.
Truncus arteriosus	Narrow pedicle, frequently accompanied by an absent thymus.
Total anomalous pulmonary venous connection (supracardiac)	"Snowman" appearance* caused by the dilated vertical vein, innominate vein, and SVC, pulmonary plethora.
Transposition of great arteries	"Egg on the side" appearance* due to the narrow pedicle created by the parallel orientation of the aorta and pulmonary artery.

**Note: The characteristic X-ray picture may not be evident in the immediate neonatal period.*

Line Positions

Umbilical arterial line:

- **High:** Between T6 and T9 thoracic vertebrae.
- **Low:** Between L3 and L4 vertebrae.

Umbilical venous line: 0.5–1 cm above the diaphragm.

Endotracheal tube tip: Between the lower border of T1 to the upper border of T2 thoracic vertebrae. (**Note:** Position of the baby's head and neck may alter ETT position).

Percutaneous central line (PICC): When inserted from the upper limb, the line must have crossed the first rib and passed medially, with the tip lying between T3 and T6 vertebrae.

Practical Tips[5]

While Doing an X-ray

- Follow aseptic precautions. Adequate hand hygiene is a must for all, including the radiographer.
- Always discuss the exposure settings with the radiographer to optimize the image quality. A rough guide is to use 30–50 kV (kilo Volts) and 4–10 mA (milliamps).
- Avoid direct contact with the X-ray plate with the baby to prevent hypothermia. Always place the X-ray plate in the tray meant for that purpose.

- In small babies, beware of hypothermia as the radiant warmer is tilted away during the X-ray and provide an additional heat source if necessary. An X-ray can be safely done through an incubator.
- Instruct healthcare providers to wear a lead apron. A safe distance of 2 meters should be maintained for healthcare professionals when an X-ray is filmed to prevent radiation hazards.
- Expose only the area of interest and remove any chest leads, tubings, etc. from the field.
- Make sure the baby is not rotated.
- As far as possible, quieten the baby to avoid swings in respiratory depth.

While Reading an X-ray[5]

- Read the X-ray schematically. Significant findings may be missed while jumping to the diagnosis.
- Correlate the findings with clinical details.
- Note the neonate's age in hours/days and interventions done before (such as surfactant administration) and after the X-ray (pulling out a deeply placed endotracheal tube).
- The use of a view box and the magnifying glass is ideal.
- Writing serial numbers chronologically on the films is helpful When multiple X-rays have been performed on the same baby. If the positions of the ET tube or central lines have been changed, the changed place should be marked.
- Neonatal X-rays should be read by the neonatologist; relying on a pediatric radiologist (who may not be reading neonatal films regularly) as a routine is not advisable.

REFERENCES

1. Deorari A, Kumar P, Murki S. Workbook on CPAP: Science, evidence and practice. ed. New Delhi: 2011. Neonatal chest X-ray interpretation; p.59–64.
2. Swischuk LE. Imaging of the newborn, infant, and young child. 5th ed. Philadelphia: Lippincott Williams and Wilkins: 2004. Respiratory system; p.1–108.
3. Northway WH, Rosan RC, Porter DY. Pulmonary disease following respirator therapy of hyaline-membrane disease. Bronchopulmonary dysplasia. N Engl J Med. 1967 Feb 16;276(7):357–68.
4. Abdulla R. Heart Diseases in Children: A Pediatrician. Respiratory system;inger: 2011. Chapter 2, Cardiac Interpretation of Pediatric Chest X-Ray; p.17–34.
5. Jones J, Bell D, Bickle I, et al. Neonatal chest radiograph in the exam setting. Reference article, Radiopaedia.org (Accessed on 17 Apr 2023) https://doi.org/10.53347/rID-16903.

CHAPTER

39

Arterial Blood Gases: Interpretation

Arterial blood gas (ABG) can be obtained directly from indwelling arterial catheters, intermittent peripheral artery punctures, or arterialized capillary samples. Preferred sites of arterial sampling include the umbilical artery and radial artery.[1,2] Blood gas analyzers measure pH, PCO_2, and PO_2 using separate analytical electrodes. The serum bicarbonate concentration is then calculated using the Henderson–Hasselbach equation.[3]

$$pH = 6.10 + \log ([HCO^{3-}] \div [0.03 \times PaCO_2])$$

Current blood gas analyzers also report lactate concentrations, hemoglobin, electrolytes, oxyhemoglobin, carboxyhemoglobin, and methemoglobin concentrations.

TERMINOLOGIES USED

The terminologies used to define acid-base disorders are based on the principles of the Henderson–Hasselbach equation.

- **Acidemia:** An arterial pH less than 7.35.
- **Alkalemia:** An arterial pH greater than 7.45.
- **Acidosis:** A process lowering the pH of extracellular fluid by low serum HCO_3^- concentration or increased $PaCO_2$.
- **Alkalosis:** A process raising the extracellular fluid pH by either elevating serum HCO_3 concentration or reducing $PaCO_2$.
- **Metabolic acidosis:** A disorder that decreases the pH and serum HCO_3^- concentration.
- **Metabolic alkalosis:** A disorder that raises pH and serum HCO_3^- concentration.
- **Respiratory acidosis:** A disorder that raises $PaCO_2$ and thus reduces the pH.
- **Respiratory alkalosis:** A disorder that decreases $PaCO_2$ and increases the pH.

- **Simple acid–base disorder:** The presence of a single condition, as mentioned above, with appropriate respiratory or renal compensation for that disorder.
- **Mixed acid–base disorder:** When more than one acid-base disorders are present concurrently. Suspect mixed acid–base disorders if there is a less- or more-than-expected compensatory (respiratory or renal) response.
- **Buffers** are substances that help attenuate the change in pH occurring if an acid or base is added to the body system. They act within minutes to bring the pH to be normal. The principal physiological buffers include bicarbonate, hemoglobin, and proteins.
- **Buffer base:** Normal BB is 48–49 mmol/L. BB is contributed by bicarbonate (50%), hemoglobin buffer (25%), and 25% by other buffers (proteins, phosphate, sulfate).

Tables 39.1 and 39.2 provide typical and targeted values of different ABG parameters in neonates.

Table 39.1: Normal ABG values in newborn

Parameter	*Normal values*
pH	7.35–7.45
$PaCO_2$	35–45 mm Hg
PaO_2	50–70 mm Hg
HCO_3^-	20–24 mEq/L
Base excess	±5

$PaCO_2$: Partial pressure of carbon dioxide in arterial blood; *PaO_2:* Partial pressure of oxygen in arterial blood; *HCO_3^-:* Bicarbonate concentration

Table 39.2: Target blood gas values in neonates[4]

	<28 weeks GA	*28–40 weeks GA*	*Term infant with pulmonary hypertension*	*Infant with BPD*
pH	>7.25	>7.25	7.30–7.45	7.35–7.45
$PaCO_2$ (mm Hg)	45–55	45–55	35–45	55–65
PaO_2 (mm Hg)	45–65	50–70	80–120	50–80

$PaCO_2$: Partial pressure of carbon dioxide in arterial blood; *PaO_2:* Partial pressure of oxygen in arterial blood; *GA:* Gestational age; *BPD:* Bronchopulmonary dysplasia

Stepwise Approach to the Interpretation of ABG[5,6]

1. Clinical evaluation
2. Assess the pH
3. Assess the primary component
4. Assess the compensation status
5. Identify the possible etiology of the acid-base imbalance
6. Assess the oxygenation status

Step 1. Clinical Evaluation

Arterial blood gases should never be interpreted without other clinical information. Various symptoms and signs, such as the patient's vital signs (indicating shock or sepsis), neurological status, gastrointestinal symptoms (vomiting, diarrhea), etc. can provide clues towards identifying the underlying acid–base disorder. Intake of certain medications like diuretics can also affect the acid–base status. Previous blood gases are also reviewed to see the trends.

Step 2. Assess the pH

Check if there is acidemia (pH <7.35) or alkalemia (pH >7.45). This is usually the primary disorder (*refer to* Figs 39.1 and 39.2).

Note: Acidosis or alkalosis may be present even if the pH is within the normal range (7.35–7.45).

Step 3. Assess the Primary Component

The next step is to identify the primary component—respiratory or metabolic. In primary respiratory disorders, the pH and $PaCO_2$ change in opposite directions (i.e. if pH increases, the $PaCO_2$ decreases), whereas in primary metabolic disorders, the pH and HCO_3 change in the same direction.

Respiratory acidosis: pH↓$PaCO_2$↑

Respiratory alkalosis: pH↑$PaCO_2$↓

Metabolic acidosis: pH↓HCO_3^-↓

Metabolic alkalosis: pH↑HCO_3^-↑

Step 4. Assess the Compensation Status

During the initial phase of acid–base disturbance (uncompensated stage), the pH and $PaCO_2$ (or HCO_3^-) are abnormal. Compensation occurs to normalize the pH, which depends on the renal system, the lungs, and the intracellular and extracellular buffers. The pH is normal in a fully compensated stage, but the $PaCO_2$ or HCO_3 are altered. In response to primary metabolic disturbance, respiratory compensation occurs within hours by changes in the respiratory rate resulting in a new steady state $PaCO_2$. In primary respiratory disturbances, metabolic balance occurs by the renal buffering system resulting in a new constant state concentration of bicarbonate, which usually takes 2–5 days.

The following formulas are used for calculating compensation:[5]

A. Calculate the projected $PaCO_2$ concentration required for compensating metabolic disorder:
   - Metabolic acidosis (Winters formula)
     - $PaCO_2 = 1.5\ (HCO_3^-) + 8 \pm 2$ mm Hg
     - Complete compensation occurs within 12–24 hours.
   - Metabolic alkalosis
     - $PaCO_2 = 0.7[(HCO_3^-) - 20] + 40 \pm 2$ mm Hg

   If the $PaCO_2$ is lesser or greater than predicted, there is superimposed respiratory alkalosis or acidosis, respectively. Complete compensation occurs within 24–36 hours.

B. Calculate the projected HCO_3^- concentration required for compensating respiratory disorder:
   - Respiratory acidosis
     - **Acute:** For every 10 mm Hg increase in $PaCO_2$ above 40 mmHg, HCO_3^- increases by 1 mmol/L.
     - **Chronic:** For every 10 mm Hg increase in $PaCO_2$ above 40 mm Hg, HCO_3^- increases by 4–5 mmol/L.
   - Respiratory alkalosis

     Acute: For every 10 mm Hg decrease in $PaCO_2$ below 40 mm Hg, HCO_3^- decreases by 2 mmol/L.

     Chronic: For every 10 mm Hg decrease in $PaCO_2$ below 40 mm Hg, HCO_3^- decreases by 4–5 mmol/L.

   If the bicarbonate is greater or lesser than predicted, there is superimposed metabolic alkalosis or acidosis.

Step 5. Identify the Possible Etiology of the Acid–base Imbalance

The next step in interpreting ABG in metabolic acidosis is to calculate the anion gap (AG). The anion gap is the difference between the charges of anions and cations and is calculated by the formula.

$$AG = Na^+ + (Cl^- + HCO_3^-)$$

Elect neutrality must be maintained *in vivo* so the difference reflects the unmeasured ions. The normal anion gap is 12 + 4 mm Hg.

Step 6. Assess the Oxygenation Status

The oxygenation status of the baby can be assessed by the following:

A. **The partial pressure of oxygen (PaO_2):** Normal values for PaO_2 in term infants are 50–70 mm Hg; in preterm are 45–65 mm Hg. PaO_2 values >90–100 mm Hg are referred to as hyperoxemia and should be avoided, especially in preterm neonates. The presence of below-normal PaO_2 levels is referred to as hypoxemia. It should be differentiated from hypoxia which is inadequate tissue oxygenation and can result from several factors apart from hypoxemia, such as anemia, heart failure, etc.
Note: Always identify whether the sample is preductal or postductal before interpreting PaO_2 values. In newborns with patent ductus arteriosus, especially in pulmonary hypertension, PaO_2 levels in preductal are higher than postductal blood.

B. **Alveolar arterial oxygen tension difference ($AaDO_2$):** The difference between partial pressure of oxygen in the alveoli and arterial blood helps distinguish the pulmonary cause of hypoxemia from extrapulmonary causes. The formula gives alveolar oxygen.

$$PAO_2 = (P_B - PH_2O) \times (FiO_2) - \frac{PaCO_2}{R}$$

PB is barometric pressure, PH_2O is water vapor pressure, FiO_2 is a fraction of inspired oxygen, and R is respiratory quotient (assumed to be 0.8). Typically the $AaDO_2$ is about 5–10 mm Hg in healthy individuals. This can be as high as 25–35 mm Hg in neonates due to higher physiological dead space. Conditions associated with high $AaDO_2$: Cyanotic congenital heart disease, meconium aspiration syndrome, chronic lung disease, pneumonia, pulmonary edema, aspiration, pulmonary embolism. Conditions with normal $AaDO_2$: Respiratory center depression (encephalitis, narcotics use), neuromuscular disorders, kyphoscoliosis.

Table 39.3 describes sources of errors found in interpreting arterial blood gases.

Table 39.3: Sources of error in arterial blood gas analysis[7,8]	
Error	*Effect*
Excess dilution with heparin flush solution	$\uparrow PaO_2$, $\downarrow PaCO_2$, $\downarrow K^+$, $\uparrow Na^+$, $\downarrow Ca^{2+}$, $\uparrow Cl^-$, $\downarrow$Glu, $\downarrow$Lac
Admixture with venous blood	$\downarrow PaO_2$, $\uparrow PaCO_2$, $\downarrow SaO_2$
Presence of air bubble	$\uparrow$pH, $\uparrow PaO_2$ (150 mm Hg), $\downarrow PaCO_2$, $\uparrow SaO_2$
Delayed processing	$\downarrow$pH, $\downarrow PaO_2$, $\uparrow PaCO_2$, $\uparrow Ca^{2+}$, $\downarrow$Glu, $\uparrow$Lac
Hemolysis	$\uparrow K^+$, $\downarrow Na^+$, $\downarrow Ca^{2+}$

PaO_2: Partial pressure of oxygen in arterial blood; *$PaCO_2$:* Partial pressure of carbon dioxide in arterial blood; *SaO_2:* Oxygen saturation of arterial blood; *K^+:* potassium ion; *Na^+:* sodium ion; *Ca^{2+}:* Calcium ion; *Glu:* glucose; *Lac:* lactate

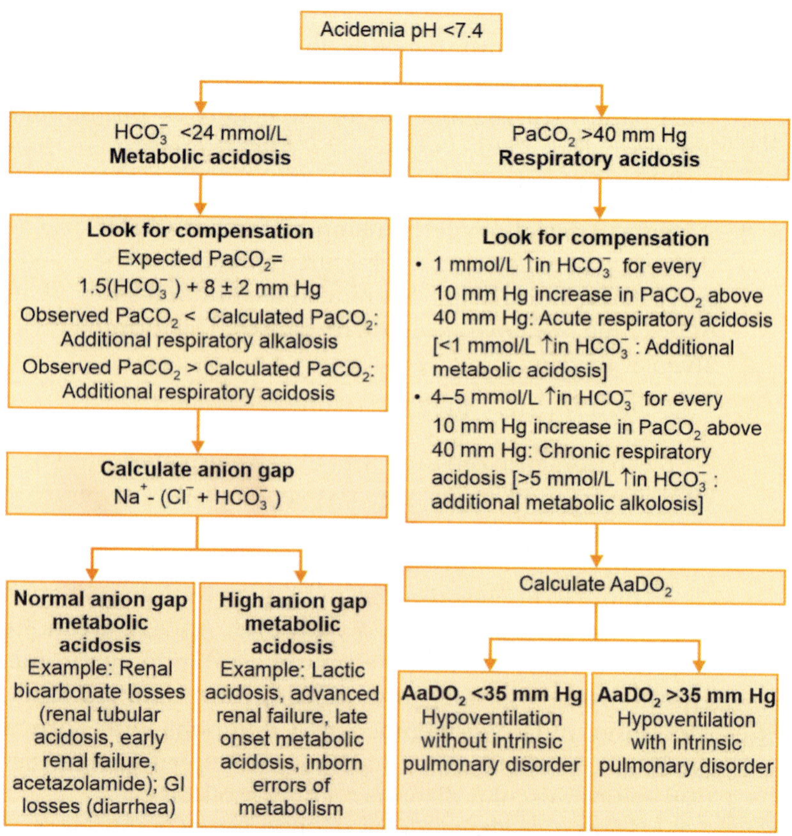

Fig. 39.1: Evaluation of acidemia

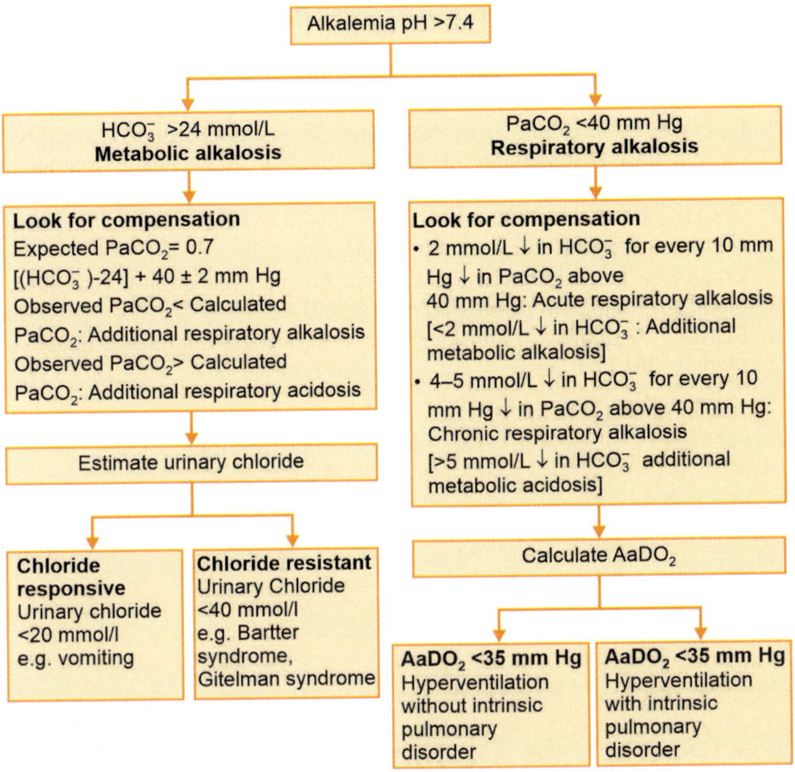

Fig. 39.2: Evaluation of alkalemia

C. **Oxygenation index:** The oxygenation index assesses the severity of hypoxemia and the response to treatment.

$$OI = \frac{MAP \times FiO_2 \times 100}{\text{Postductal } PaO_2}$$

Where MAP is mean airway pressure; OI >25: Indication for inhaled nitric oxide; OI >40: Indication for ECMO (extracorporeal membrane oxygenation)

REFERENCES

1. Smith AD. Arterial blood sampling in neonates. Lancet. 1975 Feb 1;1(7901):254–5.
2. Shaw JC. Arterial sampling from the radial artery in premature and full-term infants. Lancet. 1968:2;389–90.

3. Gomez H, Kellum JA. Understanding Acid-Base Disorders. Crit Care Clin. 2015:31;849–60.
4. Goldsmith J, Karotkin E, Keszler M, Suresh G. Assisted ventilation of the neonate. Philadelphia, PA: Elsevier. 2017.
5. Berend K, de Vries APJ, Gans ROB. Physiological Approach to Assessment of Acid–Base Disturbances. Ingelfinger JR, editor. New England Journal of Medicine. 2014:371;1434–45.
6. Sood P, Paul G, Puri S. Interpretation of arterial blood gas. Indian Journal of Critical Care Medicine. 2010:14;57–64.
7. Wennecke, G. and Knudby, M. Avoiding preanalytical errors - in capillary blood gas testing. Brønshøj: Radiometer. 2011.
8. Baird G. Preanalytical considerations in blood gas analysis. Biochemia Medica. 2013:23;19–27.

CHAPTER

40

Blood Culture and CSF Examination

BLOOD CULTURE

Blood culture remains the gold standard for the diagnosis of sepsis. It identifies the causative pathogen and its sensitivity to antibiotics. Proper blood sampling is critical to ensure the optimum growth of the pathogenic organism and prevent the growth of contaminants.[1]

A. **Blood sampling**
   - Select the appropriate vein for sampling.
   - Wear sterile gloves.
   - A 5 cm skin patch at the proposed venipuncture site is disinfected with 70% isopropyl alcohol, povidone-iodine, and isopropyl alcohol.
   - The skin should be allowed to dry for at least 60 sec before taking the sample.
   - The arterial sample offers no added advantage and is hence avoided.
   - Taking a sample from a freshly inserted peripheral venous cannula is acceptable. However, culture should be taken from a fresh venipuncture for patients with indwelling vascular lines. Additional samples for blood culture can be sent from the vascular catheter in cases of suspected catheter-related bloodstream infection (CRBSI).
   - The sample must be taken before the 1st antibiotic dose.
   - Clean the top of the blood culture bottle with an antiseptic.
   - Changing the needle between venipuncture and injecting it into the culture bottle is not recommended.

B. **Volume of blood**
   - At least 1 ml sample should be taken for blood culture in neonates, although the minimum volume specified in some pediatric blood culture systems is 0.5 ml.[2] Infectious

Disease Society of America (IDSA) recommends a minimum volume of 2 ml.

- All attempts should be made to obtain an adequate amount of blood.
- A blood-to-broth dilution ratio of 1:5 to 1:10 is considered optimal, even though it has not been consistently proven. The dilution ratio enables the dilution of the antibacterial agents in the blood and the binding of the residual antibiotics by the resins.

C. **Blood culture system**

- Brain heart infusion (BHI) broth has been used as the standard media for blood culture, with pediatric culture bottles having smaller amounts of broth to ensure an appropriate blood-to-broth ratio. Automated blood culture systems are increasingly being used, such as BACTEC and BACT/ALERT. These systems are based on the principle of detecting CO_2 produced by growing organisms by utilizing carbohydrate substrates in the culture medium. These systems estimate the CO_2 level (based on pH, colorimetry, or fluorescence) every 10–15 minutes and can detect microbial growth within 12–24 hours of inoculation.[3]
- Once culture broth is inoculated with the blood sample, it should be kept in an incubator at 37°C. If an incubator is not available, some automated culture bottles can be kept at room temperaturefor up to 36 hours after inoculation. Never put the inoculated culture bottle in the refrigerator.
- Once growth is indicated, subcultures are obtained and inoculated on culture media. Gram's staining is done from the subculture. Timely Gram's stain results can enable the administration of more targeted antibiotics.
- All blood cultures should be observed for at least 72 hours, preferably 120 hours, before reporting it as sterile.
- Evidence suggests that over 95% of blood cultures obtained in cases of early-onset neonatal sepsis before initiating antibiotics show growth within the first 24 hours.[4]
- Only aerobic cultures are routinely sent in the case of neonates. However, in cases where an anaerobic growth is likely, such as necrotizing enterocolitis, cellulitis, and maternal chorioamnionitis, it may be preferable to send separate anaerobic cultures too.

D. **Interpretation**

- In the presence of compatible clinical symptoms, the growth of even a single pathogenic organism in the blood culture suggests sepsis.
- However, the possibility of the growth of a contaminant organism may be kept in cases with clinical presentation not compatible with the diagnosis of sepsis, common contaminant organisms like coagulase-negative *Staphylococcus* species (CONS), and delayed growth in the culture medium.
- On the other hand, the growth of an organism within 48 hours, with a higher colony count, or with the growth of organisms like *Neisseria* or *Candida,* is usually taken as clinically significant.
- It is vital to have good communication between the clinical and the microbiology teams, with prompt reporting of any growth in blood culture.
- Antibiotic sensitivity is ascertained most commonly by the disc diffusion method. Commercially available antibiotic discs are used. Based on the size of the "zones of inhibition," the organism is classified into susceptible, intermediate, or resistant to a given antibiotic. "Susceptible" implies that the organism is inhibited by the usually achievable antibiotic concentration in the body by administering the usual dosage. "Intermediate" category drugs may achieve inhibition, but with poor response rates, while "resistant" antimicrobials would not inhibit the agent in usually achievable concentration.
- In addition, some organisms are intrinsically resistant to certain classes of antimicrobials, for example, Pseudomonas aeruginosa to amoxicillin, cefotaxime, tigecycline, cotrimoxazole, etc.
- Despite a poor blood culture positivity rate in clinical sepsis in neonates, it is essential to send blood culture in all suspected cases of sepsis.
- A positive blood culture with antimicrobial sensitivity can guide targeted antibiotic therapy, while a negative blood culture can enable early discontinuation of antibiotic therapy. Trends of positive cultures and their antimicrobial sensitivity also helps in determining empirical antimicrobial choice at a given center.

Practice tip
At least 1 mL sample should be taken for blood culture in neonates.

CEREBROSPINAL FLUID (CSF) EXAMINATION

The incidence of neonatal meningitis in resource-poor countries varies from 0.8 to 6.1 per 1000 live births. It increases with increasing postnatal age and is associated with significant mortality (40–58%) and long-term neuromorbidities.[5] However, it may be clinically silent or present with non-specific signs, especially in the first week of life, precluding reliance on clinical diagnosis alone. Hence, the CSF exam is included as an essential investigation in the evaluation of neonatal sepsis. Lumbar puncture is an invasive procedure with a risk of complications, necessitating a careful selection of neonates requiring a lumbar puncture.

A. **Indications and contraindications**
   - The indications and contraindications for performing a lumbar puncture for evaluation of neonatal meningitis have been depicted in Table 40.1.[6]
   - LP may be safely omitted in case of initiation of antibiotics solely based on risk factors, with no symptoms of sepsis and in preterm neonates with respiratory distress only but no other systemic signs.

B. **Patient position**
   - Various patient positions have been described for performing a lumbar puncture, including lateral recumbent with or without hip flexion and sitting position with or without hip flexion.
   - Lateral recumbent position with hip flexion has been used most commonly for neonatal lumbar puncture.

Table 40.1: Indications and contraindications for lumbar puncture[6]

Indications of LP	*Contraindications for LP*
• Clinical features suggestive of sepsis.	• Coagulopathy and/or thrombocytopenia (platelet count <50,000/mm^3).
• Blood culture positive	• Increased intracranial pressure
• Late-onset neonatal sepsis	• Cardiorespiratory instability
• Clinical deterioration or failure to show an improvement despite 48–72 hours of antibiotics therapy	• Local infection at the LP site

- Sitting position with hip flexion provides the maximum interspinous distance and may be equivalent or superior to lateral recumbent position, with equivalent clinical safety.[7]
- Ultrasound-guided lumbar puncture has also been successfully used to provide real-time guidance in challenging cases.[8] Our unit uses a lateral recumbent position with maximum hip flexion.

C. **Normative ranges for CSF parameters**
- Various studies have evaluated the normal values of CSF parameters in term and preterm neonates (Table 40.2).[9]
- A combination of CSF protein, glucose, and WBC count values provides a higher diagnostic yield than any individual parameter. Broadly, a CSF WBC count of 20 cells/mm^3 (both term and preterm) and CSF protein level of 170 mg/dl (in preterm) and 120 mg/dl (in term) has a reasonable diagnostic accuracy.
- With increasing postnatal age, CSF protein level decreases, CSF glucose remains similar, while CSF TLC shows a less predictable trend.[10]
- NNF India Clinical Practice Guidelines 2021 recommend using CSF WBC count and protein estimation, but not CSF glucose, for the diagnosis of suspected meningitis in neonates.[11] CSF culture remains the gold standard test for diagnosis of meningitis. Around 30–40% of CSF culture-positive meningitis may have sterile blood culture.
- Around 30–46% of the lumbar punctures done in neonates may be traumatic.[10] However, correcting the WBC count in case of traumatic LP is not recommended. CSF protein increases by around 1.9 mg/dl for every 1000 RBCs in CSF and does not require correction.

Table 40.2: Normal CSF parameters

CSF components	*Term neonates*	*Preterm neonates*
WBC counts (cells/mm^3) [mean (range)]	8 (0–32)	9 (0–29)
Protein (mg/dl) [mean (range)]	90 (20–170)	115 (65–150)
Glucose (mg/dl) [mean (range)]	52 (34–119)	50 (24–63)

- Although even a few hours of antibiotic exposure may result in sterile CSF cultures, CSF biochemistry can still enable a diagnosis of meningitis. CSF WBC counts remain the most reliable parameter in such a scenario, followed by CSF protein level, which decreases but usually remains above the cut-off range. CSF glucose may normalize rapidly after antibiotic exposure. Lumbar puncture should not be omitted because of prior antibiotic therapy.[10,11]
- Gram's stain is a highly specific test for meningitis but has limited sensitivity. Given the low cost and rapidity of results, Gram's staining of the CSF sample is recommended in every case.
- CSF Latex agglutination has modest sensitivity and good specificity. It may be considered in cases of negative Gram stain and/or in patients who have received prior antibiotics.[12] Recently, broad-range CSF PCR which primarily detects conserved regions of the bacterial 16S RNA gene, has been made available. This method has a sensitivity and specificity approaching 100%. Cost and availability remain limiting, especially in resource-poor settings. Other emerging markers, including CSF procalcitonin, IL-1β, lactate, lipocalin 2, NGAL, etc. are yet to find a routine clinical application.

REFERENCES

1. Buttery J. Blood cultures in newborns and children: optimising an everyday test. Arch Dis Child Fetal Neonatal Ed. 2002 Jul;87(1):F25–8.
2. Huber S, Hetzer B, Crazzolara R, Orth-Höller D. The correct blood volume for paediatric blood cultures: a conundrum? Clin Microbiol Infect Off Publ Eur Soc Clin Microbiol Infect Dis. 2020 Feb;26(2):168–73.
3. Kirn TJ, Weinstein MP. Update on blood cultures: how to obtain, process, report, and interpret. Clin Microbiol Infect Off Publ Eur Soc Clin Microbiol Infect Dis. 2013 Jun;19(6):513–20.
4. Marks L, de Waal K, Ferguson JK. Time to positive blood culture in early onset neonatal sepsis: A retrospective clinical study and review of the literature. J Paediatr Child Health. 2020 Sep;56(9):1371–5.
5. Thaver D, Zaidi AKM. Burden of neonatal infections in developing countries: a review of evidence from community-based studies. Pediatr Infect Dis J. 2009 Jan;28(1 Suppl):S3–9.
6. Aleem S, Greenberg RG. When to Include a Lumbar Puncture in the Evaluation for Neonatal Sepsis. NeoReviews. 2019 Mar;20(3):e124–34.

7. Hart C, Thompson A, Moriarty P. QUESTION 2: Is the lateral decubitus position best for successful paediatric lumbar puncture? Arch Dis Child. 2016 Aug 1;101(8):774–7.
8. Muthusami P, Robinson AJ, Shroff MM. Ultrasound guidance for difficult lumbar puncture in children: pearls and pitfalls. Pediatr Radiol. 2017 Jun;47(7):822–30.
9. Sarff LD, Platt LH, McCracken GH. Cerebrospinal fluid evaluation in neonates: comparison of high-risk infants with and without meningitis. J Pediatr. 1976 Mar;88(3):473–7.
10. Srinivasan L, Harris MC, Shah SS. Lumbar puncture in the neonate: challenges in decision making and interpretation. Semin Perinatol. 2012 Dec;36(6):445–53.
11. Diagnosis and Management of Neonatal Sepsis. NNF India Evidence-based Clinical Practice Guidelines December 2021.
12. Tunkel AR, Hartman BJ, Kaplan SL, Kaufman BA, Roos KL, Scheld WM, et al. Practice Guidelines for the Management of Bacterial Meningitis. Clin Infect Dis. 2004 Nov 1;39(9):1267–84.

CHAPTER

41

Umbilical Cord Blood Sampling

Umbilical cord arterial blood (UCAB) normally reflects fetal acid base balance while venous blood reflects a combination of maternal acid–base status and placental function. Paired umbilical artery and venous samples should ideally be taken for optimal interpretation as it gives insights into the etiology of acidosis. Practically, however, we take UCAB for knowing fetal acid–base balance.

INDICATIONS

American College of Obstetricians and Gynecologists (ACOG) and American Academy of Pediatrics (AAP) recommends UCAB to be taken in all high-risk deliveries.[1] We take UCAB in following neonates:

1. Gestation below 32 weeks.
2. Evidence of fetal distress such as fetal heart abnormalities, meconium-stained liquor.
3. Sentinel events such as cord prolapse and antepartum hemorrhage.
4. Requiring positive pressure ventilation.

Umbilical cord gas and neonatal outcomes: What is the evidence?

In a meta-analysis (51 studies, 4, 80,000 neonates), a pH threshold of 7.0 had a strong association with neonatal morbidity (OR 12.5, 95% CI 6.1– 25.6), and a pH threshold of 7.1 with mortality (OR 7.1, 95% CI 3.3–15.3).[1]

In a case control study (*n* = 174 infants), moderate to severe encephalopathy occurred in 10% Of neonates with umbilical arterial base deficit between 12–16 mmol/L and in 40% of those with base deficit >16 mmol/L.[2]

In a retrospective review (n= 56,574 infants), the combined outcome of death or cerebral palsy was 3%,10% and 40% at lowest pH of 6.9–6.99, 6.8–6.89 and <6.8 respectively; and 8%, 14% and 59% at base deficit of 12–15.9, 16–19.9 and 20.0 mmol/L or more, respectively.[3]

PROCEDURE (FIG. 41.1)

- Immediately after the birth, approximately 20 cm of the cord should be isolated between two sets of clamps. The baby is then handed over to the newborn team for post-birth care.

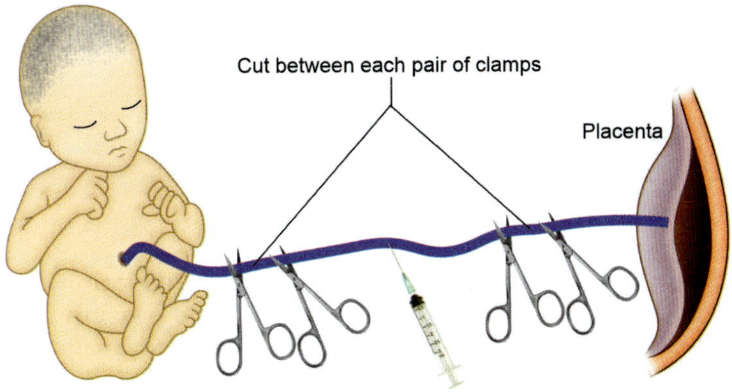

Fig. 41.1: Site for umbilical arterial blood sampling

- The blood in this segment of the cord is reflective of fetal acid base status that is not affected by postnatal changes in the neonate or the mother.
- The sample must be taken from both umbilical artery and umbilical vein. Umbilical vein is large and easy to sample whereas the umbilical artery is thin and difficult to sample. When a single sample is obtained due to sampling difficulty, it is likely to be venous.
- Blood is sampled into a pre-heparinized syringe. Use one mL syringe with a 21-gauge needle. Draw one drop of heparin in it, move the plunger up and down expelling residual heparin.
- Withdraw a minimum of 0.2 ml blood. Expel all air bubbles and cap the syringe before mixing the sample.
- Label the syringe and process the sample within 30 minutes. Document in records.

INTERPRETATION

- The normal values for umbilical cord gases are given in Table 41.1. Umbilical venous blood gas has higher pH and lower pCO_2 than arterial blood. The venous-arterial pH difference ranges from 0.02 to 0.49 units, median 0.09, while the PCO_2 difference ranges from 0.5 to 9.9 kPa; median 1.9 kPa.[4] Progressive widening of umbilical arterial and venous blood gas values is seen in restriction of umbilical blood flow (nuchal cord), whereas, the difference is small in impairment of placental perfusion (abruption).[2]

Table 41.1: Normal values for umbilical cord blood gases[5,6]		
pH	*7.18–7.38*	*7.25–7.45*
PO_2 (mm Hg)	5.6–30.4	17.4–41.0
PCO_2 (mm Hg)	32.4–66.0	27.0–49.4
BDECF (mmol/L)*	4.79 (3.46)	4.0 (3.5)

**Ranges based on mean ± 2 SD*

- Umbilical cord arterial pH varies with gestational age. It decreases with increasing gestational age possibly due to increased placental oxygen consumption with advancing age.
- The current evidence states that cord arterial pH of <7.0 and base deficit of >12 mmol/L is associated with increased risk of adverse neurological outcomes and hence these values are taken to be indicative of fetal hypoxia significant enough to cause neurological deficit.
- Isolated respiratory acidosis (elevated pCO_2) is seldom associated with adverse outcomes and is usually due to short lived impairment in circulation.
- Delayed cord clamping has small or no effect on cord blood acid base balance.[3]

REFERENCES

1. ACOG Committee on Obstetric Practice. ACOG Committee Opinion No. 348, November 2006: Umbilical cord blood gas and acid-base analysis. Obstet Gynecol 2006;108(5):1319–22.
2. Armstrong L, Stenson BJ. Use of umbilical cord blood gas analysis in the assessment of the newborn. Arch Dis Child Fetal Neonatal Ed 2007;92(6):F430–4.
3. Nudelman MJR, Belogolovsky E, Jegatheesan P, Govindaswami B, Song D. Effect of Delayed Cord Clamping on Umbilical Blood Gas Values in Term Newborns: A Systematic Review. Obstet Gynecol 2020;135(3):576–82.
4. Westgate J, Garibaldi JM, Greene KR. Umbilical cord blood gas analysis at delivery: a time for quality data. Br J Obstet Gynaecol. 1994 Dec;101(12):1054–63.
5. Yeomans ER, Hauth JC, Gilstrap LC, Strickland DM. Umbilical cord pH, PCO_2, and bicarbonate following uncomplicated term vaginal deliveries. Am J Obstet Gynecol 1985;151(6):798–800.
6. Wiberg N, Källén K, Olofsson P. Base deficit estimation in umbilical cord blood is influenced by gestational age, choice of fetal fluid compartment, and algorithm for calculation. Am J Obstet Gynecol 2006;195(6):1651–6.

CHAPTER

42

Central Vascular Access

The commonly used central vascular catheter (CVC) includes umbilical venous catheter (UVC), umbilical artery catheter (UAC), and peripherally inserted central catheter (PICC). Though not a CVC, we have also included peripheral arterial cannulation here.

UMBILICAL ARTERY CATHETERIZATION

Indications

1. Continuous monitoring of arterial blood pressure in sick and ventilated babies.
2. Arterial blood gas (ABG) analysis in ventilated babies.
3. Isovolumetric exchange blood transfusion (in unstable neonates).

Contraindications

1. Omphalitis/omphalocele.
2. Vascular compromise in lower limbs.
3. Necrotising enterocolitis.
4. Age >3 days (beyond day 1, UAC insertion is technically challenging).

Length of Insertion

Table 42.1 provides formulae for estimating the length of insertion.

As the formulae give a rough estimate, always confirm the tip position by chest X-ray, including the abdomen and upper thighs. UAC is seen as having a looping course in the abdomen on the X-ray film.

Two Positions

1. **High:** The tip of the catheter lies between T6 and T9 vertebrae. A high position is preferred due to a lower incidence of vascular complications.

Table 42.1: UAC insertion length (cm)*	
Methods	
Dunn	Measure shoulder umbilical length (SUL; the distance from the tip of the shoulder to a point vertically below till the level of the umbilicus.[1]
Shukla and Ferrera	[3 x weight (kg)] + 9 cm (Preferred in infants with birth weight >1500 g)[2]
Wright	[4 x weight (kg)] + 7 cm (Preferred in infants with birth weight ≤1500 g)[3]

**Add umbilical stump length to the estimated insertion length.*

2. **Low position:** The tip of the catheter lies between the L3 and L4 vertebrae.

The high position of UAC: What is the evidence[4]?

A high position compared to a low position of UAC is associated with a lower incidence of clinical vascular complications (RR 0.53, 95% CI 0.44–0.63) but no difference in intraventricular hemorrhage, death rates, and necrotizing enterocolitis.

Recommended Catheter Size

- Infants ≤1.2 kg: 3.5 Fr
- Infants >1.2 kg: 5 Fr

Catheter Type and Material

End-hole catheters are preferred to the side-hole to decrease the risk of complications. No clinically relevant differences exist between standard polyvinyl chloride (PVC) catheters and other materials like polyurethane.

Practical tip

- Attempt UAC insertion first (followed by UVC, if required) unless it is an emergency.
- Dilate the artery lumen for around 60 seconds using iris forceps[3] before attempting the insertion of a catheter (Fig. 42.1)
- If one gets a "Popping" sensation rather than relaxation during insertion:
  - UAC may have created a false channel; remove the catheter and use the second artery.

(Contd.)

(*Contd.*)

- Resistance may be felt after ~ 6–8 cm catheter insertion as the umbilical artery angles around the bladder towards the internal iliac artery. Applying gentle and steady pressure for 30–60 sec, flexing the hip, and tilting the infant to the side of the catheterized artery may help.
- Never advance an *in situ* catheter.
- If it is low for the high position (between T10 and L2), withdraw an equal length of the catheter by measuring the distance between the actual and appropriate position on the radiograph.
- Once the correct position is confirmed, secure the catheter.
- Run a low-dose heparin infusion (0.5–1.0 U/ml) at 0.5 ml/hour to maintain the patency of the catheter. Account for this fluid volume in total, particularly in ELBW neonates.
- Document the date and time, indication, number of attempts, depth of insertion, and position on X-ray.

Recommended duration: 5–7 days

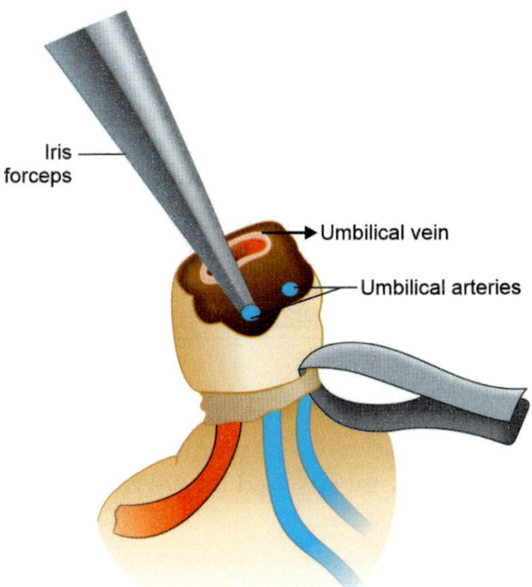

Fig. 42.1: Umbilical arteries are smaller, thick walled and may protrude slightly from cut surface. Umbilical veins are larger, thin walled seen usually at 12 o'clock position at the base of the stump.

Complications

1. Vascular complications (most common)
   a. Arterial vasospasm leads to blanching and cyanosis of the buttocks, legs, fingers, and toes. If the leg blanches,

rewarm the opposite leg with a warm (not hot) towel, which causes reflex vasodilatation. Apply topical nitroglycerine (2% ointment; ribbon length of 4 mm/kg) 1–2 cm proximal to the ischemic site. If there is no return of normal color within 5 minutes, remove the catheter.[5]

  b. Thromboembolism involving renal, mesenteric, iliac, and other vessels presenting as NEC, hypertension, hematuria, renal failure, pallor/coldness of extremities. The catheter should be removed in all such cases. It is seen days or weeks after insertion.
  c. Aortic thrombus, aneurysm
2. Creation of false passage, hematoma, peritoneal perforation, and vessel perforation
3. Catheter breakage
4. Infection (cellulitis, omphalitis, sepsis)
5. Line migration

Removal of the Catheter

1. Remove once the catheter is no more needed. Any complication may require catheter removal earlier.
2. Stop heparinized saline infusion 30 min before removal. Pull the catheter slowly with gentle traction over 30–60 seconds to avoid bleeding.

UMBILICAL VENOUS CATHETERIZATION (UVC)

Indications

1. Emergency vascular access during resuscitation at birth.
2. Central venous pressure (CVP) monitoring (the UVC must pass through the ductus venosus, and the tip must rest in the inferior vena cava).
3. Exchange transfusion.
4. Administration of TPN, blood products, and hyperosmolar solutions.

Contraindications

1. Omphalitis/omphalocele
2. Necrotizing enterocolitis
3. Age > 5 days (beyond 24 hours as in UAC, technically challenging to place. Use of saline-soaked gauze may facilitate ease of insertion)

Table 42.2: Methods to estimate the UVC insertion length (cm)	
Formula	
Dunn	By measuring shoulder umbilical length (SUL)[1]
Shukla	$\frac{[3 \times \text{weight (kg)}]}{2} + 1 + 9$
Verheij	$\frac{[3 \times \text{weight (kg)}] + 9}{2}$
Real-time ultrasonography (RT-USG)[6]	**Probe:** Small sectorial probe 7–8 MHz **View:** Subcostal longitudinal view **Procedure:** Visualize the tip as it passes through the umbilical vein, the ductus venosus, and the IVC. It is followed until it reaches the junction of IVC and the right atrium. A normal saline flush (0.5–1 ml) can improve the visualization.

**For exchange transfusion and emergency vascular access, the catheter is advanced until the point of good blood flow (usually 2–5 cm).*

Length of Insertion

UVCs often get malpositioned due to complex portal venous anatomy. The formulae based on the length and birth weight have a low success rate for UVC. Real-time ultrasonography (RT-USG) has yielded better success rates in the proper position. RT-USG is accurate, safe, and cost-effective but needs significant training (Table 42.2).

Confirmation of Tip Position

1. **X-ray:** The UVC tip position should be confirmed with an anteroposterior chest X-ray, including the abdomen. The preferred catheter tip position is 0.5–1 cm above the right diaphragm (UVC tip at thoracic vertebrae T8–T9 corresponds to cavo-atrial junction) (Fig. 42.2).
2. **RT-USG:** Helps in accurate localization of catheter tip and reduces radiation exposure. If using RT-USG, the catheter should pass beyond the ductus venosus and at the junction of the inferior vena cava (IVC) and right atrium.[7]

Catheter Size

- Infant's birth weight ≤1.5 kg: 3.5 Fr
- Infant's birth weight >1.5 kg: 5 Fr

Recommended duration of UVC: 10–14 days

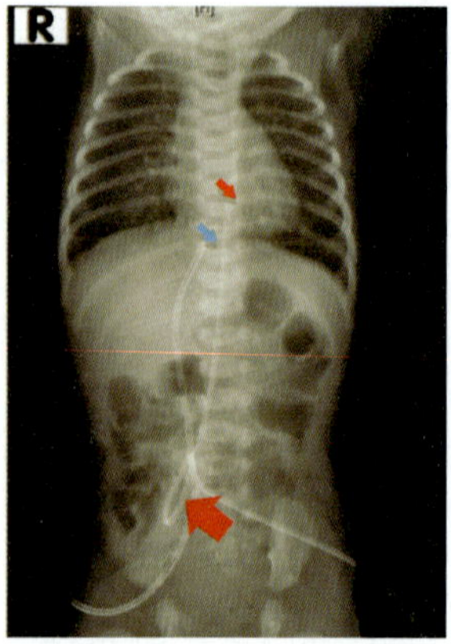

Fig. 42.2: Anteroposterior radiograph of chest and abdomen showing satisfactory position of UAC (red arrow) and UVC (blue arrow). UAC can also be identified by its looping course (block arrow).

Practice tip

- Identify the umbilical vein by its 12 o'clock location in the umbilical cord cut section and by its thinner wall and wider lumen.
- "Popping" sensation during insertion may indicate the catheter entering the portal venous system. Do the following:
  - Withdraw the catheter for about 2–3 cm, and push it again while rotating the catheter clockwise to get through ductus venosus
  - Double catheter technique: Passing a new catheter into the same vessel, leaving a misdirected catheter in situ (avoid in ELBW neonates due to risk of vessel damage)
  - Placing the neonate in the right lateral decubitus position.
- Secure catheter
- Never advance an in situ catheter
- Avoid infusion of hypertonic solutions if the catheter tip is not in IVC.
- Document the date & time, indication, number of attempts, insertion depth, and position on the X-ray.

Complications

1. Infection (most common): Sepsis, cellulitis, omphalitis, endocarditis, septic emboli, liver abscess. Any evidence of central line-associated blood stream infection (CLABSI) warrants catheter removal.
2. Line malposition
   a. **Heart and major vessels:** Pericardial effusion, cardiac tamponade, arrhythmia, endocarditis, left atrial thrombus. Cardiac complications are rare but life-threatening.

   b. **Portal system:** Portal vein thrombosis, NEC, hepatic necrosis, hepatic abscess.[6]
3. Blood loss
   a. From umbilical stump
   b. Accidental UVC disconnection
4. Thromboembolism can happen to the lungs, liver, or systemic circulation. It can present as pulmonary edema, pulmonary hemorrhage, hepatic necrosis, abscess, and calcification. Removal of the catheter is indicated.
5. Catheter breakage

Percutaneously Inserted Central Catheter

A percutaneously inserted central catheter (PICC) is a soft, flexible catheter inserted into a peripheral vein and directed into the central vein. Neonatal PICC are small bore catheters (1–2.7 Fr) suitable for low flow infusion rates in neonates (1–3 ml/min).

Indications

1. Preterm neonates needing parenteral nutrition when UVC is contraindicated (refer above).
   a. All neonates <1000 g and not on significant feeds.
   b) Birth weight 1000–1499 g and not likely to receive significant feeds for 3 or *more days*.
   c. Birth weight more than 1500 g and not likely to receive significant feeds for 5 or more days.
2. Prolonged intravenous access (usually more than 5–7 days) in gastrointestinal/surgical disorders, congenital cardiac conditions, etc.
3. Hyperosmolar intravenous fluid/medication (dopamine, dobutamine, calcium gluconate) administration.
4. Difficult intravenous access.

Vein Selection

Upper limb: Cephalic, basilic, median cubital, or axillary vein.
Lower limb: Saphenous vein, popliteal vein.

Scalp veins (temporal and posterior auricular veins)and external jugular veins can rarely be used.

Length of Insertion

The desired insertion length for PICC is calculated using surface landmarks for both upper and lower limbs (Table 42.3).

Table 42.3: Estimation of length of insertion for PICC	
Estimating distance of insertion	*Optimum tip position*
Upper limb: Measure the distance from the insertion point along the venous pathway to the suprasternal notch to the right 3rd intercostal space (Fig. 42.3).	PICC tip is considered to be correctly positioned if it meets all of the following three parameters: First, it crosses the first costochondral junction of the same side, second after crossing the first costochondral junction, it should have progressed medially and downwards and should have stayed above the heart base. The point where the right atrial hump straightens towards SVC on contrast radiography was considered the heart base (Fig. 42.4).
Lower limb: Measure the distance from the point of insertion to the umbilicus and then to the xiphisternum.	The inferior vena cava (IVC) is below the diaphragm (T9–T10) and above the L4–L5 vertebrae level.

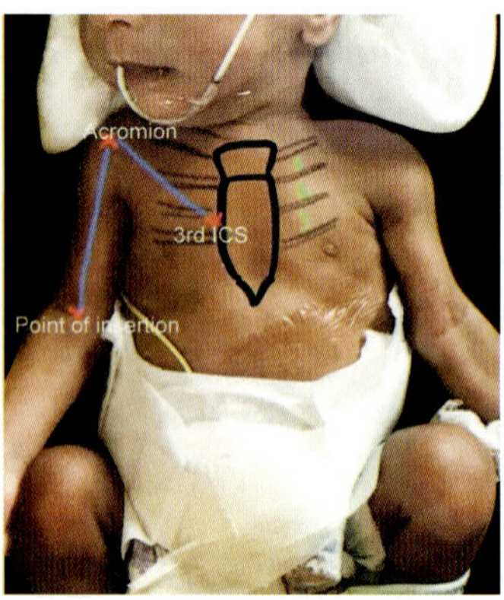

Fig. 42.3: Estimating the desired length of PICC insertion in upper limb.

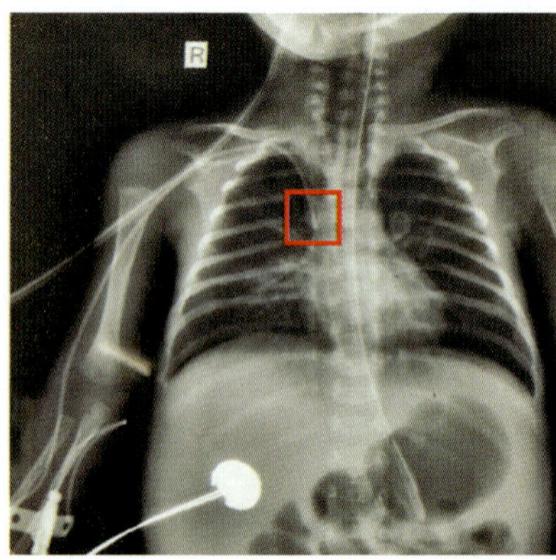

Fig. 42.4: Anteroposterior radiograph of chest showing satisfactory position of PICC line (red box) inserted in the right upper limb.

The malposition rate is high when anatomical landmarks are used for calculating the length to be inserted, with a tendency to overestimate the actual length.

Confirmation of PICC Tip Position

1. **X-ray:** Always confirm the tip position of the catheter by an X-ray (see above); preferably, both anteroposterior and lateral views are

to be taken in case of lower limb PICC for better visualization. Radio-opaque contrast (0.3–0.5 ml) helps assess the location of the catheter tip in small-size catheters.

2. **Real-time ultrasound (RT-USG):** High parasternal, subcostal, bicaval, and apical views can be used to localize the PICC tip during the procedure. The tip should be manipulated to lie at the SVC – RA junction.[6]

Recommended Catheter Size

- Infant's birth weight ≤1.0 kg: 1 Fr (28 G)
- Infant's birth weights >1.0 kg: 2 Fr (24 G)

Practical tip

- Prefer upper limb PICC as they are associated with fewer complications.
- Do not use PICC for blood sampling or central venous pressure monitoring.
- Packed cell transfusions should be avoided due to the risk of catheter occlusion.

PICC Maintenance

1. Use transparent occlusive dressings to allow easy visualization of the catheter site. Change the dressing only when visibly soiled, damp, or loosened. For optimum sterility, two persons should change the dressing.
2. Assess the catheter site and review the need for a central catheter daily. Remove the catheter at the earliest when it is no longer needed.
3. Always "scrub the hub" for at least 15 seconds before initiating any infusion to prevent contamination of the central line.
4. For surveillance, use quality indicators such as catheter dwell time and central line-associated bloodstream infections (CLABSI). Use CLABSI Bundle (Table 42.4).

Table 42.4: A bundled approach for prevention of CLABSI[8]

1. Proper hand hygiene is the single most crucial intervention.
2. Best CVC practices: optimal insertion using a checklist, daily maintenance, timely removal.
3. Real-time surveillance and reporting of infection.

Complications

1. **Catheter-related sepsis:** Higher chance of multiple insertion attempts, hub manipulation, etc. Coagulase-negative staphylococci are the most common pathogen. It is also the most common healthcare-associated infection in NICU. Bundled care approach helps in reducing CLABSI; Table 42.5).
2. **Line migration:** Cardiac arrhythmia, pericardial effusion, pericardial tamponade, tissue extravasation, pleural effusion. Ascending lumbar vein (ALV) migration is a common complication of lower limb PICCs.
3. **Thrombosis (more in lower extremity lines):** It includes deep venous thrombus, renal vein thrombus, and intracardiac thrombus. It is responsible for 90% of venous thromboembolic events in neonates.
4. Catheter breakage or dysfunction
5. Phlebitis

In rare situations when PICC placement is not possible, and there is no other venous access, central venous access can be established by centrally inserted central catheters (CICC) (using internal jugular vein (IJV), subclavian vein and femoral vein)

PERCUTANEOUS ARTERIAL CATHETERIZATION

Indications

1. Continuous monitoring of invasive blood pressure in critically sick babies.
2. Need for frequent samplings, such as the need for repeated arterial blood gases in ventilated babies.
3. Inability to insert a UAC/removal of UAC due to complications.

Table 42.5: Central: line-associated bloodstream infection (CLABSI) definition

Presence of all

1. Occurrence of laboratory-confirmed bloodstream infection (LCBI).
2. Duration of central line (CL) or umbilical catheter (UC) for 2 or more calendar days on the occurrence of CLABSI, with a day of catheter insertion being the first day.
3. The line must be in place either on the day of CLABSI or the day before.

The term catheter related blood stream infection (CRBSI) is used when the same organism is recovered from percutaneous blood culture and from culture of catheter tip with a 3-fold colony count in the latter.

Preferred Site

Radial artery or posterior tibial artery as they have good collateral circulation. The axillary artery, femoral artery, dorsalis pedis artery, and temporal artery should be avoided.

Practical tip

- Perform modified Allen's test (Table 42.6) before cannulation of the radial artery to establish patency of ulnar artery circulation.
- Use transillumination with a cold light for better visualization of the artery (Fig. 42.5).
- Always fix the cannula allowing good visibility of fingers and toes.
- Maintain patency of catheter using low-dose heparin infusion(0.5 U/ml).

Complications

1. Vascular—vasospasm/thrombosis/embolism: Most common; can lead to blanching of extremity, skin necrosis, gangrene, and loss of digits. The catheter should be removed immediately once evidence of ischemia is seen.
2. Hemorrhage/hematoma at the puncture site
3. Infection
4. Air embolism

Table 42.6: Modified Allen test

- Apply pressure on the palm and fingers of the infant to blanch.
- Apply pressure using your fingers to both the radial and ulnar arteries of the infant to obstruct blood flow.
- Release the occlusive pressure only on the ulnar artery.
  - Positive test If hand flushes within 5–15 seconds (good flow in the ulnar artery).
- Negative test - If the hand does not flush within 5–15 seconds, there is poor flow in the ulnar artery. Do not puncture the radial artery puncture in such cases.

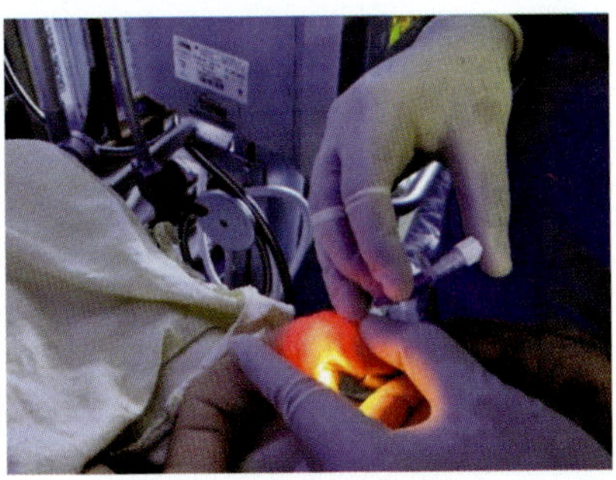

Fig. 42.5: Radial artery cannulation using transillumination

REFERENCES

1. Dunn PM. Localization of the umbilical catheter by post-mortem measurement. Arch Dis Child. 1966;41(215):69–75.
2. Shukla H, Ferrara A. Rapid estimation of insertional length of umbilical catheters in newborns. Am J Dis Child. 1986 Aug;140(8):786–8.
3. Wright IM, Owers M, Wagner M. The umbilical arterial catheter: a formula for improved positioning in the very low birth weight infant. Pediatr Crit Care Med. 2008 Sep;9(5):498–501.
4. Barrington KJ. Umbilical artery catheters in the newborn: effects of position of the catheter tip. In: The Cochrane Collaboration, ed. Cochrane Database of Systematic Reviews. Chichester, UK: John Wiley & Sons, Ltd; 1999. doi:10.1002/14651858.CD000505.
5. Samiee-Zafarghandy S, van den Anker JN, Ben Fadel N. Topical nitroglycerin in neonates with tissue injury: A case report and review of the literature. Paediatr Child Health. 2014 Jan;19(1):9–12.
6. Barone G, Pittiruti M, Biasucci DG, Elisei D, Iacobone E, La Greca A, Zito Marinosci G, D'Andrea V. Neo-ECHOTIP: A structured protocol for ultrasound-based tip navigation and tip location during placement of central venous access devices in neonates. J Vasc Access. 2021 Apr 5:11297298211007703.
7. Kishigami M, Shimokaze T, Enomoto M, Shibasaki J, Toyoshima K. Ultrasound-Guided Umbilical Venous Catheter Insertion With Alignment of the Umbilical Vein and Ductus Venosus. J Ultrasound Med. 2020 Feb;39(2):379–83.
8. Butler-O'Hara M, D'Angio CT, Hoey H, Stevens TP. An evidence-based catheter bundle alters central venous catheter strategy in newborn infants. J Pediatr. 2012;160(6):972-7.e2. doi:10.1016/j.jpeds.2011.12.004.

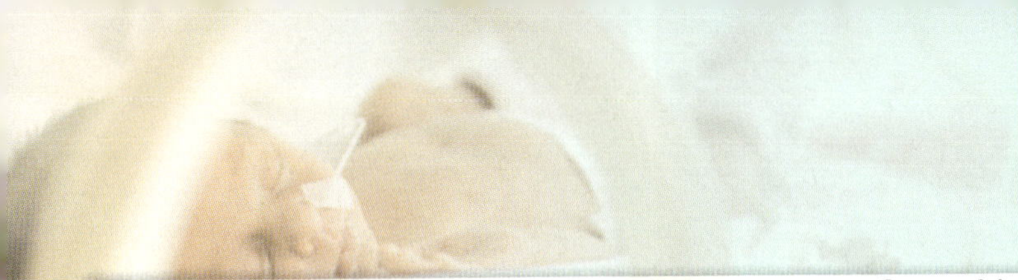

Section

12

Therapeutic Modalities

CHAPTER

43

Oxygen Saturation Policy in the NICU

Oxygen is a drug and oxygen toxicity can have significant adverse effects in preterm infants including bronchopulmonary dysplasia (BPD) and retinopathy of prematurity (ROP). Each NICU should have a policy for targeting oxygen saturation in neonates and implementation of such guidelines has shown reduction in the incidence of severe ROP.[1]

Evidence on oxygen saturation targeting

Five major randomized controlled trials, the SUPPORT Study, the Benefits of Oxygen Saturation Targeting (BOOST II) trial and the Canadian Oxygen Trial (COT) compared two SpO_2 target ranges—low (85–89%) vs. high (91–95%)—involving around 5000 preterm neonates of <28 weeks of gestation. The results have been pooled in a meta-analysis called the NEOPROM[2] project which showed no significant difference between the lower and higher SpO_2 target range on the primary composite outcome of death or major disability at a corrected age of 18–24 months. However, neonates randomized to the lower SpO_2 target range had a higher risk of death and necrotizing enterocolitis, but a lower risk of retinopathy of prematurity. This study suggests that an SpO_2 target range of 91–95% may be safer compared to 85–89% in extremely preterm infants due to a higher risk of death associated with the lower range.

IMPLICATIONS FOR PRACTICE

- The National Neonatology forum (NNF) clinical practice guidelines (CPG) recommend an oxygen saturation target of 91–95% in all neonates (both 34 weeks and >34 weeks of gestational age) requiring respiratory support.[3]
- The NNF-CPG also recommends a similar oxygen saturation target (91–95%) for preterm neonates with evolving or established BPD and requiring respiratory support.
- Oxygen therapy should always be administered based on pulse oximeter based continuous SpO_2 monitoring.

- The alarm limits should be set no more than 1 or 2% above or below the chosen target range and should always be 'on'. The upper alarm limit should always be 95% and it can be increased to 100% if the neonate is on 21% FiO_2 on respiratory support to decrease alarm fatigue.[4]
- The alarm delay should not be longer than 20 sec to ensure that significant events are not missed.
- Small incremental changes (1–5%) in FiO_2 are preferred to avoid fluctuations in SpO_2 unless oxygen saturation is below 70% or associated with apnea or bradycardia.
- Routine preoxygenation (up to 100%) for procedures such as endotracheal suction, venous cannulation, or other painful procedures should be avoided.
- When hypoxia or hyperoxia is indicated by the monitor, respond to the neonate first and the monitor next. The evaluation should include:
  - Ascertaining if there is bradycardia, apnea, or cyanosis by a clinical examination, which may warrant immediate intervention.
  - Assessing air-way patency and clear secretions, if any.
  - Ensuring if the pulse oximeter probe is attached correctly and there are no motion artifacts.
  - Adjusting the FiO_2 in small incremental steps to achieve the target saturation and
  - Addressing the underlying disease problem.
- Discuss the percentage time spent within and outside the target SpO_2 range if oxygen saturation histograms are downloadable from pulse oximeters and the frequency of desaturations over the preceding 24-hour period with the healthcare providers during daily rounds.
- Quality improvement initiatives targeting caregiver education, implementation of guidelines for oxygen administration and targeting, bedside availability of histograms, and event review during rounds can result in better oxygen saturation targeting and improved clinical outcomes.[4]

REFERENCES

1. Lau YY, Tay YY, Shah VA, Chang P, Loh KT. Maintaining optimal oxygen saturation in premature infants. Perm J. 2011;15(1):e108–13.
2. Askie LM, Darlow BA, Finer N, Schmidt B, Stenson B, Tarnow-Mordi W, et al. Neonatal Oxygen-ation Prospective Meta-analysis (NeOProM) Collaboration.

Association Between Oxygen Satu-ration Targeting and Death or Disability in Extremely Preterm Infants in the Neonatal Oxygena-tion Prospective Meta-analysis Collaboration. JAMA. 2018;319(21):2190–201.

3. NNF India Evidence-based Clinical Practice Guidelines. Oxygen therapy in neonates. December 2021. Available at: https://www.nnfi.org/assests/upload/usefull-links-pdf/Oxygen_therapy_in_neonates_NNFI_CPG_Dec2021.pdf Accessed 18-04-2023.
4. Shivananda S, Thomas S, Dutta S, Fusch C, Williams C, Gautham KS. Care Bundle to Improve Oxygen Maintenance and Events. Pediatr Qual Saf. 2023;8(2):e639.

CHAPTER

44

Surfactant Replacement Therapy in Neonates

Respiratory failure secondary to surfactant deficiency is a significant cause of morbidity and mortality in preterm neonates. Exogenous surfactant therapy substantially reduces mortality and respiratory morbidities in them.

SURFACTANTS (Table 44.1)

Dosage

Term infants usually have a surfactant storage pool of approximately 100 mg/kg, whereas preterm infants have an estimated pool of only 4–5 mg/kg at birth. Exogenous surfactant therapy rapidly increases pool size and improves pulmonary gas exchange until endogenous surfactant is released. A minimum of 100 mg/kg of surfactant should

Table 44.1: Commonly used surfactant preparations

Natural	*Minced lung extract*	1. Beractant (Survanta®) 2. Poractantalfa (Curosurf®) 3. Surfactant TA (Surfacten®)
	Lung lavage extract	1. Bovine LipidExtract Surfactant (BLES) 2. Calfactant (Infasurf®) 3. SF-RI1 (Alveofact®)
Newer synthetic	New synthetic (protein analogs)-second generation	1. Lucinactant (Surfaxin)-SPB analogues, Sinapultide 2. rSP-C surfactant (Venticute)-SPC analogues, Lusupultide
	Third generation	CHF 5633 (SP-B and SP-C enriched synthetic surfactant)

1. Bovine minced lung extracts contain less than 10% of the SP-B found in the bovine lung lavage extracts.
2. Synthetic surfactants do not have the theoretical concerns associated with animal-derived surfactants like transmission of microorganisms, exposure to animal proteins and inflammatory mediators, and susceptibility to inactivation.
3. First-generation protein-free synthetic surfactants are no longer used.

Table 44.2: Common brands of surfactant available in India and dosage			
Surfactant preparations	*Survanta (Abbvie)*	*Curosurf (Nicholas)*	*Neosurf (Cipla)*
Dose Phospholipids	4 ml/kg (100 mg/kg)	2.5 ml/kg (200 mg/kg)	5 ml/kg (135 mg/kg)
Available formulation	4 ml and 8 ml	1.5 ml and 3 ml	3 ml and 5 ml
Cost	INR 8800 and 14500	INR 11780 and 20790	INR 4900 and 7950

be administered to preterm infants with RDS. Doses of 50 mg/kg to 200 mg/kg have been studied. A higher dose of poractant (200 mg/kg) has been found to be superior in reducing mortality and BPD compared to low-dose poractant or beractant (Table 44.2).

Indications for Surfactant Therapy

Surfactant replacement is done mainly for RDS. But it can be used in other conditions where the surfactant is inactivated, such as meconium aspiration syndrome, pneumonia, pulmonary hemorrhage, congenital diaphragmatic hernia, and acute respiratory distress syndrome.

In extreme or very preterm neonates, the surfactant can be administered prophylactically or as rescue therapy (Fig. 44.1).

1. **Prophylactic surfactant:** Surfactant is administered within 15–30 min of birth, irrespective of the signs of RDS. Prophylactic surfactant therapy should be used with caution as recent evidence suggests an increased risk of BPD/mortality compared to selective surfactant administration. It may be considered only in neonates born before 28 weeks of gestation with no/incomplete antenatal steroids or required intubation and mechanical ventilation immediately after birth.[1–5]

   Rationale: Administration of surfactant to a previously unventilated or minimally ventilated lung will diminish acute lung injury. Acute lung injury results in alveolar-capillary damage, leakage of proteinaceous fluid into the alveolar space, and release of inflammatory mediators, resulting in decreased response to surfactant replacement.

2. **Early rescue:** Surfactant is administered in an infant with features of RDS within 2 hours. Early administration of surfactant is

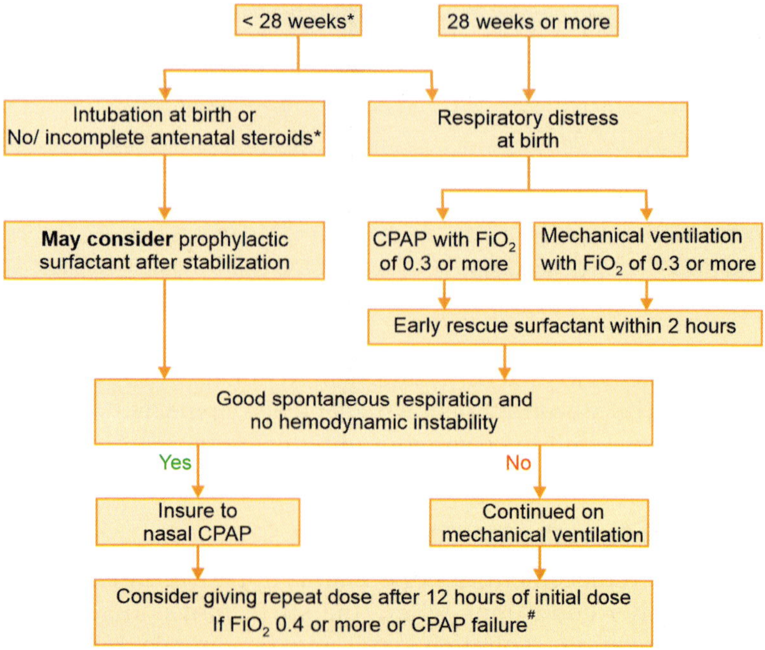

*Individualised decision to be taken for giving prophylactic surfactant in this group
#Duration might vary based on the preparation

Fig. 44.1: Surfactant replacement therapy

advantageous as the presence of lung fluid helps in the uniform distribution of the surfactant. It also ensures that surfactant is administered before widespread atelectasis develops in the lungs. Early rescue surfactant therapy following a trial of CPAP is preferred over prophylactic treatment because it reduces the amount of surfactant used with comparable immediate outcomes.

3. **Late rescue:** Surfactant is administered in an infant with features of RDS after 2 hours. It is usually done in outborn neonates who are transported late to referral centers.

Procedure for Surfactant Administration via InSurE

The standard method of surfactant administration is through the endotracheal tube after intubation of the infant (Table 44.3).

Methods of Surfactant Administration

Surfactant preparations must spread uniformly throughout the lung into the air-liquid interface once instilled in the proximal airways.

Table 44.3: Procedure for surfactant administration

1. A physician or a nurse experienced in surfactant administration should administer the surfactant.
2. Warm the surfactant prior to administration (for 8 minutes if the vial is held between the palms of the hands or for 20 minutes at room temperature.) The vial should not be heated, and it should not be kept on radiant warmer. It should not be kept in room air for morc than 30 min as it increases viscosity.
3. Do not shake the surfactant.
4. Intubate the baby with appropriate size endotracheal tube.
5. Assess breath sounds for equality. Chest X-ray is not mandatory for confirmation of ET tube position.
6. Infant should be connected to a pulse oximeter and oxygen saturation and heart rate must be monitored throughout the procedure.
7. Administer the surfactant through the feeding tube inserted in the ET tube or through the side port of the ET tube (if available).
8. Surfactant is given as bolus instillation in four aliquots of the total dose.
9. Connect the infant to ventilator or the T-piece resuscitator with set PIP and PEEP and ventilate carefully till saturation and heart rate stabilizes before administering the next aliquot.
10. Consider increasing PIP by 10% for about 5 min after surfactant administration if chest rise is inadequate.
11. No position change of the infant is required between the aliquots.
12. Suctioning of ET tube should be avoided for at least 2 hours following surfactant administration

**Strict asepsis should be carried out throughout the procedure*

1. **Slow infusion versus rapid bolus administration:** Surfactant can be administered either by slow tracheal infusion or rapid bolus administration. Natural surfactant works best if given by a rapid bolus into the lungs as it leads to the homogeneous distribution of surfactant and results in rapid improvement in oxygenation. On the other hand, it can also cause ET tube obstruction, transient bradycardia, hypotension, and changes in cerebral blood flow. Slow infusion results in nonhomogenous distribution of surfactant. Currently, the rapid bolus technique is the recommended method of surfactant administration.
2. **Through endotracheal tube (InSurE-Intubate – Surfactant – Extubate to CPAP):** InSurE comprises intubation, surfactant administration, a brief period of ventilation (usually <1 hour), and rapid extubation to nasal CPAP to prevent ventilation induced lung injury (VILI). In infants with signs and symptoms of RDS, InSurE to nasal CPAP results in a decreased duration of

mechanical ventilation, air leak, and less incidence of BPD. InSurE technique may not be successful in neonates with severe birth asphyxia, lack of complete course of antenatal steroids, extreme prematurity, delayed administration of surfactant, and shock.

3. **Through a thin catheter (Less invasive surfactant administration [LISA]/Minimally invasive surfactant therapy [MIST]):** Due to the risks associated with ET tube placement and ventilation, newer techniques with less invasive surfactant therapy have emerged. LISA involves the administration of surfactant through a feeding tube (4–5 Fr catheter) inserted into the trachea using Magill forceps under direct laryngoscopy without intubation. In contrast, in MIST, a slightly stiff catheter (e.g. surfcath, angiocath 16G) is used to administer surfactant without using Magill forceps. CPAP is continued during surfactant administration to facilitate alveolar recruitment, which helps distribute surfactant and avoids positive pressure ventilation. LISA technique, as compared to InSurE, has been shown to reduce the risk of death or BPD, the need for mechanical ventilation, and pneumothorax. Nowadays, dedicated LISA catheters have become available. Personnel practicing LISA should be adequately trained regarding the use of Magill forceps and the depth of insertion of the catheter. Poractant is preferable for LISA/MIST as the volume instilled is lesser than beractant.
4. **Through laryngeal mask airway:** A few trials that used LMA for surfactant therapy in infants of more than 1000 g showed less need for mechanical ventilation. Surfactant reflux and coughing are more frequently seen in these infants. There is a lack of solid evidence to recommend using LMA for surfactant administration in preterm neonates.
5. **Nebulized surfactant delivery:** It is a genuinely noninvasive technique. Practical issues like loss of surfactant in the upper airway/esophagus, inactivation of surfactant, and nonhomogenous distribution need to be addressed before nebulized surfactant can be adopted in routine clinical practice.

Repeat Dose of Surfactant

Multiple doses of surfactant have a more significant effect than a single dose on air leaks. Repeat doses of surfactant may be required in an infant if the administered surfactant is inhibited by edema fluid, soluble proteins, or inflammatory mediators present in the alveoli after lung injury due to mechanical ventilation, delayed surfactant administration, or sepsis. Using a higher threshold for re-treatment with surfactant is as effective as a low threshold and can result in significant cost savings. Infants may require repeat dose(s) of surfactant if they require FiO_2 of 0.4 or more on CPAP and mechanical ventilation to maintain target saturation. Infants with lower gestational age, male sex, lack of antenatal steroids, and initial requirement of higher FiO_2 might require repeated doses of surfactant. Administering more than three doses has not been shown to have a benefit.

Poor Response to Surfactant

Some infants may not show the expected response to the surfactant administered ('RDS plus'). These non-responders usually have lung injury either before birth (infection) or after delivery but prior to treatment (volutrauma and barotrauma), asphyxia, sepsis/pneumonia, meconium aspiration, the severity of disease, pulmonary hypoplasia, or hemodynamic instability (shock).

Intratracheal Administration of Corticosteroids and Surfactant

Corticosteroids (systemic and inhaled) have been used to prevent and treat BPD. Early intratracheal administration of corticosteroids (especially budesonide) has been hypothesized to reduce the incidence of BPD by suppressing lung inflammation. But trials on intratracheal administration of steroids alone have not shown any proven benefit. Meta-analysis of trials comparing intratracheal steroids with surfactant as a vehicle compared to surfactant alone have shown to decrease the risk of BPD and BPD/mortality at 36 weeks. But due to the heterogeneity of trials, additional cost, and feasibility of preparing the mixture, intratracheal administration of steroids with surfactant is currently not recommended.

Adverse Reactions of Surfactant Administration

Surfactant replacement therapy is much safer, and side effects are usually transient. Hypoxia and bradycardia can occur during surfactant instillation due to acute airway obstruction. Other less common acute adverse effects are reflux of surfactant into the pharynx, increased PCO_2, gagging, and mucous plugging of the ET tube. There is an increase in the risk of pulmonary hemorrhage following surfactant therapy which is more common with natural surfactants (5–6%) than with newer-generation synthetic surfactants (1–3%). Pulmonary hemorrhage typically occurs within 72 hours and is due to improved lung compliance after surfactant therapy, which promotes an increase in left-to-right shunt through the PDA, resulting in increased blood flow and congestion. Evidence suggests that surfactant therapy reduces the risk of mortality, air leak, or BPD.

LONG-TERM OUTCOMES

Improved or equivalent results on pulmonary function testing but no significant differences in the long-term neurodevelopmental outcomes have been reported in infants treated with surfactant compared to those treated with placebo.

Evidence[6–13]

Prophylactic versus selective surfactant

Studies conducted prior to the routine application of CPAP demonstrated a decrease in the risk of air leak and neonatal mortality associated with prophylactic administration of surfactant. However, when all studies were evaluated together, no benefits of prophylactic surfactant could be demonstrated and there is higher incidence of BPD or death in prophylactic surfactant group (RR1.13; 95% CI 1.02–1.25) (Cochrane 2012).

Early rescue versus late rescue surfactant

Early rescue surfactant reduces the risk of neonatal mortality (RR 0.84; 95% CI 0.74–0.95), BPD (RR 0.69; 95% CI 0.55–0.86), and overall air leak syndromes (RR 0.61; 95% CI 0.48–0.78) (Cochrane 2012).

InSurE

InSurE compared with surfactant administration followed by continued mechanical ventilation and extubation from low respiratory support was associated with a lower incidence of need for mechanical ventilation [RR 0.67, 95% CI 0.57–0.79], air leak syndromes [RR 0.52, 95% CI 0.28–0.96] and BPD [RR 0.51, 95% CI 0.26–0.99] (Cochrane 2007).

Surfactant replacement therapy (SRT) in LMIC

Systematic review on SRT in preterm with RDS from LMICs showed a significant reduction in mortality (RR 0.67; 95% CI 0.57–0.79) and air leaks (RR0.51; 95% CI 0.29–0.90).

New synthetic versus animal-derived surfactant

Protein containing synthetic surfactant compared with animal-derived surfactant did not demonstrate any significant reduction in risk of mortality (RR0.81, 95% CI 0.64–1.03) or BPD (RR 0.99, 95% CI 0.84–1.18) (Cochrane 2007).

Single dose versus multiple doses of surfactant

Repeat dose of surfactant administration results in a lower incidence of pneumothorax (RR 0.51, 95% CI 0.30–0.88) and a decreased trend towards mortality (RR0.63, 95% CI 0.39–1.02) (Cochrane 2009).

(Contd.)

(*Contd.*)

Less Invasive Surfactant Administration (LISA)
Metanalysis of 6 trials comparing the LISA technique with intubation for surfactant delivery demonstrated the reduced composite outcome of death or BPD at 36 weeks (RR 0.75; 95% CI 0.59–0.94), BPD at 36 weeks (RR 0.72; 95% CI 0.53–0.97) or need for mechanical ventilation anytime during NICU stay (RR 0.66; 95 % CI 0.47–0.93).

REFERENCES

1. Polin RA, Carlo WA, Committee on Fetus and Newborn, American Academy of Pediatrics. Surfactant replacement therapy for preterm and term neonates with respiratory distress. Pediatrics. 2014 Jan;133(1):156–63.
2. Ng EH, Shah V. Guidelines for surfactant replacement therapy in neonates. Paediatr Child Health. 2021;26:35–49.
3. Sweet DG, Carnielli V, Greisen G, Hallman M, Ozek E, te Pas A, et al. European Consensus Guidelines on the Management of Respiratory Distress Syndrome - 2019 Update. Neonatology. 2019 Jun;115(4):432–50.
4. Abiramalatha T, Ramaswamy VV, Bandyopadhyay T, Somanath SH, Shaik NB, Pullattayil AK, et al. Interventions to Prevent Bronchopulmonary Dysplasia in Preterm Neonates: An Umbrella Review of Systematic Reviews and Metaanalyses. JAMA Pediatrics. 2022.
5. National Neonatology Forum India Clinical Practice Guidelines [Dec 2021 update]. Surfactant Replacement therapy in neonates. Available from www.nnfi.org/cpg.
6. Rojas-Reyes MX, Morley CJ, Soll R. Prophylactic versus selective use of surfactant in preventing morbidity and mortality in preterm infants. Cochrane Database Syst Rev. 2012 Mar 14;(3):CD000510.
7. Bahadue FL, Soll R. Early versus delayed selective surfactant treatment for neonatal respiratory distress syndrome. Cochrane Database Syst Rev. 2012 Nov 14;11:CD001456.
8. SUPPORT Study Group of the Eunice Kennedy Shriver NICHD Neonatal Research Network, Finer NN, Carlo WA, Walsh MC, Rich W, Gantz MG, et al. Early CPAP versus surfactant in extremely preterm infants. N Engl J Med. 2010 May 27;362(21):1970–9.
9. Stevens TP, Harrington EW, Blennow M, Soll RF. Early surfactant administration with brief ventilation vs. selective surfactant and continued mechanical ventilation for preterm infants with or at risk for respiratory distress syndrome. Cochrane Database Syst Rev. 2007 Oct 17;(4):CD003063.
10. Sankar MJ, Gupta N, Jain K, Agarwal R. Efficacy and safety of surfactant replacement therapy for preterm neonates with respiratory distress syndrome in low- and middle-income countries: a systematic review. J Perinatol. 2016;36 Suppl 1:S36–48.

11. Pfister RH, Soll RF, Wiswell T. Protein containing synthetic surfactant versus animal derived surfactant extract for the prevention and treatment of respiratory distress syndrome. The Cochrane Database Syst Rev. 2007(4):CD006069.
12. Soll R, Ozek E. Multiple versus single doses of exogenous surfactant for the prevention or treatment of neonatal respiratory distress syndrome. Cochrane Database Syst Rev. 2009 Jan 21;(1):CD000141.
13. Aldana-Aguirre JC, Pinto M, Featherstone RM, Kumar M. Less invasive surfactant administration versus intubation for surfactant delivery in preterm infants with respiratory distress syndrome: a systematic review and meta-analysis. Arch Dis Child Fetal Neonatal Ed. 2017;102(1):F17-F23.

CHAPTER

45

Fluid and Electrolyte Management

The goal of fluid and electrolyte management is to maintain fluid homeostasis, which can be altered by the physiological immaturity of organ systems involved in maintaining homeostasis or various systemic illnesses in neonates.

Adaptation to extrauterine life consists of three phases of fluid balance. In the first week of life, there is a decrease in the total body water by shrinkage of the extracellular fluid (ECF) compartment.[1] Loss of the excess ECF and evaporative water loss from immature skin results in physiological weight loss during this period. This phase of transition ends with maximum weight loss. Since the ECF compartment is larger in more preterm neonates, the weight loss is greater in preterm neonates. During the second phase, the insensible water loss reduces as the skin barrier matures, urine volume falls to less than 2 ml/kg/hour, and sodium excretion becomes low. The third phase consists of stable growth characterized by continuous weight gain with a positive net balance for water and sodium.

RENAL FUNCTION

Neonates have a limited capacity to excrete either concentrated (due to immaturity of the distal nephron with an anatomically shortened loop of Henle) or diluted urine (due to physiologically low glomerular filtration rate). The physiological range of urine osmolality varies from a lower limit of 50 mmol/L to upper limits of 600 mmol/L in preterm neonates and 800 mmol/L in term neonates[2,3] An acceptable osmolality range of 300–400 mmol/L corresponds to a daily urine output of 2–3 ml/kg/hr.

SODIUM BALANCE

Neonatal kidneys have a limited capacity to excrete or conserve sodium. The maturity of sodium handling depends on the gestation and postnatal age.[4] Normally, there is salt and water diuresis in the first 48–72 hours of life. Therefore, sodium supplementation should be started after ensuring initial diuresis or at least 5–6% weight loss. Preterm neonates have a limited tubular capacity to reabsorb sodium due to tubular immaturity and reduced responsiveness to aldosterone and hence have increased urinary losses.[5] Failure to supplement sodium after the first week of life can result in low body stores of sodium and poor weight gain.[3,6] Very low birth weight infants on exclusive breastfeeding may need sodium supplementation in addition to breast milk till 32–34 weeks corrected age.[7,8]

FLUID LOSSES

In addition to water loss by the kidneys and gastrointestinal system ('sensible' loss), additional water losses occur due to evaporation from the skin and respiratory tract. This water loss is termed insensible water loss (IWL). IWL tends to be higher in preterm infants (Table 45.1).

Evaporative loss through the skin usually contributes to 70% of IWL.[1] The remaining 30% is contributed by losses from the respiratory tract. The fluid management of neonates should focus on prevention rather than replacement of increased IWL.

The strategies to reduce insensible water loss include the following:

- Antenatal corticosteroids aid in accelerated skin maturation in preterm babies.[9]
- Double-wall incubators with humidification.
- Covering the bassinette of the radiant warmer with cling wrap.[10]
- Covering the head and extremities with caps and socks.
- Topical application of emollient or coconut oil or safflower oil (50%).[11,12]
- Use of warm and humidified inspiratory gas for babies on respiratory support.

Table 45.1: Insensible water loss according to birth weight on day 1

Birth weight (g)	*Insensible water loss (ml/kg/day)*
<1000	60–80
1000–1500	40–60
>1500	20

Guidelines for Fluid and Electrolyte Therapy

First week of postnatal life: The goals for fluid and electrolyte administration during the first week are to:

a. Allow contraction of ECF (without compromising intravascular fluid volume and cardiovascular function) with a negative fluid balance of not more than 10%.
b. Allow a negative net balance for sodium of 2–5 mmol/kg/day to maintain normal serum electrolyte concentrations.
c. Avoid oliguria (0.5–1.0 ml/kg/hour) for longer than twelve hours, and
d. Avoid excessive transepidermal water loss. Once the transition period is over, the goals are to attain a weight gain of 15–20 g/kg/day and progressively increase oral feeds.

The amount of actual fluid intake to be prescribed from the recommended range for each day (Table 45.2) is decided based on the clinical examination and laboratory parameters—the neonate should have physiological (not excessive) weight loss, normal tissue perfusion, normal serum electrolytes, and adequate urine output (see below).

Physiological Basis for Fluid Requirements in the First Week of Life

Term and Preterm Neonates with a Birth Weight of 1500 g or more

Day 1: These neonates must excrete a solute load of about 15 mOsm/kg/day through the kidneys. To excrete this solute load at a urine osmolarity of 300 mOsm/kg/day, they need a minimum of 50 ml/kg of free water. Allowing for an additional IWL of 20 ml/kg, the initial fluids should be 60–70 ml/kg/day.

Day 2–7: As the neonate grows and receives enteral milk feeds, the solute load presented to the kidneys increases, and the infant requires more fluid to excrete the solute load. Water is also needed for fecal losses and growth purposes. Therefore, the fluid requirements increase by 15–20 ml/kg/day up to 150 ml/kg/day.

Preterm Very Low Birth Weight Neonates

Day 1: The urine output in these neonates is likely to be similar to that of term neonates. However, their fluid requirement will be higher due to increased IWL and weight loss (extracellular fluid loss). Using caps, socks, and plastic barriers (cling wrap) under the radiant warmer is recommended to reduce the IWL rather than

Table 45.2: Parenteral fluid and electrolyte requirements during the first week after birth

	Parenteral fluid in ml/kg/day *Day after birth*						
	1	*2*	*3*	*4*	*5*	*6*	*7*
Term neonates AND Preterm neonates with birth weight >1500 g	60–80	80–100	100–120	120–140	140–160	140–160	140–160
Preterm neonates with birth weight <1500 g	80–90	100–110	120–130	130–150	140–160	150–170	150–180

Electrolyte requirement (mEq/kg)*	
Sodium	3–4 (careful adjustment needed in neonates weighing <1000 g)
Potassium	1–2 (start after the onset of diuresis)
Chloride	3–4

**No electrolyte supplementation is required in the initial 48 hours of life.*

NB:
- Dextrose infusion should be maintained at 4–6 mg/kg/min; ELBW neonates are at high risk of hyperglycemia—blood glucose should be monitored frequently to titrate the glucose infusion rate.
- Calcium may be used in a dose of 4 ml/kg/day (40 mg/kg/day) of calcium gluconate for the first 3 days in certain high-risk situations (see the protocol on 'hypocalcemia').

unduly increase the fluid intake. With the measures to reduce IWL (see above), managing VLBW neonates with a fluid intake of 80 mL/kg/day on day 1 of life is possible. The fluid requirement on the first day of life in extremely preterm neonates is discussed below (*see* 'Specific clinical conditions').

Day 2–7: As the skin matures in preterm neonates, the IWL progressively decreases and becomes like that of term neonates by the end of the first week. Hence, their fluid requirement is not different from that of term neonates during this period. Fluid intake needs to be increased by 15–20 ml/kg/day up to 150–180 ml/kg/day.

After the First Postnatal Week

The goals in stable neonates after the first week of life are to maintain water and electrolyte homeostasis and provide enough additional fluids and electrolytes to build new tissue at intrauterine growth rates (Table 45.3).

Restricted fluids in preterm neonates: what is the evidence?

A review of five randomized studies with different levels of fluid intake during the first week of life concluded that fluid restriction reduces the risk of patent ductus arteriosus and necrotizing enterocolitis with trend towards reduction in risk of bronchopulmonary dysplasia, intracranial hemorrhage, death, and increased risk of dehydration.[13]

MONITORING OF FLUID AND ELECTROLYTE STATUS

Body weight: Serial weight measurements can be used to estimate the fluid deficit in neonates. Term neonates lose 1–2% of their weight daily, with a cumulative loss of 7–10% in the first week of life. Preterm neonates lose 2–3% of their birth weight daily, with a cumulative loss of 10–15% in the first week of life. Failure to lose weight in the first week of life indicates the need for possible fluid restriction. On the other hand, excessive weight loss in the first 7 days would merit additional fluids to ensure normal fluid homeostasis.

Clinical examination: The usual physical signs of dehydration are unreliable in neonates. Neonates with 10% (100 ml/kg) dehydration may have sunken eyes and fontanelle, cold and clammy skin, poor skin turgor, and oliguria. Those with 15% (150 ml/kg) or more dehydration would have signs of shock (hypotension, tachycardia, and weak pulses) in addition to the abovementioned features. Dehydration warrants the correction of fluid and electrolytes gradually over the next 24–48 hours.

Serum biochemistry: Serum sodium and plasma osmolarity help assess the hydration status. Serum sodium values should be

Table 45.3: Parenteral fluid and electrolyte requirements after the first postnatal week

	Fluid (ml/kg/day)	*Sodium (mmol/kg/day)*	*Potassium (mmol/kg/day)*
Term neonates	140–160	2–3	1–3
Preterm neonates	150–180	3–5 (up to 7)	4

maintained between 135–145 mEq/L. Hyponatremia with weight loss suggests sodium depletion and merits sodium replacement. Hyponatremia with weight gain indicates water excess and necessitates fluid restriction. Hypernatremia with weight loss suggests dehydration and the need for fluid correction over 48 hours. Hypernatremia with weight gain suggests salt and water overload and the need for fluid and sodium restriction.

Urine output, specific gravity (SG), and osmolarity: The capacity of the newborn kidneys to either concentrate or dilute urine is limited. Nevertheless, the estimation of urine SG helps guide fluid therapy. The acceptable ranges of urine output, specific gravity, and osmolarity are 1–3 ml/kg/hour, 1.005–1.012, and 100–400 mOsm/L, respectively. Specific gravity can be checked by a dipstick or by a hand-held refractometer. Osmolarity is estimated by a freezing point osmometer.

Blood gas analysis: Blood gases are not needed routinely for fluid management. However, they are helpful in the acid-base management of neonates with poor tissue perfusion and shock. Hypoperfusion is associated with metabolic acidosis.

LABORATORY GUIDELINES FOR FLUID AND ELECTROLYTE THERAPY

Fluid intake should be increased in the presence of:

a. Increased weight loss (>3%/day or a cumulative loss >15–20%).
b. Increased serum sodium (Na>145 mEq/L).
c. Increased urine specific gravity (>1.020) or urine osmolality (>400 mOsm/L), or
d. Decreased urine output (<1 ml/kg/hour).

Fluids should be restricted in the presence of:

a. Decreased weight loss (<1%/day or a cumulative loss <5%).
b. Decreased serum sodium (Na <130 mEq/L) in the presence of weight gain.
c. Decreased urine specific gravity (<1.005) or urine osmolality (<100 mOsm/L), or
d. Increased urine output (>3 ml/kg/hour).

Specific Clinical Conditions

Extreme prematurity (gestation <28 weeks): They have extremely high insensible water loss (IWL) in the initial few days of life, which may be 10–15 times that of term neonates. Moreover, there is a considerable variation in the IWL, making it necessary to rely on frequent monitoring instead of assumptions alone. The fluid requirement can be minimized considerably by implementing strategies to reduce IWL (see above). Most guidelines recommend administering around 90–120 ml/kg/day fluids on day 1 of life, with frequent revision of fluid rate in the subsequent days based on urine output, change in weight, and serum sodium level (which predominantly depends on fluid status rather than sodium intake in the first week of life). It is desirable to allow around 2% weight loss per day, with a cumulative weight loss of 6–12%, to allow physiological contraction of extracellular fluid. Sodium supplementation is not recommended in the initial 24–48 hours of life and is added at 3–4 mEq/kg/day thereafter. After the first week of life, a higher sodium intake of around 5–7 mEq/kg/day is recommended to maintain a positive sodium balance. Potassium should be added at 2–3 mEq/kg/day after 48 hours of life. Hyperkalemia of prematurity (serum potassium up to 6.5 mEq/L) is relatively common till 72 hours of life and does not usually require treatment. The stratum corneum of these neonates matures rapidly in 1–2 weeks; therefore, fluid requirements become comparable to larger infants by the end of the second week.

Perinatal asphyxia: Perinatal asphyxia may be associated with the syndrome of inappropriate ADH (SIADH) secretion and renal failure. However, fluid restriction (e.g. two-thirds of daily intake) is not routinely recommended. It should be done only in the presence of oliguric hyponatremia. Renal parenchyma injury from perinatal asphyxia may result in acute tubular necrosis (ATN) accompanied by oliguria or anuria. In case of oliguric renal failure, fluid intake should be restricted to replenishing IWL and metabolic water requirement (400 ml/m^2 or 40 ml/kg) and any other losses (urine output, gastric secretions, etc.). During the recovery phase of ATN, there can be large urinary sodium and potassium losses, which should be estimated and replaced.

Diarrhea: Neonates develop dehydration quickly because of the limited concentrating ability of their kidneys. The fluid deficit is corrected over 24 hours in neonates with diarrhea. Ongoing losses need to be assessed and corrected 6–8 hourly.

REFERENCES

1. Bell EF, Oh W. Fluid and electrolyte management. In: Avery GB, Fletcher MA, MacDonald MG, eds. Neonatology: Pathophysiology of the Newborn. 5th ed. Philadelphia: Lippincott Williams and Wilkins; 1999:345–61.

2. Chevalier RL. Developmental renal physiology of the low birth weight preterm newborn. J Urol 1996;156:714–9.
3. Modi N. Renal function, fluid and electrolyte balance, and neonatal renal disease. In: Rennie JM, Roberton NRC, eds. Textbook of Neonatology. 3rd ed. Edinburgh: Churchill Livingstone; 1999:1009–36.
4. Nakamura KT, Paul Matherne G, McWeeny OJ, Smith BA, Robillard JE. Renal Hemodynamics and Functional Changes during the Transition from Fetal to Newborn Life in Sheep. Pediatr Res 1987.
5. Bueva A, Guignard JP. Renal function in preterm neonates. Pediatr Res 1994;36(5):572–7.
6. Al-Dahhan J, Haycock GB, Nichol B, Chantler C, Stimmler L. Sodium homeostasis in term and preterm neonates. III. Effect of salt supplementation. Arch Dis Child 1984;59:945–50.
7. Ayisi RK, Mbiti MJ, Musoke RN, Orinda DA. Sodium supplementation in very low birth weight infants fed on their own mother's milk I: Effects on sodium homeostasis. East Afr Med J 1992;69:591–5.
8. Segar DE, Segar EK, Harshman LA, Dagle JM, Carlson SJ, Segar JL. Physiological Approach to Sodium Supplementation in Preterm Infants. Am J Perinatol 2018.
9. August D, Kandasamy Y. The effects of antenatal glucocorticoid exposure on fetal and neonatal skin maturation. J Perinat Med 2017;45(8):969–75.
10. Kaushal M, Agarwal R, Aggarwal R, et al. Cling wrap, an innovative intervention for temperature maintenance and reduction of insensible water loss in very low-birthweight babies nursed under radiant warmers: a randomized, controlled trial. Ann Trop Paediatr 2005;25:111–8.
11. Nangia S, Paul VK, Chawla D, Agarwal R, Deorari AK, Sreenivas V. Topical coconut oil application reduces trans-epidermal water loss (TEWL) in very low birth weight (VLBW) neonates: A randomized clinical trial. In: Pediatric Academic Society. Toronto; 2007:7933.21.
12. Lane AT, Drost SS. Effects of repeated application of emollient cream to premature neonates' skin. Pediatrics 1993;92:415–9.
13. Bell EF, Acarregui MJ. Restricted versus liberal water intake for preventing morbidity and mortality in preterm infants. Cochrane Database Syst Rev 2014.

CHAPTER

46

Continuous Positive Airway Pressure

Continuous positive airway pressure (CPAP) refers to the application of positive pressure to the airway of a spontaneously breathing infant throughout the respiratory cycle. CPAP predominantly helps by preventing the collapse of the alveoli. Preterm infants have difficulty establishing and maintaining lung volumes due to surfactant deficiency, muscle hypotonia, slow clearance of lung fluid, and a compliant chest wall. CPAP results in the recruitment of alveoli, thus increasing the functional residual capacity (FRC) and preventing alveolar collapse.[1]

COMPONENTS

The components of a CPAP system are:

1. **Gas source:** To provide a continuous supply of warm, humidified, and blended gases, i.e. air and oxygen.
2. **Pressure generator:** To create positive pressure in the circuit.
3. **Patient interface/delivery system:** To connect the CPAP circuit to the infant's airway.

Devices Used for Pressure Generation

The pressure sources of CPAP can be broadly grouped into two types (Fig. 46.1):[2] We use continuous flow CPAP by both conventional ventilators and bubble CPAP devices in our unit.

Devices Used for CPAP Delivery (Patient Interface)

Various devices used for CPAP delivery include:

1. Nasal prongs (single/double or binasal)
2. Long (or) nasopharyngeal prongs
3. Nasal cannula
4. Nasal masks

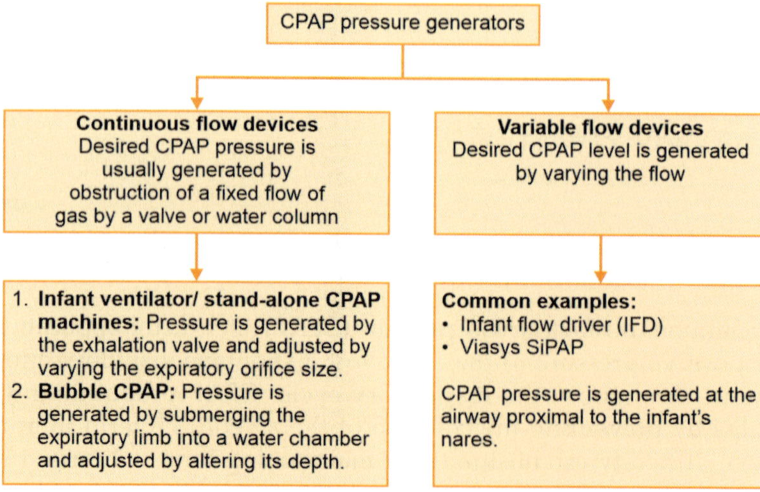

Fig. 46.1: Surfactant replacement therapy

Hudson, Argyle, IFD prongs, and RAM cannula are the commonly used short binasal prongs in neonates. A study comparing RAM cannula, Hudson prongs, and nasal masks found that the nasal masks delivered oropharyngeal pressure closer to the set CPAP.[3] Also, nasal masks may reduce the risk of treatment failure and nasal injury compared to nasal prongs.[4] On the other hand, the ToNIL study revealed that leakages are common for both masks and prongs, but the degree of the leak was significantly higher with prongs. Leakage can be significantly decreased using corrective measures such as adjusting the interface seal by external pressure, closing the mouth, changing interface size, and adjusting the cap and patient position.[5] *We use Argyle prongs, RAM cannula, or nasal masks to deliver CPAP.*

INDICATIONS FOR CPAP

The common clinical indications of CPAP have been listed in Table 46.1.

We use CPAP predominantly in preterm infants (<35 weeks and birth weight <1800 g) with respiratory distress, apnea of prematurity, delayed adaptation, and pneumonia; also, we extubate VLBW infants to CPAP routinely. We occasionally use CPAP in late preterm and term infants with respiratory distress secondary to TTNB, pneumonia, meconium aspiration syndrome, etc.

Table 46.1: Indications for CPAP
Common indications
1. Respiratory distress syndrome (RDS)
2. Apnea of prematurity
3. Post-extubation in preterm VLBW infants
4. Transient tachypnea of the newborn (TTNB)
Other indications
1. Pneumonia
2. Meconium aspiration/other aspiration syndromes
3. Pulmonary edema/pulmonary hemorrhage
4. Laryngomalacia/tracheomalacia/bronchomalacia

CONTRAINDICATIONS OF CPAP

The important contraindications for CPAP include:

1. Progressive respiratory failure with $PaCO_2$ levels >60 mm Hg or inability to maintain oxygenation (PaO_2 <50 mm Hg).
2. Congenital malformations of the airway (choanal atresia, cleft palate, tracheoesophageal fistula, congenital diaphragmatic hernia, etc.)
3. Severe cardiovascular instability (hypotension).
4. Poor respiratory drive not improved by CPAP.

GUIDELINES FOR CPAP THERAPY

When to Initiate Cpap?

Early CPAP: It is important to note that CPAP helps mainly by preventing an alveolar collapse in preterm neonates with surfactant deficiency. Once atelectasis and collapse have occurred, CPAP might not help much. Therefore, all preterm infants (<35 weeks of gestation) with any sign of respiratory distress (tachypnea/chest in-drawing/grunting) should be started immediately on CPAP. Infants of 32–34 weeks of gestation can have a little higher threshold (say, silverman score of at least 3–4 or RR of 70 bpm+) for initiating CPAP than infants <32 weeks of gestation (in whom CPAP must be started early for any distress or tachypnea).

Prophylactic CPAP: The Cochrane review that compared prophylactic CPAP with supportive care in preterm infants (mostly 29–32 weeks of gestation) concluded that there is insufficient evidence for any additional benefit with prophylactic CPAP.[7]

However, in preterm neonates born at or before 28 weeks of gestation, prophylactic CPAP administered immediately after birth in the delivery room (i.e. delivery room CPAP) has been found to reduce the need for mechanical ventilation and surfactant and also reduce the incidence of BPD when compared to intubation and mechanical ventilation.[6]

We do not practice prophylactic CPAP for preterm infants born after 28 weeks of gestation. However, we generally employ delivery room CPAP in preterm infants born at or before 28 weeks.

PROTOCOL FOR CPAP THERAPY

Table 46.2 outlines the protocol for CPAP therapy in the three most common neonatal conditions.

MONITORING WHILE ON CPAP

The following parameters need to be monitored while the infant is on CPAP:

1. Regular monitoring of respiratory rate, heart rate, SpO_2
2. Serial monitoring of:
   a. Severity of respiratory distress by using Downe's or Silverman score.
   b. Arterial blood gases (ABGs).
   c. Perfusion—CFT, BP, peripheral pulses, urine output.
   d. Abdominal girth.
   e. Nasal injury

During CPAP therapy, the target saturation and blood gases are SpO_2 90–95%; PaO_2 50–70 mm Hg; $PaCO_2$ 40–50 mm Hg.

HAZARDS/COMPLICATIONS OF CPAP

CPAP, though less invasive and generally safer than IMV, is not free of side effects.

1. Nasal irritation, damage to the septal mucosa, or skin damage and necrosis from the fixing devices are the most common adverse effects of CPAP. A nasal injury scoring system helps monitor skin integrity, septum, and other anatomic structures. Use of appropriate-size nasal prongs and proper nursing care, including frequent instillation of saline drops in the nostrils, ensuring an adequate gap between the prongs and the

Table 46.2: Protocol for CPAP therapy in the three common neonatal conditions

	Indications		
	RDS	*Apnea of prematurity*	*Post extubation*
Initiating CPAP			
Pressure	• Start at 5–6 cm H_2O	• Start at 4 cm H_2O	• Start at 4–5 cm H_2O
FiO_2	• 0.3–0.5 (titrate based on SpO_2)	• 0.21–0.4 (as decided by SpO_2)	• Same or 0.05 above the pre-extubation FiO_2
What to do if there is no improvement?			
Pressure	• Increase in steps of 1–2 cm H_2O to reach a maximum of 8 cm H_2O	• Increase up to 5 cm H_2O (further increase is not warranted usually -may lead to hyperinflation)	• Increase in steps of 1–2 cm H_2O to reach a maximum of 7–8 cm H_2O
FiO_2	• Increase in steps of 0.05 (if oxygenation is still compromised) up to a maximum of 0.6	• FiO_2 increase does not help much	• Increase in steps of 0.05 to a maximum of 0.6
	Worsening respiratory distress, as indicated by Silverman scoring, hypoxemia (PaO_2 <50 mm Hg), or hypercarbia ($PaCO_2$ >60 mm Hg) despite CPAP pressure of 7–8 cm H_2O and FiO_2 of 0.5–0.6	Recurrent episodes of apnea requiring PPV	Same as for RDS

(*Contd.*)

Table 46.2: Protocol for CPAP therapy in the three common neonatal conditions (*Contd.*)

	Indications		
	RDS	*Apnea of prematurity*	*Post extubation*
Failure of CPAP	Likely to occur in infants with severe RDS with delay in initiation of CPAP/ administration of surfactant, associated sepsis, and in ELBW infants who have not received ANS[10,11]	Likely to occur in infants with central apnea and apnea secondary to sepsis/pneumonia	Likely to occur in ELBW infants and sepsis/pneumonia, PDA, metabolic acidosis, and collapse
Weaning from CPAP			
• When to wean?	• When there is no respiratory distress and SpO_2/blood gases are normal	• No episodes of apnea/ desaturation/bradycardia for at least 12–24 hours	• Same as for RDS
• How to wean?	• Reduce FiO_2 in steps of 0.05 to 0.3, then decrease pressure in steps of 1 cm H_2O every 24 hrs until 4 cm H_2O (infant's clinical condition will guide the speed of weaning). • Recent data suggest that in very preterm neonates sudden wean and pressure wean (decreasing pressure by 1 cm every 24 hours till 4 cm H_2O) were equally good choices. However, pressure wean is preferred in neonates <28 weeks of gestation.[12]	• Same as for RDS	

columella, and maintaining optimal humidity and temperature in the circuit would help minimize nasal injury. In some infants, protective barriers such as 'cannulaide,' hydrocolloid dressing, and alternating between nasal masks and prongs might also be considered to reduce the risk of injury.[7]

2. Pulmonary air leaks are the most severe adverse effects of CPAP.[8] They occur following over-distension of the lungs caused by inappropriately set high pressures.
3. Decreased cardiac output due to reduced venous return, decreased right ventricular stroke volume, and altered dispensability of the left ventricle.[9]
4. Impedance of pulmonary blood flow with increased pulmonary vascular resistance (with inappropriately high CPAP pressure).
5. Gastric distension and 'CPAP belly syndrome.' Routine use of an orogastric tube minimizes the risk.

REFERENCES

1. Sankar MJ, Deorari AK. CPAP – A gentler mode of ventilation. J Neonatol 2007; 21:160–5.
2. Courtney SE, Barrington KJ. Continuous positive airway pressure and noninvasive ventilation. ClinPerinatol. 2007;34:73–92.
3. Sharma D, Murki S, Maram S, Pratap T, Kiran S, Venkateshwarlu V, et al. Comparison of delivered distending pressures in the oropharynx in preterm infant on bubble CPAP and on three different nasal interfaces. Pediatr Pulmonol. 2020 Jul;55(7):1631–9.
4. Prakash R, De Paoli AG, Oddie SJ, Davis PG, McGuire W. Masks versus prongs as interfaces for nasal continuous positive airway pressure in preterm infants. Cochrane Database Syst Rev. 2022 Nov 14;11(11): CD015129.
5. Falk M, Gunnarsdottir K, Baldursdottir S, Donaldsson S, Jonsson B, Drevhammar T. Interface leakage during neonatal CPAP treatment: a randomized, cross-over trial. Arch Dis Child Fetal Neonatal Ed. 2021 Nov;106(6):663–7.
6. Subramaniam P, Ho JJ, Davis PG. Prophylactic nasal continuous positive airway pressure for preventing morbidity and mortality in very preterm infants. Cochrane Database Syst Rev. 2016 Jun 14;(6): CD001243.
7. Alsop EA, Cooke J, Gupta S, et al. Nasal trauma in preterm infants receiving nasal continuous positive airway pressure. Archives of Disease in Childhood 2008; 93:n23.
8. Hall RT, Rhodes PG: Pneumothorax and pneumomediastinum in infants with idiopathic respiratory distress syndrome receiving CPAP. Pediatrics 55:493, 1975.

9. Tittley JG, Fremes SE, Weisel RD, Christakis GT, Evans PJ, Madonik MM, et al. Hemodynamic and myocardial metabolic consequences of PEEP. Chest 1985;88:496–502.
10. Pillai MS, Sankar MJ, Mani K, Agarwal R, Paul VK, Deorari AK. Clinical prediction score for nasal CPAP failure in pre-term VLBW neonates with early onset respiratory distress. J Trop Pediatr2011;57:274–9.
11. Murki S, Kandraju H, Oleti T, Saikiran, Gaddam P. Predictors of CPAP Failure-10 years' Data of Multiple Trials from a Single Center: A Retrospective Observational Study. Indian J Pediatr. 2020 Nov;87(11):891–6.
12. Jensen CF, Sellmer A, Ebbesen F, et al. Sudden vs. Pressure Wean From Nasal Continuous Positive Airway Pressure in Infants Born Before 32 Weeks of Gestation: A Randomized Clinical Trial. JAMA Pediatr. 2018;172(9):824–31.

CHAPTER

47

Heated Humidified High Flow Nasal Cannula Therapy

In recent years, the heated, humidified high-flow nasal cannula (HFNC) has emerged as an alternative to CPAP among neonates. Its popularity is related to ease of application and maintenance, less nasal trauma, better infant tolerance, and, most importantly, better access to neonates for caregiving, skin-skin care, and feeding.[1]

HFNC therapy refers to administering blended oxygen and air to neonates via nasal cannula at higher flow rates (>1 L/minute)—typically between 2 and 8 L/minute. Just as a CPAP, the delivery of gas flow rates between 2 and 10 L/minute to the nasopharynx has been shown to develop positive distending pressure in both preterm and term infants. However, the pressure delivered is unpredictable depending on the size of the nasal cannula, gas flow rate, size of the patient's airway, and the amount of air egress around the nares and mouth.

MECHANISMS OF ACTION

1. The washout of nasopharyngeal dead space is an important mechanism that promotes alveolar ventilation and improves CO_2 elimination.
2. Higher gas flow rates provide CPAP to the airway, recruit alveoli and stabilize both the alveoli at end-expiration, maintaining the FRC. This, in turn, improves oxygenation and decreases the work of breathing.
3. Splints the pharynx and upper airways.
4. The heated and humidified gas decreases the metabolic work of breathing and reverses the dryness and mucosal injury that would otherwise occur at high gas flow rates.

EQUIPMENT

Optiflow Junior (Fisher & Paykel, New Zealand) and the *Precision Flow* (Vapotherm, Exeter, NH, USA) are the common devices used. The essential parts of a Fisher and Paykel HFNC system are described below.

1. Oxygen and air source.
2. Blender: FiO_2 can be adjusted in increments of 1% from 21 to 100%.
3. Flow meter: standard 0–15 L/minute flow meter is used. In HFNC systems, circuit flow is adjusted according to the level of respiratory distress, and in neonates, the maximum flow used is 8 L/minute. Although a pressure relief valve is used in some circuits, the internal circuit pressure is not routinely measured.
4. Humidifier: Should be set at 37°C. The length of the circuit from temperature probe to nares will result in temperatures dropping to a comfortable level while maintaining optimal humidity. At flow rates of 1–4 L/minute, both Optiflow and Vapotherm devices achieve an oro-pharyngeal temperature of 33–34°C and relative humidity (RH) of >96%. At high flow rates, the temperature and RH achieved by these devices are less than bubble CPAP or ventilator CPAP.[4]
5. Circuit tubing to attach to the humidifier.
6. Nasal cannula (prongs): The nasal cannula of HFNC is small and thin, does not occlude the nostrils, and mandatorily has a leak around it.
7. Water bag for the humidifier.

INDICATIONS

1. **Post-extubation support:** This is a common indication for HFNC use. Studies comparing HFNC versus CPAP for post-extubation support in preterm infants showed no significant differences in treatment failure rates, reintubation, death, or BPD.[2] Neonates treated with HFNC had reduced nasal trauma rates by 36%. Though the treatment failure rate was similar across different gestational groups, relatively few extremely preterm neonates were enrolled in the studies.

2. **To aid in weaning from CPAP in preterm neonates:** Although the best way to wean CPAP is to take the neonate off CPAP and to reinstate the therapy if indicated, HFNC has been used in the interim as a bridge to transition neonates to room air. Two studies (149 infants) found that preterm infants randomized to HFNC had a reduced duration of hospitalization compared with infants who remained on CPAP with no difference in weaning success or other morbidities.[2]

3. **As an alternative to CPAP in stable preterm neonates** at risk of or have established nasal trauma or for better nursing care to promote mother–infant bonding, kangaroo care, and oral feeding.
4. **As a primary mode of support in preterm neonates with RDS:** A recent systematic review that included 10 studies (1830 infants) noted 1.34-fold higher treatment failure than CPAP but no difference in intubation rates and lesser nasal trauma.[3] In our unit, we prefer CPAP as the primary mode of respiratory support in preterm neonates with RDS.[4] If HFNC is to be considered as the primary support due to nasal trauma or ease of care, its use should be restricted to neonates above 28 weeks of gestation, and the units should have access to CPAP or NIPPV to manage treatment failures.[5]

CONTRAINDICATIONS

Severe RDS, neonates with recurrent apnea, pneumothorax, and cranial and airway anomalies

Initiation, Escalation, and Weaning of HFNC[6]

1. **Choosing an appropriately sized nasal cannula:** Nasal cannula should occupy less than 50% of the area of the nostril aperture to allow ample egress of expired gas. A snugly fitting or tight nasal cannula can lead to inadvertently high distending pressures in the nasopharynx.
2. **Setting flow rates:** An initial flow rate of 4–6 L/minute is recommended. Our unit policy is to begin flows based on the current weight of the neonate as follows: for 1000–1999 g = 3 L/minute, for 2000–2999 g = 4 L/minute, and ≥3000 g = 5 L/minute.
3. **FiO_2:** Begin at 30% or FiO_2, similar to ventilatory or CPAP settings. A pulse oximeter should be used to titrate FiO_2 to target oxygenation.
4. **Conditioning of respiratory gases:** The humidifier should be set at 37°C in the invasive mode. However, if there is condensation in the circuit at flow rates < 4 L/minute, it may be necessary to lower the set temperature to 34–35°C.
5. **Monitoring during therapy:** A neonate on HFNC requires the same level of monitoring as a neonate on CPAP. Monitoring should include respiratory rate, heart rate, chest retractions, and degree of chest-in drawing. The use of an objective scoring system like the Silverman and Anderson score is recommended.

6. **Escalation of therapy:** Flow rates can be increased in increments of 1 L/minute up to a maximum of 8 L/minute in response to increased chest retractions, tachypnea, and higher FiO_2 requirement.
7. **Failure of HFNC:** Increasing FiO_2 requirement >50%, respiratory acidosis (pH 7.2 and PCO_2 > 60 mm Hg), or recurrent episodes of apnea requiring positive pressure ventilation should be considered as a failure of HFNC and alternative respiratory support (CPAP/intubation) is mandated.
8. **Weaning of HFNC:** One can consider weaning when the neonate is stable on HFNC for 12–24 hours. FiO_2 is weaned down to 30% or lower, and then the flow rate in decrements of 1 L/minute every 12 or 24 hours guided by work of breathing. Once a flow rate of 2 L/minute is reached, HFNC can be discontinued. Neonates requiring minimal oxygen before discontinuation may need to be placed on low-flow titrated oxygen therapy.

REFERENCES

1. Manley BJ. Nasal high flow: going viral? Arch Dis Child Fetal Neonatal Ed. 2016;101:F282–3.
2. Wilkinson D, Andersen C, O'Donnell CP, De Paoli AG, Manley BJ. High flow nasal cannula for respiratory support in preterm infants. Cochrane Database Syst Rev. 2016;2(2):CD006405.
3. Bruet S, Butin M, Dutheil F. Systematic review of high-flow nasal cannula versus continuous positive airway pressure for primary support in preterm infants. Arch Dis Child Fetal Neonatal Ed. 2022 (1):56–9.
4. Non-invasive respiratory support for newborns. NNF India. Evidence-based Clinical Practice Guidelines. January 2020. Available at: http://www.nnfi.org/assests/pdf/cpg-guidelines/NIV-CPAP.pdf. Last accessed 25–04–2023.
5. Sweet DG, Carnielli VP, Greisen G, Hallman M, Klebermass-Schrehof K, Ozek E, Te Pas A, Plavka R, Roehr CC, Saugstad OD, Simeoni U, Speer CP, Vento M, Visser GHA, Halliday HL. European Consensus Guidelines on the Management of Respiratory Distress Syndrome: 2022 Update. Neonatology. 2023;120(1):3–23.
6. Roehr CC, Yoder BA, Davis PG, Ives K. Evidence Support and Guidelines for Using Heated, Humidified, High-Flow Nasal Cannulae in Neonatology: Oxford Nasal High-Flow Therapy Meeting, 2015. Clin Perinatol. 2016; 43:693–705.

CHAPTER

48

Nasal Intermittent Positive Pressure Ventilation

Nasal intermittent positive pressure ventilation (NIPPV) is a noninvasive mode of respiratory support that provides a continuous positive end-expiratory airway pressure (CPAP or PEEP) along with intermittent higher pressures delivered using nasal masks or nasal prongs. NIPPV is also called nasal intermittent mandatory ventilation (N-IMV) or noninvasive pressure support ventilation (NI-PSV).

PHYSIOLOGIC EFFECTS[1]

- Like CPAP, NIPPV stabilizes the alveoli, maintains alveolar recruitment, and prevents airway collapse. It also supports the inspiratory work of breathing, splints the nasopharynx, and improves both central and obstructive apneic events.
- The application of peak inspiratory pressure (PIP) in NIPPV is postulated to promote better ventilation by delivering positive pressure breaths to the lower airways. However, the pressure delivered at the nasopharynx is highly variable and does not consistently reach lower airways or produce a chest rise. In the non-synchronized mode, a tidal volume increase is noted only when the PIP was delivered during the infant's spontaneous inspiratory effort.
- Additional mechanisms of action include triggering an augmented inspiratory reflex (Head's paradoxical reflex) in preterm infants to support spontaneous breathing, chest wall splinting, and better thoracoabdominal synchrony.

EQUIPMENT

Any mechanical ventilator can be used to provide nonsynchronized NIPPV. When the peak pressure is delivered synchronized with the infant's inspiration, it is called synchronized NIPPV. Most neonatal ventilators can provide a wide range of set peak pressures

(10–25 cm H_2O) at variable rates (10–60 per minute) and variable inflation times (0.3–0.5 seconds).

Bilevel positive airway pressure (BiPAP), also called biphasic CPAP system, delivers alternating high and low levels of CPAP pressure. The flow-driver SiPAP and Infant Flow Driver Advance (Care Fusion, USA) are examples of devices that can deliver BiPAP. *See* Table 48.1 for differences between BiPAP and NIPPV.

Nasal interface: The most common interface used to deliver both NIPPV and BiPAP breaths is the short binasal prongs, with the other interfaces being nasal masks and long nasopharyngeal tubes.

SYNCHRONIZATION IN NIPPV

The peak pressure delivered in the NIPPV device can be synchronized with the infant's respiratory efforts, similar to synchronization in a ventilator. Synchronization can be achieved using a pneumatic capsule, pneumotachograph (flow-trigger), respiratory inductance plethysmography, or diaphragmatic electromyogram (Table 48.2). Synchronized NIPPV was available with the Infant Star ventilator, which is currently no longer in production, and newer ventilators like Giulia (Giulia Neonatal Nasal Ventilator, Ginevri Medical Technologies, Italy). In this ventilator, synchronization is achieved using a fixed orifice pneumotachograph placed between the nasal prongs and Y-piece. Another ventilator, Maquet Servo-n from Getinge provide synchronized NIPPV with help of Neurally adjusted ventilator assist (NAVA) technology (Table 48.2).

INDICATIONS FOR NIPPV

NIPPV can be considered in the following situations:

1. **Preterm neonates with RDS:** The standard strategy involves early use of CPAP with early selective surfactant administration. NIPPV can be used as the primary mode of respiratory support, in place of CPAP, in neonates less than 6 hours of age with RDS. NIPPV has been compared to CPAP as the primary mode.[2] An updated meta-analysis suggested a 37% relative reduction in respiratory failure needing mechanical ventilation in the first week of life.[3] The benefits were found to be greater with ventilator-derived NIPPV. There was also a reduction in mortality, BPD (22% relative reduction), and risk of air leaks compared to CPAP (Table 48.3).[4]

Table 48.1: Differences between BiPAP and NIPPV

Bilevel CPAP or BiPAP	*Nasal intermittent positive pressure ventilation*
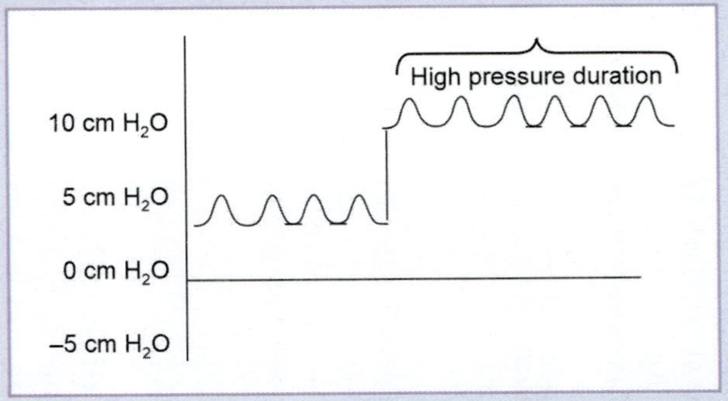	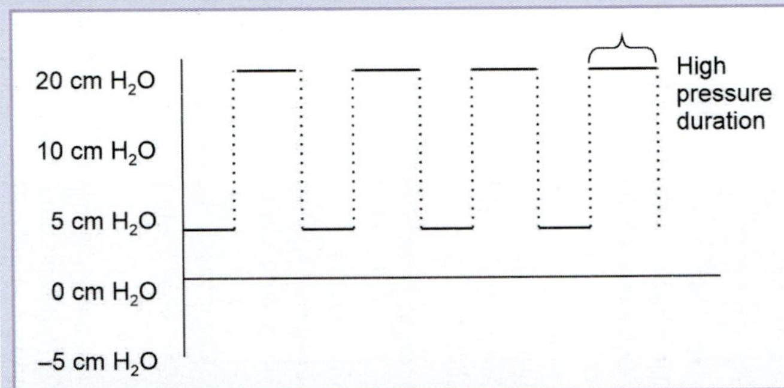
BiPAP provides two nasal CPAP levels, over which the infant breathes independently.	NIPPV mimics invasive ventilation in its setting.
The high-pressure duration is longer (0.5–1.0 s).	The inflation times (0.3–0.5 s) are shorter.
The rates used are low (10–30/min). The rate refers to cycle between high and low CPAP pressures.	The rates are variable from 10 to 60/min (generally 45/min)
The maximum high pressure that can be delivered in BiPAP depends on the machine – 11 cm H_2O for the infant flow driver, and 11–15 cm H_2O for the SiPAP.	Peak pressures and positive end expiratory pressure can be used similar to that of invasive ventilation (PIP of 20–22 cm H_2O and PEEP of 5–8 cm H_2O)

Table 48.2: Devices for synchronization in NIPPV

Devices for synchronization	*Mechanism*
Pneumotachograph	This device measures inspiratory flow when the gases flowing across a fixed resistance tube creates a pressure difference. In NIPPV, leaks at the mouth and nose can interfere with the accuracy. The device requires frequent calibration and changes in gas temperature, humidity, and water condensation can affect performance.
Graesby capsule	It is a pneumatic capsule that detects outward abdominal movement due to diaphragmatic contraction. Ventilators (Infant star) using these capsules are no longer commercially available. The SiPAP device uses a similar abdominal capsule. Disadvantages: some breaths may be missed in neonates with tachypnea and abdominal distension
Respiratory inductance plethysmography	Measures respiration from body surface movements using abdominal and chest bands
Neurally adjusted ventilator assist (NAVA)	NAVA uses a diaphragmatic electromyogram. It synchronises inflations with inspiratory effort and provides pressure support proportional to the infant's inspiratory effort. It requires nasogastric insertion, and its sensors are expensive.

Table 48.3: Summary of evidence for NIPPV in neonates

- NIPPV is superior to CPAP as a primary mode in neonates with RDS and for post-extubation in preterm neonates. NIPPV reduces the risk of treatment failure and the need for additional ventilator support. NIPPV also reduces mortality, BPD, and air leaks. In both scenarios, the observed benefits were attributed to ventilator-generated, synchronized NIPPV.
- Ventilator derived NIPPV is superior to BiPAP. It is unknown if one would get the same benefits if the mean pressures generated by a CPAP device could match the mean pressures of NIPPV.
- No harm was noted with NIPPV use in neonates. However, care should be taken to avoid nasal injury from the interface.

2. **Prevention of post-extubation failure:** When used after extubation in preterm neonates, NIPPV resulted in a 22% reduction of respiratory failure and less need for re-intubation within the first week compared to CPAP.[4,5]

3. **Treatment of apnea of prematurity:** Studies that evaluated the role of NIPPV in apnea of prematurity found beneficial effects in short-term outcomes, namely the incidence of apnea, desaturations, and bradycardia episodes. However, there was no difference in the need for intubation and mechanical ventilation. NIPPV may augment the beneficial effects of CPAP in preterm infants with frequent or severe apnea and can be considered before initiating mechanical ventilation.
4. **CPAP failure:** NIPPV may be instituted as a bridge before shifting to intubation and mechanical ventilation in neonates with CPAP failure.

Although evidence favors synchronized NIPPV over CPAP as a primary mode in neonates with RDS and after extubation from invasive ventilation, it is challenging to implement it because of the lack of availability of equipment providing synchronized NIPPV and the need for more careful monitoring (compared to CPAP). We do not routinely use NIPPV in all preterm neonates. *We use unsynchronized NIPPV preferentially in extreme preterm or extremely low birth weight neonates at high risk of mortality and BPD.*

SETTINGS AND MONITORING FOR PROVIDING NIPPV SUPPORT

1. **NIPPV settings:** The typical settings are provided in Table 48.4.
2. **Monitoring:** Monitor respiratory rate, Silverman score, SpO_2, and heart rate. Blood gas and chest X-ray should be done if there is worsening respiratory distress.

Table 48.4: NIPPV settings in various scenarios

Parameter	*Settings when used as the primary mode*	*Settings for post-extubation*
PIP	10 cm H_2O above PEEP (Maximum 30)	2–4 cm H_2O more than PIP of ventilator at the time of extubation
PEEP	5–6 cm H_2O (Maximum 8)	Same as PEEP of ventilator at extubation
Rate	10–40/min (Maximum 50)	20–30/min
Inspiratory time (Ti)	0.3–0.5	0.35–0.4 sec
Flow	8–12 L/min	8–12 L/min
FiO_2	Titrate to maintain SpO_2 91–95%; maximum FiO_2 is 60–70%	

3. **Failure criteria (indication for reintubation):**
    a. **Clinical:** Severe and recurrent apnea (>4 apnea/hr requiring tactile stimulation or >2 episodes requiring bag and mask ventilation in a day), Silverman score >6, shock requiring inotropes.
    b. FiO_2 >60% to maintain target saturation.
    c. Blood gas: pH <7.2 with $PaCO_2$ >60 mm Hg.
4. Weaning
    a. Gradually decrease FiO_2 by 3–5% while maintaining target SpO_2 in the range of 91–95% until it reaches 30%.
    b. If there is no worsening of distress, taper PIP by 1–2 cm of H_2O till PIP is 15 cm H_2O.
    c. Rates are kept at 40/min until PIP is weaned and then decreased in steps to 20/min.
    d. Wean to nasal CPAP if settings are PIP 14 cm of H2O, PEEP 5 cm H_2O, rate 20 bpm, and FiO_2 30%.

SAFETY OF NIPPV

Although studies have not shown severe complications like gastrointestinal perforation or necrotizing enterocolitis, most were small studies and were not sufficiently powered to detect adverse effects. Similarly, nasal injury due to NIPPV use has not been adequately studied.

REFERENCES

1. Owen LS, Manley BJ. Nasal intermittent positive pressure ventilation in preterm infants: Equipment, evidence, and synchronization. Semin Fetal Neonatal Med. 2016;21(3):146-53.
2. Lemyre B, Laughon M, Bose C, Davis PG. Early nasal intermittent positive pressure ventilation (NIPPV) versus early nasal continuous positive airway pressure (NCPAP) for preterm infants. Cochrane Database Syst Rev. 2016;12(12): CD005384.
3. Rüegger CM, Owen LS, Davis PG. Nasal Intermittent Positive Pressure Ventilation for Neonatal Respiratory Distress Syndrome. Clin Perinatol. 2021;48(4):725–44.
4. Ramaswamy VV, More K, Roehr CC, Bandiya P, Nangia S. Efficacy of non-invasive respiratory support modes for primary respiratory support in preterm neonates with respiratory distress syndrome: Systematic review and network meta-analysis. Pediatr Pulmonol. 2020;55(11):2940–63.
5. Lemyre B, Davis PG, De Paoli AG, Kirpalani H. Nasal intermittent positive pressure ventilation (NIPPV) versus nasal continuous positive airway pressure (NCPAP) for preterm neonates after extubation. Cochrane Database Syst Rev. 2017 Feb 1;2(2): CD003212.

CHAPTER

49

Parenteral Nutrition

The goal of nutrition management in neonates, especially very low birth weight (VLBW) infants, is achieving postnatal growth at a rate that approximates the intrauterine growth of a fetus and ensuring optimal long-term neurodevelopment.[1] This is best achieved by enteral nutrition. However, parenteral nutrition (PN) is required when enteral nutrition is inadequate or contraindicated. PN is especially crucial for extremely low birth weight neonates and neonates with congenital gastrointestinal anomalies.

INDICATIONS

Parenteral nutrition (PN) should be considered in neonates who are not expected to be on significant enteral feeds for more than 3–5 days or are anticipated to receive less than 50% of the total energy requirement in the next 7 days (Table 49.1).

MACRONUTRIENTS

Energy

The total energy is provided by a combination of macronutrients that include carbohydrates, fats, and proteins. It is preferable

Table 49.1: Indications of parenteral nutrition

- Birth weight less than 1000 g: TPN to be started on day 1 (MEN to be started along with TPN if hemodynamically stable and no contraindication for feeding like A/REDF).
- Birth weight 1000–1499 g and anticipated to be not on significant feeds for 3 or more days.
- Birth weight more than 1500 g and anticipated to be not on significant feeds for 5 or more days.
- Surgical conditions: necrotizing enterocolitis, gastroschisis, omphalocele, tracheoesophageal fistula, intestinal atresia, malrotation, short bowel syndrome, meconium ileus, and others that prevent the initiation of enteral feeds.

to have a balance of energy from carbohydrates (60–75%), fats (25–40%), and proteins (10–15%).[2]

A daily energy intake of 110–120 kcal/kg is needed to meet the metabolic demands of a healthy preterm neonate and to allow for a growth rate comparable to the intrauterine growth rate.[3,4] Energy requirement of term neonates is 90–100 kcal/kg/day. The energy intake of sick neonates (e.g. those with acute respiratory illness, chronic lung disease, necrotizing enterocolitis) is not precisely known; it is likely to be near the upper limits of the energy requirement of preterm infants.

Each gram of dextrose and lipid provides 3.4 kcal and 9 kcal, respectively. If the non-protein energy is insufficient, amino acids are catabolized for energy production. An adequate balance between nitrogen and non-protein energy sources (protein/energy ratio: 3–4 g/100 kcal) is needed to promote protein accretion.[5] However, if the dextrose infusion is initiated at the physiological rate (4–6 mg/kg/minute), starting with even 3–3.5 g/kg/day of amino acids in the first few days of life may be beneficial. There is no concrete evidence for monitoring the P: E; however, pragmatic studies show the benefit of starting with higher amino acids in better achieving lean body mass. A balance between carbohydrates and fat is needed to prevent excessive fat deposition and excessive production of CO_2.

Carbohydrates

Carbohydrates are the primary energy substrate for neonates receiving PN. The amount of carbohydrate delivered as dextrose is commonly initiated at the endogenous hepatic glucose production and utilization rate of 4–6 mg/kg/min. This provides an energy intake of 40–50 kcal/kg/d and preserves carbohydrate stores. Once the glucose infusion rate (GIR) supports acceptable serum glucose values, it is advanced in a gradual, stepwise fashion (2 mg/kg/min/day) to a suggested maximum glucose oxidative rate for neonates of 12–13 mg/kg/min to support growth and maintained there unless serum glucose values change significantly. In the first week of life, it is advisable to be cautious in advancing GIR due to reduced insulin sensitivity and glucose tolerance. Table 49.2 summarizes the GIR recommendations as per various nutrition guidelines:

Insulin infusion should not be routinely used to increase the GIR. However, it can be started if the infant develops high glucose levels despite a GIR of 4–6 mg/kg/minute.

Table 49.2: GIR recommendation as per various nutrition guidelines			
	Day 1 (mg/kg/min)	*Advancement (mg/kg/min)*	*Maximum rate (mg/ kg/min)*
NICE	Preterm and term: 4–6.25	–	6.25–11.1
ESPGHAN	Preterm: 4–8 Term: 2.5–5	Advance over 2–3 days	Preterm: 5–10 (max 12) Term: 8–10 (max 12)
ASPEN	Preterm: 6–8 Term: 6–8	Advance over 7–10 days	10–14 (max 14–18)

NICE: National Institute for Health and Excellence; *ESPGHAN:* European Society for Pediatric Gastroenterology, Hepatology, and Nutrition; *ASPEN:* American Society for Parenteral and Enteral Nutrition

Carbohydrates in PN: Evidence

Excessive carbohydrate delivery above the amount that can be oxidized for energy and glycogen storage can increase basal metabolic rate, fat deposition, cholestasis, or hepatic steatosis.[6–8] Use of insulin to achieve a higher glucose infusion rate and promote growth has been associated with lactic acidosis.[9]

LIPIDS

Fats are provided as intravenous lipid emulsions and should be started on the first day at a dose of 1.5 g/kg/d and then increased gradually by 0.5–1.0 g/kg/day stepwise to reach 3.5 g/kg/day.[4] Evidence suggests that early initiation of lipids within the first 48 hours is well tolerated and improves cerebellar volume and retinal growth, in addition to improving the nitrogen balance and linear growth in preterm infants.

Specific concerns with the use of lipids have been observed, including PNALD (parenteral nutrition associated liver disease) and IFALD (intestinal failure associated liver disease). The newer combined lipids with fish oil (SMOF) have been postulated to reduce the associated hepatic damage. In preterm neonates with hyperbilirubinemia in the range of exchange transfusion threshold, lipids may be restricted to minimum amounts (1 g/kg/day) to provide only the essential fatty acids.[10]

Intravenous lipid emulsions are available in two strengths: 10% and 20% (*see* Appendix of this chapter). Using 20% lipid emulsions is preferable to decrease the risk of hypertriglyceridemia, hypercholesterolemia, and hyperphospholipidemia.[11] When lipids are exposed to light, they form potentially toxic lipid hydroperoxides. Hence lipid syringes and tubing should be covered by wrapping them in aluminum foil.

Lipids in PN: Evidence

Even a short delay of 3–7 days in supplying lipids to parenterally fed preterm infants leads to biochemical EFA deficiency.[12]

Type of Lipid Infusions

There have been three generations of intravenous lipid emulsions which have been used to date:

First-generation lipid emulsions: The main component of these lipids (e.g. IntraLipid by Fresenius Kabi) is soyabean oil or safflower oil containing long-chain triglycerides (LCT), defined as having 16–18 carbon atoms. The risk of adverse effects (steatosis, cholestasis) with these long-chain lipids mandated better preparations. The concern of sepsis was also high with these lipid emulsions.

Second-generation lipid emulsions: They were marketed with the intent of reducing the LCT content. These emulsions contain 50% of medium-chain triglycerides (MCT) with 6–12 carbon atoms. These emulsions do not require carnitine to enter the mitochondria and are oxidized easily. Lipofundina (soybean oil and medium-chain triglycerides), Clinoleic (soybean and olive oil), and Structolipid (structured lipids) are some of the lipid emulsions of this generation. None of these is being used in India.

Third-generation lipid emulsions: The main constituent of this generation is the omega-3 fatty acids. Compared to omega-6, omega-3 fatty acids have better immunomodulatory and immunosuppressive effects. SMOFLipid (Fresenius Kabi; Soyabean oil, medium chain triglycerides, olive oil, and fish oil), Omegaven (100% refined fish oil emulsion), and Lipoplus (MCT, soyabean oil, and fish oil) are included in this generation of lipid emulsions. Of these, SMOFlipid is available in India.

SMOFlipid vs. Intralipid: Evidence

A meta-analysis of 14 studies, of which 9 studies compared different types of lipid emulsions, concluded that emulsions that are not purely soyabean oil based might be associated with a lower incidence of sepsis.[13–16] Beneficial effects on growth could not be shown. Some retrospective studies show a lesser incidence of parenteral nutrition-associated liver disease (PNALD), but large-scale RCTs are warranted. The use of SMOF in PNALD has been shown to increase the resolution of abnormal liver function tests compared to soyabean-based emulsions; however, its role in the prevention of PNALD is yet uncertain (Cochrane 2019).

Amino Acids

PN should provide 3.0–3.5 g/kg/day of amino acids (AA). An optimal amino acid solution should contain essential (valine, leucine, isoleucine, methionine, phenylalanine, threonine, lysine, and histidine) and conditionally essential (cysteine, tyrosine, glutamine, arginine, proline, glycine and taurine) amino acids, should not have an excess of glycine and methionine, and should not contain sorbitol. Depending on practical feasibility, the amino acid infusion should be started on the first day of birth, preferably soon after birth. Providing adequate proteins since day one not only contributes to fat-free mass but also helps in normalizing insulin secretion in ELBW neonates, in whom insulin levels are low.[2]

Proteins in PN: Evidence

The amount started on day 1 of PN has varied from 0.5–3.0 g/kg/day in different studies. A higher intake of 3-3.5 g/kg/day can be safely administered starting from the first day of birth.[2] Early provision of protein is critical to attaining positive nitrogen balance and accretion, as premature babies lose about 1% of their protein stores daily.

MICRONUTRIENTS AND MINERALS

Sodium, potassium, chloride, calcium, magnesium, and phosphorus must be provided in PN solution as their daily needs (Table 49.3). All these minerals are readily available for administration in neonates except for phosphate. Sodium, potassium, and chloride are essential to life, and their requirements depend on obligatory losses, abnormal losses, and amounts necessary for growth. Calcium, phosphorus, and magnesium are the most abundant minerals in the body. They are closely interrelated to each other in metabolism, the formation of tissue structure, and function. Estimated and advisable intakes (Table 49.3) are based on accretion studies and urinary and fecal losses from balance studies.[17]

Calcium and phosphate supplementation: The current recommendation is to provide early and appropriate supplementation of calcium gluconate and phosphate (on day 1) to prevent metabolic bone disease. To promote the highest retention of these minerals, the ideal ratio of calcium: phosphorus (mg: mg) for parenteral nutrition should be 0.8–1.1 on Day 1 and 1.3–1.7:1, subsequently in the neonatal period.[18]

An ideal phosphate preparation (should not precipitate when combined with intravenous calcium preparation) is difficult to procure in India. Many units administer intravenous phosphorus

Table 49.3: Daily requirement of minerals[18]	
Mineral	*Requirement*
Sodium	0–3 mEq/kg/day (1st week of life) 2–3 mEq/kg/day (beyond 1st week in term neonates) 3–5 mEq/kg/day (beyond 1st week in preterm neonates)
Potassium	0–2 mEq/kg/day (1st week of life) 1–3 mEq/kg/day (beyond 1st week)
Chloride	2–3 mEq/kg/day
Calcium	2–4 mEq/kg
Magnesium	0.3–0.5 mEq/kg
Phosphorus	1–2 mEq/kg

(Injection Potphos; NEON Laboratories Ltd; 15 ml ampoule; 89 INR per ampoule) and intravenous calcium gluconate in separate syringes in alternate 4–6 hours cycles to avoid precipitation.

VITAMINS

Vitamins are essential cofactors and coenzymes needed for the metabolism of macronutrients and should be added to PN solution to meet the daily requirement (Table 49.4). Preparations

Table 49.4: Recommended vitamin intake[18]			
Vitamin	*Term (daily dose)*	*Preterm (dose/kg/day)*	*Available MVI (per 1 ml)*
Vitamin A (IU)	2300	1640 (700–1500)	1000
Vitamin D (IU)	400	160 (80–400)	100
Vitamin E (IU)	7	2.8 (2.8–3.5)	0.50 mg
Vitamin K (μg)	200	10	
Vitamin B_6 (mg per kg)	1000	0.15–2	1500
Vitamin B_{12} (μg)	1	0.3	
Vitamin C (mg)	80	15–25	50 mg
Biotin (μg)	20	5–8	
Folic acid (μg)	140	56	
Niacin (mg)	17	4–6.8	10
Pantothenic acid (mg)	5	2.5	2.50
Riboflavin (mg)	1400	0.15–2	1400
Thiamin (mg)	1200	0.35–0.5	5 mg

of fat-soluble and water-soluble vitamins suitable for neonates are not available in India. Multivitamin injection (MVI), when added in a dose of 1.5 ml/kg to lipid solution, meets the need for vitamin A and most other vitamins. Intravenous vitamin delivery may be less due to photodegradation of vitamins A, D, E, K, B_2, B_6, B_{12}, C, and folic acid and adsorption of vitamins A, D, and E into the vinyl delivery bags and tubing. Vitamin K needs to be given separately as weekly intramuscular injections. Although vitamin B_{12} is absent in MVI, its deficiency is not manifested unless the neonate is on long-term PN. The total vitamin E dose from multivitamin infusion should not exceed 11 mg/day.

TRACE ELEMENTS

Eight trace elements (zinc, copper, chromium, iron, manganese, selenium, molybdenum, and iodine) should be part of PN solutions in neonates.[4] Zinc is universally recommended from day one of TPN, whereas the other trace minerals are generally provided after two weeks of TPN without any appreciable enteral feeding. Copper, selenium, molybdenum, and iron can be delivered separately also. Zinc is a critical micronutrient, and zinc deficiency is known if not supplemented, especially in preterm neonates with excessive GI and urinary losses. The dosage is 150–400 microgram/kg/day, but a suitable preparation is difficult to find in the Indian market. Enteral iron is the preferred mode, and the parenteral route for iron is to be considered only in prolonged parenteral nutrition (beyond three weeks). Manganese and chromium are usually present in many parenteral nutrition solutions and need not be replaced. Selenium and molybdenum are required only if prolonged PN beyond 3 weeks is administered. Recommended daily doses of parenteral trace elements are provided in Table 49.5.

WEANING AND DISCONTINUING TPN

There are no clear recommendations on when to start weaning TPN—it depends on the underlying cause of initiating TPN and the neonate's clinical condition. TPN can be gradually weaned off once 50% of total daily needs are tolerated as enteral feeds. Sudden stoppage of GIR may be associated with rebound hypoglycemia. The other components of TPN can be stopped without tapering also. Parenteral nutrition can be stopped once enteral feeds are tolerated at 140–150 ml/kg/day in neonates less than 28 weeks of gestation and 120–140 ml/kg/day in neonates born at or after 28 weeks of gestation (NICE guidelines 2020).

Table 49.5: Recommended daily doses of parenteral trace elements[18]

Trace element	*Preterm*	*Term*	*Maximum dose per day*
Zinc (µg per kg)	400–500	100–250	5 mg
Copper (µg per kg)	40	20	0.5 mg
Chromium (µg per kg)	0.05–0.3	0.2	5 µg
Iron (µg per kg)	200–250	50–100	5 mg
Manganese (µg per kg)	<1	<1	50 µg
Selenium (µg per kg)	7	2–3	100 µg
Molybdenum (µg per kg)	1	0.25	5 µg
Iodine (µg per kg)	1–10	1	–

SUMMARY: RECOMMENDATIONS

Evidence-based recommendations for the use of PN constituents are summarized in Table 49.6.

DISPENSING PN SOLUTION

In developed countries, the PN solution is prepared by a central pharmacy and delivered ready for use. This facility is usually unavailable in most Indian hospitals, and physicians and nurses must chart and prepare PN. The steps for calculation and preparing PN are as follows (a PN chart is provided in the appendix):

1. Determine the total fluid requirement for the day.
2. Subtract the amount of fluid used for medications (e.g. diluting and infusing antibiotics) and enteral feeds.
3. Plan amino acids, intravenous lipids, and glucose to be given over 24 hours.
4. Load intravenous lipid (IVL) suspension in one syringe and add multivitamins (MVI).
5. Mix amino acids, dextrose, electrolytes, and trace elements in the second syringe.
6. IV L+MVI suspension is infused separately from AA-glucose-minerals solution, although they can be mixed using a three-way adapter at the infusion site.

Osmolarity of PN: Weak and conditional evidence recommends that the osmolarity of PN should not exceed 900 mOsm/L to avoid the potential risk of thrombophlebitis in neonates.

Table 49.6: Evidence-based recommendations for parenteral nutrition	
Component	*Recommendations*
Fluids	Day 1: 60–80 ml/kg/day (*See* the protocol on 'Fluid and electrolyte management'). Postnatal weight loss up to 3% per day to a maximum of 10–15% is acceptable. This is achieved by progressively increasing the fluid intake to 150 ml/kg/d by the end of first week of life.
Energy	The goal is 100–120 kcal/kg/day (higher in infants with BPD). An intake of 50 kcal/kg/day is sufficient to match ongoing expenditure but it does not meet the additional requirements of growth.
Protein	The optimal parenteral amino acid intake is 3.5 g/kg/day. Parenteral amino acids can begin from day 1 at 1.5–2 g/kg/day.
Carbohydrates	From day one, 6 mg/kg/min can be infused, increased by 2 mg/kg/min every day to 12–14 mg/kg/min, and adjusted to maintain euglycemia. Insulin is only used in infants who continue to have hyperglycemia associated with glycosuria and osmotic diuresis even after the glucose intake has been reduced to 4–6 mg/kg/min. Insulin is given as a continuous infusion commencing at a rate of 0.05 units/kg/h, increasing as required for persistent hyperglycemia.
Fat	Intravenous fat, 1.5 g/kg/d can be started from day 1, at the same time as when intravenous amino acids are started. This is increased to 2 g/kg/day and 3 g/kg/day over the next two days, maximum of 3.5 g/kg/day. It is delivered as a continuous infusion of 20% intravenous fat via a syringe pump, separate from the infusate containing the amino acids and glucose. The syringe and infusion line should be shielded from ambient light.
Minerals and trace elements	Minerals should include sodium, chloride, potassium, calcium, phosphorus, magnesium. Trace elements should include zinc, copper, selenium, manganese, iodine, chromium, iron and molybdenum.
Vitamins	Vitamins must be added to the fat emulsion to minimize loss during administration due to adherence to tubing and photodegradation.

ROUTE OF ADMINISTRATION

PN can be delivered through **peripheral or central venous lines**. Short-term PN can be given through the peripheral venous line.

Peripheral access offers the advantage of a lower risk of infection due to the greater distance of the catheter from the central circulation and fewer mechanical complications.

However, nutrition delivery is limited with peripheral lines due to constraints created by a solution's osmolarity. The limiting factor in deciding the delivery route is the AA-glucose solution's osmolarity, which depends on dextrose concentration. A dextrose concentration greater than 12.5% has an acidic pH and causes irritation to the peripheral veins. In addition to dextrose, electrolytes and minerals added to the solution also increase the osmolarity. Hypertonic solutions should ideally be administered through the central venous line.

The use of peripherally inserted central catheters (PICC) has facilitated the administration of PN while avoiding many potential complications of surgically inserted central lines. Another attractive option in neonates is a central line inserted through the umbilical vein. An umbilical venous catheter can be used for up to 14 days, after which the risk of complications increases.[15,16]

MONITORING AND COMPLICATIONS

Meticulous **monitoring** is needed in a neonate receiving PN (Table 49.7). Monitoring should be more frequent in the initial stages. Once a steady metabolic stage has been achieved, monitoring can be reduced to once a week.

Complications of PN can be nutrient-related or venous access-related.

Nutrient-related complications include hypoglycemia (plasma sugar <50 mg/dl) and hyperglycemia (plasma sugar >150 mg/dl), azotemia and metabolic acidosis (protein-related), hypertriglyceridemia (triglyceride >200 mg/dl; lipid-related), cholestasis, and trace element deficiency. Most of these complications can be avoided by adequately monitoring and providing nutrients.

Parenteral nutrition-associated liver disease (PNALD) is a commonly encountered complication of prolonged parenteral nutrition. The most widely used definition of PNALD requires a direct bilirubin (DB) concentration of 2 mg/dl with no other cause of liver disease. It presents initially with biochemical evidence of cholestasis, clinical evidence of jaundice, and failure to thrive. The reported incidence of PNALD varies from 25% to 60% in infants receiving long-term PN, depending on the criteria used to diagnose PNALD.

Table 49.7: Monitoring schedule for a neonate on parenteral nutrition

Parameter	*Frequency*
Blood sugar	2–3 times a day while increasing glucose infusing rate Once a day while on stable glucose infusion rate
Urine sugar	Once per nursing shift
Serum electrolytes	Twice a week initially, then weekly
Blood urea	Twice a week initially, then weekly
Calcium, magnesium and phosphorous	Weekly
Packed cell volume	Weekly
Liver function tests	Weekly
Serum triglycerides	Weekly
Anthropometry	
Weight Head circumference Length	Daily at the same time Weekly Weekly
Nutrient intake calculation	Energy in kcal per kg day Proteins in grams per kg per day

Management strategies include two methods: Lipid replacement and lipid restriction. Soyabean-based lipid composition (Intralipid) contains phytosterols which are implicated in PNALD. Replacing Intralipid with SMOFlipid has been shown to have liver-protecting properties in older children receiving PN; however, lipid restriction and lipid replacement in neonates with PNALD is still controversial and requires further studies.[19,20] There are currently no recommendations for restricting the amino acid component of the TPN. The best protective strategy for PNALD would be to minimize the duration of parenteral fluids and switch over to enteral feeds as early as possible.

Intestinal failure-associated liver disease (IFALD):[21] Preterm neonates with gastrointestinal pathologies like necrotizing enterocolitis (NEC) or surgical intestinal conditions and are on PN are predisposed to develop IFALD. The clinical and pathological features are similar to PNALD, with progressive cholestasis, biliary fibrosis, and steatohepatitis. The etiology is multifactorial, with genetics, the role of soyabean oil in PN, and alteration of gut microbiome being implicated to a certain extent in the development of IFALD. Restriction of soyabean oil based PN and transition to enteral feeds have been associated with a gradual reduction of symptoms of IFALD in some reports.

Neonatal refeeding syndrome:[18] Inappropriate rates of minerals, electrolytes, and amino acids (low electrolytes and high amino acids) can lead to increased uptake of phosphate, potassium, and magnesium into cells for energy and protein synthesis, thus leading to the neonatal refeeding syndrome characterized by low serum phosphate, potassium, and magnesium and high serum calcium, glucose, and sodium. This can trigger white matter injury and chronic lung disease.

Venous access-related complications include occlusion, dislodgement, and infection.

PREVENTION OF INFECTION[22–24]

Healthcare-associated infection (HAI) is a significant complication of PN. All efforts should be made to avoid HAI:

- Aseptic precautions during the preparation of PN
- Use of laminar flow for preparation of parenteral fluid solutions
- No compromise on disposables
- Trained staff
- No reuse of the PN solutions
- No interruption of the venous line carrying PN
- Use of bacterial filter

APPENDIX

See Tables 49.8 and 49.9

Table 49.8: Sources of parenteral solutions

Component	*Commercial preparation*	*Concentration*
Proteins	Aminoven Primene	10% (0.1 g/ml)
Lipids	Intralipid	10% (0.1 g/ml) 10% PLR (phospholipids reduced) 20% (0.2 g/ml)
Glucose	Dextrose	5% (0.05 g/ml) 10% (0.1 g/ml) 25% (0.25 g/ml) 50% (0.5 g/ml)

(Contd.)

Table 49.8: Sources of parenteral solutions (*Contd.*)		
Component	*Commercial preparation*	*Concentration*
NaCl	NaCl	0.9% (0.009 g/ml = 0.15 mEq/ml) 3% (0.03 g/ml = 0.5 mEq/ml)
KCl	KCl	15% (0.15 g/ml = 2 mEq/ml)
Calcium	Calcium gluconate	10% (9 mg/ml of elemental calcium)
Multivitamin	Adult MVI	–
Trace elements	Celcel 4 (Claris) Celcel 5 (Claris)	–
Magnesium sulfate	Magnesium sulfate	50% (0.5 g/ml = 4 mEq)

Table 49.9: Cost and availability of common parenteral fluids			
Name of the fluid	*Concentration (%)*	*Manufacturer*	*Cost (INR)*
Aminoven	6 10	Fresenius Kabi	220 (100 ml) 280 (100 ml)
Primene (Amino acid)	10	Baxter	288 (100 ml)
Intralipid	10 20	Fresenius Kabi	255 (100 ml) 520 (250 ml)
SMOF lipid emulsion	20	Fresenius Kabi	690 (250 ml)
Calcium gluconate	10	Biostan	12 (10 ml)
Magnesium sulphate	50	Ravi Pharma	8 (2 ml)
MVI	–	Psychotropics India (Multizac) NBZ Pharma Infuvite Pediatric (Baxter)	15 (10 ml)

REFERENCES

1. Vlaardingerbroek H, van Goudoever JB, van den Akker CH. Initial nutritional management of the preterm infant. Early Hum Dev 2009;85:691–5.
2. te Braake FW, van den Akker CH, Riedijk MA, van Goudoever JB. Parenteral amino acid and energy administration to premature infants in early life. Semin Fetal Neonatal Med 2007;12:11–8.
3. Hulzebos CV, Sauer PJ. Energy requirements. Semin Fetal Neonatal Med 2007;12:2–10.
4. Koletzko B, Goulet O, Hunt J, Krohn K, Shamir R. 1. Guidelines on Paediatric Parenteral Nutrition of the European Society of Paediatric Gastroenterology, Hepatology and Nutrition (ESPGHAN) and the European Society for Clinical

Nutrition and Metabolism (ESPEN), Supported by the European Society of Paediatric Research (ESPR). J Pediatr Gastroenterol Nutr 2005;41 Suppl 2:S1–87.

5. Ziegler EE, Thureen PJ, Carlson SJ. Aggressive nutrition of the very low birthweight infant. Clin Perinatol 2002;29:225–44.
6. Kanarek K, Santeiro M, Malone J. Continuous infusion of insulin in hyperglycemic low-birth weight infants receiving parenteral nutrition with and without lipid emulsion. J Parenter Enteral Nutr 1991;15:417–20.
7. Henry B. Pediatric Parenteral Nutrition Support. . In: Nevin-Folino N, ed. Pediatric Manual of Clinical Dietetics: Faulhabes; 2003:495–514.
8. Shulman RJ. New developments in total parenteral nutrition for children. Curr Gastroenterol Rep 2000;2:253–8.
9. Poindexter BB, Karn CA, Denne SC. Exogenous insulin reduces proteolysis and protein synthesis in extremely low birth weight infants. J Pediatr 1998;132:948–53.
10. Aba-Sinden A, Bollinger R. Challenges and controversies in the nutrition support of the preterm infant. Support Line 2002;2:2–15.
11. Haumont D, Deckelbaum RJ, Richelle M, et al. Plasma lipid and plasma lipoprotein concentrations in low birth weight infants given parenteral nutrition with twenty or ten percent lipid emulsion. J Pediatr 1989;115:787–93.
12. Gutcher GR, Farrell PM. Intravenous infusion of lipid for the prevention of essential fatty acid deficiency in premature infants. Am J Clin Nutr 1991;54:1024–8.
13. Waitzberg DL, Torrinhas RS, Jacintho TM. New parenteral lipid emulsions for clinical use. JPEN J Parenter Enteral Nutr.2006;30:351–67.
14. Wanten GJ, Calder PC. Immune modulation by parenteral lipidemulsions. Am J Clin Nutr. 2007;85:1171–84.13.
15. Calder PC. Hot topics in parenteral nutrition. Rationale forusing new lipid emulsions in parenteral nutrition and a reviewof the trials performed in adults. Proc Nutr Soc. 2009;68:252–60.
16. Manzanares W, Dhaliwal R, Jurewitsch B, Stapleton RD, Jee-jeeboy KN, Heyland DK. Parenteral fish oil lipid emulsions inthe critically ill: a systematic review and metaanalysis. JPEN.2014;38:20–8.
17. Ziegler EE, O'Donnell A, Nelson S. Body composition of the reference fetus. Growth 1976;40:320–41.
18. Groh-Wargo S, Barr SM. Parenteral Nutrition. Clin Perinatol. 2022 Jun;49(2):355-79. doi: 10.1016/j.clp.2022.02.002. PMID: 35659091.
19. Zugasti Murillo A, Petrina Jáuregui E, Elizondo Armendáriz J. Parenteral nutrition-associated liver disease and lipid emulsions. *Endocrinología y Nutrición (English Edition)* 2015;62(6):285–9.
20. Nandivada P, Fell GL, Gura KM, Puder M. Lipid emulsions in the treatment and prevention of parenteral nutrition-associated liver disease in infants and children. Am J Clin Nutr. 2016 Feb;103(2):629S–34S.
21. Lee WS, Chew KS, Ng RT, Kasmi KE, Sokol RJ. Intestinal failure-associated liver disease (IFALD): insights into pathogenesis and advances in

management. Hepatol Int. 2020 May;14(3):305-16. doi: 10.1007/s12072-020-10048-8. Epub 2020 Apr 30. PMID: 32356227.

22. Puangco MA, Nguyen HL, Sheridan MJ. Computerized PN ordering optimizes timely nutrition therapy in a neonatal intensive care unit. J Am Diet Assoc 1997;97:258–61.
23. O'Grady NP, Alexander M, Dellinger EP, et al. Guidelines for the prevention of intravascular catheter-related infections. The Hospital Infection Control Practices Advisory Committee, Center for Disease Control and Prevention, U.S. Pediatrics 2002;110:e51.
24. Butler-O'Hara M, Buzzard CJ, Reubens L, McDermott MP, DiGrazio W, D'Angio CT. A randomized trial comparing long-term and short-term use of umbilical venous catheters in premature infants with birth weights of less than 1251 grams. Pediatrics 2006;118:e25–35.

CHAPTER

50

Peritoneal Dialysis

INDICATION

The indications for kidney replacement therapy in neonates include hyperkalemia, hyponatremia with volume overload (pulmonary edema, severe hypertension), metabolic acidosis (pH<7.20 despite medical management), hypocalcemia, hyperphosphatemia refractory to therapy, and uremic encephalopathy.

While anuria and the above are absolute indications for initiating kidney replacement therapy, dialysis should begin early to prevent catastrophic metabolic complications. In addition, dialysis is indicated for removing dialyzable toxins, especially ammonia, in the case of inborn errors of metabolism.

Fluid accumulation per se increases vulnerability for AKI and often predates it. It can also worsen AKI by increasing venous pressure and causing abdominal hypertension and interstitial edema. Overall, evidence suggests >10–20% fluid overload may represent a critical threshold at which outcomes are adversely impacted, and targeted interventions should be considered.[1]

Therefore, additional indications for the initiation of kidney replacement are the following:

- Fluid overload >10–20%.
- Inability to provide adequate nutrition due to fluid restriction.

Kidney replacement can be implemented by acute peritoneal dialysis (PD), intermittent hemodialysis (IHD), or continuous kidney replacement therapy (CKRT). Factors dictating the mode of kidney replacement include the urgency of fluid and solute removal, hemodynamic stability, the feasibility of vascular access, whether the peritoneal membrane is intact for dialysis, and resources available at a given institution.

MODE OF KIDNEY REPLACEMENT (PERITONEAL DIALYSIS)

Peritoneal dialysis is the preferred mode of kidney replacement in neonates chiefly due to its technical simplicity, lack of hemodynamic compromise, and requirement of vascular access.

Principle: The two purposes of kidney replacement are dialysis (removal of solutes) and ultrafiltration (removal of water). Dialysis occurs by removing plasma solutes by diffusion down their concentration gradient across the peritoneal lining. Instilling hypertonic dialysate into the peritoneal cavity creates a transmembrane osmotic gradient, allowing fluid removal by ultrafiltration. Therefore, PD allows a slow continuous exchange of fluid and solutes.

Peritoneal dialysis catheters: Peritoneal access in most institutes is achieved by a stiff catheter, but when used beyond 48–72 hours, infection rates are high. The Acute Disease Quality Initiative (ADQI) conference for neonatal AKI recommended cuffed catheters (Tenckhoff catheters made of silicone polymer of methyl-silicate) for prolonged PD due to its low risk of infection and visceral injury (Fig. 50.1).[2] Limitations of soft Tenckhoff catheter include its long intraperitoneal length and relatively larger width for use in tiny babies with sparse subcutaneous fat, with possible risks of catheter migration and pressure skin necrosis.[3]

Procedure for peritoneal dialysis by stiff catheter:

- Empty the bladder by catheterization.
- Clean and drape the abdomen with the neonate supine.
- Create a fluid-filled reservoir by infusing 20–30 ml/kg of warmed dialysate into the peritoneum using a 22G cannula in the midline at the junction of the upper one-third and lower two-thirds of the distance between the umbilicus and pubic symphysis.

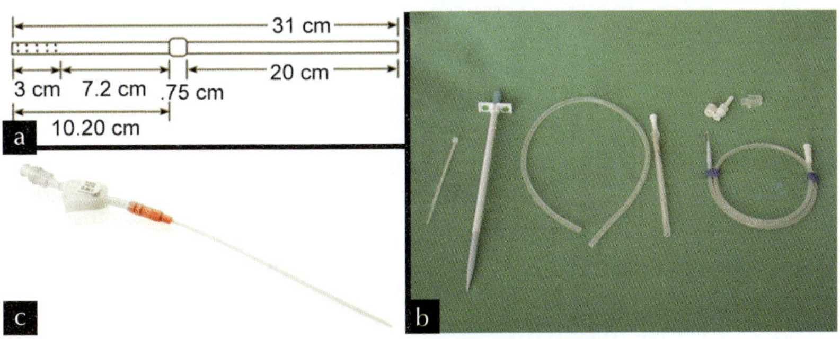

Fig. 50.1: Peritoneal dialysis catheters: Soft Tenckhoff catheters (a and b) have single or double cuffs and side holes (3 cm). Introducer set (items in b) is required for insertion by the Seldinger technique. These catheters require approximately 10 cm of the catheter to be inserted into the abdomen (a), limiting utility in very tiny neonates, in which case a stiff 12 Fr single-lumen femoral catheter (c) may be used.

- Insert the PD catheter into the peritoneal cavity after placing a small vertical nick using a 15 no. blade and connect it to a three-way cannula. The common insertion sites are in the midline below the umbilicus (midline approach) and the right or left lower quadrant of the abdomen (paramedial approach). The exit site should be out of the diaper region to prevent soiling and placed on the side of the abdomen contralateral to any stoma. It is helpful to place to grasp the catheter between the thumb and index finger at a point just above the skin to control excessive penetration.
- The dialysate fluid is connected to a pediatric burette set, and its terminal end is connected to one of the ports of the three-way cannula. The remaining three-way port is connected to the IV set, the end of which is let into a sterile container (empty IV fluid bottle).
- The abdomen is filled with 20–30 ml/kg of dialysis fluid infused over 10 min. A 15–30 min dwell time is used before draining the fluid over 10 min. Peritoneal dialysis can be continued till the desired effect is obtained.
- Hypothermia must be prevented by using pre-warmed dialysis fluid.

PD fluid: The PD prescription includes dialysate type and composition, number of exchanges, fill volume, inflow, dwell, and outflow times, ultrafiltration volume and the number of exchanges, or PD cycles, per day.

Composition of PD fluid[4]
Osmotic agent: Dextrose 1.4–3.9 g/dl
Base: Lactate 35–40 mEq/L or bicarbonate 34 mEq/L
Sodium 132–134 mEq/L, calcium 1.25–1.75 mM/L,
Magnesium 0.25–0.75 mM/L, chloride 95–103.5 mEq/L

- The box above shows the composition of standard commercially available PD fluids. The dialysate fluid contains 1.7% dextrose as an osmotic agent with lactate/bicarbonate as a base. If a higher gradient is required, as in the case of fluid overload, a 3% dextrose solution can be used.[4] This can be prepared by adding 25 ml of 50% dextrose to one liter of 1.7% PD fluid.
- Lactate-free, bicarbonate-based solutions are more biocompatible and are available commercially or may be made in-house. Babies with liver failure, as in asphyxia, may be unable to metabolize lactate quickly and benefit from using such fluids.[4]

- The higher the fill volume, the greater is the ultrafiltration and clearance. The initial fill volume recommended is 10–20 ml/kg (300–600 ml/m^2), increased gradually up to 30 ml/kg (800 ml/m^2)[5]. Limited evidence shows that even low fill volumes (10 ml/kg) with rapid exchanges can achieve adequate ultrafiltration and clearance.[6]
- Initial dwell times are 15–30 min, with 16–20 cycles daily being the norm. The fluid balance and biochemical abnormalities determine the dwell time; a shorter dwell time is used for rapid urea, fluid, and potassium clearance.
- Dialysate inflow time should be restricted to 10–15 min for efficient dialysis, with outflow times ranging from 20–30 min. Complete drainage of effluent should be ensured to avoid elevated intra-abdominal pressure.
- If baby becomes hypokalemic during the procedure, add 3–4 mEq of potassium to 1 L to dialysate fluid.
- Heparin 250–1000 U/L should be added if hemorrhagic effluent is present to avoid catheter-related clotting.
- Prophylactic use of a single dose of IV vancomycin (10 mg per kg) given 60 min before the procedure decreases the rate of peritonitis.[7]

Monitoring: Neonates require careful clinical and biochemical monitoring (Table 50.1).

Nutrition: Measures for the provision of adequate nutrition in babies with PD include the following:

- Monitoring of serum sodium and supplementation to compensate for PD losses(approximately 13 mEq for every 100 ml of ultrafiltrate).[8]
- Total calorie intake should be calculated accounting for ~10 kcal/kg/day obtained from dextrose within the dialysate.[8]
- Accounting for protein losses by PD by providing 1.8 g/kg/day of dietary protein.[5]

Table 50.1: Monitoring of neonates on peritoneal dialysis

Parameter	*Frequency of monitoring*
Clinical assessment of fluid balance	6–12 hourly
Blood sugar, sodium, potassium and bicarbonate	6 hourly
Serum creatinine	24–48 hourly
Peritoneal fluid cell count	24–48 hourly
Catheter tip and the fluid culture	End of procedure

Contraindications: Absolute contraindications include necrotizing enterocolitis, diaphragmatic hernia, recent intra-abdominal surgery, and intra-abdominal malignancy. A relative contraindication is a severe respiratory compromise, as it may worsen with abdominal distension. The latter may be circumvented with smaller volume cycles.

Complications: PD is an invasive procedure, and the following complications need to be remembered[9–11]

- Electrolyte imbalance is the commonest complication, including hypokalemia (57–76%) and hyperglycemia (6–47%), especially when a higher glucose concentration is used.
- Peritonitis is defined as the presence of >*100 cells/mm*^{3} or >50% neutrophils in the PD fluid after a dwell time of 2 hours. It occurs in 4–12.9% of cases with soft catheters. The common organisms are *S. aureus* and gram-negative bacteria. Peritoneal fluid cell count should be monitored every 24–48 hours. If suggestive of peritonitis, empirical intraperitoneal antibiotics (loading doses of ceftazidime 500 mg/L and vancomycin1g/L) should be initiated with a PD dwell time of 4–6 hours while awaiting peritoneal fluid culture. Antibiotics should be modified based on culture; recommended duration is 21 days for *S. aureus* and 14 days for other organisms. Removal of PD catheter should be considered, based on the patient's overall condition, in case of fungal peritonitis or failure of the PD fluid effluent to clear despite 5–7 days of appropriate antibiotics.
- Adhesion of catheter tip to omentum causing catheter malfunction may occur. A systematic review showed catheter-related complications, including catheter leakage and obstruction, occurred in 21% of ELBW and VLBW infants.[11]
- Bleeding due to catheter and perforation of abdominal viscera are uncommon complications (2–6%).

HEMODIALYSIS

Challenges of hemodialysis in the neonatal age group include the need for large extracorporeal volumes causing excessive fluid shifts and impairing thermic control, technical difficulty in establishing adequately sized vascular access, and calibration of machines not designed for neonates.

Without access to neonatal blood tubings, the minimum extracorporeal volume achieved at our center is approximately 80 mL with the smallest possible dialyzer (FxPaed, Fresenius) and pediatric bloodlines. Hence, hemodialysis in the Indian context is currently possible only for neonates weighing at least 3 kg.

CONTINUOUS KIDNEY REPLACEMENT THERAPY (CKRT)

Continuous kidney replacement therapy (CKRT) helps manage neonatal AKI in hemodynamically unstable patients, especially if peritoneal dialysis is not feasible. The solutes are cleared by hemofiltration and hemodiafiltration. Systemic anticoagulation and placement of optimally sized vascular access are necessary. CRRT machines are not designed to treat small infants requiring low and accurate blood flow rates with minimal ultrafiltration error.

REFERENCES

1. Selewski DT, Gist KM, Nathan AT, et al. The impact of fluid balance on outcomes in premature neonates: a report from the AWAKEN study group. Pediatr Res. 2020;87:550–7.
2. Harer MW, Selewski DT, Kashani K, et al. Improving the quality of neonatal acute kidney injury care: neonatal-specific response to the 22nd Acute Disease Quality Initiative (ADQI) conference. J Perinatol. 2021;41:185–95. Kaddourah A, Goldstein SL.
3. Spector BL, Misurac JM. Renal Replacement Therapy in Neonates. Neoreviews. 2019;20:e697-e710.
4. Kaddourah A, Goldstein SL. Renal replacement therapy in neonates. Clin Perina.
5. Fischbach M, Warady BA. Peritoneal dialysis prescription in children: bedside principles for optimal practice. Pediatr Nephrol. 2009;24:1633–42; quiz 1640,1642.
6. Golej J, Kitzmueller E, Hermon M, Boigner H, Burda G, Trittenwein G. Low-volume peritoneal dialysis in 116 neonatal and paediatric critical care patients. Eur J Pediatr. 2002;161:385–9.
7. Nourse P, Cullis B, Finkelstein F, et al. ISPD guidelines for peritoneal dialysis in acute kidney injury: 2020 Update (paediatrics). Perit Dial Int. 2021;41:139–57.
8. Hölttä THC RK. Peritoneal dialysis during infancy. Warady BA, Schaefer F, Alexander SR, eds. Pediatric Dialysis. 2nd ed. New York, NY: Springer; 2012; chap 13.
9. Kara A, Gurgoze MK, Aydin M, Taskin E, Bakal U, Orman A. Acute peritoneal dialysis in neonatal intensive care unit: An 8-year experience of a referral hospital. Pediatr Neonatol. 2018;59:375–9.
10. Hakan N, Aydin M, Zenciroglu A, et al. Acute peritoneal dialysis in the newborn period: a 7-year single-center experience at tertiary neonatal intensive care unit in Turkey. Am J Perinatol. 2014;31:335–8.
11. Bellos I, Karageorgiou V. Peritoneal dialysis in very low and extremely low birthweight infants: A pooled analysis. Perit Dial Int. 2021:8968608211059888.

CHAPTER

51

Blood Component Therapy

Blood component therapy is one of the common interventions in NICUs. Approximately 40% of VLBW and 95% of ELBW neonates would receive a packed red blood cells (PRBC) transfusion to correct anemia during the NICU stay. The decision to transfuse needs to be judicious because oxidative damage associated with blood component transfusion has been implicated in the pathogenesis of adverse neonatal outcomes like bronchopulmonary dysplasia (BPD), retinopathy of prematurity (ROP), and necrotizing enterocolitis (NEC).[1]

BLOOD COMPONENT SPECIFICATION AND PRETRANSFUSION TESTING[2–4]

In contrast to adults and older children, neonates constitute a vulnerable age group because of the small circulating blood volume and neurological and immunological immaturity.

i. **Donor specification:** The donor should be negative for all mandatory microbiological markers (HIV, Hepatitis B and C, syphilis, and malaria) and preferably have had at least one prior donation in the previous two years.

ii. **Multiple donor exposure:** Pedi packs/satellite packs (previously separated product units containing about one-quarter of the typical unit volume in smaller storage bags) should be considered for top-up transfusions to minimize multiple donor exposure.

iii. **CMV seronegativity:** Recommended for intrauterine transfusions (IUTs) and neonates up to 44 weeks postmenstrual age.

iv. **Use fresh blood** (<5 days; collection day taken as day '0' and component to be transfused before midnight of day 5) to minimize the risk of hyperkalemia. This is recommended for red cell IUTs, neonatal exchange transfusion, and large volume transfusion (equivalent to at least a single circulating blood volume—about 80 ml/kg for neonates over 24 hours or 50% of the circulating volume within 3 hours). For routine top-up transfusions, irradiated red cells may be used up to 14 days.

v. **Pretransfusion testing:** Antibody screening of a neonate represents the maternal antibody status rather than the fetal/ neonatal antibody status because of the active transport of maternal IgG antibodies across the placenta and poor red cell antibody production within the first four months of life. Both mother's (within 3 days predelivery or post-delivery) and neonate's samples should be obtained for initial ABO and D (Rhesus) group determination. If the maternal sample is unavailable, details of the maternal group, antibody status, and transfusion history of both mother and baby should be obtained; antibody screening and crossmatch compatibility with neonatal blood should be performed (Table 51.1).

vi. **In neonates** with a history of transfusion, there is no need to repeat ABO typing or to perform crossmatch compatibility testing if the antibody screen is negative and the neonate has received either group O, ABO identical, or ABO compatible RBCs as well as compatible D (Rh) type.

vii. **In emergencies**, when unable to meet all neonatal specifications, the following hierarchy may be considered for the issue of component:
   1. ABO compatibility with mother and neonate.
   2. Antigen-negative for maternal antibodies.
   3. Age of unit.
   4. Irradiation status.
   5. CMV negativity or leukocyte reduction (LR).

Table 51.1: Investigations on the maternal and fetal/neonatal sample

Maternalsample	*Fetal/neonatal sample*
i. ABO and D group/type	i. ABO and D group/type
ii. Antibody screening	ii. Direct antiglobulin test (DAT)—to be performed when hemolysis/ hemolytic disease of the newborn (HDN) is suspected or when the mother has significant red cell antibodies
iii. Identification of the antibody/antibodies if the antibody screen (+)	iii. Antibody screening of plasma in the absence of maternal sample

The preferred blood group component in different conditions is shown in Tables 51.2 and 51.3.

Table 51.2: Blood component selection for transfusion

Component	*Preferred group*	*Comment*
Packed red cells (PRBC)	Compatible with maternal and neonatal ABO group and Rh type	
Double volume exchange transfusion (DVET) 1. Rh isoimmunization 2. ABO incompatibility	• Rh -ve blood of baby's ABO type compatible with maternal plasma (1st choice) • O-ve whole blood (2nd choice) • Blood group 'O' and Rh compatible suspended in AB plasma and cross-matched with baby's and mother's blood	• D (Rhesus) -ve and K (Kell) -ve • Fresh blood (≤5 days) • Irradiated blood if prior IUT • CPD instead of SAGM to prevent mannitol toxicity
Platelets	• ABO and D identical or compatible with recipient • HPA compatible with maternal platelet antibody for neonates with NAIT (as for IUT platelets)	• Avoid use of group O platelets for non-O patients as much as possible. • Platelets should be compatible for D. • If a patient requires HLA matched platelets, HLA match takes precedence over ABO group.
FFP and cryoprecipitate	• ABO compatible plasma should be selected as far as possible. • Group O plasma must only be given to O recipient.	• Reserve AB plasma for emergency transfusions/patient's group is unknown.

Table 51.3: Choice of ABO components in neonate ABO compatible with mother				
Neonatal Group	*Choice*	*Choice of ABO group for transfusion*		
		RBC	*Platelet*	*FFP*
O	1st	O	O	O
	2nd	–	AB or A or B	AB or A or B
A	1st	A	A	A
	2nd	O	AB	AB
B	1st	B	B	B
	2nd	O	AB	AB
AB	1st	AB	AB	AB
	2nd	O or A or B	Plasma free A or B	–

Packed Red Blood Cells (PRBC)

PRBCs are prepared from the whole blood by centrifugation under a closed system within 8 hours of collection. They must be stored at 2–6°C irrespective of the preservative used. PRBCs are often subjected to further modifications to make PRBC transfusion safer in neonates (Table 51.4):

Indications of Blood Component Therapy[2,3]

a. PRBC Transfusion

PRBC transfusion is mainly indicated for resolving symptomatic anemia and to improve tissue oxygenation (which depends on cardiac output, oxygen saturation, and hemoglobin concentration). The thresholds for transfusion vary according to gestational age (GA), postnatal age, respiratory support, and the presence of congenital heart disease. Clinical factors like severity of illness, symptoms of anemia (lethargy, difficulty in suckling, poor growth, tachycardia, and tachypnea), rate of fall of Hb, anticipated blood loss, and nutritional status also guide the decision to transfusion (Tables 51.5 and 51.6). Evaluating the degree of reticulocyte response is also essential: a reticulocyte count $>100 \times 10^3/\mu l$ indicates adequate bone marrow compensation. Though there is a paucity of evidence on transfusion thresholds in moderate to late preterm and term infants, recent multicentric trials have tried to evaluate the optimum transfusion threshold in very preterm neonates. Clinicians may consider these thresholds used in preterm and term neonates (Tables 51.5 and 51.6).

Table 51.4: Packed red blood cell modification

Modification type	*Method*	*Comments*
Leucocyte reduction (LR)	• Universal LR recommended before storage • At least 3-log reduction in leukocytes depending on the method used, like buffy coat removal, red cell washing, and leukofiltration • Pre-storage LR preferred	Prevents • Transmission of leukotropic viruses (CMV, EBV, and HTLV-1) • Non-hemolytic febrile transfusion reactions (NHFTR) • Transfusion-related acute lung injury (TRALI)
Irradiation (Gamma or X-rays)	• Dose of 25–50 gray • Inactivates donor T cells • Recommended in susceptible patient groups (preterm neonates <1200 g, cellular immune deficiency, transfusion from blood relations, HLA/cross-matched platelets)	• Only available method to prevent transfusion-associated graft versus host disease (TA-GVHD) • Irradiated blood to be used within 24 hours • Reduces shelf life of PRBCs to 28 days • Risk of hyperkalemia
CMV reduced RBCs	• By preselecting CMV negative donors or LR or a combination of both • A blood component containing $<5 \times 10^6$ leukocytes per unit is considered safe (NB: fresh frozen plasma does not transmit CMV infection)	• Preferred in neonates weighing ≤1,500 g at birth or born at or before 30 weeks of gestation (because they are at the greatest risk of CMV infection) • Viremia in the initial latent phase of infection can still transmit CMV even if leukoreduced/ CMV negative donor
Washed RBCs	• Removes most of the plasma and anticoagulant preservative solution from RBC • Helps to reduce potassium in the RBC.	Preferred for • IUTs, exchange transfusion, and large volume transfusions (more than 20 ml/kg) • IgA deficiency (five times washing advisable) • Recurrent allergic reactions (two times washing advisable)

CMV: Cytomegalovirus; *EBV:* Epstein Barr virus; *HTLV-1:* Human T-lymphotropic virus 1; *HLA:* Human leukocyte antigen; *IUT:* Intrauterine transfusion

Table 51.5: Packed red blood cells transfusion thresholds in preterm neonates			
Postnatal age	*Suggested transfusion threshold: Hb in g/dl (Hct)*		
	Ventilated	*On oxygen or CPAP/ NIPPV*	*No supplemental oxygen*
First 24 hours	<12 (35)	<12 (35)	<10 (30)
Days 2–7	<12 (35)	<10 (30)	<10 (30)
Days 8–14	<10 (30)	<9.5 (28)	<7.5–8.5 (23–25)*
Day 15 onwards	<10 (30)	<8.5 (25)	<7.5 (23)*

**Use clinical judgment and consider transfusion at a higher threshold of <8.5*

Table 51.6: Packed red blood cells transfusion thresholds in term neonates	
Condition	*Suggested transfusion threshold: Hb in g/dl (Hct)*
Severe pulmonary disease (Defined as MAP >8 cm H_2O and FiO_2 >0.4 on conventional ventilation or MAP >14 and FiO_2 >0.4 on HFV)	<10 (30)
Moderate pulmonary disease (Defined as MAP ≤8 cm H_2O and/or FiO_2 ≤0.4 on a conventional ventilator, or MAP <14 and/or FiO_2 <0.4 on HFV)	<8 (24)
Severe cardiac disease	<10 (30)
Major surgery	<10 (30)
Symptomatic anemia 1. ≥24 hours of tachycardia (HR >180 bpm) or tachypnea (RR >60) 2. Doubling of the oxygen requirement in the previous 48 hours 3. Serum lactate ≥2.5 mEq/L or an acute metabolic acidosis (pH <7.2) 4. Weight gain <10 g/kg/day over the previous four days while receiving ≥120 kcal/kg/day	<7 (21)

Hb: Hemoglobin; *Hct:* Hematocrit; *HR:* Heart rate; *RR:* Respiratory rate

For acute blood loss, transfusions should generally be considered when there is blood volume loss of 10% with symptoms of decreased oxygen delivery or when acute blood volume loss is >20%.

Restrictive threshold for packed red blood cell transfusion. What is the evidence?

Two recent multicentric trials—'Effect of Transfusion Thresholds on Neurocognitive Outcomes' of ELBW infants (ETTNO) and 'Transfusion of Prematures' (TOP) trial—which randomized 2837 (1013 in ETTNO and 1824 in TOP) neonates of <30 weeks' gestation into liberal and restrictive thresholds (28–41% vs. 21–34% in ETTNO and 32–38% vs. 21–32% in TOP) showed no difference in mortality or neurodevelopmental impairment at 24 months corrected age. A significant limitation of both trials is that neonates were randomised to the most restrictive Hct levels only after 3 weeks of postnatal age.

Practice tip: PRBC transfusion

1. What is the recommended rate and volume of PRBC transfusion?
   Rate: 5 ml/kg/hour
   Volume: Prefer smaller volume (10–15 ml/kg)—no benefit with higher volumes.
   DVET: The aliquot exchanged each time should be about 5 ml/kg, and the rate should not exceed 2–3 ml/kg/min
2. Is it mandatory to use diuretics during blood transfusion?
   The decision to use should consider known adverse effects with uncertain benefits. Studies have found no difference in clinical respiratory, ventilatory, or hemodynamic parameters with the use of furosemide compared to placebo after elective RBC transfusion in preterm infants except for minimal increase in post-transfusion FiO_2.
3. What are the strategies to reduce or prevent PRBC transfusion in neonates?
   - Limiting phlebotomy losses by using point-of-care devices, minimizing unnecessary laboratory testing, in-line arterial testing, and optimizing frequency and volume of blood draws; umbilical cord blood can also be made use for sampling.
   - Delayed cord clamping (≥ 30 seconds to 180 seconds)

Studies have also evaluated the role of recombinant human erythropoietin (rh-EPO) in reducing the number of PRBC transfusions in preterm neonates. EPO stimulates erythropoiesis and reduces the number (early and late EPO) and volume (early EPO) of RBC transfusions. However, a multicentric study (Preterm Erythropoietin Neuroprotection Trial; PENUT) found no significant impact of EPO on mortality or severe neurodevelopmental impairment at two years of age and no effect on neonatal morbidities, including ROP, IVH, sepsis, NEC, BPD. So, routine use of rh-EPO is not recommended.

b. Platelet Transfusion

Platelet components used in neonates include random donor platelets (RDP) and single donor platelets (SDP). The SDP unit has a higher platelet concentration (3×10^{11} per unit) than RDP (0.5×10^{10} per unit). SDP is not recommended for routine neonatal transfusion except when prolonged and severe thrombocytopenia is anticipated. Neonates, particularly high-risk neonates, have a favorable outcome when a lower platelet count threshold is used for transfusion (Table 51.7).

c. Fresh Frozen Plasma (FFP) and Cryoprecipitate Transfusion

Cryoprecipitate contains fibrinogen (150–250 mg), factor VIII (80–120 IU), Factor XIII (40–60 IU), fibronectin (30–60 mg), and vWF (100 IU). Given the paucity of evidence-based guidelines, plasma

Table 51.7: Suggested thresholds of platelet count for neonatal platelet transfusion

Platelet Count	*Condition*
<25,000/mm^3	Neonates with no bleeding (including neonates with NAIT if no bleeding and no family history of ICH)
<50,000/mm^3	• Neonates with bleeding • Current coagulopathy • Before surgery • NAIT if previously affected sibling with ICH
<1,00,000/mm^3	Major bleeding e.g. significant IVH Major surgery

NAIT: Neonatal alloimmune thrombocytopenia; *ICH:* Intracranial hemorrhage; *IVH:* Intraventricular hemorrhage

Practice tip: Platelet therapy

1. Recommended volume and rate
   Rate: 10–20 ml/kg/hour.
   Start the infusion slowly; if there are no reactions, gradually increase the rate to complete the transfusion within 1 hour.
   Volume: 10–20 ml/kg
2. Whole blood derived platelets contain ~10×10^9 platelets in 10 ml; 10 ml/kg dose may increase platelet count by 100×10^9/L or more. Studies have shown that 15 ml/kg of platelets increase platelet count by ~$30–90 \times 10^9$/L in sick neonates with ongoing platelet consumption, e.g. NEC and sepsis
3. No role for routine use of platelet transfusion for PDA closure in thrombocytopenic preterm neonates with hs-PDA.

Table 51.8: Indications for FFP and cryoprecipitate transfusion	
FFP	*Cryoprecipitate*
1. Disseminated intravascular coagulation (DIC)	1. Congenital factor VIII deficiency#
2. Vitamin K deficiency associated bleeding (VKDB)	2. Congenital factor XIII deficiency#
3. Neonates with ongoing bleeding and significant coagulopathy*	3. Afibrinogenemia and dysfibrinogenemia with active bleeding or while undergoing an invasive procedure
4. Neonates with significant coagulopathy* who must undergo invasive procedures with a risk of significant bleeding	4. von Willebrand disease (vWD) with active bleeding when a. Diamino-D-arginine vasopressin is contraindicated, not available, or does not elicit a response. b. Virus inactivated plasma-derived factor VIII concentrate is not available.

**Significant coagulopathy (PT or aPTT significantly above the normal gestational and postnatal age-related reference ranges)*
#In the absence of factor concentrate

Practice tip: FFP transfusion
1. Recommended rate: 10–20 ml/kg/hour; volume: 15–20 ml/kg. 2. No role of prophylactic FFP in non-bleeding neonates receiving therapeutic hypothermia and having deranged coagulation parameters.

therapy is often misused in NICU. There is no role for routine coagulation profile screening for neonates admitted to the NICU (Table 51.8).

Cryoprecipitate may be used if there is persistent hypofibrinogenemia (<1.0 g/L) despite FFP transfusion, rapidly falling fibrinogen or significant hemorrhage in DIC.

Adverse Transfusion Reactions[5–9]

Transfusion of blood products is not without its inherent risks. The adverse reactions associated with transfusions can be classified as acute and delayed transfusion reactions (Table 51.9).

Acute

1. **Allergic reactions:** Caused by preformed immunoglobulin E antibody against an allergen in the transfused plasma. It occurs infrequently and responds to antihistamines.

Table 51.9: Adverse transfusion reactions	
Acute	*Delayed*
Allergic transfusion reactions	Transfusion transmitted infections
Febrile non-hemolytic transfusion reaction (FNHTR) (rare in neonates)	Transfusion associated graft-versus-host disease (TA-GVHD)
Pulmonary transfusion reaction • TAD • TACO • TRALI	Delayed serologic (DSTR) and delayed hemolytic transfusion reaction (DHTR) (rare in neonates)
Hypotensive transfusion reaction	RBC alloimmunisation (rare in neonates)
Acute hemolytic transfusion reaction (AHTR)	

2. **Pulmonary reactions:** Range from transfusion-associated dyspnea (TAD) to transfusion-associated circulatory overload (TACO) and transfusion-related acute lung injury (TRALI). TACO and TRALI are syndromes of acute respiratory distress that occur within 6 hours of blood transfusion.
   i. **TRALI:** Characterized by non-cardiogenic pulmonary edema. Onset usually within 2 hours and presents with respiratory distress, severe hypoxemia, and fever, with or without hypotension. Examination findings include crackles or diminished breath sounds without evidence of fluid overload. X-ray chest might reveal bilateral alveolar and interstitial infiltrates. TRALI is common with transfusion of plasma-rich components like fresh frozen plasma, apheresis platelets, and stored cellular blood components. Treatment includes ventilatory and hemodynamic support. Diuretics are not helpful. The prognosis is usually good, with the resolution within 96 hours.
   ii. **TACO:** TACO is characterized by pulmonary hydrostatic (cardiogenic) edema. Clinical improvement after treatment with a diuretic or an inotropic agent is characteristic of TACO but not TRALI. Other findings suggestive of TACO include persistent hypertension, a post-transfusion brain natriuretic peptide (BNP) level of at least 100 pg/ml, and a post-transfusion:pre-transfusion BNP ratio of 1.5.
3. **Hypotensive transfusion reaction:** Not well defined in neonates.
4. **AHTR:** Rare in neonates and mainly occur following RBC transfusion in 'mis-transfusion' situations: Either sample

misidentification ('wrong blood in tube') or patient misidentification. It presents as increased pallor, free hemoglobin in the plasma, hemoglobinuria, increased serum potassium levels, and acidosis. Treatment is mainly supportive.

5. **Metabolic complications:** Include hypocalcemia, hyperkalemia, hypomagnesemia, and hypo/hyperglycemia.

Delayed

1. **TA-GVHD:** Rare but fatal complication occurring 2 days to 6 weeks after a transfusion mediated by donor lymphocytes. Fetuses requiring intrauterine transfusions, neonates receiving exchange transfusions, and those with potentially undiagnosed immunodeficiencies are at particular risk for TA-GVHD.
2. **Transfusion-transmitted infections (TTI):** It includes human immunodeficiency virus (HIV), hepatitis B and C viruses, cytomegalovirus (CMV), bacterial infections, parasites (malaria), and prions. In India, it is mandatory to test every unit of blood collected for hepatitis B, hepatitis C, HIV, syphilis, and malaria. There still exists a risk of transmission of HBV, HCV, and HIV due to the window period infections and mutant strains that evade detection in testing.

Others

1. **Iron overload:** Occurs following repeated RBC transfusions. It can lead to cardiac, hepatic, and endocrine complications.
2. **Transfusion-associated acute gut injury (TRAGI)/Transfusion-associated NEC (TANEC):** Conflicting evidence with numerous observational studies associating transfusion and NEC. TRAGI/TANEC denotes a spectrum of severe gastrointestinal reactions observed after a blood transfusion. Proposed etiological mechanisms include inflammatory substances in PRBC units, oxidative stress, gut immaturity, possible pre-transfusion small bowel hypoxia, and mesenteric blood flow disturbances secondary to transfusion. Reports also suggest that severe anemia rather than transfusion leads to NEC. The precise etiology remains unclear and is likely to be multifactorial.
3. **Risk of ROP and BPD**
   - **ROP:** PRBC transfusion is an independent risk factor for ROP, with an adjusted OR of 2.4 (95% CI: 1.4–4.) following two or more transfusions compared to none. It is possibly related to

adult hemoglobin (HbA) in the PRBCs with lower O_2 affinity and a greater capacity to release O_2.

- **BPD:** The numerous pro- and anti-inflammatory mediators in stored RBCs could play a role in the pathophysiology of BPD.

REFERENCES

1. Zerra PE, Josephson CD. Transfusion in Neonatal Patients: Review of Evidence-Based Guidelines. Clin Lab Med. 2021;41:15–34.
2. New HV, Berryman J, Bolton-Maggs PH, Cantwell C, Chalmers EA, Davies T, Gottstein R, Kelleher A, Kumar S, Morley SL, Stanworth SJ; British Committee for Standards in 2016;175:784–828.
3. Tewari VV, Pandita A, Taligasalam V, Kumar A, Gupta G. Use of Blood Components in newborns. In: Kumar P, Kabra NS, Gupta G, Chawla D, Bhatia BD, Sankar MJ, Shah S, editors. In: Evidence-based clinical practice guidelines. New Delhi: National Neonatology Forum of India; 2019. p. 99–128.
4. Reece JT, Sesok-Pizzini D. Inventory Management and Product Selection in Pediatric Blood Banking. Clin Lab Med. 2021;41:69–81.
5. Sostin N, Hendrickson JE. Pediatric Hemovigilance and Adverse Transfusion Reactions. Clin Lab Med. 2021;41:51–67.
6. Girelli G, Antoncecchi S, Casadei AM, Del Vecchio A, Isernia P, Motta M, Regoli D, Romagnoli C, Tripodi G, Velati C. Recommendations for transfusion therapy in neonatology. Blood Transfus. 2015;13:484–97.
7. Mo YD, Delaney M. Transfusion in Pediatric Patients: Review of Evidence-Based Guidelines. Clin Lab Med. 2021;41:1–14.
8. Jackson ME, Baker JM. Hemolytic Disease of the Fetus and Newborn: Historical and Current State. Clin Lab Med. 2021;41:133–51.
9. Villeneuve A, Arsenault V, Lacroix J, Tucci M. Neonatal red blood cell transfusion. Vox Sang. 2021;116:366–78.

CHAPTER

52

Kangaroo Mother Care

Kangaroo mother care (KMC) is a method of care for preterm or low birth weight (LBW) infants by placing them in skin-to-skin (STS) contact with the mother or other caregiver to ensure their optimum growth and development.[1,2] Initially devised as an alternative to conventional technology-based care, KMC is now considered the standard of care for LBW infants in all settings.

COMPONENTS[2]

The four components of KMC are

1. Kangaroo position (skin-to-skin contact) between the mother and the infant in a vertical position, between the mother's breasts, and under her clothes. The provider must keep herself in a semi-reclining position to avoid gastric reflux in the infant. The mother can share this responsibility with the father and other relatives.
2. Exclusive or nearly exclusive breastfeeding.
3. Early discharge from health facilities.
4. Continued follow-up: Mothers at home require adequate support and follow-up; hence, a follow-up program and access to emergency services must be ensured.

BENEFITS

KMC is a simple, cost-effective intervention with numerous benefits for the infant and the community.[3] A recent systematic review[4] that included studies done both in health facilities and in community settings (27 studies and 12,000 neonates) shows that KMC when compared with conventional neonatal care:

- Reduces the risk of death during birth hospitalization or 28 days of age (RR 0.68; 95% CI 0.53–0.86). This reduction in mortality is noted irrespective of gestational age or weight at enrolment, time of initiation, and setting (hospital or community).
- Reduces severe infection till the latest follow-up.

- Reduces the risk of hypothermia by 68%.
- Results in better gain in anthropometric parameters, namely weight gain per day and length and head circumference gains per week.
- Results in higher exclusive breastfeeding rates at discharge and 28 days of life.

KMC of at least 8 hours per day was found to have greater mortality benefits than shorter-duration of KMC. Long-term benefits of KMC are difficult to ascertain due to additional influences from parental nurturing, optimal home environment, and external factors on development. Follow-up studies from a single RCT showed that the risk of cerebral palsy, Griffith Quotients at 12 months of corrected age, or IQ scores at 20 years of age were not different between KMC and conventional care infants.[5] The most vulnerable infants (birth weight <1800 g) who received KMC demonstrated significantly reduced school absenteeism and reduced hyperactivity, aggressiveness, and externalization at 20 years of age.

WHEN TO INITIATE KMC?

Most units wait until infants become clinically stable and are weaned from respiratory support and parenteral nutrition to initiate KMC. Four recent studies explored the benefits of early initiation of KMC before 24 hours of age compared to later initiation until neonates were deemed hemodynamically stable. Three of these studies, including the large immediate KMC (iKMC) multi-country study,[6] were conducted in low- and middle-income countries. In all the studies, neonates in the early KMC group received KMC within 24 hours of birth, even when on noninvasive respiratory support. The only exclusions were inability to breathe at birth, invasive ventilation, shock, seizures, severe jaundice, or major congenital malformations requiring immediate management. The meta-analysis of these studies showed that early-initiated KMC, compared to later initiation:

- Reduces neonatal mortality by 22% (RR 0.78, 95% CI 0.66–0.92).
- Reduces the incidence of hypothermia and clinical sepsis till 28-days of life.
- Results in higher rates of the exclusive breastfeeding at discharge.

Post-hoc analysis of the iKMC study data further showed that the babies immediately initiated on KMC have no significant difference in heart rate, respiratory rate, oxygen saturation as compared to babies in control arm further demonstrating the safety of immediate KMC initiation.[7]

Based on recent evidence, the WHO recommendations for the care of preterm or low-birthweight infants advocate the following:

- Kangaroo mother care (KMC) is recommended as routine care for all preterm or LBW infants. KMC can be initiated in the healthcare facility or at home and should be given 8–24 hours per day (as many hours as possible). (Strong recommendation, high-certainty evidence).
- KMC should be started as soon as possible after birth. (Strong recommendation, high-certainty evidence).

REQUIREMENTS FOR KMC IMPLEMENTATION

KMC is feasible everywhere because it does not require any equipment to implement. Also, it is advantageous for the organization of health services provided the following requirements are met:

1. Health facility or home setting.
    a. The health facility should always allow entry of the parents to the neonatal unit.
    b. Mother-neonatal intensive care unit (Mother-NICUs), wherein the bed of mother is beside the incubator/warmer of preterm baby, wherever feasible can further help to promote early KMC (as done in an Indian centre for iKMC study). Such an undertaking will require interdepartmental coordination.
    c. Reclining chairs in the nursery and postnatal wards and beds with adjustable backrests (Fig. 52.1) help mothers to practice KMC for long hours.
    d. Mother can also provide KMC at home, sitting on an ordinary chair or in a semi-reclining posture on a bed with the help of pillows.

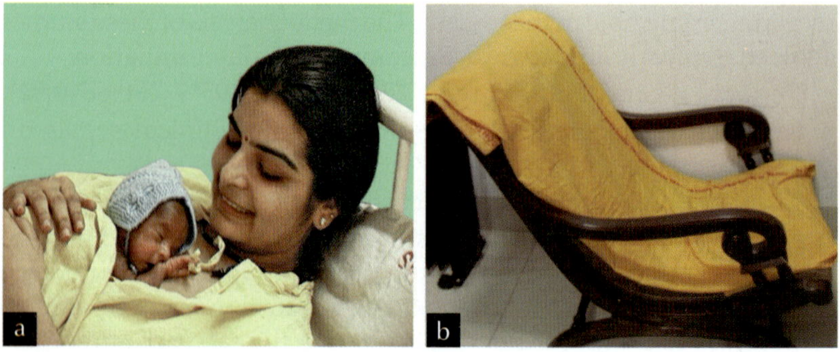

Fig. 52.1: Mother practicing KMC in reclining posture (a) and KMC chair (b)

2. Supporting staff and family members.
   a. In hospital settings, a trained nurse is indispensable in assisting mothers with KMC.
   b. Staff should receive adequate training on KMC, including the nutrition of LBW infants. Additional training is needed on the expression and storage of breast milk, using alternate feeding methods, and daily monitoring of the growth of LBW infants. The training could be done by exposing them to units already practicing KMC.
   c. Educational material such as information sheets, posters, and video films on KMC in the local language should be available to mothers, families, and the community.
   d. At home, a supportive family who can also share the responsibility of providing KMC is essential.
3. Follow-up.
   a. Ensure continued KMC at home. Arrange follow-up to track growth and development.
4. Institutional, social, and community support
   a. The requirement for a successful KMC program can be summarized in three words: Communication, sensitivity, and education.
   b. Apart from supporting the mother, family members should also be encouraged to provide KMC when the mother wishes to rest.
   c. The mother would need her family's cooperation to handle her conventional household chores and responsibilities until the baby requires KMC.
   d. Community awareness about the benefits should be created. This is particularly important when there are social, economic, or family constraints.

CRITERIA FOR ELIGIBILITY OF KMC

1. **Neonate**
   - All preterm and LBW neonates are eligible for KMC.
   - KMC can be initiated as soon after birth in spontaneously breathing infants, even if they are on respiratory support (i.e. non-invasive ventilation).
   - KMC can be provided while the baby receives intravenous fluids or is fed via an orogastric tube.
   - Apnea is not a contraindication for KMC. On the contrary, KMC helps decrease apneic episodes, probably related

to the prone position of the infant that is associated with better ventilatory mechanics and the rhythmic kinaesthetic stimulation from the mother. A systematic review showed that KMC resulted in a 60% reduction in apnoea episodes (RR 0.41; 95% CI 0.22, 0.78).[8]

- Contraindications: hemodynamic instability (shock), severe respiratory distress, seizures, asphyxia, or other medical conditions that need priority management of airway, breathing, or circulation.

2. **Caregivers:** Mothers and close family members can provide KMC, irrespective of age, parity, education, culture, and religion. The following points must be taken into consideration when counseling for KMC:
   a. **Willingness:** The mother must be willing to provide KMC. Healthcare providers should counsel and motivate her. Once the mother realizes the benefits of KMC for her baby, she will learn and undertake KMC.
   b. **General health and nutrition:** The mother should be free from serious illness to be able to provide KMC. She should receive an adequate diet and supplements recommended by her physician.
   c. **Hygiene:** The mother should maintain good hygiene: daily bath/sponge, change of clothes, hand washing, and short and clean fingernails.

INITIATION OF KMC

1. **Counseling:** When the neonate is ready for KMC, arrange a convenient time for the mother and her baby. Demonstrate to her the KMC procedure in a caring and gentle manner and with patience. Answer her queries and allay her anxieties. Encourage her to bring her mother/mother-in-law, husband, or any other family member. It helps build a positive attitude in the family and ensures family support to the mother, which is particularly crucial for post-discharge home-based KMC.[9] It is helpful that the mother starting KMC interacts with someone already practicing KMC for her baby.
2. **Mother's clothing:** The mother can wear any front-open dress per local culture. This may include a sari, a blouse, a front open gown, a suit, or a simple shirt (Fig. 52.2). KMC can be done

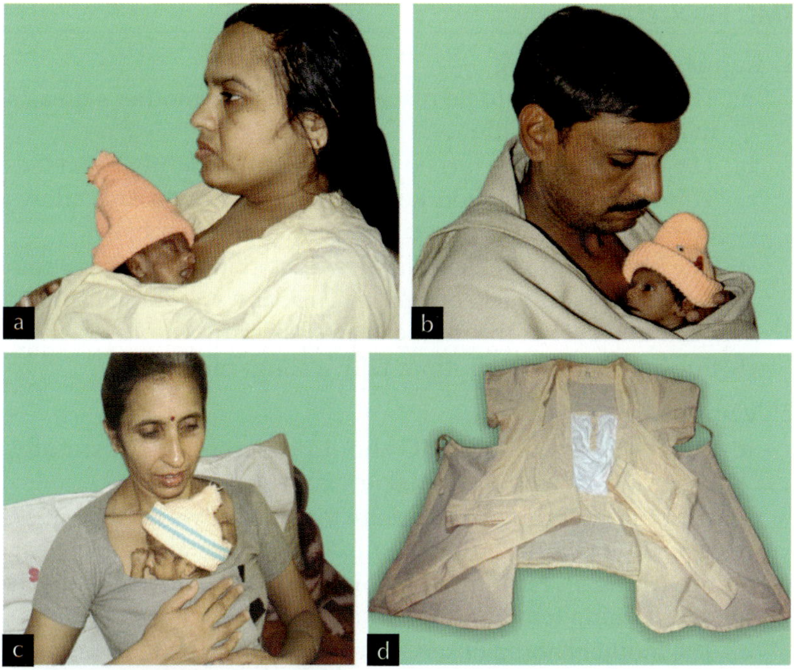

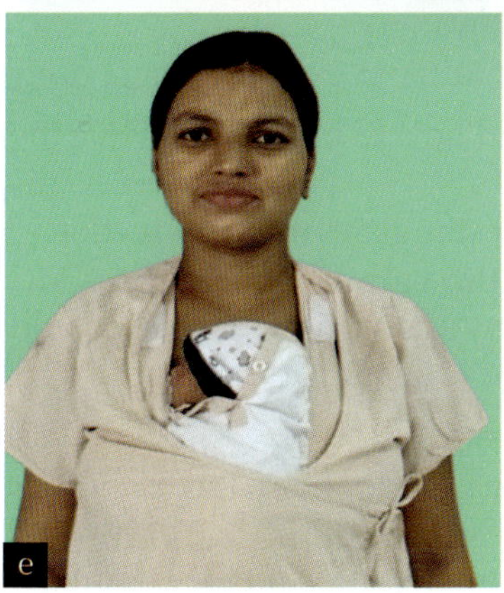

Fig. 52.2: Mother (a) and father (b) practicing KMC in a front-open gown and shawl. Mother performing KMC using AIIMS KMC jacket (c). IIT-AIIMS KMC Jacket (d) and mother performing KMC using IIT-AIIMS KMC jacket (E).

with special apparel (such as the KEM bag or AIIMS KMC jacket) designed to suit the needs of mothers. Any other suitable clothing that can retain the baby for an extended period can be adapted locally.

3. **Neonate's clothing:** Neonate is dressed in a cap, socks, nappy, and front-open sleeveless shirt.

KMC PROCEDURE

1. **Kangaroo positioning**
   a. The neonate should be placed between the mother's breasts in an upright position.
   b. The head should be turned to one side and slightly extended. This extended position keeps the airway open and allows eye-to-eye contact between the mother and her baby.
   c. The hips should be flexed and abducted in a "frog" position; the arms should also be flexed. The baby's abdomen should be at the level of the mother's epigastrium.
   d. Support the baby's bottom with a sling/binder.
2. **Monitoring**
   a. Neonates receiving KMC should be monitored carefully, especially during the initial few days.
   b. Nursing staff should make sure that the baby's neck position is neither too flexed nor too extended, the airway is clear, breathing is regular, the color is pink, and the baby is maintaining temperature.
   c. The mother should observe the baby during KMC so that she can continue monitoring at home.
3. **Feeding**
   a. The mother should be explained how to breastfeed while the baby is in the KMC position.
   b. Holding the baby near the breast stimulates milk production.[5,6]
   c. She may express milk while the baby is still in the KMC position. Depending on the baby's condition, the baby could be fed with a paladai, spoon, or orogastric tube.
4. **Duration**
   a. Skin-to-skin contact should start gradually in the nursery.
   b. The length of skin-to-skin contact should be gradually increased up to 24 hours a day, interrupted only for changing diapers.

Discharge Criteria

The unit's standard policy for hospital discharge should be followed. Generally, the following criteria are accepted at most centers:[9]

- The baby's general health is good.

- Gaining weight (at least 15–20 g/kg/day for three consecutive days).
- Able to maintain body temperature satisfactorily for at least three consecutive days at room temperature.
- Feeding well and receiving exclusively or predominantly breast milk.
- The mother and family members are confident in taking care of the baby.

WHEN TO DISCONTINUE KMC?

If the mother and baby are comfortable, KMC is continued at the hospital and at home for as long as possible. Often this is desirable until the baby's gestation reaches term or the weight is around 2500 g. Once the neonate starts wriggling to show that she is uncomfortable, pulls her limbs out, cries, and fusses whenever put in skin-to-skin contact, the mother can wean the baby from KMC.

POST-DISCHARGE FOLLOW-UP

Close follow-up is a fundamental prerequisite of KMC practice. Baby is followed once or twice a week till 37–40 weeks of gestation or until the baby reaches 2.5–3 kg. After that, a follow-up once in 2–4 weeks may be enough till 3 months of postmenstrual age. The baby should gain adequate weight (15–20 g/kg/day up to 40 weeks of postmenstrual age and 10 g/kg/ day subsequently). More frequent visits should be made if the baby is not growing well or his/her condition demands.

REFERENCES

1. Charpak N, Ruiz-Pelaez JG, Charpak Y. Rey-Martinez Kangaroo Mother Program: an alternative way of caring for low birth weight infants? One year mortality in a two cohort study. Pediatrics 1994; 94(6 Pt 1):804–10.
2. World Health Organization. Kangaroo mother care: a practical guide. Department of Reproductive Health and Research, WHO, Geneva.2003.
3. Conde-Agudelo A, Belizán JM, Diaz-Rossello J, Jose L. Kangaroo mother care to reduce morbidity and mortality in low birthweight infants. Cochrane Database Syst Rev. 2016 August 16; (3):CD002771.
4. Sivanandan S, Sankar MJ. Kangaroo mother care for preterm or low birth weight infants: A systematic review and meta-analysis. *BMJ Global Health* 2023;1–13. doi: bmjgh-2022–010728.

5. Charpak N, Tessier R, Ruiz JG, Hernandez JT, Uriza F, Villegas J et al. Twenty-year Follow-up of Kangaroo Mother Care Versus Traditional Care. Pediatrics. 2017;139(1):e20162063.
6. Immediate "Kangaroo Mother Care" and Survival of Infants with Low Birth Weight. N Engl J Med. 2021 May 27;384(21):2028–38.
7. Linnér A, Westrup B, Rettedal S, Kawaza K, Naburi H, Newton S, et al. Immediate skin-to-skin contact for low birth weight infants is safe in terms of cardiorespiratory stability in limited-resource settings. Global Pediatrics. 2023 Mar;3:100034.
8. Montealegre-Pomar A, Bohorquez A, Charpak N. Systematic review and meta-analysis suggest that Kangaroo position protects against apnoea of prematurity. Acta Paediatr. 2020 Jul;109(7):1310–6.
9. Chan GJ, Labar AS, Wall S, Atun R. Kangaroo mother care: a systematic review of barriers and enablers. Bull World Health Organ. 2016;94(2):130–141J.

CHAPTER

53

Pain Assessment and Management

Neonates admitted to NICU undergo several painful procedures per day, and they communicate their pain and stress through various autonomic, motor, and behavioral cues. The caregivers in NICU must recognize these cues and modify the environment to reduce stress and pain and facilitate self-regulatory mechanisms to promote the infant's comfort.

Four subsystems need continuous positive environmental influence and synchronized functioning to optimize well-being and growth in neonates. Table 53.1a to d lists the subsystems and the associated organized and disorganized behavior.

Pain prevention is essential from a humanitarian perspective because pain is associated with long-term neurobehavioral consequences. Every healthcare facility caring for neonates should implement a comprehensive pain prevention program, including routine assessment of pain, minimizing procedures that can cause pain, effective use of nonpharmacological and pharmacological techniques to prevent pain during common procedures, and complete pain relief during major surgeries.[1]

Table 53.1a: Organized and disorganized behavior in autonomic and visceral subsystem

Parameter	*Organized behavior*	*Disorganized behavior*
Respiratory rate	Stable	Very fast/very slow or with pauses
Heart rate	Stable	Very fast or very slow
Skin color	Pink	Blanching
Oxygen saturation	Normal	Gasping/ cyanosis
Other signs	Absent	Yawning, startles, tremors, twitches, sneezing, coughing drooling, spitting, vomiting, gagging, straining as if passing bowel

Table 53.1b: Organized and disorganized behavior in motor subsystem		
Parameter	*Organized behavior*	*Disorganized behavior*
Tone	Normal	Flaccidity in trunk, extremities, stiffening or arching and hyperextension
Posture	Maintains flexed posture	All limbs are extended
Movement	Slow regulated, controlled smooth movements	Jerky movements/ very slow movements, flailing movements of the arms and legs
Other signs	Nil	Arching body, finger splay, foot splay, fisting of hands, salute, high arm guard, sitting on air, tongue protrusion

Table 53.1c: Organized and disorganized behavior in attention and interactive sub-system	
Organized behavior	*Disorganized behavior*
Neonate is in deep sleep or quiet and alert, maintains eye contact, mouth pursing, cooing, smiling, consolable	Neonate is in a diffused sleep state, twitching, fussy, frowning, grimacing, irritable, crying, eyes rolling upwards, averting eye gaze, gaping, sleepless

Table 53.1d: Behavior in self-regulatory subsystem*	
Organized behavior	*Disorganized behavior*
This system helps the preterm infant to calm and soothe themselves in stressful situations. An infant who can self-regulate will have a longer duration of undisturbed sleep; have better-organized learning and coping mechanisms during different painful experiences. *Self-regulatory signs are finger clasping, clasping of blanket or sheet, fingers in the mouth with or without sucking, foot clasp, and feet against the bassinet for support.*	Neonate will be fussy, irritable, and unable to interact with the environment positively.

**Observing an infant over a period is crucial. These cues indicate whether the infant is ready for the activity, needs to be calmed before the activity is continued, or is unprepared to engage. The older the infant, the more they use self-calming or self-regulatory techniques to organize themselves.*

PAIN ASSESSMENT

- Use Premature Infant Pain Profile: Revised (PIPP-R; Table 53.2) for assessment of acute pain.[2]
- ComfortNeo pain scale may be used to assess the degree of prolonged pain and its response to analgesics.[3]

Table 53.2: Premature Infant Pain Profile: Revised (PIPP-R)

S.N.	*Parameters*	*Score*			
		0	*+1*	*+2*	*+3*
1.	Change in heart rate (bpm) from baseline	0–4	5–14	15–24	>24
2.	Decrease in oxygen saturation (%) from baseline	0–2	3–5	6–8	>8 or increase in O_2
3.	Brow bulge (sec)	None (<3)	Minimal (3–10)	Moderate (11–20)	Maximal (>20)
4.	Eye squeeze (sec)	None (<3)	Minimal (3–10)	Moderate (11–20)	Maximal (>20)
5.	Naso-labial furrow (sec)	None (<3)	Minimal (3–10)	Moderate (11–20)	Maximal (>20)
		Subtotal score: (1 + 2 + 3 + 4 + 5)			
6.	Gestational age (weeks)	>36 weeks	32 – 35 + 6 weeks	28 – 31 + 6 weeks	<28 weeks
7.	Baseline behavioral state	Active and awake	Quiet and awake	Active and asleep	Quiet and asleep
		Total score:			

Instructions:

- Observe the infant for 15 sec at rest to determine baseline vital signs.
- Observe the infant for 30 sec after the procedure to assess changes in the vital parameters.
- If infants require an increase in FiO_2 during a procedure, give a score of 3 in the O_2 saturation score.
- If the subtotal score > 0, add gestational age and behavioral state scores.
- Total score = Sub-total score + GA score + BS score
- Maximum score = 21
- Score 7–12: non-pharmacological measures; score >12: pharmacological analgesia

PREVENTING OR REDUCING PAIN

General Measures

Pain is managed most effectively by preventing, limiting, or avoiding noxious stimuli. The following measures in combination are followed to minimize pain:

- Keep ambient light and sound levels minimum; avoid strong perfumes and pungent odours.
- Close incubator doors gently and optimize alarm limits and alarm sounds.
- Limit the number of painful procedures and handling by clustering the care activities.
- Encourage parental involvement and interaction.
- 'Sensorial stimulation': gently stimulate audiovisual, gustatory, and tactile systems simultaneously.
- Swaddling, facilitated tucking, distraction measures like talking, music, etc.

Nonpharmacological Measures

The nonpharmacological measures include sucrose (24% solution), dextrose (20–30% solution), breastfeeding or breastmilk through pacifiers, skin-to-skin contact, and sensorial stimulation. These measures have been best studied for acute mild-to-moderate procedural pain, including pain during heel lance, venipuncture, adhesive removal, intramuscular injections, etc. These measures are more effective when used simultaneously. No significant adverse effects have been described, though the long-term effects have yet to be well-studied. Table 53.3 summarizes the evidence supporting nonpharmacologic analgesics.

The sucrose/dextrose solution is given orally by a syringe/ pacifier 2–3 min before the procedure and may be repeated 1–2 min afterward. The effect lasts around 4–6 minutes. Intragastric administration has no analgesic effect. The usual dose is 0.1–0.5 ml for preterm (<32 weeks neonates) and 0.2–1 ml for late preterm and term neonates.

Pharmacological Measures

The pharmacological measures can be broadly divided into:

- Local anesthetic agents
- Systemic agents: opioids, paracetamol

Table 53.3: Evidence supporting nonpharmacological analgesic measures in neonates

Agent	*Evidence*	*Major findings and conclusions*
Sucrose (24%)	Cochrane meta-analysis[4] (74 studies, 7049 infants)	• Reduction in pain scores (PIPP) during heel lance, venipuncture, and intramuscular injections, in both preterm and term infants. • Inconclusive benefits during other painful procedures. • No major adverse effects. • Combination of sucrose with other nonpharmacological measures may augment the analgesic effect.
Dextrose (20–30%)	Systematic review and meta-analysis[5] (38 studies, 3785 infants)	• Reduction in pain scores during heel lance and venipuncture.
Breast milk and breastfeeding	Cochrane meta-analysis[6] (20 studies)	• Breastfeeding reduces pain during heel lance and venipuncture. • Supplemental breastmilk has uncertain benefits. • Glucose/sucrose have similar effectiveness as breastfeeding.
Skin-to-skin contact	Cochrane meta-analysis[7] (25 studies, 2001 infants)	• Reduction in composite pain indicators (both physiological and behavioral). • Insufficient evidence regarding additive effect with other interventions.

Nonsteroidal anti-inflammatory agents (NSAIDs) are generally not used as analgesics in newborns.

Local Anesthetics

Local anesthesia is helpful for the management of acute procedure-related pain. It can be either topically applied on intact skin or injected subcutaneously. The common preparations include EMLA (eutectic mixture of local anesthetics), lidocaine (2%) injection, and tetracaine (4%). Proparacaine eye drops are used for topical anesthesia during ROP examination.

The dose of EMLA is 0.5–2 g with a contact period of 30 min to 1 hour. Apply the cream over a 2–3 cm^2 area with 1–2 mm thickness and cover with transparent (Tegaderm) dressing. For maximal analgesic effect, topical anesthetics should be combined with other nonpharmacological measures like sucrose analgesia or breast milk supplementation. The clinical effect of EMLA is modest, with good efficacy for lumbar puncture and no or minimal benefit for heel lance and venipuncture. The major drawback is the delayed onset of action and a contact period of at least 1 hour before the procedure, making it unsuitable for emergent procedures. Though EMLA is approved for use in only infants older than three months, it has been used off-label in neonates.[8] There is a possible risk of methemoglobinemia with EMLA cream; it is recommended to test for MetHb levels if multiple doses of EMLA are used.

For emergent procedures (e.g. chest drain insertion), subcutaneous local anesthetic injection (2% lidocaine hydrochloride) is preferred over topical creams.

Opioids

Opioid drugs are the mainstay in managing severe pain, including mechanical ventilation, endotracheal intubation, and post-surgical pain in neonates. The two most used agents are morphine and fentanyl. The common adverse effects of opioids include respiratory depression, hypotension, urinary retention, reduced intestinal motility, bronchospasm, and chest wall rigidity (fentanyl). Also, their pharmacokinetics have not been well-described in preterm neonates, underscoring the need for cautious use. Tolerance and withdrawal are common with prolonged use. Fentanyl is the preferred opioid among neonates. Short-acting opioids like Sufentanil, Remifentanil, etc. have been used for brief procedures like endotracheal intubation and short surgeries.

Special considerations for fentanyl and morphine:

- Avoid morphine (and prefer fentanyl) in case of hypotension, gestation <27 weeks, acute kidney injury, and reduced gastrointestinal motility.[9]
- Avoid fentanyl in neonates who have undergone abdominal surgery or are at risk of increased intraabdominal pressure and during ECMO (circuit sequestration of fentanyl).[10,11]

Analgesia for Specific Procedures

Table 53.4 enumerates the recommended analgesia measures in routine bedside procedures.

Table 53.4: Analgesia measures for routine bedside procedures

Procedure	*Analgesia measure recommended*			
	General measures	*Sucrose analgesia**	*Breast milk**	*Skin-to-skin contact/sensorial stimulation*
Venipuncture Sampling#	+	+	+	+
Heel prick#	+	+	+	+
Subcutaneous/IM injection	+	+	+	+
Adhesive tape removal$	+	±	±	+
IV cannulation	+	+	+	+
Urinary catheterization	+	+	+	–
Echocardiography	+	+	+	–

*Either sucrose analgesia or breastfeeding can be adopted depending on the availability and feasibility; for slightly longer procedures, sucrose analgesia is preferred over breast milk/breastfeeding

#Venipuncture should be the preferred mode of blood sampling as heel lance is more painful; automated lancets are superior to conventional lancets for the heel prick

$Use adhesive removal solution

NON-EMERGENCY INTUBATION

Endotracheal intubation is a stressful procedure and may be associated with bradycardia, hypoxia, hypertension (both systemic and pulmonary), and increased intracranial pressure. In all non-emergent intubations, premedications are recommended to blunt the stress response, decrease the risk of adverse events, and facilitate successful intubation. These drug regimens generally consist of the following:

A. A sedative-analgesic (e.g. fentanyl, morphine) to decrease pain and stress.
B. A vagolytic (e.g. atropine, glycopyrrolate) to counter bradycardia and decrease secretions.
C. A muscle relaxant (e.g. vecuronium, rocuronium) to allow adequate visualization (Table 53.5).

The AAP recommends the following for all non-emergency neonatal intubations:[12]

- Analgesic agents or anesthetic doses of a hypnotic drug should be given.
- Vagolytic agents and rapid-onset muscle relaxants should be considered.

Table 53.5: Analgesia-sedation for non-emergency intubation*			
S.No.	*Drug*	*Dose*	*Timing*
1	Inj Fentanyl	1–4 μg/kg IV	Slowly over 3–5 minutes
2	Inj Atropine	0.02 mg/kg IV (minimum dose 0.1 mg)	1–2 min prior to intubation
3	Inj Vecuronium#	0.1 mg/kg IV	2–3 minutes prior to intubation

*Preferred regimen includes the above three-drug combination.

#Avoid using paralytic agents (vecuronium) if an experienced person is unavailable for intubation.

- Use of sedatives alone, such as benzodiazepines without analgesic agents, should be avoided.
- A muscle relaxant without an analgesic agent should not be used.

Mechanical Ventilation

Mechanical ventilation is a painful and uncomfortable experience that may adversely affect the course of acute illness and long-term neurodevelopment.

- There is no role for routine opioids in mechanically ventilated neonates. Consider opioids only in the following situations:
  1. Chest tube insertion, post-surgery, planned intubation/reintubation.
  2. Significant ventilator dyssynchrony that is not attributable to improper/inadequate ventilator settings or secretions. Note that inadequate ventilatory setting is a more common cause of ventilator dyssynchrony than lack of sedation-analgesia.
  3. Documented pain (document PIPP-R pain score at baseline and 30 minutes after dose)
  4. PPHN requiring mechanical ventilation and not improving with environmental measures alone.
- Assess the requirement of opioids daily and document the same in case records.
- Consider early de-escalation.
- In neonates with expected short duration of mechanical ventilation (e.g. preterm infants with respiratory distress syndrome), use intermittent boluses of opioids only if required to ensure lower cumulative doses:
  - **Fentanyl:** 1–2 μg/kg IV slowly over 5 minutes.
  - **Morphine:** 10–50 μg/kg IV over 15–30 minutes.

- Emergency intubation and resuscitation kit (including IV naloxone: 0.1 mg/kg/dose) should be ready bedside while administering a bolus dose of opioids.
- In neonates with an expected longer duration of ventilation, continuous infusion of opioids is preferred over intermittent boluses, but only in defined indications cited above.
- Avoid opioids in extremely preterm neonates due to uncertain safety and pharmacokinetic profile.

Analgesia/sedation in ventilated neonates: what is the evidence?

A Cochrane review (2021), including 23 studies and 2023 neonates (both term and preterm), examined the role of opioids during mechanical ventilation in neonates. It found no significant benefit of using opioids over placebo in terms of PIPP score 12–48 hours after starting the infusion, duration of mechanical ventilation, IVH, BPD, neurodevelopmental impairment at 18–24 months and 5–6 years, and mortality. The authors recommended selective use of opioids in neonates based on pain assessment using validated tools.[14]

Table 53.6 enlists the recommended analgesia measures for other procedures in the NICU.

Table 53.6: Analgesic measures for specific procedures[13]

Procedure	*Measures*
Arterial puncture/ cannulation Lumbar puncture PICC line placement	• Sucrose/dextrose analgesia • EMLA cream locally (esp for LP) • General measures
Chest tube placement	• Inj Fentanyl* 0.5–1 µg/kg 2–3 min prior • Local infiltration with lignocaine 2% • Sucrose/ dextrose analgesia
Chest drain removal	• Sucrose/dextrose analgesia • General measures
ROP screening	• Local anesthetic eye drops • Sucrose/dextrose analgesia • General measures
Laser photocoagulation for ROP**	• Inj Fentanyl 2 µg/kg bolus followed by 2–5 µg/kg/hr infusion till the procedure lasts • Local anesthetic eye drops • Sucrose analgesia • General measures • Post-procedure paracetamol 15 mg/kg q 6 hourly for 1–2 days

(Contd.)

Table 53.6: Analgesic measures for specific procedures[13] (Contd.)	
Procedure	*Measures*
CT/ MRI for sedation	**Intubated:** • Inj Fentanyl 0.5–1 µg/kg IV 2–3 min prior • Inj Midazolam 0.1–0.2 mg/kg IV **Non-intubated:** • Oral Trichlophos 20–30 mg/kg or chloral hydrate 50–100 mg/kg, 20–30 min prior • Inj Midazolam 0.1–0.2 mg/kg

**In non-ventilated babies while using opioids, watch for apnea/respiratory depression; IV Naloxone should be kept ready and used in case of respiratory depression or apnea (0.1 mg/kg or 0.25 ml/kg IV)*

***Even ventilated patients on opioid infusion during procedures need additional analgesic measures*

Table 53.7 depicts the dosages and common adverse effects of different analgesic agents used in the NICU.

Opioid Tolerance

- Tolerance leads to reduced efficacy of the drug and may require dose escalation. Tolerance is rare, with a duration of therapy of less than 4 days. Other causes of increased pain, such as worsening primary disease, opioid-related hyperalgesia, and ventilator asynchrony, must be considered and ruled out.
- Consider escalating the dose after about 4 days of fentanyl infusion or 14 days of morphine infusion, based on pain scores.
- Opioid rotation, i.e. switching to an equianalgesic dose of a different opioid, may help counter tolerance and decrease the need for dose escalation.
- While switching from one opioid to another, reduce the equianalgesic dose of the new opioid by 20–30% to adjust for a probable lack of cross-tolerance.
- To convert intravenous fentanyl to an equivalent intravenous morphine dose, multiply the fentanyl dose (in µg/kg/hour) by 10–20, reduce it by 25%, and continue that dose as morphine infusion (in µg/kg/hour).
- When very high doses of opioid analgesics are required or sedation is desirable, adding agents like midazolam (to be used cautiously in preterm infants), dexmedetomidine, or ketamine may help decrease the opioid doses.

Table 53.7: Drugs and dosages of analgesic/sedative medications commonly used in NICU

Drug	*Dose*	*Preparation/administration*	*Pharmacology*	*Adverse effects*
Morphine	Bolus: 25–100 μg/kg slow IV Infusion: 7–50 μg/kg/hour IV	1 ml = 15 mg Dilute in NS/10D/5D to make a maximum concentration of 5 mg/ml Incompatible with phenytoin, phenobarbitone	Narcotic analgesic Onset: 5–15 min Duration of action: 3–5 hours Not recommended in neonates <28 weeks	Respiratory depression, bradycardia, hypotension ileus, urinary retention; naloxone can reverse effects
Fentanyl	Bolus 1–4 μg/kg IV slow over 3–5 minutes Infusion: 1–4 μg/kg/hour (≥32 weeks); start at 0.5 μg/kg/hour in neonates <32 weeks during 1st week of life	1 ml = 50 μg Dilute in NS/5D/10D Incompatible with phenytoin, phenobarbitone	50–100 times more potent than morphine Onset: immediate Duration of action 30–60 min	Respiratory depression, chest wall rigidity (esp with rapid push), urinary retention, hypotension; naloxone can reverse effects
Midazolam	• Bolus: 0.05–0.1 mg/kg slow IV • IV Infusion: 0.25–1 μg/kg/min • Intranasal: 0.2–0.3 mg/kg may also be used	1 ml = 1 mg Dilute in NS/ 5D/10D Incompatible with $NaHCO_3$, fat emulsion	Short acting benzodiazepine Sedation only, no analgesic effect Onset: 1–5 min (iv), Duration of action: 20–30 min (iv) Not recommended in preterm neonates	Apnea, CNS depression, myoclonic jerks, hypotension; flumazenil can reverse effects

(*Contd.*)

Table 53.7: Drugs and dosages of analgesic/sedative medications commonly used in NICU

Drug	*Dose*	*Preparation/administration*	*Pharmacology*	*Adverse effects*
Paracetamol	10–15 mg/kg/dose PO 6–8 hourly 30 mg/kg/ dose per rectal	Syrup 5 ml = 125 mg Drops 1 ml = 100 mg Suppositories 80 mg	Rectal route has an erratic absorption	Avoid in hepatic dysfunction
EMLA cream	0.5–2 g for 30–60 minutes	Lidocaine (2.5%) and prilocaine (2.5%) in 1:1 ratio (e.g. Oint Prilox available in India) 5 g/30 g with transparent dressing	Onset: 30–60 min Duration of action: 2–4 hours	Methemoglobinemia

Withdrawal and Opioid Tapering

- Withdrawal symptoms may be seen with rapid tapering of opioids and present with features similar to those seen in neonatal abstinence syndrome, such as irritability, poor sleep, diarrhea, vomiting, jitteriness, tremors, tachycardia, sweating, fever, mottling, seizures, excessive sucking. Certain factors like prematurity, male gender, longer duration of therapy, lower initial dose of opioids, use for post-operative pain, and concomitant use of sedatives have been associated with a higher risk of opioid withdrawal.[14]
- Assess the need for opioids daily, and start de-escalating the dose as early as possible.
- If the neonate has received opioids for less than 5 days, initially decrease the original dose by 30–50% and then by 20–30% every 6–8 hours.
- If the neonate has received opioids for 5 or more days, decrease the original dose by 20% and then by 10% every 12 hours.[14]
- Document modified Finnegan score before starting tapering and then every 4 hours subsequently.

If the score is 8 or more, pause the tapering. Increase the dose to the previous higher dose if the score is 12 or more.

In case of a prolonged tapering regimen, switching from IV fentanyl or morphine to oral morphine may help obviate the need for IV access (Table 53.8).

Table 53.8: Algorithm for converting IV dose of opioid to equianalgesic oral dose of opioids

Current intravenous agent	*Usual maintenance infusion rate*	*Equivalent oral opioid dose*
IV fentanyl	1–5 μg/kg/hour	Multiply hourly fentanyl dose (in μg/kg/hour) by 0.1; Administer as oral morphine (in mg/kg/dose) q 4 hours
IV fentanyl	1–5 μg/kg/hour	Multiply hourly fentanyl dose (in μg/kg/hour) by 0.05–0.1; Administer as oral methadone (mg/kg/dose) q 6 hours
IV morphine	7–50 μg/kg/hour	Multiply hourly morphine dose (in μg/kg/hour) by 0.01; Administer as oral morphine (in mg/kg/dose) q 4 hours

REFERENCES

1. Committee On Fetus And Newborn And Section On Anesthesiology And Pain Medicine. Prevention and Management of Procedural Pain in the Neonate: An Update. Pediatrics. 2016;137:e20154271.
2. Stevens BJ, Gibbins S, Yamada J, Dionne K, Lee G, Johnston C, et al. The premature infant pain profile-revised (PIPP-R): initial validation and feasibility. Clin J Pain. 2014;30:238–43.
3. van Dijk M, Roofthooft DWE, Anand KJS, Guldemond F, de Graaf J, Simons S, et al. Taking up the challenge of measuring prolonged pain in (premature) neonates: the COMFORTneo scale seems promising. Clin J Pain. 2009;25:607–16.
4. Stevens B, Yamada J, Ohlsson A, Haliburton S, Shorkey A. Sucrose for analgesia in newborn infants undergoing painful procedures. Cochrane Database Syst Rev. 2016;7:CD001069.
5. Bueno M, Yamada J, Harrison D, Khan S, Ohlsson A, Adams-Webber T, et al. A systematic review and meta-analyses of nonsucrose sweet solutions for pain relief in neonates. Pain Res Manag. 2013;18:153–61.
6. Shah PS, Herbozo C, Aliwalas LL, Shah VS. Breastfeeding or breast milk for procedural pain in neonates. Cochrane Database Syst Rev. 2012;12:CD004950.
7. Johnston C, Campbell-Yeo M, Disher T, Benoit B, Fernandes A, Streiner D, et al. Skin-to-skin care for procedural pain in neonates. Cochrane Database Syst Rev. 2017;2:CD008435.
8. Weise KL, Nahata MC. EMLA for painful procedures in infants. J Pediatr Health Care Off Publ Natl Assoc Pediatr Nurse Assoc Pract. 2005;19:42–7.
9. Hall RW, Kronsberg SS, Barton BA, Kaiser JR, Anand KJS, NEOPAIN Trial Investigators Group. Morphine, hypotension, and adverse outcomes among preterm neonates: who's to blame? Secondary results from the NEOPAIN trial. Pediatrics. 2005;115:1351–9.
10. Koehntop DE, Rodman JH, Brundage DM, Hegland MG, Buckley JJ. Pharmacokinetics of fentanyl in neonates. Anesth Analg. 1986;65:227–32.
11. Shekar K, Roberts JA, Mcdonald CI, Fisquet S, Barnett AG, Mullany DV, et al. Sequestration of drugs in the circuit may lead to therapeutic failure during extracorporeal membrane oxygenation. Crit Care. 2012;16:R194.
12. Kumar P, Denson SE, Mancuso TJ; Committee on Fetus and Newborn, Section on Anesthesiology and Pain Medicine. Premedication for nonemergency endotracheal intubation in the neonate. Pediatrics. 2010;125:608-15.
13. Hall RW, Shbarou RM. Drugs of choice for sedation and analgesia in the neonatal ICU. Clin Perinatol. 2009;36:15–26.
14. Ancora G, Lago P, Garetti E, Merazzi D, Savant Levet P, Bellieni CV, et al. Evidence-based clinical guidelines on analgesia and sedation in newborn infants undergoing assisted ventilation and endotracheal intubation. Acta Paediatr Oslo Nor 1992. 2019;108:208–17.

CHAPTER

54

Donor Human Milk

INTRODUCTION

Preterm neonates are vulnerable and have feeding issues due to immature gut. They are more at risk of developing necrotizing enterocolitis (NEC) and sepsis. Direct breastfeeding may not be possible in such neonates. Expressed breast milk (EBM) from their own mothers is provided to them. In case of absence of mother's own milk (MOM), donor human milk is the second-best option for a preterm neonate.

DONOR HUMAN MILK

Donar human milk (DHM) is the milk expressed and voluntarily donated by lactating women other than the biological mother of the recipient baby. This donor human milk is pasteurized using the Holder pasteurization method (pasteurized donor human milk; PDHM) and dispensed for use of the recipient.

Donation should be free and without any monetary benefit. The recipient should also be provided the DHM free of cost.

Advantages

World Health Organization (WHO)[1] and National Neonatology Forum (NNF)[2], India recommends DHM as the preferred choice if mother's own milk is not available for feeding of preterm or low-birthweight (LBW) infants, including very preterm (<32 weeks' gestation) or very LBW (<1.5 kg) infants. The acceptance of PDHM among preterm neonates is increasing globally. DHM is species-specific and contains various bioactive and immunomodulatory factors that has a beneficial and protective effect.[3] However, pasteurization affects the nutritive content of DHM. Hence, PDHM does not provide nutritional and non-nutritional benefits equivalent to mother's own milk. In addition, the nutritive content of DHM is variable and may be affected by the duration of lactation.

Studies have shown the protective effect of DHM against NEC (particularly severe NEC with ≥Bell's stage 2), late-onset sepsis, BPD.[4] Systematic review with meta-analysis published in 2018 examined and compared the effect of human milk vs preterm formula on NEC, late-onset sepsis, retinopathy of prematurity (ROP), bronchopulmonary dysplasia (BPD) and neurodevelopment among preterm neonates with gestation ≤28 weeks and/or birth weight ≤1500 grams. The results showed clear protective effect of human milk against NEC, and a possible reduction in LOS, severe ROP and severe NEC.[5] Another systematic review was conducted to investigate the role of DHM in duration of hospital stay, and it was seen that DHM and preterm infant formula had comparable duration of hospital stay. The incidence of NEC was however reduced, further validating the protective role of DHM among VLBW neonates.[6]

Nevertheless, more studies need to be conducted to understand the long-term and neurodevelopment outcomes among neonates, also how the nutritive value of DHM is affected on pooling, pasteurization and storage.

Comprehensive Lactation Management Centre (CLMC)

Many lactating mothers have surplus breastmilk left even after feeding their own baby. In such cases, mothers can donate the extra milk for other neonates who do not have access to their own mother's milk due to various reasons.

In CLMC, lactation counseling and support is provided regarding early initiation of breastfeeding, proper positioning, and attachment of the baby to the breast, and also helps in resolving breastfeeding issues like engorgement, cracked nipple, flat or inverted nipple. CLMC also provides facilities for collection, screening, processing, storage and dispensing of DHM to babies who do not have access to their own mother's milk.

First human milk bank was opened in Vienna, Austria in 1909. In India, Sneha, founded by Dr Armida Fernandez, was the first milk bank started at SION, Mumbai in 1989.

In 2017, the Ministry of Health and Family Welfare, Government of India issued 'National guidelines on lactation management centres in public health facilities'.[7]

Process of Screening the Donor Mothers and Consent

Who can donate milk: Donor mothers are healthy lactating mothers, voluntarily willing to give their extra breastmilk for other babies, without compromising the needs of their own baby.

Mothers of the babies who are admitted in NICU, attend OPD or immunization clinic, lactating staff working in the hospital, mothers who have lost their babies or cannot give milk to their own babies and lactating mothers motivated by community and other awareness means can donate milk. Mothers should be tested negative (within 6 months prior to donating milk) for HIV, VDRL, hepatitis B and hepatitis C. If tests were done earlier, fresh blood tests will be required to be done before the mother can be accepted as a donor.

For eligible mothers it is essential to obtain a written informed consent before milk donation.

Milk Expression, Storage and Processing

Breastfeeding is when the baby is latched and fed directly from the breast. But in preterm babies, direct breastfeeding may not be possible. In such babies, mothers may express the milk either manually or through breast pumps, and then feed their babies using palade or *katori* and spoon.

Expression protocol: Mother should wash their hands properly using soap and water. Breast should be wiped with a swab moist with water. Place a clean container below the breast to collect the milk. The breast should be massaged gently towards the nipple. The mother should place the thumb and index finger opposite each other outside the areola, and squeeze to express the milk. Breast pumps may also be used for expression.

Storage and processing of DHM: The collected milk is first properly labelled with mother's details and date of collection, and then stored in –80 deep freezer. Pasteurization needs to be done within 3 months of collection of milk. Batches are prepared, milk thawed and pooled before pasteurization. Prepasteurization, culture testing is done from each batch and counts should be $<10^5$ CFU/ml for total viable organisms. Pasteurization is done using Holder method, i.e. milk is gently heated at 62.5°C in a shaking water bath for 30 minutes. It virtually eliminates HIV, HTLV, CMV and mycobacteria. Post-pasteurization, again the microbiology culture testing from each batch needs to be done and it should not show any growth. PDHM is then stored in the freezer in clean, dry, and sterilized bottles that are properly labeled.

A unit can have its own PDHM dispersal policy. PDHM should be preferably dispersed to the preterm neonates of less than 32 weeks or <1500 g at least for a span of first 14 days of life, after taking consent from the parents.

Comprehensive Lactation Managment Centre (CLMC): Process and Activities (Fig. 54.1)

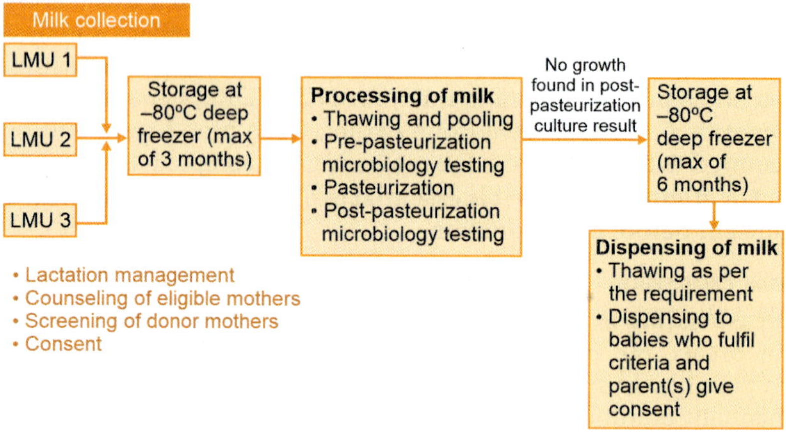

Fig 54.1: Comprehensive lactation management centre

REFERENCES

1. WHO recommendations for care of the preterm or low birth weight infant. Geneva: World Health Organization; 2022. Licence: CC BY-NC-SA 3.0 IGO.
2. Clinical Practice Guidelines. Feeding of low-birth weight neonates: National Neonatology Forum, India 2020.
3. Bertino E, Giuliani F, Baricco M, Nicola PD, Peila C, Vassia C, Chiale F, Pirra A, Cresi F, Martano C, Coscia A. Benefits of donor milk in the feeding of preterm infants. Early human development 2013; 89 (2): S3–S6.
4. Villamor-Martínez E, Pierro M, Cavallaro G , Mosca F, Kramer BW, Villamor E. Donor Human Milk Protects against Bronchopulmonary Dysplasia: A Systematic Review and Meta-Analysis. Nutrients 2018, 10, 238:2–16.
5. Miller J, Tonkin E, Damarell RA , McPhee AJ , Suganuma M, Suganuma H, Middleton PF, Makrides M, Collins CT. A Systematic Review and Meta-Analysis of Human Milk Feeding and Morbidity in Very Low Birth Weight Infants. Nutrients 2018, 10: 707. doi:10.3390/nu10060707.
6. Yang R, Chen D, Deng O, Xu X. The effect of donor human milk on the length of hospital stay in very low birthweight infants: a systematic review and meta-analysis. International Breastfeeding Journal 2020; 15, 89 https://doi.org/10.1186/s13006–020–00332–6.
7. National guidelines on lactation management centres in public health facilities 2017. National Health Mission, Child health division, Ministry of Health and Family welfare, Government of India.

CHAPTER

55

Developmentally Supportive Care

The period of maximum cognitive development of an extremely preterm infant (third trimester of pregnancy and first 3 months after birth) is spent in the neonatal intensive care unit (NICU) in an environment that is not conducive to optimal growth and development. The constant exposure to the harmful and overstimulating environment of the NICU leaves these infants fussy, irritable, and exhausted.

Developmentally supportive care (DSC) is a systematic, structured process that begins when an infant is brought into NICU and continues until discharge and beyond that. Though guided by a protocol, the DSC activities may not strictly conform to a set routine. All members of the NICU family—healthcare providers, parents, therapists, and support staff—must consciously provide a structured healing environment to every infant that is customized for her needs. Table 55.1 lists the standard terms used in DSC.

Developmentally supportive care has seven components[1] (Fig. 55.1).

A. Safeguarding Sleep

Kangaroo mother care, containment, nesting, swaddling, non-nutritive sucking, placing the infant in the lateral position, and cluster care aid undisturbed sleep. Each infant deserves adequate 'quiet time' when no medical intervention or routine caregiving activities are provided. Dimming the lights, reducing noise, and appropriately handling the baby during feeding would help the infant sleep without disturbances.

B. Partnering with Families

Partnering with families involves the family and the parents in the decision-making and caregiving of the infants. The family communicates its concerns and fears with the treatment team if

Table 55.1: Definitions of terms used in DSC[1,2]

- **Containment:** Holding and calming a baby during a painful procedure. One hand of the caregiver is placed firmly yet gently on the head of the baby, while the other hand can be placed on the lower back, buttocks, or soles.
- **Swaddling:** Wrapping the baby in a sheet around in such a way that the infant feels safe, secure, and contained.
- **Nesting/creating a boundary:** Creating a nest-like oval boundary around the infant using sheets.
- **Healing environment:** An environment that supports the infant's appropriate growth and development while minimizing the pain and stress caused by continuous exposure to unwanted and harsh stimuli during their NICU stay.
- **Protected sleep:** Modifying the environment and infant's cue-based care to ensure undisturbed sleep.
- **Family-centered care:** Family works together closely, making informed decisions regarding their infant's medical and developmental well-being.
- **Activities of daily living:** Caregiving activities that are important for the infant's growth, development, hygiene, and general well-being, e.g. dressing and undressing, diaper change, sponging, massage, skincare, and feeding.
- **Non-nutritive sucking (NNS):** Sucking opportunities provided to the infants in the form of sucking their own fingers, the mother's fingers, a gauze lollipop dipped in mother's milk or even mother's breast. NNS helps the infant to self-regulate, stay calm and organize self during painful medical and other stressful situations in the NICU.

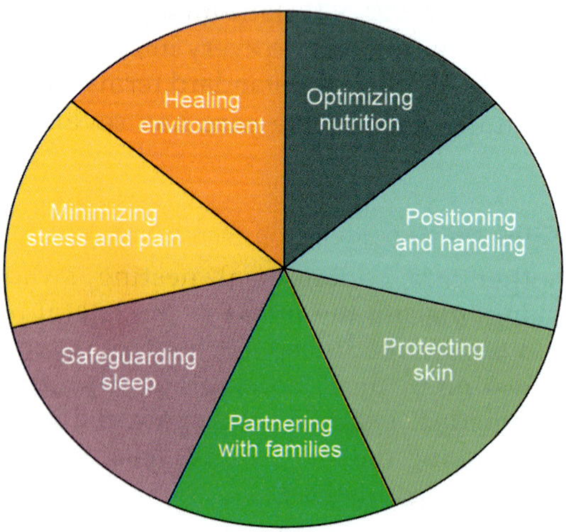
Healing environment
Optimizing nutrition
Positioning and handling
Protecting skin
Partnering with families
Safeguarding sleep
Minimizing stress and pain

Fig. 55.1: Seven core components of developmentally supportive care[1,3]

approached with respect and a non-judgmental attitude. This empowers the family members to participate in the activities of daily living actively.

C. Minimizing Stress and Pain

Infants communicate their pain and stress through several cues that caregivers can observe and measure. Care during the medical intervention and activities of daily living should respect these cues and adjust and modify the environment to reduce stress and pain and facilitate self-regulatory mechanisms to promote the optimal organization of the infant.

D. Healing Environment

Simple modifications in the NICU enhance the quality of care and development of preterm and sick infants. These modifications are listed below:

1. Spacing

- The distance between the bassinettes should be adequate to allow caregiving and medical interventions without disturbing the other infants.

2. Visual Stimulation

- Minimise light unless required for a procedure.
- Cover the incubator with a thick cloth to prevent daylight from directly reaching the infant's eyes.
- Cover and shield the eyes of the infant during phototherapy.
- Limited visual stimulation, e.g. only a brief exposure of the mother's face, is what the infant will tolerate. The mother's face should be 20–25 cm from the infant's face.
- Avoid talking while encouraging eye contact.
- Ensure the infants do not arch and extend their heads upwards to look at the overhead light.

3. Auditory Stimulation

- Sound intensity of up to 45 dB is considered safe for neonates.
- Healthcare providers and caregivers should talk softly near the infant's bassinet or move slightly away while medical intervention is being discussed.
- Mother's speaking or singing comforts the infant.
- Attend to telephone rings and alarms of the monitor quickly. Reduce the volume of alarms/keep only visual alarms, if appropriate.

- Refrain from speaking loudly from across the room.
- Do not drag chairs or close the incubator doors loudly.
- Avoid musical toys over the bassinettes.

4. Olfactory and Gustatory Sensation

- Avoid opening pungent-smelling alcoholic wipes, perfumes, or oils near the infant.

5. Vestibular Sensation

- Gently roll the infant from one position to another during routine postural change.
- Swaddle the baby during transfers and transportation.
- Providers should bend forward while lifting or placing the infant on the mother's lap or bassinet.

6. Tactile Sensation

- Club medical interventions together with caregiving activities to reduce the frequency of contact with the infant.
- Use gentle yet firm touch (not feathery or tickling) to calm the infant.
- Do cleaning, sponging, massaging, dressing, and undressing or removal of adhesives with care and caution.

7. Positioning a Preterm Infant in NICU

- The position of the neonate should be changed regularly.
- **The prone position** facilitates flexion and the development of early head control. The baby is positioned with some pelvic elevation so that the legs are weight-bearing through the anterior knee and lower legs, and the hips are not flexed more than 90°.
- **Supine position** promotes the development of visual skills, and appropriate and adequate support would allow the knees and elbows to be supported off the cot surface to reduce hip and shoulder abduction. Potential disadvantages include neck extensor muscle tightness and arching.
- **Side-lying/lateral position** is the closest to the fetal position maintained in the womb, with minimized hip abduction and retraction of shoulders. Side-lying position encourages flexion and symmetry. The hands can be placed near the mouth for self-regulation.

E. Optimising Nutrition

Human milk is the ideal source of nutrition for a preterm neonate but may not be able to meet their complex nutrition requirements and hence the need of optimising feeding practices.

- While feeding with *paladai* or spoon infant must be awake and not asleep.
- Swaddle the infant and support the 'head, neck, and trunk with the caregiver's arm or body.
- Do not wake infants by pinching, tickling, pulling, or flicking their ears or soles.
- Do not sing or talk to the infant while feeding.

F. Positioning and Handling

Activities of daily living should be carried out according to the baby's readiness and not be protocol driven. During these activities, care should be taken to position the preterm infant to ensure that it supports symmetric development.

Sponging

- Lukewarm water should be used for sponging the infant. Check the temperature of the water before sponging.
- Start from the head and sponge down to the legs (clean to unclean).
- Stop sponging and calm the newborn if stress signs are seen.
- Do not leave the infant in the middle of sponging to get cloth for drying, clean diapers, and clothes.

Massaging

- Apply oil for very preterm and extremely low birth weight infants.
- In supine, prone and side-lying positions, start massaging from the head and move to the face, the chest, the abdomen, and the limbs.
- Fingers should be placed flat on the infant's body, and the massage should be done with moderate pressure using long, firm, yet gentle strokes.
- Gentle extending and flexing of limbs can be done during the massage.

Diaper Change

- Make sure clean diapers and wet cotton swabs are ready and near the infant.

- Open the dirty nappy and pick up both the legs of the infant, flexing them towards the abdomen, clean from front to back in gentle strokes.
- Make sure all the folds are cleaned and dried thoroughly. The touch should be firm and gentle. Stretch the infant's lower limbs one at a time and beyond their flexibility.

Changing Clothes

Some important points to remember during changing clothes:

- Gently change clothes taking care of wires and tubes attached to the infant.
- Cover the head and hands of preterm and extremely low birth weight infants with caps and mittens.

Transfers and Transportation

- Care should be taken when transporting premature, sick, and fragile infants to prevent exposure to sudden movements or change in position and temperature.

G. Protecting Skin

- Avoid using lotions and soap.
- Protect the skin surface during the removal or application of adhesive products.
- Care is to be taken to avoid pressure and device-related sores.

REFERENCES

1. Altimier L, Phillips R. The Neonatal Integrative Developmental Care Model: Advanced Clinical Applications of the Seven Core Measures for Neuroprotective Family-centered Developmental Care. Newborn and Infant Nursing Reviews. 2016;16:230–44.
2. Lubbe W, Van der Walt CS, Klopper HC. Integrative literature review defining evidence-based neurodevelopmental supportive care of the preterm infant. J Perinat Neonatal Nurs. 2012;26:251–9.
3. Bruton C, Meckley J, Nelson L. NICU Nurses and Families Partnering to Provide Neuroprotective, Family-Centered, Developmental Care. Neonatal Netw. 2018 Nov;37(6):351-7. doi: 10.1891/0730-0832.37.6.351. PMID: 30567884.

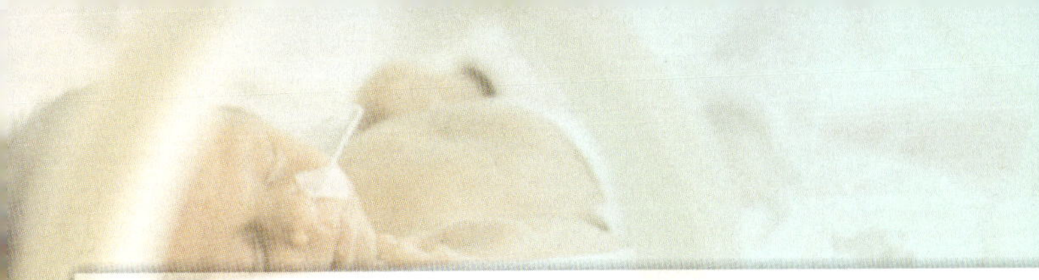

Annexures

1. Drug Dosages
2. Medication Use in G6PD Deficiency
3. Drug Dose Modification in Acute Kidney Injury
4. Immunization Schedule

ANNEXURE 1

Drug Dosages

1. Adrenaline

Resuscitation, and bradycardia:

- **Intravenous/Intraosseous:** 0.01–0.03 mg/kg with 0.1 mg/ml solution.
- **Endotracheal:** 0.05–0.1 mg/kg via endotracheal tube with 0.1 mg/ml solution.
- **Continuous IV infusion:** 0.1–1 µg/kg/min.

Septic shock, and fluid refractory shock: 0.05–0.3 µg/kg/minute.

- **Solution compatibility:** 5% dextrose, 10% dextrose, and normal saline.
- **Solution incompatibility:** Ampicillin, aminophylline, and sodium bicarbonate.

2. Amikacin

Dose: IV infusion in syringe pump over 30–60 minutes.

- **Dose interval**

  PMA: 29 weeks or lesser
  - 0–7 days: 14 mg/kg/dose every 48 hours
  - 8–28 days: 12 mg/kg/dose every 36 hours
  - 29 days or older: 12 mg/kg/dose every 24 hours

  PMA: 30–34 weeks
  - 12 mg/kg/dose every 36 hours for 0–7 postnatal days.
  - 12 mg/kg/dose every 24 hours for 8 postnatal days.

  PMA: ≥35 weeks
  - 12 mg/kg/dose every 24 hours for all postnatal days.
- **Solution compatibility:** 5% dextrose, 10% dextrose, and normal saline.
- **Solution incompatibility:** Ampicillin, amphotericin B, heparin (>1 unit/L), azithromycin, imipenem/cilastatin, oxacillin, and phenytoin.

3. Aminophylline

Dose, and administration:

- **Loading:** 8 mg/kg over 30–60 min IV or can be given orally.
- **Maintenance:** 1.5–3 mg/kg/dose orally or IV slow push every 8–12 hours (maintenance dose 8–12 hours after the loading dose).
- **Solution compatibility:** 5% dextrose, 10% dextrose, and normal saline.
- **Solution incompatibility:** Ciprofloxacin, dobutamine, adrenaline, insulin, cefepime, ceftriaxone, and penicillin G.

4. Ampicillin

Dose: Slow IV push or IM

- **Dose interval**

  PMA ≤29 weeks
  - 0–28 days: 25–50 mg/kg/dose every 12 hours.
  - 29 days or more: 25–50 mg/kg/dose every 8 hours.

  PMA: 30–36 weeks
  - 0–14 days: 25–50 mg/kg/dose every 12 hours.
  - 15 days or older: 25–50 mg/kg/dose every 8 hours.

  PMA: 37–44 weeks
  - 0–7 days: 25–50 mg/kg/dose every 12 hours.
  - 8 days or more: 25–50 mg/kg/dose every 8 hours.

  PMA: ≥45 weeks
  - 25–50 mg/kg/dose every 6 hours.
- **Solution compatibility:** 5% dextrose, normal saline, and sterile water.
- **Solution incompatibility:** Amikacin, dopamine, adrenaline, gentamicin, midazolam, sodium carbonate, and tobramicin.

5. Amphotericin B

Dose: 1–1.5 mg/kg every 24 hours IV infusion over 2–6 hours.

- **Solution compatibility:** 5% dextrose, and 10% dextrose.
- **Solution incompatibility:** Normal saline, Lipid emulsion, amikacin, calcium gluconate, ciprofloxacin, dopamine, fluconazole, gentamicin, meropenem, penicillin G, piperacillin-tazobactam, and tobramycin.

6. Liposomal Amphotericin B

Dose: 2.5–7 mg/kg per dose every 24 hours iv infusion by syringe pump over 2 hours.

- **Solution compatibility:** 5%, 10%, and 20% dextrose.
- **Solution incompatibility:** Amino acid, and normal saline.

7. Acyclovir

Dose: IV infusions by syringe pump over 1 hour.

- **Dose interval**
  PMA: <30 weeks; 20 mg/kg/dose every 12 hours.
  PMA: 30 weeks; 20 mg/kg/dose every 8 hours.
- **Duration:**
  - Localized HSV infection: 14 days.
  - Disseminated HSV infection OR CNS disease: 21 days.

  (Continue IV therapy for seven more days if repeat DNA PCR done between 19–21 days after treatment is positive).
- **Solution compatibility:** 5% dextrose, and normal saline
- **Solution incompatibility:** Amino acid, fat emulsion, caffeine citrate, dobutamine, dopamine.
- **Monitoring:** RFT at baseline, and at least once weekly in patients with renal dysfunction on prolonged therapy.

8. Caffeine Citrate

Dose: Loading of 20–25 mg/kg of caffeine citrate IV (over 30 min) or oral.

- **Maintenance:** 5–10 mg/kg of caffeine (slow IV or oral), to be started 24 hours after loading dose.
- **Mechanism of action:** CNS stimulant (stimulates central inspiratory drive).
- **Solution compatibility:** 5% dextrose.
- **Solution incompatibility:** Furosemide, acyclovir, lorazepam, oxacillin, and ibuprofen.

9. Cefoperazone Sulbactam

Dose: 30–40 mg/kg/dose of cefoperazone (not combined cefoperazone-sulbactam). Infuse over 30–60 minutes every 8 hours.

- **Solution compatibility:** Normal saline, 5% dextrose, and 10% dextrose.

10. Cefotaxime

Dose: IM injection, IV push, or Intermittent IV infusion over 10–30 minutes.

- **Sepsis:**
  PNA: Less than 7 days: 50 mg/kg/dose IV every 12 hours.
  PMA: < 32 weeks.
  - 7 days or older: 50 mg/kg/dose IV every 8 hours.

  PMA: ≥ *32 weeks.*
  - 7 days or older: 50 mg/kg/dose IV every 6 hours.
- **Meningitis:**
  PNA: 7 days: 100–150 mg/kg/day IV every 8–12 hours, 8 days: 150–200 mg/kg/day IV every 6–8 hours.
- **Disseminated gonococcal infection:** 25 mg/kg/dose IV or IM every 12 hours for 7 days, for meningitis 10–14 days.
- **Solution compatibility:** 5% dextrose, 10% dextrose, and normal saline.
- **Solution incompatibility:** Sodium bicarbonate, vancomycin, fluconazole, and azithromycin.

11. Ceftazidime

Dose: IV infusion over 30 min.

PMA: 29 weeks or lesser
- 0–28 days: 30 mg/kg/dose every 12 hours.
- 29 days or older: 30 mg/kg/dose every 8 hours.

PMA: 30–36 weeks
- 0–14 days: 30 mg/kg/dose every 12 hours.
- 15 days or older: 30 mg/kg/dose every 8 hours.

PMA: 37–44 weeks
- 0–7 days: 30 mg/kg/dose every 12 hours.
- 8 days or older: 30 mg/kg/dose every 8 hours.

PMA: 45 weeks or greater
- 30 mg/kg/dose every 8 hours.

- **Meningitis:**
  0–7 days: 100–150 mg/kg/day IV every 8–12 hours.
  8–28 days: 150 mg/kg/day IV every 8 hours.
- **Solution compatibility:** 5% dextrose, 10% dextrose, and normal saline.
- **Solution incompatibility:** Erythromycin, phenytoin, midazolam, fluconazole, and Vancomycin.

12. Ceftriaxone

Dose: IV infusion over 60 minutes

- Sepsis: 50 mg/kg every 24 hours; meningitis: 100 mg/kg loading dose followed by 80 mg/kg every 24 hours.
- Gonococcal infection prophylaxis, and Uncomplicated Gonococcal Ophthalmia: 25–50 mg/kg/dose as a single dose
- Disseminated Gonococcal infection: 25–50 mg/kg/dose IV/IM single dose for seven days, for meningitis 10–14 days

- **Contraindications:** Premature infants, Neonatal Hyperbilirubinemia (Increased risk of Kernicterus), along with calcium-containing solution.
- **Solution compatibility:** 5% dextrose, 10% dextrose, and normal saline.
- **Solution incompatibility:** Aminophylline, calcium chloride, calcium gluconate, azithromycin, fluconazole, and vancomycin.

13. Ciprofloxacin

Dose: IV infusion over 30–60 minutes

PMA:

- 32–37 weeks:10 mg/kg/dose every 12 hours.
- 38 weeks or more: 15 mg/kg/dose every 12 hours.

- **Solution compatibility:** 5% dextrose.
- **Solution incompatibility:** Antacids, and divalent salts.

14. Calcium Gluconate

Dose

- Acute symptomatic hypocalcemia: 100–200 mg/kg/dose 10% calcium gluconate to be diluted and infused IV over 10–30 minutes.
- Maintenance dose: 200–800 mg/kg/day for 3–5 days. Oral and IV to be given in the same dose (2–8 ml/kg/day, equivalent to 20–80 mg/kg elemental calcium).

- **Solution compatibility:** Normal saline, 5% dextrose, and 10% dextrose.
- **Solution incompatibility:** Amphotericin B, ceftriaxone, fluconazole, indomethacin, meropenem, metoclopramide, sodium bicarbonate, lipid emulsions, phosphate, and magnesium salts.

15. Cloxacillin

Dose: 25–30 mg/kg/dose IV or orally every 6–8 hours.

- **Solution compatibility:** 5% dextrose and normal saline.

- **Solution incompatibility:** Aminoglycosides, tetracycline, and erythromycin.

16. Colistin

Dose as per renal function:

GFR (ml/min/1.73 m²)	*Amount (Colistin-based activity)*
≥80 ml/min	5 mg/kg/day in 2–3 divided doses
50–79 ml/min	2.5–3.8 mg/kg 12 hourly
30–49 ml/min	2.5 mg/kg/ q 24 hourly/1.25 mg/kg 12 hourly
10–29 ml/min	1.5 mg/kg q 36 hourly
Hemodialysis Continuous renal replacement therapy	1.5 mg/kg 24–48 hourly 2.5 mg/kg 12–24 hourly

1 mg of colistin base activity = 30,000 IU colistin

- **Solution compatibility:** 5% dextrose, 10% dextrose, 0.9% normal saline, and ringer lactate
- **Solution incompatibility:** Incompatible with erythromycin and hydrocortisone sodium succinate.

17. Dexamethasone

Dose

- For extubation and airway edema: 0.25–0.5 mg/kg/dose; may repeat eight hourly, max of 4 doses IV.
- For prevention of BPD: 0.15 mg/kg per day for three days, 0.10 mg/kg per day for three days, 0.05 mg/kg per day for two days, and 0.02 mg/kg per day for two days; a total of 0.89 mg/kg over 10 days (DART regimen)
- Solution compatibility: 5% dextrose, 10% dextrose, and normal saline.

- **Solution incompatibility:** Midazolam, glycopyrrolate, and Vancomycin.
- **Monitoring:** Blood sugar, Blood pressure, and intraocular pressure.

18. Digoxin

Dose: Loading dose given for treating arrhythmias and acute congestive heart failure IV slowly over 15–30 min, administered as three divided doses eight hourly. It is not to be administered as an IM injection.

- **Loading dose**
  PMA 29 weeks: IV–15 μg/kg; oral–20 μg/kg.
  - *PMA 30–36 weeks:* IV–20 μg/kg; oral–25 μg/kg
  - *PMA 37–48 weeks:* IV–30 μg/kg; oral–40 μg/kg
  - *PMA 49 weeks:* IV–40 μg/kg; oral–50 μg/kg
- **Maintenance dose**
  - *PMA 29 weeks:* IV–4 μg/kg; oral–5 μg/kg every 24 hours.
  - *PMA 30–36 weeks:* IV–5 μg/kg; oral–6 μg/kg every 24 hours.
  - *PMA 37–48 weeks:* IV–4 μg/kg; oral–5 μg/kg every 12 hours.
  - *PMA 49 weeks:* IV–5 μg/kg; oral–6 μg/kg every 12 hours.
- **Solution compatibility:** 5% dextrose, 10% dextrose, normal saline, and sterile water.
- **Solution incompatibility:** Dobutamine, furosemide, meropenem, midazolam, milrinone , and propranolol.

19. Dopamine

Dose: 2–20 μg/kg/minute as continuous infusion. Start at less than 10 μg/kg/minute for fluid refractory shock. Use a large vein for IV.

- **Solution compatibility:** 5% dextrose, 10% dextrose, normal saline, and ringer lactate.
- **Solution incompatibility:** Ampicillin, furosemide, indomethacin, penicillin G, insulin, and sodium bicarbonate.

20. Dobutamine

Dose: 2–25 μg/kg/minute as a continuous infusion.

- **Solution compatibility:** 5% dextrose, 10% dextrose, normal saline, and ringer lactate.
- **Solution incompatibility:** Aminophylline, cefepime, digoxin, ibuprofen, indomethacin, phenytoin, piperacillin—tazobactam, and sodium bicarbonate.

21. Domperidone

Dose: 0.2–0.4 mg/kg per dose, 8 hourly orally

22. Furosemide

Dose: 1 mg/kg/dose IV, IM, or can be given orally. Maximum of 2 mg/kg/dose IV or 6 mg/kg/dose orally.

- **Dose interval:** Preterm infants–24 hourly. Term infants–12 hourly. Term infant older than one month 6–8 hourly. Consider alternate-day therapy for long-term use.
- **Contraindications:** Anuria and hypersensitivity to furosemide.

- **Monitoring:** Serum, and urine electrolytes, RFT periodically during therapy.
- **Solution compatibility:** 5% dextrose, 10% dextrose, normal saline, and sterile water.
- **Solution incompatibility:** Ciprofloxacin, dopamine, dobutamine, erythromycin, gentamycin, midazolam, and netilmicin.

23. Fluconazole

Dose: Invasive candidiasis 12–25 mg/kg as a loading dose, then 6–12 mg/kg per dose IV infusions by syringe pump over 30 minutes or orally. Thrush 6 mg/kg on day 1, then 3 mg/kg per dose every 24 hours orally. Prophylaxis 3–6 mg/kg per dose via IV infusion twice weekly or orally for 6 weeks (considered in VLBW infants at high risk of fungal disease).

- **Dosing interval for invasive candidiasis:**
  PMA: 29 weeks or lesser
  - 0–14 days: every 48 hours
  - 15 days or older: every 24 hours

  PMA: 30 weeks or older
  - 0–7 days: every 48 hours
  - 8 days or older: every 24 hours
- **Solution compatibility:** 5% dextrose, 10% dextrose.
- **Solution incompatibility:** Amphotericin B, ampicillin, calcium gluconate, cefotaxime, ceftazidime, ceftriaxone, chloramphenicol, piperacillin, clindamycin, digoxin, erythromycin, furosemide, and imipenem.

24. Fentanyl

Dose:
- Sedation – 0.5–4 µg/kg per dose IV slow push. Infusion rate- 1–5 µg/kg/hour.
- Analgesia – 0.5–3 µg/kg per dose IV slow push. Infusion rat- 0.5–2 µg/kg/hour.

- **Solution compatibility:** 5% dextrose, 10% dextrose, and normal saline.
- **Drug incompatibility:** Azithromycin, phenobarbitone, and phenytoin.

25. Fosphenytoin

Dose:
- Loading dose: 15–20 mg PE/kg IM or IV over at least 10 min (IV route is preferred).

- Maintenance dose 4–8 mg PE/kg every 24 hours; PE= Phenytoin equivalents.
- Fosphenytoin 1 mg PE= phenytoin 1 mg.

- **Monitoring:** ECG, blood pressure, and respiratory function during infusion and 10–20 min after infusion.
- **Solution compatibility:** Normal saline, 5% dextrose, and 10% dextrose.
- **Solution incompatibility:** Midazolam.

26. Gentamicin

Dosage and route of administration: Slow IV infusion over 30 minutes

- **Prolonged serum half-life** in neonates undergoing hypothermia for HIE.

PMA: 29 weeks or lesser
- 0–7 days: 5 mg/kg/dose every 48 hours.
- 8–28 days: 4 mg/kg/dose every 36 hours.
- 29 days or older: 4 mg/kg/dose every 24 hours.

PMA: 30–34 weeks
- 0–7 days: 4.5 mg/kg/dose every 36 hours.
- Eight days or older: 4 mg/kg/dose every 24 hours.

PMA: 35 weeks or older
- 4 mg/kg/dose every 24 hours.

- **Solution compatibility:** 5% dextrose, 10% dextrose, and normal saline.
- **Solution incompatibility:** Ampicillin, furosemide, heparin, and indomethacin.

27. Ganciclovir

Dose: 6 mg/kg per dose every 12 hours IV infusion over 1 hour. Treatment for a minimum of 6 weeks if possible.

- **Monitoring:** CBC every 2–3 days during the first three weeks of therapy, weekly after that if stable.
- **Solution compatibility:** 5% dextrose, normal saline, and Ringer's lactate.
- **Incompatibility:** Lipid emulsions, aztreonam, cefepime, and piperacillin/tazobactam.

28. Hydrocortisone

Dose:
- Hypoglycemia: 10 mg/kg/day IV or PO in 2 divided doses. Taper after a few days once the blood glucose levels stabilize.

- Physiologic replacement: 7–9 mg/m^2 per day IV or orally every 8–12 hours.
- Shock:

Day	*Dose (mg/kg)*	*Interval (hrs)*
Day 1	1	8 hours ×3 doses*
Day 2	0.5	12 hours ×2 doses
Day 3	0.25	12 hours ×2 doses
Day 4	0.125	24 hours ×1 dose

**The BP response is evident as early as 2 hours after hydrocortisone treatment. If efficacy is noted, the dose can be repeated every 8 hours for 2–3 days. Slow dosage weaning after that*

- **Chorioamnionitis-exposed ELBW infants to decrease the risk of CLD:** 0.5 mg/kg/dose IV every 12 hours for 12 days, followed by 0.25 mg/kg IV every 12 hours for 3 days.
- **Solution compatibility:** 5% dextrose, 10% dextrose, and normal saline.
- **Solution incompatibility:** Midazolam, phenobarbitone, and phenytoin.

29. Intravenous Immunoglobulin

Dose:

- Usual Dosage: 500–1000 mg/kg per dose over 2–6 hours; may repeat in 12 hours if necessary.
- For neonatal alloimmune thrombocytopenia: 1g/kg/dose IV every day for two doses.
- Most studies have used a single dose, although additional doses have been given at 24-hour intervals.

- The rate of administration varies by product

30. Ibruprofen

Dose: 1st dose 10 mg/kg, 2nd dose, and 3rd dose is 5 mg/kg 24 hourly.

- **Contraindications:** In patients who have experienced asthma, urticaria, and allergic-type reactions after aspirin or other NSAIDs.
- **Solution compatibility:** Normal saline, and 5% dextrose.
- **Solution incompatibility:** Caffeine citrate, and dobutamine

31. Indomethacin

Dose: 3 doses per course maximum 2 courses. 12–24 hourly intervals.

- Age <48 hours: 0.2 mg/kg on day 1; 0.1 mg/kg on day 2, and day 3.

- Age 2–7 days: 0.2 mg/kg once a day for 3 days.
- Age 8 days or more: 0.2 mg/kg on day 1, 0.25 mg/kg on days 2 and 3.

- **Contraindications:** Active bleeding, significant thrombocytopenia or coagulation defects, NEC, impaired renal function.
- **Monitoring:** Urine output, serum electrolytes, glucose, and platelet count.
- **Solution compatibility:** 5% dextrose, and normal saline.
- **Solution incompatibility:** Calcium gluconate, dobutamine, dopamine , and gentamicin.

32. Insulin

Dose: 0.1–0.2 unit/kg subcutaneously every 6–12 hours.

- **Continuous infusion:** 0.01–0.1 unit/kg/hour.
- **Solution compatibility:** 5% dextrose, 10% dextrose, and normal saline.
- **Solution incompatibility:** Aminophylline, dopamine, phenobarbitone, and phenytoin.

33. Lorazepam

Dose: 0.05–0.1 mg/kg per dose IV slow push. Avoid intra-arterial administration and Perivascular extravasation.

- **Solution compatibility:** Normal saline, 5% dextrose, and sterile water.
- **Solution incompatibility:** Lipid emulsion, caffeine, micafungin, nafcillin, and imipenem.

34. Levetiracetam

Dose: Loading 20–150 mg/kg/day IV every 24 hours, maintenance dose: 41.7–65 mg/kg/day IV every 12 hours.

- **Solution compatibility:** 5% dextrose, 10% dextrose, normal saline, Ringer lactate.

35. Metronidazole

Dose

- Loading dose: 15 mg/kg/dose orally or IV infusion over 30 to 60 minutes.
- Maintenance dose: Orally or IV infusions over 30–60 minutes.
  - PMA: 24–25 weeks – 7.5 mg/kg/dose every 24 hours.
  - PMA: 26–27 weeks – 10 mg/kg/dose every 24 hours.
  - PMA: 28–33 weeks – 7.5 mg/kg/dose every 12 hours.

- PMA: 34–40 weeks – 7.5 mg/kg/dose every 8 hours.
- PMA >40 weeks – 7.5 mg/kg/dose every 6 hours.

- **Solution compatibility:** 5% dextrose, and normal saline.
- **Solution incompatibility:** Aztreonam, and meropenem.

36. Midazolam

Dose: 0.05–0.15 mg/kg over 5 min every 2–4 hours IV. Decreased dose requirement with concurrent use of narcotics. Can be used intranasally, sublingual, and orally.

- **Continuous infusion:** 10–60 μg/kg/hour.
- **Anticonvulsant:**
- **Loading dose:** 0.15 mg/kg IV followed by maintenance dose.
- **Maintenance infusion:** 0.06–0.4 mg/kg/hour (1–7 μg/kg/min).
- **Solution compatibility:** 5% dextrose, sterile water, and normal saline.
- **Solution incompatibility:** Ceftazidime, dexamethasone, furosemide, hydrocortisone, and sodium bicarbonate.

37. Morphine

Dose: 0.05–0.2 mg/kg per dose IV, IM or subcutaneous over 5 min repeat every 4 hours.

- **Continuous infusion:** Loading dose 0.1 mg/kg over 1 hour followed by 0.01–0.02 mg/kg/hour. Dose reduction required in neonates undergoing Therapeutic hypothermia for HIE.
- **Neonatal abstinence syndrome:** 0.03–0.1 mg/kg per dose orally every 3–4 hours. Maximum dose 0.2 mg/kg. Wean dose by 10–20% every 2–3 days based on abstinence scoring.
- **Contraindications:** Respiratory depression, acute or severe bronchial asthma, suspected GI obstruction including paralytic ileus.
- **Solution compatibility:** 5% dextrose, 10% dextrose, and normal saline.
- **Solution incompatibility:** Phenytoin, azithromycin, and cefepime.

38. Meropenem

Dose:

- Sepsis: 20 mg/kg/dose IV infusion over 30 minutes.
  PMA: Less than 32 weeks; 0–14 days: every 12 hours, and 15 days or older: every 8 hours.

PMA: 32 weeks; 0–7 days: every 12 hours, and 8 days: 30 mg/kg IV every 8 hours.

- Meningitis, and infections caused by *Pseudomonas* species 40 mg/kg per dose.
  PMA: <32 weeks; 0–14 days: every 12 hours 15 days: every 8 hours.
  PMA: 32 weeks—every 8 hours.

- **Solution compatibility:** 5% dextrose, 10% dextrose, and normal saline.
- **Solution incompatibility:** Acyclovir, amphotericin-B, calcium gluconate, metronidazole, and zidovudine.

39. Magnesium Sulfate

Dose:

- Resuscitation (pulseless torsades) 25–50 mg/kg IV/rapid intraosseous infusion.
- Hypomagnesemia 25–50 mg/kg infusion over 30–60 minutes. Daily maintenance (TPN) 0.25–0.5 mEq/kg/day IV.
- **Antidote:** Calcium chloride.
- **Solution compatibility:** 5% dextrose, sterile water, and normal saline.
- **Solution incompatibility:** Fat emulsion, amiodarone, amphotericin B, cefepime , and sodium bicarbonate.

40. Milrinone

Dose: Loading dose: 50 μg/kg IV over 15 minutes or 75 μg/kg IV infused over 60 minutes, immediately followed by maintenance infusion: 0.3–0.75 μg/kg/minute.

- **Premature infants less than 30 weeks GA:** Loading dose: 135 μg/kg intravenous over 3 hours, immediately followed by maintenance infusion 0.2 μg/kg/minute.
- **Solution compatibility:** 5% dextrose, 10% dextrose, normal saline, ringer lactate.
- **Solution incompatibility:** Furosemide, imipenam, cilastin , and procainamide.

41. Noradrenaline

Dose: Septic shock 0.2–0.5 μg/kg/minute of nor-adrenaline base as IV.

- **Solution compatibility:** 5% dextrose, 10% dextrose, normal saline, and half normal saline.
- **Solution incompatibility:** Aminophylline, phenobarbitone, phenytoin, and sodium bicarbonate.

42. Naloxone

Dose: 0.1 mg/kg IV push, the amount needed to reverse narcotic-induced depression may be as low as 0 .01 mg/kg.

- **Monitoring:** Respiratory effort, and neurologic status. Monitor 24 hours for relapse.
- **Solution compatibility:** Normal saline, and 5% dextrose.
- **Solution incompatibility:** Heparin, amphotericin, and alkaline solution.

43. Netilmycin

Dose: IV infusion over 30 minutes

PMA ≤29 weeks

- 0–7 days: 5 mg/kg/dose every 48 hours
- 8–28 days: 4 mg/kg/dose every 36 hours
- 29 days or older: 4 mg/kg/dose every 24 hours

PMA 30–34 weeks

- 0–7 days: 4.5 mg/kg/dose every 36 hours
- 8 days or more: 4 mg/kg/dose every 24 hours

PMA ≥35 weeks

- 4 mg/kg/dose every 24 hours

- **Solution compatibility:** 5% dextrose, 10% dextrose, and normal saline.
- **Solution incompatibility:** Ampicillin, furosemide, heparin, and penicillin G.

44. Paracetamol (Acetaminophen)

Dose:

- For PDA: 15 mg/kg/dose 6 hourly for 12 doses
- For pain, and fever:
  Oral loading dose 20–25 mg/kg followed by maintenance 12–15 mg/kg per dose.
  Maintenance intervals: Term infants- every 6 hours, preterm infants greater than or equal to 32 weeks PMA- every 8 hours, and preterm infants less than 32 weeks PMA- every 12 hours.

- **Solution compatibility:** 5% dextrose, Normal saline.
- **Solution incompatibility:** Diazepam.

45. Phenobarbitone

Dose:

- Loading dose of 20 mg/kg IV slowly over 10–15 minutes.

- Refractory seizures: Additional 10 mg/kg /dose, up to a total of 40 mg/kg.
- Maintenance dose: 3–5 mg/kg/day beginning 12–24 hours after the loading dose q 24 hours.
- VLBW, preterm neonates: Lower loading doses of less than 15 mg/kg IV Followed by a single injection of less than 3 mg/kg/day 24 hours later.

- **Contraindications:** Patients with manifest or latent porphyria, marked liver function impairment, or respiratory depression.
- **Solution compatibility:** 5% dextrose, 10% dextrose, and normal saline.
- **Solution incompatibility:** Lipid emulsion, hydrocortisone, insulin, and Vancomycin.

46. Phenytoin

Dose:

- Loading: 15–20 mg/kg IV infusion over at least 30 minutes.
- Maintenance: 4–8 mg/kg every 24 hours IV slow push or orally.

- **Monitoring:** ECG, blood pressure, and respiratory function during infusion, and 15 minutes to 1 hour after infusion.
- **Solution compatibility:** Normal saline only.
- **Solution incompatibility:** 5% dextrose, 10% dextrose, amino acid solutions, amikacin, ceftazidime, dobutamine, heparin, insulin, morphine, dobutamine, sodium bicarbonate, hydrocortisone, and sodium bicarbonate.

47. Piperacillin Tazobactum

Dose: 50–100 mg/kg/dose of piperacillin IV infusion over 30 minutes.

PMA ≤29 weeks

- 0–28 days: every 12 hours
- 29 days or more: every 8 hours

PMA: 30–36 weeks

- 0–14 days: every 12 hours
- 15 days or older: every 8 hours

PMA: 37–44 weeks

- 0–7 days: every 12 hours
- 8 days or more: every 8 hours

PMA ≥45 weeks every 8 hours

- **Solution compatibility:** 5% dextrose, 10% dextrose, and normal saline.
- **Solution incompatibility:** Amikacin, dobutamine, gentamicin, netilmicin, gentamicin, tobramycin, azithromycin, amphotericin B, and vancomycin.

48. Prostaglandin E1

Dose:
- Initial: 0.05–0.1 μg/kg/min by continuous IV infusions, titrate to infants response.
- Maintenance: may be as low as 0.01 μg/kg/min.
- The initial dose depends on duct size. If PDA is significant, therapy can be started at a low dose of 0.01 μg/kg/min. If the duct is restrictive, the initial dose can be started at 0.05 μg/kg/min.

- **Solution compatibility:** 5% dextrose, and normal saline.
- **Solution incompatibility:** Aminophylline, ampicillin, caffeine citrate, calcium chloride, cefotaxime, dopamine, dobutamine, furosemide, gentamicin, metronidazole, penicillin G, tobramycin, and vancomycin.

49. Sildenafil

Dose:
- Loading: 0.4 mg/kg IV infusion over 3 hours.
- Maintenance: 1.6 mg/kg every 24 hours (0.067 mg/kg/hour).
- Oral: 0.5–1 mg/kg/dose orally three times daily.

- **Monitoring:** Blood pressure, and oxygenation.
- **Solution compatibility:** Dextrose, and sterile water.

50. Vancomycin

Dose: 10–15 mg/kg/dose every 6–18 hours IV infusion over 30 minutes. Meningitis: 15 mg/kg/dose, bacteremia: 10 mg/kg/dose.

PMA ≤29 weeks PMA
- 0–14 days: every 18 hours
- 15 days or older: every 12 hours

PMA: 30–36 weeks
- 0–14 days: every 12 hours
- 15 days or older: every 8 hours

PMA: 37–44 weeks
- 0–7 days: every 12 hours
- 8 days or more: every 8 hours

PMA $\geq$*45 weeks*

- every 6 hours

- **Solution compatibility:** 5% dextrose, 10% dextrose, and normal saline.
- **Solution incompatibility:** Cefepime, cefotaxime, ceftriaxone, ceftazidime, dexamethasone, heparin, phenobarbitone, piperacillin-tazobactam, and ticarcillin.

51. Vitamin K

Dose: At birth: <1.5 kg–0.5 mg IM, >1.5 kg–1 mg IM

b. Hemorrhagic disease: 1–10 mg slow IV push

- **Monitoring:** Check prothrombin time when treating clotting abnormalities.
- **Solution compatibility:** 5% dextrose, 10% dextrose, and normal saline.
- **Solution incompatibility:** Dobutamine, and phenytoin.

52. Vecuronium

Dose: 0.1 mg/kg (0.03–0.15 mg/kg) IV push. The usual dosing interval is 1–2 hours.

- **Solution compatibility:** 5% dextrose, Ringer lactate, and normal saline.
- **Solution incompatibility:** Diazepam, furosemide, ibuprofen, and micafungin.

53. Albumin

Dose:

- Hypotension, and septic shock: 0.5 g/kg of 5% albumin IV over 30 min. may repeat up to a maximum of 3 doses.

- **Contraindications:** Severe anemia or cardiac failure with normal or increased intravascular volume.
- **Solution compatibility:** 5% dextrose, 10% dextrose, and dextrose normal saline.
- **Solution incompatibility:** Amino acid mixtures, protein hydrolysates, alcohol-containing solutions.

54. Heparin

Dose:

- Maintaining patency of central, and peripheral vascular catheters: 0.5 units/kg/hour

- Thrombosis: Loading dose: 75 units/kg IV over 10 min (Avoid IM injection as there is a risk of hematoma formation)
- Continuous infusion: 28 units/kg/hour

- **Contraindications:** Intracranial or GI bleed, thrombocytopenia.
- **Specific monitoring:** aPTT measured 4 hours after initiating therapy, and the dose adjusted to achieve a PTT of 60–85 sec.
- **Solution compatibility:** 5% dextrose, 10% dextrose, and normal saline.
- **Solution incompatibility:** Amikacin, amiodarone, phenytoin, diazepam, Vancomycin.

55 Nevirapine

Dose: Perinatal HIV transmission:

- For prophylaxis – 3 doses; the first dose within 48 hours of birth, the second dose 48 hours after the first dose, and the third dose 96 hours after the second dose. It must be administered with Zidovudine.
- Birth weight: 1.5–2 kg – 8 mg/dose, > 2 kg – 12 mg/dose

HIV treatment:

- *PMA: 34–37 weeks*
  - 0–7 days – 4 mg/kg/dose orally twice daily.
  - Older than 7 days – 6 mg/kg/dose orally twice daily.
  - Older than 4 weeks – 200 mg/m^2 orally twice daily.
- *PMA: 38 weeks or greater*
  - Younger than one month – 6 mg/kg/dose orally twice daily.
  - Older than four weeks – 200 mg/m^2 orally twice daily.

- **Contraindication:** Moderate-to-severe hepatic impairment.

56. Potassium Chloride

Dose: IV infusion over 1 hour or orally. Maximum concentration for peripheral infusion 60–80 mEq/L.

- **Contraindications:** Renal failure.
- **Adverse effects:** GI irritation—diarrhea, vomiting, and bleeding.
- **Specific monitoring:** Continuous ECG monitoring during infusion.
- **Solution incompatibility:** Amphotericin B, diazepam , and Phenytoin.

ANNEXURE

2

Medication Use in G6PD Deficiency

AVOID

1. Anti-malarial, e.g. primaquine, pamaquine, tafenoquine.
2. Anti-bacterials, e.g. fluroquinolones, nitrofurantoin, nalidixic acid, dapsone, mafenide cream.
3. Analgesics, e.g. phenacetin, acetanilid, phenazopyridine (pyridium).
4. Sulfonylureas, e.g. chlorpropamide, glipizide, glyburide, glibenclamide.
5. Miscellaneous, e.g. flutamide (eulexin), methylene blue, rasburicase.
6. Chemical exposures: Fava beans, henna compounds, naphthalene, phenylhydrazine, RUSH (isobutyl nitrite).

SAFE[1]

1. Anti-malarial, e.g. quinine, chloroquine and hydroxychloroquine.
2. Anti-bacterials, e.g. chloramphenicol, streptomycin, sulfa-containing drugs (sulfacetamide, sulfadiazine, sulfamethoxazole, trimethoprim-sulfamethoxazole, sulfanilamide, sulfisoxazole), pyrimethamine, trimethoprim.
3. Antifungals, e.g. clotrimazole.
4. Analgesics, e.g. acetaminophen, aspirin (acetylsalicylic acid).
5. Miscellaneous, e.g. antazoline (antihistamine), ascorbic acid (vitamin C), colchicine,diphenhydramine (Benadryl), isoniazid, levodopa (L-dopa), para-aminosalicylic acid, para-aminobenzoic acid (PABA),phenylbutazone,phenytoin,probenecid, procainamide, vitamin K.

REFERENCE

1. Youngster I, Arcavi L, Schechmaster R, Akayzen Y, Popliski H, Shimonov J, Beig S, Berkovitch M. Medications and glucose-6-phosphate dehydrogenase deficiency: an evidence-based review. Drug Saf. 2010 Sep 1;33(9):713–26.

ANNEXURE

3 Drug Dose Modification in Acute Kidney Injury

EXAMPLE

A preterm (32 weeks; 1600 g; length 45 cm) neonate develops lethargy and poor feeding on day 5 of life. Due to clinical sepsis, the treating team initiates antibiotics (piperacillin-tazobactam and amikacin). On postnatal day seven, the infant develops oligo-anuria and deranged renal function (serum creatinine 1.5 mg/dl; baseline of 0.3 mg/dl). How will you make renal dose adjustments for this baby?

Answer (Table A3.1)

1. Calculate the eGFR to define the category K (0.33)* Length (45)/ S Creatinine (1.5 mg/dl).*
2. eGFR ~10 ml/1.73 m^2/min.
   a. Inj piperacillin-tazobactam (70% of recommended dose)- 110 mg/kg/dose q 8 hourly.
   b. Inj amikacin (5–7.5 mg/kg/day)—12 mg in 10 ml NS over 30 mins to 1 hour as an infusion

**K is 0.45 for term infants*

Table A3.1: Dose modification of common neonatal drugs in renal failure[1–3]

Medication	*Dose in normal renal function (in neonates >35 weeks, per dose)*	*Dose with impaired renal function (GFR mL/min/1.73 m^2)*			*Supple-mental dose with peritoneal dialysis*
		30–50	*10–29*	*<10*	
Amikacin	15 mg/kg q 24 hours	5–7.5 mg/kg q 12–18 hours	5–7.5 mg/kg q 24 hours	5–7.5 mg/kg q 48–72 hours	Yes

(Contd.)

Table A3.1: Dose modification of common neonatal drugs in renal failure (*Contd.*)

Medication	*Dose in normal renal function (in neonates >35 weeks, per dose)*	*Dose with impaired renal function (GFR mL/min/1.73 m²)*			*Supplemental dose with peritoneal dialysis*
		30–50	*10–29*	*<10*	
Amphotericin	1–1.5 mg/kg q 24 hours	No change	No change	No change	No
Ampicillin	25–50 mg/kg q 8–12 hours	No change	Reduce dose to 25% of normal	Reduce dose to 15% of normal	No
Cefotaxime	50 mg/kg q 8–12 hours	50 mg/kg q 8–12 hours	50 mg/kg q 12 hours	50 mg/kg q 24 hours	No
Ceftazidime	30 mg/kg q 8–12 hours	30 mg/kg q 12 hours	30 mg/kg q 24 hours	30 mg/kg q 48 hours	No
Ceftriaxone	50–80 mg/kg q 24 hours	No change	No change	Reduce dose by 25–50%	No
Cefoperazone + sulbactam	30–40 mg/kg q 8 hours	No change	50% of dose of sulbactam	25% of dose of sulbactam	No
Ciprofloxacin	10 mg/kg q 12 hours	No change	Reduce dose to 50% of normal	Reduce dose to 25% of normal	No
Fluconazole	6–12 mg/kg q 24 hours	Reduce dose to 50% of normal	Reduce dose to 50% of normal	Reduce dose to 25% of normal	No
Meropenem	30–40 mg/kg q 8 hours	10–20 mg/kg q 12 hours	10–20 mg/kg q 12 hours	10–20 mg/kg q 24 hours	NA
Piperacillin-tazobactam	50–100 mg/kg of piperacillin q 8–12 hours	Reduce dose by 30%; q 8 hours	Reduce dose by 30%; q 8 hours	Reduce dose by 30%; q 8 hours	No

(*Contd.*)

Table A3.1: Dose modification of common neonatal drugs in renal failure (*Contd.*)

Medication	*Dose in normal renal function (in neonates >35 weeks, per dose)*	*Dose with impaired renal function (GFR mL/min/1.73 m²)*			*Supplemental dose with peritoneal dialysis*
		30–50	*10–29*	*<10*	
Phenobarbitone	1.5–2 mg/kg q 12 hours	No change	No change	Reduce the dose to 50% of normal	Yes

Footnote: Dose modifications given above are approximate and guided by features of drug toxicity and, if feasible, drug levels; Loading dose, wherever applicable, remains the same as for neonates with normal renal function. GFR Glomerular filtration rate.

REFERENCES

1. Stoops C, Stone S, Evans E, Dill L, Henderson T, Griffin R, et al. Baby NINJA (Nephrotoxic Injury Negated by Just-in-Time Action): Reduction of Nephrotoxic Medication-Associated Acute Kidney Injury in the Neonatal Intensive Care Unit. J Pediatr. 2019 Dec;215:223–8.e6.
2. Girardi A, Raschi E, Galletti S, Allegaert K, Poluzzi E, De Ponti F. Drug-induced renal injury in neonates: challenges in clinical practice and perspectives in drug development. Expert Opin Drug MetabToxicol. 2017 May;13(5):555–65.
3. Hanna MH, Askenazi DJ, Selewski DT. Drug-induced acute kidney injury in neonates.CurrOpinPediatr. 2016 Apr;28(2):180–7.

ANNEXURE

4

Immunization Schedule

Age	*National Immunization Schedule*	*IAP Schedule*
Birth	BCG, OPV, Hepatitis B	BCG, OPV, Hepatitis- B1
6 weeks	Pentavalent-1, Rota-1, PCV-1, OPV-1, fIPV-1	DTwP/DTaP-1, Hib-1, Hepatitis B-2(Pentavalent), Rotavirus-1, PCV-1, IPV-1 (No OPV)
10 weeks	Pentavalent-2, Rota-2, OPV-2	DTwP/DTaP-2, Hib-2, Hepatitis B-3 (Pentavalent), Rotavirus-2, PCV-2, IPV-2 (No OPV)
14 weeks	Pentavalent-3, Rota-3, PCV-2, OPV-2, fIPV-2	DTwP/DTaP-3, Hib-3, Hepatitis B-4 (Petavalent), Rotavirus-3, PCV-3, IPV-3 (No OPV)
6 months	–	Influenza vaccine (IIV)-1
7 months	–	Influenza vaccine (IIV)-2
6–9 months	–	Typhoid conjugate vaccine (TCV)
9 months	9–12 months MR-1, JE-1 (Endemic districts), PCV- Booster (selected states) fIPV-3	MMR-1 No PCV booster
12 months	–	Hepatitis A-1
15 months	–	MMR-2, Varicella-1, PCV- Booster
16–24 months	MR-2, JE-2 (Endemic districts), DPT Booster-1, OPV Booster	16–18 months DTwP/DTaP-B1, Hib-B1, IPV-B1(No OPV)
18–19 months	–	Hepatitis A-2, Varicella-2
5–6 years	DPT Booster	4–6 years DTwP/DTaP-B2, IPV-B2,MMR-3
10 years	Td	10–12 years Tdap,HPV

Recommendations and overview of availability of immunogenicity and safety of recommended vaccinations for preterm and LBW infants ≤12 months of age.

Vaccine	*Recommended by WHO*	*India (IAP)*	*Included in National Immunization Program*	*Age (chronological age) recommendation in India*	*Immunogenicity/ Effectiveness*		*Safety*	
					Preterm (<37 weeks)[a]	*LBW (<2,500 g)*	*Preterm (<37 weeks)*	*LBW (<2500 g)*
BCG	Yes	Yes	Yes	At birth or as early as possible till one year of age	Yes	Yes	Yes	Yes
Hepatitis B	Yes	Yes	Yes	First dose at birth or as early as possible within 24 hours	Yes	Yes	Yes	Yes
OPV – 0	Yes	Yes	Yes	At birth or as early as possible within the first 15 days	Yes	NA	Yes	NA

(*Contd.*)

Recommendations and overview of availability of immunogenicity and safety of recommended vaccinations for preterm and LBW infants ≤12 months of age. *(Contd.)*

Vaccine	*Recommended by WHO*	*India (IAP)*	*Included in National Immunization Program*	*Age (chronological age) recomm-endation in India*	*Immunogenicity/ Effectiveness*		*Safety*	
					Preterm (<37 weeks)[a]	*LBW (<2,500 g)*	*Preterm (<37 weeks)*	*LBW (<2500 g)*
OPV – 1, 2, 3	Yes	Yes, at 6 and 14 weeks, in case IPV NA	Yes	At 6, 10 and 14 weeks (OPV can be given till 5 years of age)	Yes	NA	Yes	NA
Fractional IPV	Yes	Yes	Yes	Two fractional doses at 6 and 14 weeks of age	Yes	.NA.	Yes	NA
Pentavalent combination (DPT-Hib-Hep B)	NA	Yes	Yes	At 6 weeks, 10 weeks and 14 weeks (can be given till one year of age)	NA	NA	NA	NA

(Contd.)

Recommendations and overview of availability of immunogenicity and safety of recommended vaccinations for preterm and LBW infants ≤12 months of age. *(Contd.)*

Vaccine	*Recommended by WHO*	*India (IAP)*	*Included in National Immunization Program*	*Age (chronological age) recommendation in India*	*Immunogenicity/ Effectiveness*		*Safety*	
					Preterm (<37 weeks)[a]	*LBW (<2,500 g)*	*Preterm (<37 weeks)*	*LBW (<2500 g)*
Hexavalent combination (DTaP- Hib-IPV-Hep B)	No		No	Yes	Yes	Yes		
PCV	Yes	Yes	Yes	At 6 and 14 weeks. Booster dose at 9–15 months of age.	Yes (PCV7, PCV10, PCV13)	Yes (PCV7, PCV10)	Yes	Yes
Rotavirus	Yes	Yes	Yes	At 6, 10 and 14 weeks (can be given till one year of age)	Yes	NA	Yes	NA
Influenza	No	Yes	No	6 months–5 years	Yes	Yes	Yes	Yes
MMR, Varicella	NA	Yes	Yes	9 –12 months	NA	NA	NA	NA

Vaccine reactions and onset interval		
Vaccine	*Reaction*	*Onset interval*
BCG	Fatal dissemination of BCG	1–12 months
OPV	Vaccine associated paralytic poliomyelitis (VAPP)	4–30 days
DTWP	Prolonged crying and seizure	0–24 hours
	Hypotonic-hyporesponsive episodes	0–24 hours
Measles	Febrile seizure	6–12 days
	Thrombocytopenia	15–35 days
	Anaphylaxis	1 hour
Rotavirus	Intussusception	3–14 days

Index